Insulin Resistance: The Metabolic Syndrome

Insulin Resistance: The Metabolic Syndrome

Edited by Frank Cohen

hayle
medical

New York

Hayle Medical,
750 Third Avenue, 9ᵗʰ Floor,
New York, NY 10017, USA

Visit us on the World Wide Web at:
www.haylemedical.com

ISBN: 978-1-63241-907-1

Cataloging-in-Publication Data

Insulin Resistance: The Metabolic Syndrome / edited by Frank Cohen.
    p. cm.
Includes bibliographical references and index.
ISBN 978-1-63241-907-1
1. Insulin resistance. 2. Metabolic syndrome. 3. Insulin antibodies. 4. Diabetes--Complications.
5. Hormone resistance. I. Cohen, Frank.
RC662.4 .I57 2020
616.46--dc23

Table of Contents

Preface IX

Chapter 1 **Alteration of JNK-1 Signaling in Skeletal Muscle Fails to Affect Glucose
Homeostasis and Obesity-Associated Insulin Resistance in Mice** 1
Martin Pal, Claudia M. Wunderlich, Gabriele Spohn, Hella S. Brönneke,
Marc Schmidt-Supprian and F. Thomas Wunderlich

Chapter 2 **Prenatal Exposure to Lipopolysaccharide Combined with Pre- and Postnatal
High-Fat Diet Result in Lowered Blood Pressure and Insulin Resistance in
Offspring Rats** 14
Xue-Qin Hao, Jing-Xia Du, Yan Li, Meng Li and Shou-Yan Zhang

Chapter 3 **Metabolic Syndrome and Fatal Outcomes in the Post-Stroke Event** 21
Eric Vounsia Balti, André Pascal Kengne, Jean Valentin Fogha Fokouo,
Brice Enid Nouthé and Eugene Sobngwi

Chapter 4 **Celastrol, an NF-κB Inhibitor, Improves Insulin Resistance and Attenuates
Renal Injury in db/db Mice** 29
Jung Eun Kim, Mi Hwa Lee, Deok Hwa Nam, Hye Kyoung Song, Young Sun Kang,
Ji Eun Lee, Hyun Wook Kim, Jin Joo Cha, Young Youl Hyun, Sang Youb Han,
Kum Hyun Han, Jee Young Han and Dae Ryong Cha

Chapter 5 **Combined Impact of Cardiorespiratory Fitness and Visceral Adiposity on
Metabolic Syndrome in Overweight and Obese Adults** 40
Sue Kim, Ji-Young Kim, Duk-Chul Lee, Hye-Sun Lee, Ji-Won Lee and Justin Y. Jeon

Chapter 6 **An Extract of *Artemisia dracunculus* L. Inhibits Ubiquitin-Proteasome Activity
and Preserves Skeletal Muscle Mass in a Murine Model of Diabetes** 46
Heather Kirk-Ballard, Zhong Q. Wang, Priyanka Acharya, Xian H. Zhang,
Yongmei Yu, Gail Kilroy, David Ribnicky, William T. Cefalu and Z. Elizabeth Floyd

Chapter 7 **Midkine, a Potential Link between Obesity and Insulin Resistance** 58
Nengguang Fan, Haiyan Sun, Yifei Wang, Lijuan Zhang, Zhenhua Xia, Liang Peng,
Yanqiang Hou, Weiqin Shen, Rui Liu and Yongde Peng

Chapter 8 **PPAR Agonist-Induced Reduction of Mcp1 in Atherosclerotic Plaques of Obese,
Insulin-Resistant Mice Depends on Adiponectin-Induced Irak3 Expression** 68
Maarten Hulsmans, Benjamine Geeraert, Thierry Arnould, Christos Tsatsanis and
Paul Holvoet

Chapter 9 **Effects of Green Tea Extract on Insulin Resistance and Glucagon-Like
Peptide 1 in Patients with Type 2 Diabetes and Lipid Abnormalities** 80
Chia-Yu Liu, Chien-Jung Huang, Lin-Huang Huang, I-Ju Chen, Jung-Peng Chiu and
Chung-Hua Hsu

Chapter 10 **Common Genetic Variants of Surfactant Protein-D (SP-D) are Associated with Type 2 Diabetes** 88
Neus Pueyo, Francisco J. Ortega, Josep M. Mercador, José M. Moreno-Navarrete, Monica Sabater, Sílvia Bonàs, Patricia Botas, Elías Delgado, Wifredo Ricart, María T. Martinez-Larrad, Manuel Serrano-Ríos, David Torrents and José M. Fernández-Real

Chapter 11 *GCKR* **Variants Increase Triglycerides while Protecting from Insulin Resistance in Chinese Children** 98
Yue Shen, Lijun Wu, Bo Xi, Xin Liu, Xiaoyuan Zhao, Hong Cheng, Dongqing Hou, Xingyu Wang and Jie Mi

Chapter 12 **Increased Plasma DPP4 Activity is an Independent Predictor of the Onset of Metabolic Syndrome in Chinese over 4 Years: Result from the China National Diabetes and Metabolic Disorders Study** 104
Fan Yang, Tianpeng Zheng, Yun Gao, Attit Baskota, Tao Chen, Xingwu Ran and Haoming Tian

Chapter 13 **Normal Weight Obesity is Associated with Metabolic Syndrome and Insulin Resistance in Young Adults from a Middle-Income Country** 111
Francilene B. Madeira, Antônio A. Silva, Helma F. Veloso, Marcelo Z. Goldani, Gilberto Kac, Viviane C. Cardoso, Heloisa Bettiol and Marco A. Barbieri

Chapter 14 **Does DNA Methylation of *PPARGC1A* Influence Insulin Action in First Degree Relatives of Patients with Type 2 Diabetes?** 120
Linn Gillberg, Stine Jacobsen, Rasmus Ribel-Madsen, Anette Prior Gjesing, Trine W. Boesgaard, Charlotte Ling, Oluf Pedersen, Torben Hansen and Allan Vaag

Chapter 15 **Associations between Serum Apelin-12 Levels and Obesity-Related Markers in Chinese Children** 128
Hong-Jun Ba, Hong-Shan Chen, Zhe Su, Min-Lian Du, Qiu-Li Chen, Yan-Hong Li and Hua-Mei Ma

Chapter 16 **Waist Circumference Independently Associates with the Risk of Insulin Resistance and Type 2 Diabetes in Mexican American Families** 136
Manju Mamtani, Hemant Kulkarni, Thomas D. Dyer, Laura Almasy, Michael C. Mahaney, Ravindranath Duggirala, Anthony G. Comuzzie, John Blangero and Joanne E. Curran

Chapter 17 **Identification of Direct and Indirect Social Network Effects in the Pathophysiology of Insulin Resistance in Obese Human Subjects** 143
Christian H. C. A. Henning, Nana Zarnekow, Johannes Hedtrich, Sascha Stark, Kathrin Türk and Matthias Laudes

Chapter 18 **The Associations between Serum Zinc Levels and Metabolic Syndrome in the Korean Population: Findings from the 2010 Korean National Health and Nutrition Examination Survey** 152
Jin-A Seo, Sang-Wook Song, Kyungdo Han, Kyung-Jin Lee and Ha-Na Kim

Chapter 19 **Regulation of Insulin Degrading Enzyme Activity by Obesity-Associated Factors and Pioglitazone in Liver of Diet-Induced Obese Mice** 162
Xiuqing Wei, Bilun Ke, Zhiyun Zhao, Xin Ye, Zhanguo Gao and Jianping Ye

Chapter 20   **Lower Fetuin-A, Retinol Binding Protein 4 and Several Metabolites after Gastric Bypass Compared to Sleeve Gastrectomy in Patients with Type 2 Diabetes** 169
Mia Jüllig, Shelley Yip, Aimin Xu, Greg Smith, Martin Middleditch,
Michael Booth, Richard Babor, Grant Beban and Rinki Murphy

Chapter 21   **Lactoferrin Dampens High-Fructose Corn Syrup-Induced Hepatic Manifestations of the Metabolic Syndrome in a Murine Model** 180
Yi-Chieh Li and Chang-Chi Hsieh

Chapter 22   **Role of Serum Vaspin in Progression of Type 2 Diabetes** 189
Weixia Jian, Wenhui Peng, Sumei Xiao, Hailing Li, Jie Jin, Li Qin, Yan Dong and
Qing Su

Chapter 23   **Whole-Body and Hepatic Insulin Resistance in Obese Children** 196
Lorena del Rocío Ibarra-Reynoso, Liudmila Pisarchyk, Elva Leticia Pérez-Luque,
Ma. Eugenia Garay-Sevilla and Juan Manuel Malacara

Permissions

List of Contributors

Index

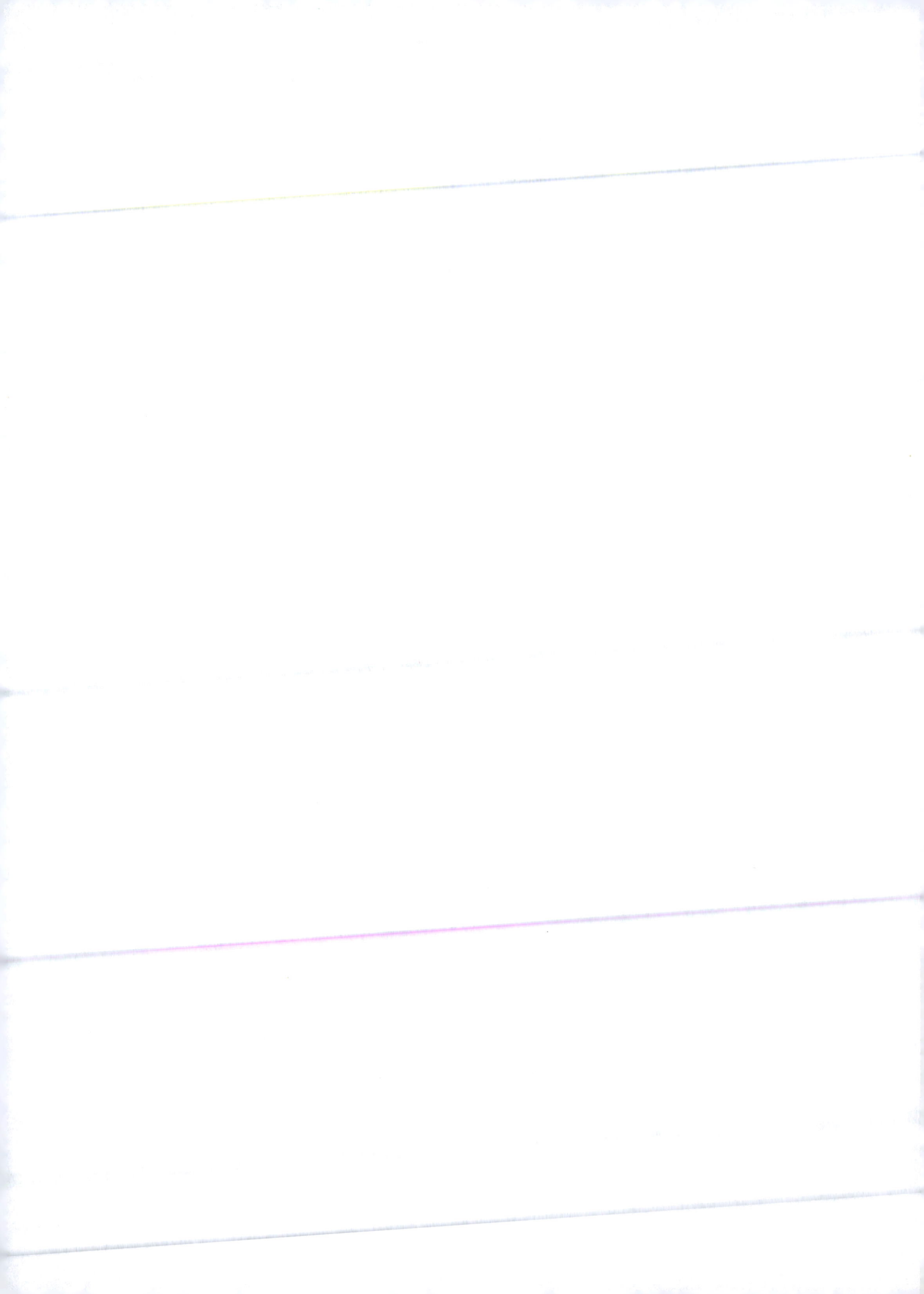

Preface

Insulin is a protein hormone which is produced by the beta cells of pancreatic islets; it is the main anabolic hormone of the body. By absorbing carbohydrate especially glucose from the blood into liver fat and skeleton muscle cell, it regulates metabolism of carbohydrate fat and protein. Main purpose of insulin is to control the glucose level in the body. Insulin resistance is a pathological condition characterized by the failure of body cells to respond normally to the hormone insulin. In insulin resistance, the cells become less effective to lower the level of glucose (sugar) in the blood. Causes of insulin resistance include molecular mechanism, sedentary lifestyle, protease inhibitors, HCV, genetics, etc. The symptoms of insulin resistance are hyperglycemia, high blood sugar level, fatigue, brain fogginess, high blood pressure, polydipsia, polyphagia etc. Risk factors associated with insulin resistance are obesity, type 2 diabetes, metabolic syndrome, liver pathologies, hemochromatosis, gastropareses, and polycystic ovary syndrome. The treatment of insulin resistance includes exercise and weight loss. This book unravels the recent studies in the field of insulin resistance. Different approaches, evaluations, methodologies and advanced studies on insulin resistance have been included in this book. It is appropriate for students seeking detailed information in this area as well as for experts.

This book has been the outcome of endless efforts put in by authors and researchers on various issues and topics within the field. The book is a comprehensive collection of significant researches that are addressed in a variety of chapters. It will surely enhance the knowledge of the field among readers across the globe.

It gives us an immense pleasure to thank our researchers and authors for their efforts to submit their piece of writing before the deadlines. Finally in the end, I would like to thank my family and colleagues who have been a great source of inspiration and support.

Editor

Alteration of JNK-1 Signaling in Skeletal Muscle Fails to Affect Glucose Homeostasis and Obesity-Associated Insulin Resistance in Mice

Martin Pal[1,9], **Claudia M. Wunderlich**[1,9], **Gabriele Spohn**[1], **Hella S. Brönneke**[2], **Marc Schmidt-Supprian**[3], **F. Thomas Wunderlich**[1]*

1 Max Planck Institute for Neurological Research, Institute for Genetics, University of Cologne and Cologne Excellence Cluster on Cellular Stress Responses in Aging-Associated Diseases (CECAD) and Center of Molecular Medicine Cologne (CMMC), Cologne, Germany, **2** Mouse Phenotyping Core Facility of Cologne Excellence Cluster on Cellular Stress Responses in Aging-Associated Diseases (CECAD), Cologne, Germany, **3** Molecular Immunology and Signaltransduction, Max Planck Institute for Biochemistry, Munich, Germany

Abstract

Obesity and associated metabolic disturbances, such as increased circulating fatty acids cause prolonged low grade activation of inflammatory signaling pathways in liver, skeletal muscle, adipose tissue and even in the CNS. Activation of inflammatory pathways in turn impairs insulin signaling, ultimately leading to obesity-associated type 2 diabetes mellitus. Conventional JNK-1 knock out mice are protected from high fat diet-induced insulin resistance, characterizing JNK-1-inhibition as a potential approach to improve glucose metabolism in obese patients. However, the cell type-specific role of elevated JNK-1 signaling as present during the course of obesity has not been fully elucidated yet. To investigate the functional contribution of altered JNK-1 activation in skeletal muscle, we have generated a ROSA26 insertion mouse strain allowing for Cre-activatable expression of a JNK-1 constitutive active construct (JNK^C). To examine the consequence of skeletal muscle-restricted JNK-1 overactivation in the development of insulin resistance and glucose metabolism, JNK^C mice were crossed to Mck-Cre mice yielding JNK^{SM-C} mice. However, despite increased muscle-specific JNK activation, energy homeostasis and glucose metabolism in JNK^{SM-C} mice remained largely unaltered compared to controls. In line with these findings, obese mice with skeletal muscle specific disruption of JNK-1, did not affect energy and glucose homeostasis. These experiments indicate that JNK-1 activation in skeletal muscle does not account for the major effects on diet-induced, JNK-1-mediated deterioration of insulin action and points towards a so far underappreciated role of JNK-1 in other tissues than skeletal muscle during the development of obesity-associated insulin resistance.

Editor: Haiyan Xu, Warren Alpert Medical School of Brown University, United States of America

Funding: This work was supported by the DFG through SFB 832 A15 to FTW and Z3 to JCB, the Center for Molecular Medicine Cologne (CMMC) (D1 to JCB, B2 to FTW), the Cluster of Excellence Cellular Stress Responses in Aging-Associated Diseases (CECAD), the European Union (FP7-HEALTH-2009-241592, EurOCHIP, to JCB), the DFG (BR 1492/7-1 to JCB), and the Competence Network for Adipositas (Neurotarget) funded by the Federal Ministry of Education and Research (FKZ01GIO845 to JCB). The funders had no role in study design, data collection and analysis, decision to publish, or preparation of the manuscript.

Competing Interests: The authors have declared that no competing interests exist.

* E-mail: Thomas.wunderlich@uni-koeln.de

⑨ These authors contributed equally to this work.

Introduction

The increasing prevalence of obesity in the population of developed countries represents a serious health problem, since obesity is a major risk factor for the development of insulin resistance, hyperglycemia, and metabolic syndrome. It is therefore important to understand the molecular mechanism that accounts for obesity-induced insulin resistance. Weight gain during the course of obesity induces low grade chronic inflammation in white adipose tissue (WAT) and liver leading to the release of pro-inflammatory cytokines such as TNF-α into circulation [1]. TNF-α inhibits insulin action in classical insulin target tissues such as skeletal muscle, liver and adipose cells, thereby resulting in impaired glucose homeostasis [2,3]. Here, TNF-stimulated activation of the cJun N-terminal kinase (JNK) and inhibitor of κB kinase (IKK) signaling pathways inhibit insulin action in a tissue-specific manner [2,4–6]. Moreover, JNK activation mediates

insulin resistance by other activators such as free fatty acids and ER stress, both of which are elevated during the course of obesity [7,8]. JNK activation leads to inhibitory serine phosphorylation of insulin receptor substrate (IRS) proteins inhibiting insulin signaling thus causing insulin resistance and ultimately contributing to the development of type 2 diabetes mellitus [9].

JNKs are expressed by three different genes, JNK-1, -2 and -3, all of which generate various JNK-isoforms by alternative splicing mechanisms [10]. JNK-1 and -2 are ubiquitously expressed, while JNK-3 expression is restricted mainly to brain and heart [11]. Recent studies identified JNK-1 as the major isoform contributing to the development of obesity-associated insulin resistance, since mouse mutants deficient for JNK-1 but not those for JNK-2 are largely protected from the development of obesity and obesity-associated insulin resistance in both diet- and genetically-induced obesity models [12,13]. However, the tissue-specific contribution of JNK-1-deficiency to the development of obesity-associated insulin resistance *in vivo* is poorly understood. While adipose-tissue-specific JNK-1-deficiency confers some protection to obesity-associated insulin resistance [14], analyses of the contribution of JNK-1-action in the hematopoetic system using bone marrow transplantation have yielded conflicting results [15,16]. On the other hand, myeloid lineage-cell-specific disruption of JNK-1 failed to protect from obesity-associated insulin resistance, ruling out a major contribution of macrophages to this phenomenon [14]. More recently, skeletal muscle-specific JNK-1 disruption reported by Sabio and colleagues revealed a potential role of JNK-1 signaling in the control of systemic insulin sensitivity in high fat diet-induced obesity [17]. Specifically, muscle-specific JNK-1-deficiency left body weight gain and glucose tolerance unaltered during the course of obesity, but ameliorated insulin sensitivity and insulin-stimulated AKT phosphorylation in liver and WAT but not in the JNK-1-deficient muscle [17]. Interestingly, another study using disruption of JNK-1 in hepatocytes demonstrated that hepatic JNK-1-signaling in lean mice is required to prevent the development of steatosis, while in diet-induced obese mice, JNK-1-deficiency was unable to further aggravate lipid accumulation in hepatocytes [18]. The most promising candidate site in which disruption of JNK-1 could largely reflect the lean phenotype of JNK-1 knock out mice was recently identified as the central nervous system. We and others could show, that neuronal and pituitary JNK-1 deficiency has significant impact on insulin sensitivity and the growth hormone/insulin like growth factor axis [19,20]. Mice carrying a central JNK-1 inactivation were small sized and had reduced body weight accompanied with increased insulin sensitivity compared to controls [19].

However, none of these mouse mutants completely phenocopied the effect observed in conventional JNK-1 knock out mice indicating that other cell types or combinations thereof are involved in mediating JNK-1's effect on insulin sensitivity. Despite the current cell type-specific knowledge about JNK-1 signaling in the development of obesity-induced insulin resistance, mimicry of JNK-1 overactivation as present in the course of obesity has not been elucidated yet. Here, we investigated mice with isolated transgenic overactivation of JNK-1 in skeletal muscle for alterations in glucose metabolism and energy homeostasis. However, besides cell type-specific aggravation of JNK-1 signaling in these organs, the impact on insulin sensitivity and glucose homeostasis was minor. To further investigate the cell type specific function of JNK-1 in obesity, we have generated conditional JNK-1 knock out mice in skeletal muscle. Strikingly, when exposed to high fat diet, obesity developed to a similar extent in JNK-1 mutants and controls and obesity induced a similar inhibition of insulin action in controls and mutants despite successful reduction of JNK-1 expression in these tissues. Taken together our data reveal, that JNK-1 action in skeletal muscle fails to affect the development of obesity and obesity-associated insulin resistance.

Materials and Methods

Animal Care

Care of all animals was within institutional animal care committee guidelines. All animal procedures were conducted in compliance with protocols and approved by local government authorities (Bezirksregierung Köln, Cologne, Germany). Animals were fed either normal chow diet (NCD) (2918 Teklad Global 18% Protein Rodent Diet, Teklad Diets, Madison, Wi., USA) containing 53.5% carbohydrates, 18.5% protein, and 5.5% fat (12% of calories from fat), or a high-fat diet (HFD) (C1057,

Altromin, Lage, Germany) containing 32.7% carbohydrates, 20% protein, and 35.5% fat (55.2% of calories from fat) starting from 3 weeks of age. All animals had access to water and food ad libitum. Body weight was measured once per week. Food intake was quantified daily over a period of 7 days. Mice were sacrificed using CO_2.

Generation of JNK^{SM-C} Mice

The JNK^C construct consisting of a JNKK-2D(MKK-7D)-JNK-1 fusion protein was created by conventional cloning techniques. Sequences encoding the JNKK2(MKK7)-JNK1 fusion protein [36] or a constitutively active MKK7D [37] were subcloned into pBluescript flanked by AscI sites. The fragment containing the S271D and T275D mutations was then excised by NotI-BsmBI from the MKK7D containing plasmid and cloned NotI-BsmBI into the JNKK2(MKK7)-JNK1 containing plasmid, yielding a MKK7D-JNK1 containing plasmid. The MKK7D-JNK1 (JNK^C) sequences were then inserted into the AscI site of the STOP-EGFP-ROSA targeting vector that additionally contained a CAG promoter. Sequences are available upon request. 10^7 Bruce4 ES cells were transfected with the targeting vector and positive clones were identified using the ROSA probe [38] in Southern Blot analysis. Positive ES cell clones were used to generate the ROSA JNK^C mouse strain, which was further crossed to Mck-Cre mice to generate JNK^{SM-C} mice. JNK^{SM-C} mice were genotyped for the presence of the JNK^C construct by performing PCR analysis using primers 5_MKK7_JNK1CA (5'-AAG-AAC-TGC-AAG-ACG-GAC-TT-3') and 3_MKK7_JNK1CA (5'- TTC-ATA-AGA-ACT-AGC-TCT-CTG-T-3').

Generation of JNK-1^{SM-KO} and JNK-1^{KO} Mice

To generate JNK-1^{SM-KO} male mice Mck-Cre mice [21] were crossed to JNK-1$^{FL/FL}$ mice [19]. Further, JNK-1$^{FL/FL}$ mice were crossed to deleter Cre mice to yield JNK-1^{KO} mice. In all experiments, littermates carrying the loxP-flanked JNK-1 allele were used as controls. Genotyping for the Mck-Cre trangene was performed by PCR by using primers mck5 (5'-GTT-CTT-AAG-TCT-GAA-CCC-GG-3'), mck3 (5'-GTC-TGG-ATG-ACA-TCG-TCC-AG-3') and Cre_intern_rev3 (5'-ATG-TTT-AGC-TGG-CCC-AAA-TGT-3'). For identifying the JNK-1$^{FL/FL}$ and the JNK-1^{KO} alleles, the primers 5J1loxNT (5'-ACA-TGT-ACC-ATG-TAC-TGA-CCT-AAG-3'), 3J1loxNT (5'-CAT-TAC-TCT-ACT-CAC-TAT-AGT-AAC-3') and 3J1deltaNT (5'-GAT-ATC-AGT-ATA-TGT-CCT-TAT-AG-3') were used.

Analysis of Body Composition

Lean mass and body fat content of live animals was determined using the NMR Analyser Minispec (Bruker Optik).

Indirect Calorimetry

Indirect calorimetry was measured in a PhenoMaster System (TSE Systems) as previously described [22,23]. After an overnight acclimatization, parameters of indirect calorimetry were measured for 48 to 72 h.

Glucose and Insulin Tolerance Test

Glucose-tolerance tests were performed on animals fasted for 16 h. Animals were injected with either 2 g/kg body weight of glucose or 0.75 units/kg body weight of insulin (Insuman Rapid, Sanofi Aventis) into the peritoneal cavity. Blood glucose concentrations were determined by using an automated glucose monitor (GlucoMen) for the indicated time points.

Insulin and Leptin Determination from Serum

Plasma insulin and leptin concentrations were examined by ELISA (mouse/rat insulin ELISA, #INSKR020, mouse leptin ELISA, #900-019, Chrystal Chem, BD Bioscience PharMingen) according to the manufacturer's protocol.

Southern Blot Analysis

For Southern blot, 15 μg of DNA isolated from embryonic stem cells was digested over night with 100 U of EcoRI. The DNA fragments were separated by agarose gel electrophoresis and transferred onto Hybond-XL™- membranes (Amersham) by alkaline capillary transfer. 80 ng DNA of the ROSA26 probe was radioactively labeled with 2.5 mCi$^{[α32P]}$dATP (Amersham) using the Ladderman™ Labeling Kit (Takara) as previously described [24].

Gene Expression Analysis

Quantitative expression for JNK^C mRNA (Hs01548508_m1, Applied Biosystems, Foster City, USA) was determined by using whole-muscle RNA isolated by TRIzol (Invitrogen). RNA was reversely transcribed with High Capacity cDNA Reverse Transcription Kit (Applied Biosystems) and amplified by using TaqMan Gene Expression Master Mix (Applied Biosystems). Relative expression of mRNAs was determined by using standard curves based on cDNA derived from the respective tissues, and samples were adjusted for total RNA content by Hprt1 (Mm00446968_m1, Applied Biosystems), Gusb (Mm00446953_m1, Applied Biosystems) and Tfrc (Mm00441941_m1, Applied Biosystems) quantitative PCR. Calculations were performed by a comparative cycle threshold (Ct) method: starting copy number of test samples was determined in comparison with the known copy number of the calibrator sample (ddCt). The relative gene copy number was calculated as 2^{-ddCt}. Quantitative PCR was performed on an ABI PRISM 7900 Sequence Detector (Applied Bioscience). Assays were linear >4 orders of magnitudes.

Insulin Signaling

Mice were anesthetized by intraperitoneal injection of ketamin (100 μg/μl, Albrecht GmbH, Germany). 5 mU of human regular insulin (Insuman Rapid, Sanofi Aventis) were injected into the inferior *vena cava*. Skeletal muscle and liver were collected 2, 5 and 7 min after injection and processed as previously described [21].

Western Blot Analysis

Muscle and liver tissues were homogenized with a polytron homogenizer (IKA Werke) in protein lysis buffer and centrifuged at 13,000 g for 1 h at 4°C. Proteins in the supernatant were electrophoresed by SDS–polyacrylamide gel electrophoresis (10%) and transferred to PVDF membranes (Bio-Rad). Membranes were probed with the following antibodies: JNK 1/3 (Santa Cruz Biotechnology Inc.), phospho-JNK (#4668, Cell Signaling Technology Inc.), AKT (pan) (#4685, Cell Signaling Technology Inc.), phospho-AKT (#9271, Cell Signaling Technology Inc.), Calnexin (#20880, Calbiochem, Germany) and goat anti-rabbit conjugated to HRP (A6154, Sigma-Aldrich).

JNK Activity Assays

JNK activity assays were performed as previously described [25]. Human cJun peptide (residues 1–79) fused to glutathione S-transferase (Biovision, USA) was bound to glutathione sepharose beads 4B (GE Healthcare, Germany) overnight. After 2 washing steps, skeletal muscle lysates from WT and JNK^{SM-C} mice were incubated overnight with the GST-c-Jun fusion beads. Kinase reaction was induced by adding 200 μM [γ-^{32}P]-ATP (3000 Ci/mmol) (Hartmann Analytic, Germany). After SDS-PAGE, phosphorylation of c-Jun was detected by using a Typhoon Trio Imager (GE Healthcare, Germany).

Statistical Analyses

Datasets were analyzed for statistical significance by using a two-tailed, unpaired Student's t test and one-or two-way analysis of variance (ANOVA) (PASW Statistics 18.0). P values <0.05 were considered significant. For visual clarity, instead of standard deviations, means +/− standard errors of the mean (SEM) are depicted in all figures.

Results

JNK is Activated in Skeletal Muscle of Obese Mouse Models

Obesity-induced JNK activation has been described to result in the development of insulin resistance in various organs by inhibitory serine phosphorylation of IRS proteins [12]. In detail, inflammatory cytokines that are elevated during the course of obesity such as TNF-α activate upstream kinases of JNK that phosphorylate JNK-1 and JNK-2 at specific Thr and Tyr residues resulting in JNK activation that can be monitored by several means. To address whether JNK is activated in response to obesity in skeletal muscle, we examined phosphorylation of JNK by using phospho-specific antibodies. Consistent with previous reports, JNK phosphorylation was increased in the muscle of mice that were exposed to high fat diet (HFD) feeding for 14 weeks when compared to organs of mice receiving normal chow diet (NCD) (Fig. 1A). Moreover, to quantify this increase in JNK activity and to prove that the elevated JNK activation under HFD conditions translates also into further downstream signaling, we elucidated JNK activity by a kinase assay using GST coupled cJun peptide as a substrate in lysates obtained from skeletal muscle of NCD- and HFD-fed mice (Fig. 1B). This analysis revealed a significant increase of JNK activity in skeletal muscle when mice were exposed to HFD feeding as revealed by quantitation of radioactively labeled cJun peptide (Fig. 1C). Thus, our data reveal a 2.8-fold increased JNK activation in skeletal muscle under obese conditions when compared to lean mice.

Successful Transgenic Mimicking of Diet-induced JNK-activation in Skeletal Muscle

Obesity-induced JNK activation has been closely linked to result in the development of insulin resistance. To mimic such JNK overactivation, we employed a novel mouse model allowing for Cre-activatable cell type-specific overactivation of JNK signaling. To this end, we generated mice carrying a constitutive active version of JNK (JNK^C) in the ROSA26 locus (ROSA JNK^C), by targeted insertion of a MKK-7D-JNK-1 fusion-gene, whose expression is prevented by a loxP-flanked transcriptional stop cassette (Fig. 1D). Upon Cre-mediated recombination, the stop cassette is excised, thus permitting the compound expression of the JNK^C construct and EGFP. The correct integration of the JNK^C transgene into the ROSA26 locus of C57BL6-derived Bruce-4 embryonic stem cells was confirmed by Southern blot analysis using the external ROSA26 probe (Fig. 1E). Correctly targeted ES cell clones were used to generate the conditional ROSA JNK^C mouse strain on a pure C57/BL6 background. By crossing the ROSA JNK^C to Mck-Cre mice, we created a mouse model with isolated skeletal muscle-specific overactivation of JNK signaling (JNK^{SM-C}).

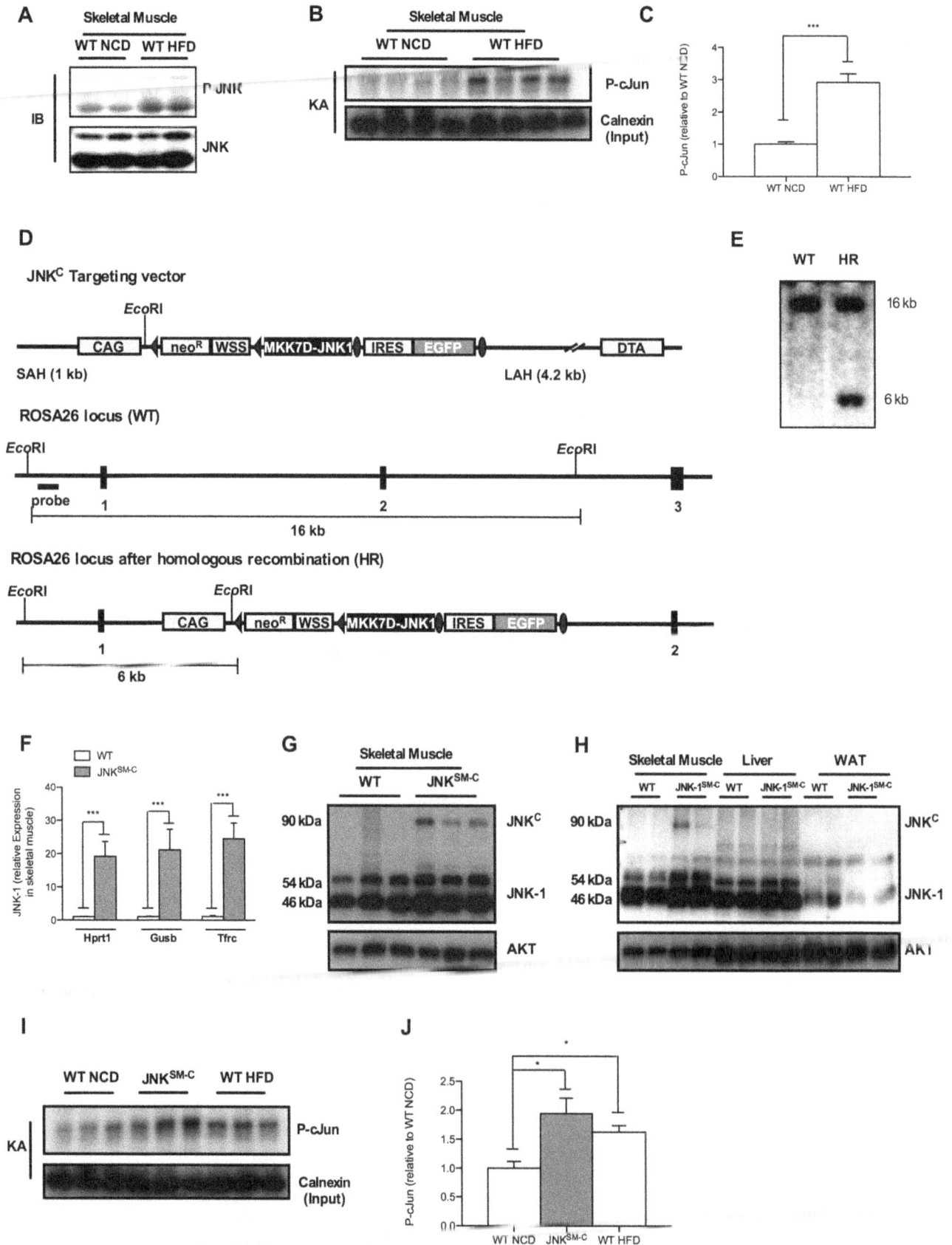

Figure 1. Muscle specific JNK overactivation. (A) Western Blot analysis (IB) of protein lysates isolated from muscles of WT mice at 20 weeks of age when exposed to NCD and HFD using P-JNK and JNK antibodies. (B) JNK-kinase assay of protein lysates isolated from muscles of WT mice at 20 weeks of age when exposed to NCD and HFD. Calnexin antibodies were used for input control. (C) Quantitation of radioactively labeled cJun peptide

in skeletal muscle of NCD fed WT and HFD WT mice. (D) Targeting strategy for the Cre-activatable JNK^C construct into the ubiquitously expressed ROSA26 locus. The CAG modified STOP-EGFP-ROSA targeting vector was described elsewhere. In the unique AscI site, a fusion cDNA between the mutant MKK7D [36] and JNK-1 [37] was inserted to generate the final ROSA JNK^C targeting vector. Homologous recombination between the homology arms and the genomic ROSA26 locus generated the targeted allele which was identified by Southern Blot analysis of EcoRI-digested clonal DNA using the ROSA probe [38] resulting in the 16 kb WT band besides the 6 kb targeted band as shown in (E). Such positive C57/BL6-derived ES cell clones were used to generate the ROSA JNK^C mouse strain. (F) Determination of relative JNK-1 mRNA expression in skeletal muscle of WT and JNK^{SM-C} mice by quantitative realtime PCR using Hprt1, Gusb and Tfrc as housekeeping genes (n = 8). (G) Western Blot analysis of protein lysates isolated from skeletal muscle of WT and JNK^{SM-C} mice using JNK-1 and AKT antibodies. (H) Expression of the JNK^C fusion protein only in skeletal muscle of JNK^{SM-C} mice indicated by Western blot analysis. (I) Functionality of the JNK^C construct in skeletal muscle of JNK^{SM-C} mice was revealed by increased phosphorylation of cJun in JNK kinase assay (KA) experiments. (J) Quantitation of radioactively labeled cJun peptide in skeletal muscle of NCD fed WT, JNK^{SM-C} and HFD WT mice. Values are means ± SEM. ***, $p \leq 0.001$.

Indeed, assessment of JNK expression in skeletal muscle revealed not only successful overexpression of the JNK^C construct on the RNA level (Fig. 1F), but also on the protein level (Fig. 1G). Of note, to exclude transcriptional regulation of the housekeeping gene by JNK, we compared and normalized relative JNK expression to the expression of Hprt1, Gusb and Tfrc genes, respectively (Fig. 1F). Nevertheless, JNK^C expression was detected exclusively in skeletal muscle but not in liver and WAT of JNK^{SM-C} mice confirming the skeletal muscle specific excision of the loxP-flanked stop cassette by the Mck-Cre transgene (Fig. 1H). The presence of the JNK^C construct in these cells clearly over-activated JNK signaling compared to NCD-fed animals as revealed by increased phosphorylation of the downstream target cJun in a kinase assay of skeletal muscle lysates whereas the transgenic JNK activity reached similar activation as detected in skeletal muscle of HFD-fed animals (Fig. 1I, J). Importantly, to exclude variation of transgenic JNK^C overactivation in skeletal muscle of individual JNK^{SM-C} mice, the densitometric quantitation of phosphorylated cJun and subsequent statistical analysis revealed similar distribution of P-cJun levels in this group (Fig. S1A, B and Fig. 1I, J). Taken together, we demonstrated that isolated JNK^C expression in skeletal muscle results in cell type-specific downstream JNK overactivation as present during the course of obesity.

Isolated JNK Overactivation in Skeletal Muscle Fails to Affect Body Composition and Energy Homeostasis

Next, we aimed to address whether JNK^C expression in skeletal muscle affects weight gain by comparing body weight of control and JNK^{SM-C} mice from 3 to 17 weeks of age. Body weight measurements in cohorts of control and JNK^{SM-C} mice revealed that skeletal muscle-specific JNK^C expression failed to affect body weight gain over this time frame when compared to controls (Fig. 2A). Moreover, body length was unaltered in the mutant mice compared to controls at the age of 17 weeks (Fig. 2B). The result of equal weighty and sized JNK^{SM-C} and control mice was also confirmed by a comparable abundance of body fat as revealed by nuclear resonance spectroscopy analysis (Fig. 2C). In line with these results, mass of epigonadal fat pads of JNK^{SM-C} mice were comparable to control fat pads (Fig. 2D), which in turn translated into equal circulating amounts of the adipose-derived hormone leptin in both cohorts of mice (Fig. 2E). Though body composition was unaltered between control and JNK^{SM-C} mice, we conducted indirect calorimetry experiments of control and JNK^{SM-C} mice to exclude any alteration in food ingestion or energy homeostasis. In line with unaltered body weight and fat mass, daily food intake (Fig. 2F), energy expenditure (Fig. 2G) and respective respiratory exchange ratio (RER) (Fig. 2H) was unchanged in the two cohorts of mice. Collectively, these results demonstrate that JNK over-activation in skeletal muscle fails to affect body composition and energy expenditure.

Overactivation of JNK in Skeletal Muscle Fails to Impair Insulin Signaling and Glucose Homeostasis in vivo

In light of the apparent lack of a major effect of skeletal muscle-specific JNK overactivation on body composition and energy expenditure, we wanted to address, whether isolated overactivation of JNK-dependent signaling in skeletal muscle (i.) causes overall alteration in whole body glucose homeostasis and (ii.) can impair insulin signaling in this organ in vivo. To this end, we performed glucose and insulin tolerance tests as well as examined circulating insulin concentrations and insulin-stimulated AKT phosphorylation as a measure of insulin sensitivity. Time-dependent glucose clearance from the blood upon intraperitoneal glucose challenge was identical between control and JNK^{SM-C} mice in glucose tolerance tests (Fig. 3A). Additionally, insulin sensitivity was unchanged in insulin tolerance tests in the two cohorts of mice (Fig. 3B). Moreover, circulating insulin concentrations were not affected by skeletal muscle specific JNK overactivation (Fig. 3C). Consistent with these observations, analysis of insulin-stimulated AKT-phosphorylation in skeletal muscle and liver of control and JNK^{SM-C} mice revealed that JNK overactivation in skeletal muscle did neither affect insulin-stimulated AKT-activation in muscle nor in liver (Fig. 3D). Taken together, these data indicate that overactivated JNK signaling in skeletal muscle as present during the course of obesity fails to impair whole body glucose homeostasis and insulin-stimulated signaling events in vivo.

Unaltered Energy Homeostasis and Body Composition in Mice Lacking JNK-1 in Skeletal Muscle

The previously published analysis of conventional JNK-1 knock out mice had revealed, that these animals are not only protected from obesity-associated insulin resistance, but that they also exhibit reduced weight gain, both after exposure to high fat diet (HFD) as well as on the background of the ob/ob genetic obesity model [12]. To directly address whether skeletal muscle specific disruption of JNK-1 contributes to this effect, we investigated our recently described mice with skeletal muscle specific disruption of JNK-1 (JNK-1^{SM-KO} mice) [26]. To this end, we exposed cohorts of control and JNK-1^{SM-KO} mice to normal chow (NCD) and high fat diet (HFD) conditions starting from 3 weeks of age and monitored parameters of adiposity as well as energy homeostasis in these animals. Though this analysis revealed that HFD-exposure significantly increased body weight, body length, body fat content, epididymal fat pad mass as well as circulating plasma leptin concentrations in control mice exposed to HFD compared to those exposed to NCD (Fig. 4A, B, C, D, E), parameters of mice with skeletal muscle specific JNK-1 deficiency were indistinguishable from control mice, both under NCD and HFD conditions. Accordingly, while unaltered food intake and energy expenditure between control and JNK-1^{SM-KO} mice was demonstrated previously [26], also food intake and energy expenditure as well as respective respiratory exchange ratios were indistinguishable

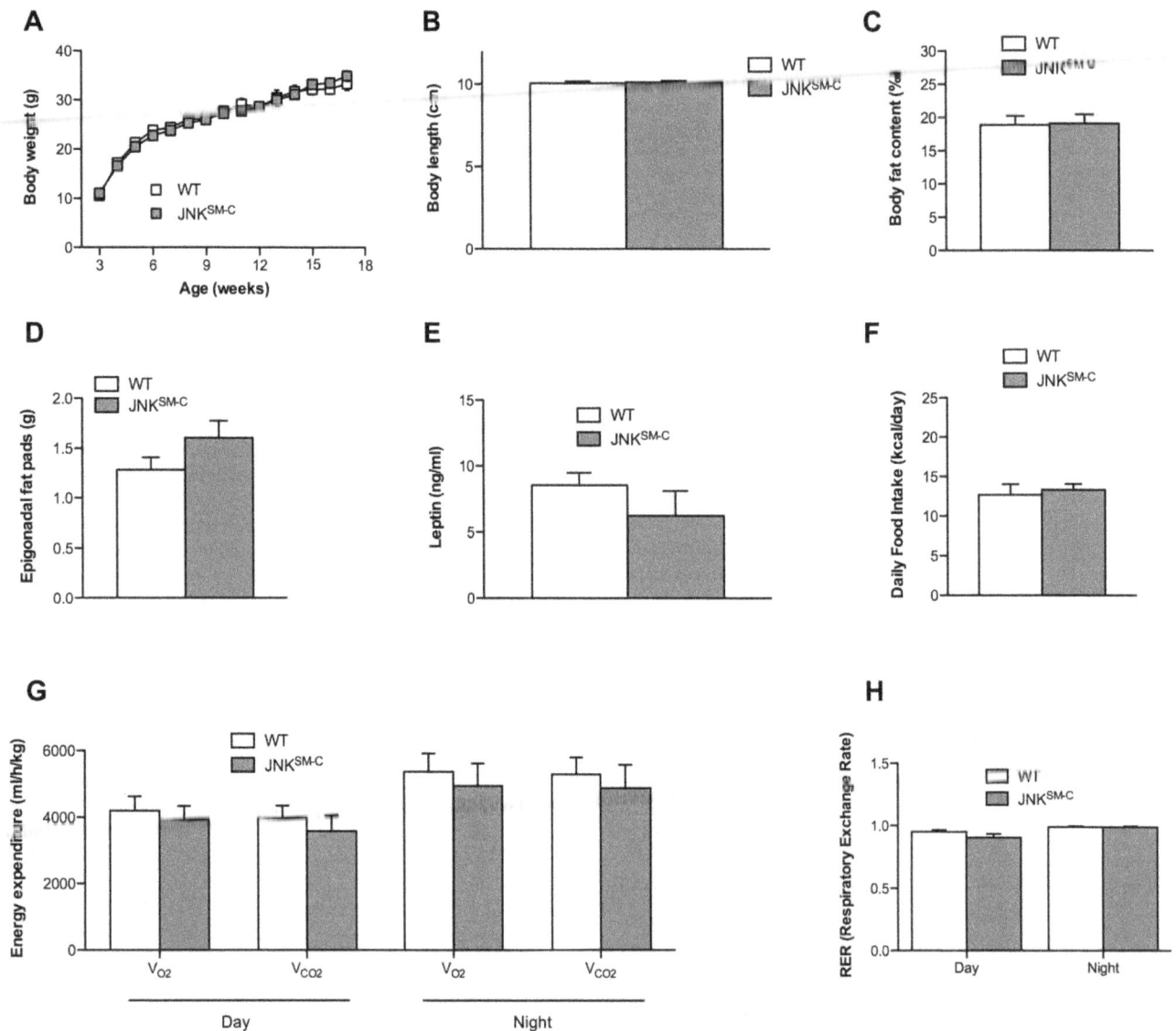

Figure 2. Unaltered body composition and energy homeostasis in JNK^{SM-C} mice. (A) The average bodyweight of control (open squares) mice was compared with JNK^{SM-C} (grey squares) mice from 3 to 17 weeks of age when feeding a NCD (n = 15). (B) Body length of control (white bar) and JNK^{SM-C} (grey bar) mice upon NCD feeding (n = 9–12). (C) Body composition of control (white bar) and JNK^{SM-C} (grey bar) mice when exposed to NCD was determined by using a Brucker minispec in week 17 (n = 10–12). (D) Weight of epigonadal fat pads from NCD fed control (white bar) and JNK^{SM-C} (grey bar) mice in week 17 (n = 9). (E) Serum leptin levels of control (white bar) and JNK^{SM-C} (grey bar) mice at the age of 17 weeks (n = 9). (F) Daily food intake of control (white bar) and JNK^{SM-C} (grey bar) mice upon NCD feeding at the age of 14 weeks (n = 5). (G) Energy expenditure revealed by the daily and nightly volume of O_2 consumption and CO_2 release of control (white bar) and JNK^{SM-C} (grey bar) mice upon NCD feeding (n = 5). (H) Respiratory exchange rate (RER) of control (white bar) and JNK^{SM-C} (grey bar) mice upon NCD feeding (n = 5). Values are means ± SEM.

between JNK-1^{SM-KO} and control mice under obese conditions (Fig. 4F, G, H). In summary, our results clearly indicate that skeletal muscle-specific disruption of JNK-1 fails to affect body composition and energy homeostasis in lean and obese mice indicating that JNK-1-dependent signaling in other organs than skeletal muscle accounts for the protective effect of JNK-1 deficiency against the development of diet-induced obesity.

Lack of JNK-1 in Skeletal Muscle does not Affect Glucose Homeostasis and Insulin Sensitivity Under Normal and Obese Conditions

While JNK-1-deficiency in skeletal muscle did not affect the development of HFD-induced obesity, we next aimed to analyze,

whether the absence of JNK-1-signaling in this organ affects the manifestation of obesity-associated insulin resistance. Exposure to HFD led to significantly impaired glucose and insulin tolerance in control mice compared to the NCD fed control cohort (Fig. 5A, B). However, when compared to the control groups of mice, glucose and insulin tolerance was unaltered in JNK-1^{SM-KO} mice both under lean and obese conditions (Fig. 5A, B). Moreover, while plasma insulin concentrations were significantly increased in obese control mice compared to NCD from 5 ng/ml to 25 ng/ml, identical results were obtained from mice with muscle specific JNK-1 deficiency (Fig. 5C). Thus, JNK-1-deficiency in skeletal muscle does not result in significant improvements of diet-induced deterioration of glucose metabolism in mice.

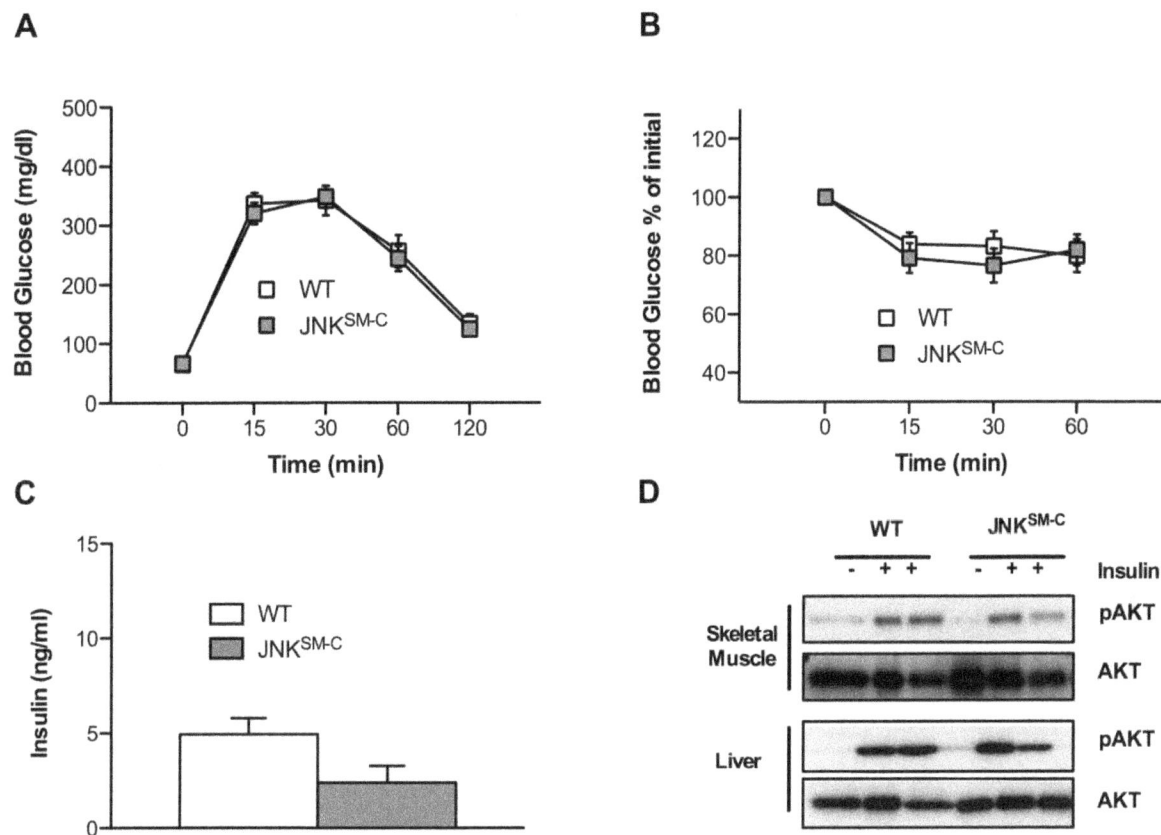

Figure 3. Unaltered glucose metabolism and insulin sensitivity in JNK^{SM-C} mice. (A) Glucose tolerance tests of control (white bar) and JNK^{SM-C} (grey bar) mice when feeding a NCD were performed at 11 weeks of age (n = 10–13). (B) Insulin tolerance tests of control (white bar) and JNK^{SM-C} (grey bar) mice upon NCD feeding were performed at 12 weeks of age (n = 13–15). (C) Insulin levels from sera isolated at week 17 from mice with the indicated genotypes upon NCD feeding determined by ELISA (n = 8–10). (D) Representative insulin-induced AKT phosphorylation of muscle and liver lysates isolated from control and JNK^{SM-C} mice when feeding NCD using Western Blot analysis with the indicated antibodies. Values are means ± SEM.

In the absence of alterations of whole body glucose metabolism in JNK-1^{SM-KO} mice compared to control mice, we next wanted to address, whether lack of JNK-1 in these organs may still lead to improved insulin signal transduction at a molecular level, which possibly fails to translate to changes in overall glucose metabolism. Thus, we assessed insulin's ability to stimulate phosphorylation of AKT, as a measure for insulin-stimulated AKT activation *in vivo*. This analysis revealed impaired insulin-stimulated AKT-phosphorylation both in skeletal muscle and liver (Fig. 5D) of control mice exposed to HFD compared to lean controls exposed to NCD. However, the lack of JNK-1 in skeletal muscle could not improve the diet-induced inhibition of insulin-stimulated AKT-phosphorylation in these organs (Fig. 5D). Thus, our experiments unequivocally demonstrate, that JNK-1 is dispensable for the development of diet-induced insulin resistance in skeletal muscle of mice.

Noteworthy, our data are not in line with a previous report that identified a role of skeletal muscle specific JNK-1 in the development of diet-induced local and systemic insulin resistance (17). To assess whether this discrepancy might be a consequence of an alternative physiological characterization, we investigated control C57/BL6 mice in the different phenotyping protocols. To this end, cohorts of C57/BL6 mice were exposed to NCD and HFD starting with 3 weeks of age (WTS3), and compared to cohorts of C57/BL6 mice receiving the different diets with 8 weeks of age (WTS8), respectively. This analysis demonstrated that HFD

exposure increased bodyweight gain, body length as well as adiposity in both protocols to a similar extent when compared to the NCD exposed control mice (Fig. S2A, B, C, D). The similar adiposity of WTS3 and WTS8 control mice exposed to HFD feeding could also be confirmed by the presence of similar circulating leptin levels as revealed by ELISA (Fig. S2E). Furthermore, while indirect calorimetry experiments revealed that WTS3 mice showed increased VO$_2$ consumption and VCO$_2$ production compared to the WTS8 counterparts mainly during the day phase under both dietary conditions, the respiratory exchange rate resulting from these data was indistinguishable (Fig. S2F, G). Nevertheless, diet-induced impairments of glucose homeostasis were similar in both protocols as revealed by glucose tolerance and insulin tolerance tests as well as increased circulating insulin concentrations (Fig. S2H, I, J, K, L). Collectively, these data demonstrate that the discrepancy between the previously published work (17) and our study is not a result of different physiological characterization protocols.

Bodywide JNK-1 Deficiency Protects against HFD-induced Glucose Intolerance and Insulin Resistance

Disruption of JNK-1 by conventional means results in decreased obesity and improved glucose metabolism [12]. To confirm this important finding with our JNK-1 allele, we inactivated JNK-1 in the whole body by crossing JNK-1$^{FL/FL}$ mice to deleter Cre mice

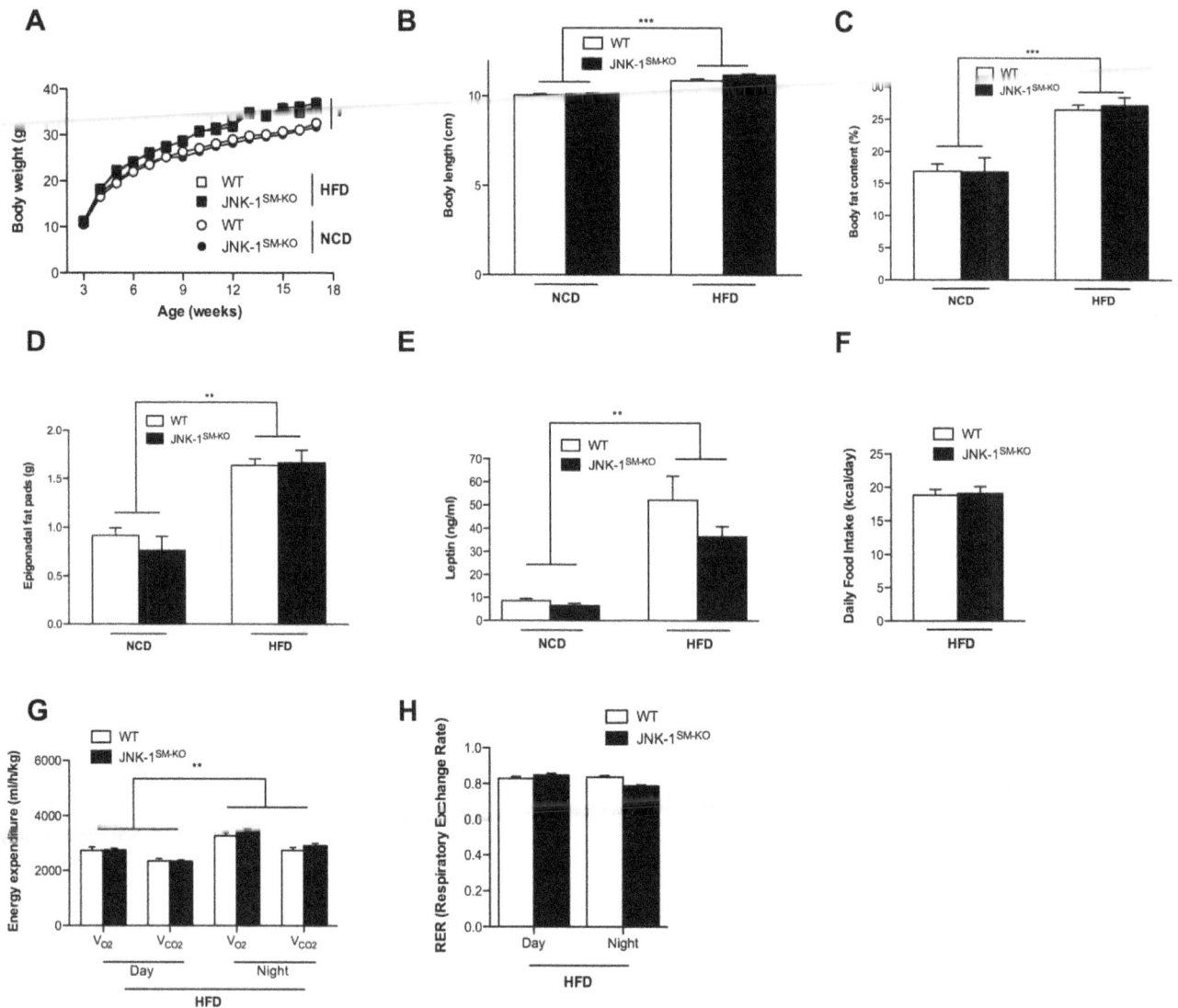

Figure 4. Unaltered body composition and energy homeostasis in JNK-1^{SM-KO} mice under normal and obese conditions. (A) The average bodyweight of control NCD fed (open circles) and HFD fed (open squares) mice was compared with JNK-1^{SM-KO} mice fed a NCD (black circles) or a HFD (black squares) from 3 to 17 weeks of age (n = 15–45). (B) Body length of control (white bar) and JNK-1^{SM-KO} (black bar) mice upon NCD and HFD feeding. (C) Body composition of control (white bar) and JNK-1^{SM-KO} (black bar) mice when exposed to NCD or HFD were determined by using a Brucker minispec in week 17 (n = 11–24). (D) Weight of epigonadal fat pads from NCD and HFD fed control (white bar) and JNK-1^{SM-KO} (black bar) mice in week 17 (n = 13–40). (E) Serum leptin levels of control (white bar) and JNK-1^{SM-KO} (black bar) mice upon NCD and HFD feeding at the age of 17 weeks (n = 8–18). (F) Daily food intake of control (white bar) and JNK-1^{SM-KO} (black bar) mice upon HFD feeding at the age of 14 weeks (n = 5–27). (G) Energy expenditure revealed by the daily and nightly volume of O_2 consumption and CO_2 release of control (white bar) and JNK-1^{SM-KO} (black bar) mice upon HFD feeding (n = 8). (H) Respiratory exchange rate (RER) of control (white bar) and JNK-1^{SM-KO} (black bar) mice upon HFD feeding (n = 8). Values are means ± SEM. **, p≤0.01; ***, p≤0.001.

(JNK-1^{KO} mice). Consistent with previously published results, JNK-1^{KO} mice on a NCD show not only unaltered bodyweight but also similar naso-anal lengths at 17 weeks of age when compared to controls (Fig. S3A, B). In line with these data, adiposity and epigonadal fat pad weights as well as circulating leptin levels and food ingestion were comparable between the two groups of mice (Fig. S3C, D, E, F). Moreover, while the parameters of energy homeostasis matched between control and JNK-1^{KO} mice (Fig. S3G, H), glucose tolerance and insulin sensitivity were largely unaffected by complete JNK-1 deficiency under normal conditions (Fig. S3I, J, K). As the beneficial effects of JNK-1 deficiency were observed under obese conditions, we assessed energy and glucose homeostasis in JNK-1^{KO} and control

mice also when exposed to HFD feeding. Indeed, determination of body weight from weaning until 17 weeks of age of WT and JNK-1^{KO} mice revealed that JNK-1^{KO} mice are protected from HFD-induced weight gain (Fig. 6A). Moreover, since mice lacking JNK-1 in the CNS show a reduction in somatic growth as a consequence of impaired growth hormone/insulin like growth factor 1 axis [19], body length of WT and JNK-1^{KO} mice was assessed, revealing a significant reduction of body length in JNK-1^{KO} mice fed a HFD (Fig. 6B). The degree of adiposity in WT and JNK-1^{KO} mice upon HFD feeding was determined by NMR analysis and by measuring the weight of the epigonadal fat pads. These analyses demonstrated that JNK-1^{KO} mice exhibit decreased body fat content when compared to WT mice as well

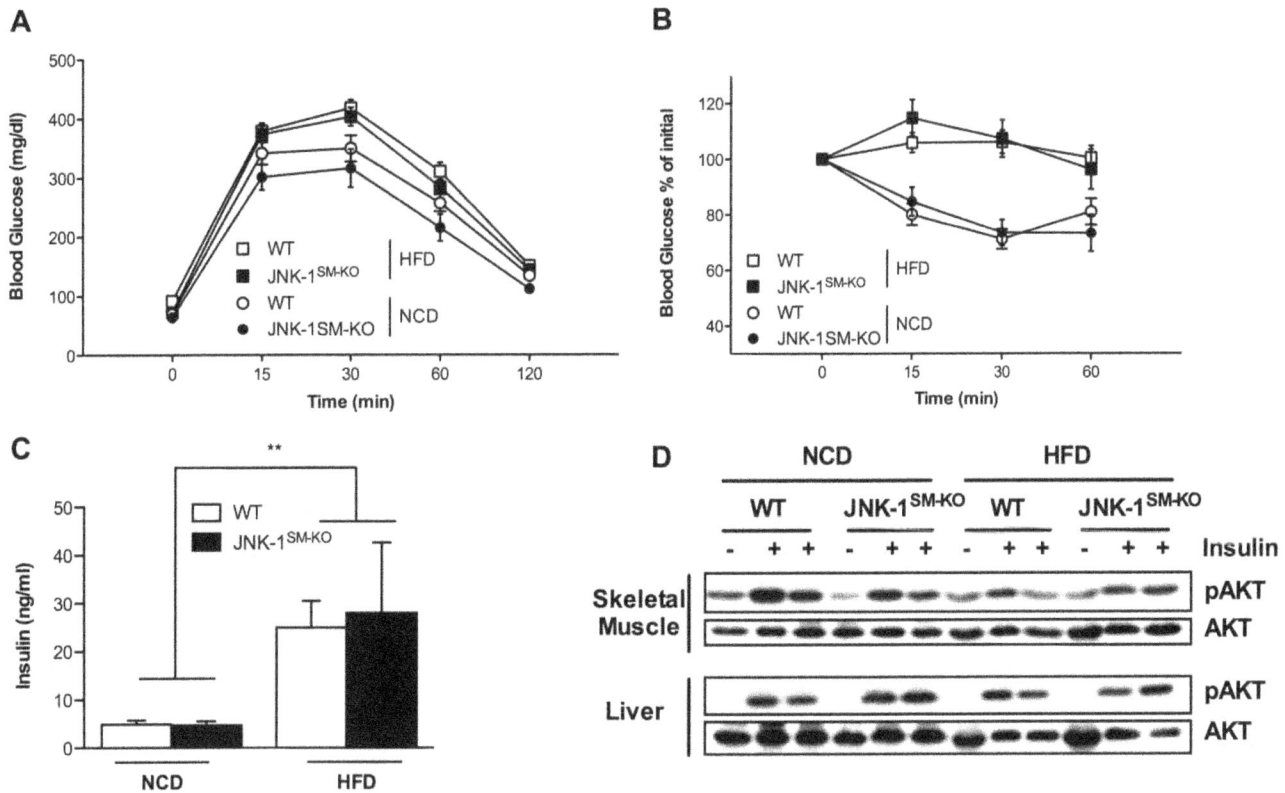

Figure 5. Unaltered glucose metabolism and insulin sensitivity in JNK-1^{SM-KO} under normal and obese conditions. (A) Glucose tolerance tests of control NCD fed (open circles) and HFD fed (open squares) mice and JNK-1^{SM-KO} mice fed a NCD (black circles) or a HFD (black squares) were performed at 11 weeks of age (n = 9–49). (B) Insulin tolerance tests of control NCD fed (open circles) and HFD fed (open squares) mice and JNK-1^{SM-KO} fed a NCD (black circles) or a HFD (black squares) were performed at 12 weeks of age (n = 5–30). (C) Insulin levels from sera isolated at week 17 from mice with the indicated genotypes upon NCD or HFD feeding determined by ELISA (n = 5–9). (D) Representative insulin-induced AKT phosphorylation of muscle and liver lysates isolated from control and JNK-1^{SM-KO} mice when feeding NCD and HFD using Western Blot analysis with the indicated antibodies. Values are means ± SEM. **, p≤0.01; ***, p≤0.001.

as reduced epigonadal fat pad weight (Fig. 6 C and D). Consistent with these findings, serum levels of leptin as an indirect measure of adiposity were reduced in JNK-1^{KO} mice when compared to WT mice (Fig. 6 E). Collectively, these results demonstrate that mice lacking JNK-1 in the whole body are protected from the development of HFD-induced adiposity. Reduced adiposity develops either in light of a reduced caloric intake or due to increases in energy expenditure or both. Noteworthy, the decreased adiposity of JNK-1^{KO} mice is a consequence of significantly reduced food intake of JNK-1^{KO} mice compared to controls (Fig. 6 F) rather than increased energy expenditure, whose means were only minor affected (Fig. 6 G). However, JNK-1^{KO} mice showed reduced HFD-induced lipid utilization as the daily and nightly RER was increased compared to controls (Fig. 6 H). Next, we wanted to address whether the reduction in adiposity in JNK-1^{KO} mice under obese conditions translates into improved glucose homeostasis. Hence, glucose and insulin tolerance tests were performed. This analysis revealed that the time-dependent glucose clearance from the blood upon an intraperitoneal glucose challenge was markedly ameliorated in JNK-1^{KO} mice when compared to control mice fed a HFD (Fig. 6 I). Moreover, insulin sensitivity as assessed by an insulin tolerance was strongly improved in JNK-1^{KO} mice when compared to WT mice (Fig. 6 J). Strikingly, JNK-1^{KO} mice were also protected from HFD-induced hyperinsulinemia as indicated by reduced circulating levels of insulin in comparison to WT mice (Fig. 6 K). In summary,

these results clearly support previous work indicating that body-wide JNK-1 deficiency protects from diet-induced weight gain and insulin resistance. Thus, our experiments assign JNK-1 activation in tissues other than skeletal muscle a critical role in the development of obesity-associated deterioration of energy and glucose homeostasis.

Discussion

The notion that obesity is associated with an increased inflammatory state, which activates numerous intracellular signaling cascades in turn inhibiting insulin action provides a unique opportunity for the development of novel therapeutic interventions to treat obesity-associated insulin resistance and diabetes. However, these novel therapeutic approaches require the exact definition of the intracellular signaling cascade activated by cytokines such as TNF-α and IL-6, ER-stress or altered lipid composition contributing to the inhibition of insulin signaling in a tissue-specific manner. Here, numerous candidate pathways activated by these stimuli have been shown to cause inhibitory serine phosphorylation of insulin receptor substrate proteins or to induce insulin resistance by other mechanisms [3,4,7,8].

Thus, obesity-induced inflammatory signaling pathways include activation of IκBα kinases (IKK), the c-Jun N-terminal kinases (JNK), atypical protein kinase C (PKC) and it has been recently recognized that altered diacylglycerol (DAG) content in skeletal

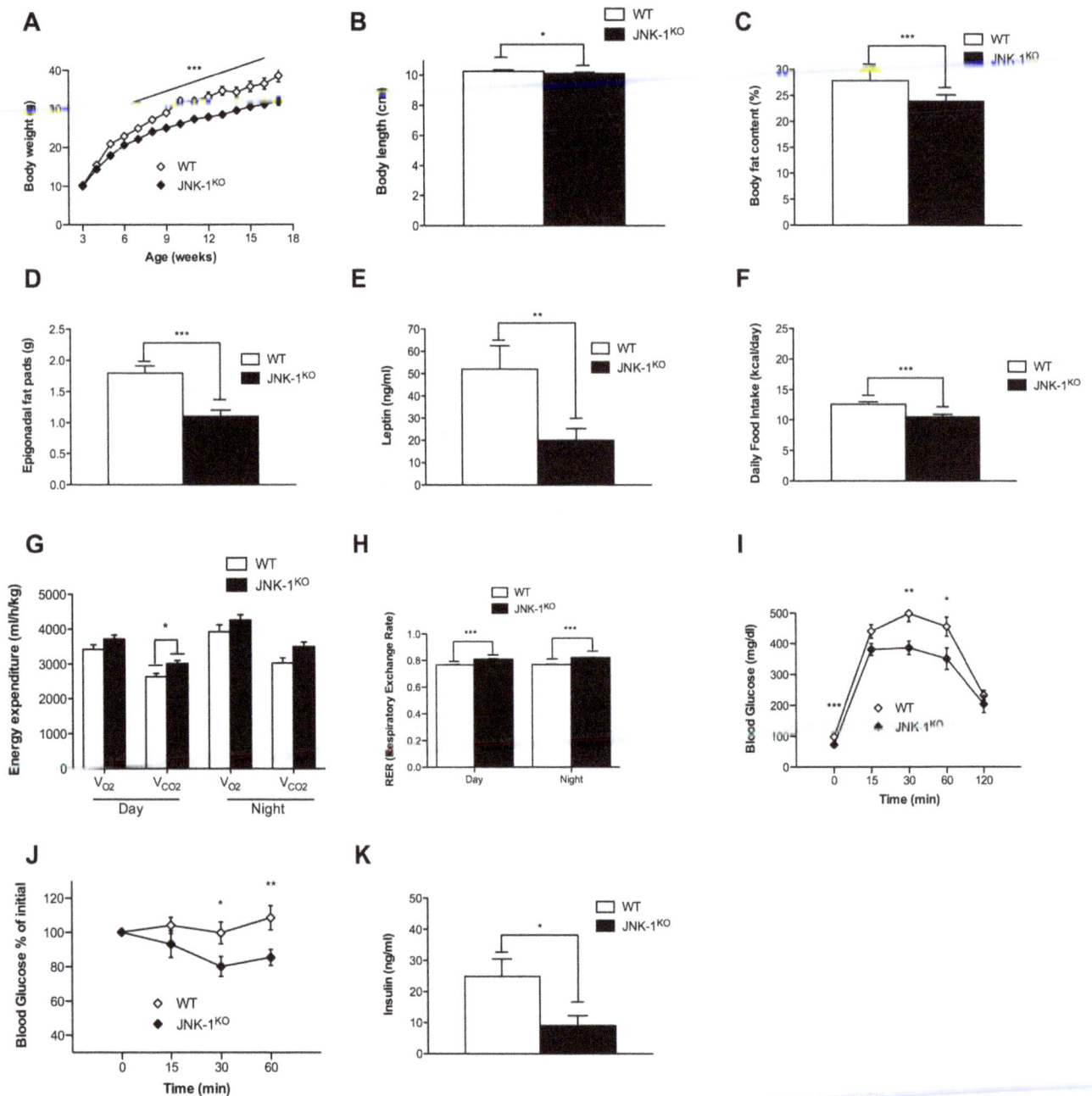

Figure 6. Complete absence of JNK-1 protects from HFD-induced obesity and insulin resistance. (A) The average body weight of WT (white diamonds) and JNK-1[KO] (black diamonds) mice fed a HFD from 3 to 17 weeks of age (n = 12–18). (B) Body length of WT and JNK-1[KO] mice upon HFD at 17 weeks age (n = 15). (C) Body composition of WT (white bar) and JNK-1[KO] (black bar) mice when exposed to HFD was determined by using a Brucker minispec in week 17 (n = 15–19). (D) Weight of epigonadal fat pads from HFD fed WT (white bar) and JNK-1[KO] (black bar) mice in week 17 (n = 10–12). (E) Serum leptin levels of WT (white bar) and JNK-1[KO] (black bar) mice at the age of 17 weeks (n = 10). (F) Daily food intake of WT (white bar) and JNK-1[KO] (black bar) mice upon HFD feeding at the age of 14 weeks (n = 17). (G) Energy expenditure revealed by the daily and nightly volume of O_2 consumption and CO_2 release of WT (white bar) and JNK-1[KO] (black bar) mice upon HFD feeding (n = 5). (H) Respiratory exchange rate (RER) of control (white bar) and JNK-1[KO] (black bar) mice upon HFD feeding (n = 5). (I) Glucose tolerance tests of WT (white diamonds) and JNK-1[KO] (black diamonds) mice when feeding a HFD were performed at 11 weeks of age (n = 14). (J) Insulin tolerance tests of WT (white diamonds) and JNK-1[KO] (black diamonds) mice upon HFD feeding were performed at 12 weeks of age (n = 14) (K) Insulin levels from sera isolated at week 17 from mice with the indicated genotypes upon HFD feeding determined by ELISA (n = 8). Values are means ± SEM, *, $p < 0.05$, **, $p < 0.01$, ***, $p < 0.001$.

muscle can induce insulin resistance via diacylglycerol kinase (DGK) activation [27].

We and others could demonstrate that in liver, IKK activation plays an important function in the development of obesity-associated insulin resistance and that both, liver-specific IKK-2 or

NEMO deficiency can protect from obesity-associated impairment of glucose tolerance [24,28]. However, deletion of IKK-2 in skeletal muscle fails to prevent the development of obesity-associated insulin resistance, underlining the tissue-specific contribution of inflammatory mediators to cause insulin resistance [29].

In light of the dramatic protection from the occurrence of obesity-associated insulin resistance in conventional JNK-1-, but not JNK-2-deficient animals, JNK-1 was predicted to play an important role - particularly in the insulin-sensitive target tissue skeletal muscle - to cause obesity-associated insulin resistance [12]. Here we demonstrate what was also reported by others that obesity increases JNK activation in skeletal muscle that could potentially impair insulin signaling accounting for the development of obesity-associated insulin resistance in this tissue [17]. To elucidate this possibility, we successfully generated a mouse strain allowing for Cre-activated expression of a JNK constitutively active construct that we crossed to Mck-Cre mice to obtain skeletal muscle specific overactivation of JNK signaling as it is present under obese conditions. However, our metabolic data using these mice eliminate the assumption that increased JNK activation under obese conditions in skeletal muscle impairs insulin signaling but instead clearly communicate the important observation that obesity-induced JNK activation fails to impair insulin action in this organ. Despite similar skeletal muscle specific JNK overactivation in these mice as it is present under obese conditions, these mice lacked any alteration in adiposity, glucose metabolism and energy homeostasis. In line with this observation, we also characterized mice with isolated JNK-1 deficiency in skeletal muscle under lean and obese conditions in which none of the assessed metabolic parameters were affected. Thus, our current finding that isolated JNK overactivation and JNK-1 deficiency in skeletal muscle fails to protect from obesity-associated disturbances in overall glucose metabolism as assessed during glucose tolerance and insulin tolerance tests is surprising. Several explanations may account for this phenomenon. An obvious possibility would be redundant signaling functions of other JNK isoforms in the absence of JNK-1. Therefore, in skeletal muscle, JNK-2 activation may compensate for the lack of JNK-1 and thereby cause development of insulin resistance upon obesity-induction. Indeed, it could be demonstrated that compound deficiency for JNK-1 and heterozygousity for a conventional JNK-2 null allele has a more profound effect to protect from diet-induced insulin resistance than isolated JNK-1 deficiency [13]. Thus, in skeletal muscle either JNK-1 and JNK-2 contribute cooperatively to the development of obesity-associated insulin resistance or alternative kinases such as atypical PKC- and DGK-activation may play a more important role in the development of obesity-induced insulin resistance in this organ [27,30]. An alternative explanation that in our settings JNK-1 deficiency in skeletal muscle fails to improve obesity-associated disorders might be the diverging gene targeting strategies used by us and others [17,19]. Though the previously described JNK-1 conventional knock out mouse replaces exon 2 of JNK-1 with a neo resistance gene [12] and we copied this strategy by flanking exon 2 of JNK-1 with loxP sites, we assessed whether the absence of JNK-1 in the whole body indeed protects from diet-induced obesity and associated disorders. Consistent with the report of Hirosoumi and colleagues [12], also our JNK-1 deficient mouse model showed protection against the development of diet-induced weight gain and showed improved insulin sensitivity.

Thus, what remains a striking observation requiring further investigation is the profound difference of the metabolic phenotype of conventional JNK-1-deficient mice and the reported phenotypes for mice with cell type-specific disruption of JNK-1 activity. While our report clearly demonstrates that skeletal muscle-specific JNK-1 deficiency is not sufficient to protect against obesity-associated insulin resistance, a recent report indicates that inactivation of JNK-1 in the adipose tissue causes some degree of protection from obesity-associated insulin resistance due to the inactivation of JNK-1 in adipose tissue [7]. In the latter study,

adipocyte-autonomous JNK-1 signaling regulates IL-6 secretion in the obese white adipose tissue that in turn inhibits hepatic insulin action through IL-6-induced SOCS-3 expression in the liver [31,32]. Noteworthy, we demonstrated recently that JNK-1 signaling in skeletal muscle controls IL-6 expression in response to exercise [26] implicating an important function of JNK-1-induced IL-6 expression also in other cell types. However, JNK-1-deficient myeloid lineage cells show unaltered IL-6 expression and JNK-1 deficiency in these cells *per se* had no effect on the development of obesity-associated insulin resistance whereas other reports on bone marrow transplantation chimeras with JNK-1-deficient hematopoetic stem cells have yielded controversial findings [14–16]. Nevertheless, neither adipocyte-specific disruption nor hematopoetic-specific JNK-1-deficiency phenocopies the effect of conventional JNK-1 deletion. In line with these reports, also JNK-1 deficiency in liver parenchymal cells has failed to affect body weight gain and insulin sensitivity, but demonstrated an important function of JNK-1 in the prevention of hepatic lipid accumulation [18]. Another candidate organ where the absence of JNK-1 could protect from diet-induced obesity is the central nervous system (CNS). The CNS plays a central role in the control of body weight and peripheral glucose metabolism [33,34]. Within the CNS, insulin action particularly in agouti-related peptide-expressing neurons of the arcuate nucleus of the hypothalamus controls peripheral glucose metabolism via inhibition of hepatic glucose production [35]. Thus, JNK-mediated inhibition of insulin signal transduction in the CNS may play an important role in deterioration of peripheral glucose metabolism. Essentially, we have demonstrated that the combined inactivation of JNK-1 in the CNS and the pituitary represents as yet the most promising approach to resemble the phenotype of conventional JNK-1 knock out mice [19]. Though in these mice adiposity is unaffected in response to HFD, systemic insulin sensitivity is improved accompanied with reduced somatic growth. Taken together, our experiments provide evidence for an important role of JNK-1 signaling in organs other than skeletal muscle in the development of obesity-associated insulin resistance and diabetes.

Supporting Information

Figure S1 Transgenic JNK^C expression in skeletal muscle enhances phosphorylation of cJun. (A) JNK-kinase assay (KA) of protein lysates isolated from muscles of WT and JNK^{SM-C} mice fed a NCD. Calnexin antibodies were used for input control of the lysates. (B) Quantitation of radioactively labeled cJun peptide in skeletal muscle of NCD fed WT and JNK^{SM-C} mice. The data were adjusted to the WT NCD data shown in figure 1 B, C. Values are means ± SEM. *, p≤0.05.

Figure S2 Physiological comparison of diet-induced obesity protocols. (A) The average bodyweight of WTS3 NCD fed (open squares) and WTS3 HFD fed (grey circles) mice was compared with WTS8 mice fed a NCD (open squares) or a HFD (grey circles) from 0 to 17 weeks on both diets, respectively (n = 10). (B) Body length of WTS3 (white bar) and WTS8 (grey bar) mice upon NCD and HFD feeding (n = 10). (C) Body composition of WTS3 (white bar) and WTS8 (grey bar) mice when exposed to NCD or HFD was determined by using a Brucker minispec in week 17 of feeding the diets (n = 10). (D) Weight of epigonadal fat pads from NCD and HFD WTS3 (white bar) and WTS8 (grey bar) mice in week 17 of feeding the diets (n = 10). (E) Serum leptin levels of WTS3 (white bar) and WTS8 (grey bar) mice upon NCD and HFD feeding after 17 weeks on both the diets (n = 10). (F) Energy expenditure revealed by the daily and nightly volume of O_2 consumption and CO_2 release of WTS3 (white bar) and WTS8 (grey bar) mice upon NCD and HFD feeding (n = 10). (G) Respiratory exchange rate (RER) of WTS3 (white bar) and WTS8 (grey bar) mice upon NCD and HFD feeding (n = 10). (H) Glucose tolerance tests of WTS3 NCD fed (open squares) and HFD fed (open circles) mice were performed after 17 weeks on either diet (n = 10). (I) Glucose tolerance tests of WTS8 NCD fed (grey squares) and HFD fed (grey circles) mice were performed after 17 weeks on either diet (n = 10). (J) Insulin tolerance tests of WTS3 NCD fed (open squares) and HFD fed (open circles) mice were performed after 17 weeks on either diet (n = 10). (K) Insulin tolerance tests of WTS8 fed a NCD (grey squares) or a HFD (grey circles) were performed after 17 weeks on either diet (n = 10). (L) Insulin levels from sera isolated after 17 weeks on either of the diets from mice with the indicated genotypes determined by ELISA (n = 10). Values are means ± SEM. **, p≤0.01; ***, p≤0.001.

Figure S3 Phenotypical analysis of bodywide JNK-1 deficiency under normal conditions. (A) The average body weight of WT (white bars) and JNK-1[KO] (black bars) mice fed a NCD at 17 weeks of age (n = 5). (B) Body length of WT and JNK-1[KO] mice upon NCD feeding at 17 weeks age (n = 5). (C) Body composition of WT (white bar) and JNK-1[KO] (black bar) mice when exposed to NCD was determined by using a Brucker minispec in week 17 (n = 5). (D) Weight of epigonadal fat pads from NCD fed WT (white bar) and JNK-1[KO] (black bar) mice in week 17 (n = 5). (E) Serum leptin levels of WT (white bar) and JNK-1[KO] (black bar) mice at the age of 17 weeks (n = 5). (F) Daily food intake of WT (white bar) and JNK-1[KO] (black bar) mice upon NCD feeding at the age of 14 weeks (n = 5). (G) Energy expenditure revealed by the daily and nightly volume of O_2 consumption and CO_2 release of WT (white bar) and JNK-1[KO] (black bar) mice upon NCD feeding (n = 5). (H) Respiratory exchange rate (RER) of control (white bar) and JNK-1[KO] (grey bar) mice upon NCD feeding (n = 5). (I) Glucose tolerance tests of WT (white diamonds) and JNK-1[KO] (black diamonds) mice when feeding a NCD were performed at 11 weeks of age (n = 5). (J) Insulin tolerance tests of WT (white diamonds) and JNK-1[KO] (black diamonds) mice upon NCD feeding were performed at 12 weeks of age (n = 5) (K) Insulin levels from sera isolated at week 17 from mice with the indicated genotypes upon NCD feeding determined by ELISA (n = 5). Values are means ± SEM, *, p<0.05.

Author Contributions

Conceived and designed the experiments: MSS FTW. Performed the experiments: MP CMW GS HB. Analyzed the data: MP CMW HB FTW. Contributed reagents/materials/analysis tools: MSS. Wrote the paper: FTW MP CMW.

References

1. Hotamisligil GS, Shargill NS, Spiegelman BM (1993) Adipose expression of tumor necrosis factor-alpha: direct role in obesity-linked insulin resistance. Science 259: 87–91.
2. Plomgaard P, Bouzakri K, Krogh-Madsen R, Mittendorfer B, Zierath JR, et al. (2005) Tumor necrosis factor-alpha induces skeletal muscle insulin resistance in healthy human subjects via inhibition of Akt substrate 160 phosphorylation. Diabetes 54: 2939–2945.
3. Hotamisligil GS, Budavari A, Murray D, Spiegelman BM (1994) Reduced tyrosine kinase activity of the insulin receptor in obesity-diabetes. Central role of tumor necrosis factor-alpha. J Clin Invest 94: 1543–1549.
4. Cai D, Yuan M, Frantz DF, Melendez PA, Hansen L, et al. (2005) Local and systemic insulin resistance resulting from hepatic activation of IKK-beta and NF-kappaB. Nat Med 11: 183–190.
5. Hotamisligil GS, Arner P, Caro JF, Atkinson RL, Spiegelman BM (1995) Increased adipose tissue expression of tumor necrosis factor-alpha in human obesity and insulin resistance. J Clin Invest 95: 2409–2415.
6. Hotamisligil GS, Peraldi P, Budavari A, Ellis R, White MF, et al. (1996) IRS-1-mediated inhibition of insulin receptor tyrosine kinase activity in TNF-alpha- and obesity-induced insulin resistance. Science 271: 665–668.
7. Solinas G, Naugler W, Galimi F, Lee MS, Karin M (2006) Saturated fatty acids inhibit induction of insulin gene transcription by JNK-mediated phosphorylation of insulin-receptor substrates. Proc Natl Acad Sci U S A 103: 16454–16459.
8. Ozcan U, Cao Q, Yilmaz E, Lee AH, Iwakoshi NN, et al. (2004) Endoplasmic reticulum stress links obesity, insulin action, and type 2 diabetes. Science 306: 457–461.
9. Aguirre V, Uchida T, Yenush L, Davis R, White MF (2000) The c-Jun NH(2)-terminal kinase promotes insulin resistance during association with insulin receptor substrate-1 and phosphorylation of Ser(307). J Biol Chem 275: 9047–9054.
10. Barr RK, Bogoyevitch MA (2001) The c-Jun N-terminal protein kinase family of mitogen-activated protein kinases (JNK MAPKs). Int J Biochem Cell Biol 33: 1047–1063.
11. Kyriakis JM, Woodgett JR, Avruch J (1995) The stress-activated protein kinases. A novel ERK subfamily responsive to cellular stress and inflammatory cytokines. Ann N Y Acad Sci 766: 303–319.
12. Hirosumi J, Tuncman G, Chang L, Gorgun CZ, Uysal KT, et al. (2002) A central role for JNK in obesity and insulin resistance. Nature 420: 333–336.
13. Tuncman G, Hirosumi J, Solinas G, Chang L, Karin M, et al. (2006) Functional in vivo interactions between JNK1 and JNK2 isoforms in obesity and insulin resistance. Proc Natl Acad Sci U S A 103: 10741–10746.
14. Sabio G, Das M, Mora A, Zhang Z, Jun JY, et al. (2008) A stress signaling pathway in adipose tissue regulates hepatic insulin resistance. Science 322: 1539–1543.
15. Solinas G, Vilcu C, Neels JG, Bandyopadhyay GK, Luo JL, et al. (2007) JNK1 in hematopoietically derived cells contributes to diet-induced inflammation and insulin resistance without affecting obesity. Cell Metab 6: 386–397.
16. Vallerie SN, Furuhashi M, Fucho R, Hotamisligil GS (2008) A predominant role for parenchymal c-Jun amino terminal kinase (JNK) in the regulation of systemic insulin sensitivity PLoS One 3: e3151.
17. Sabio G, Kennedy NJ, Cavanagh-Kyros J, Jung DY, Ko HJ, et al. Role of muscle c-Jun NH2-terminal kinase 1 in obesity-induced insulin resistance. Mol Cell Biol 30: 106–115.
18. Sabio G, Cavanagh-Kyros J, Ko HJ, Jung DY, Gray S, et al. (2009) Prevention of steatosis by hepatic JNK1. Cell Metab 10: 491–498.
19. Belgardt BF, Mauer J, Wunderlich FT, Ernst MB, Pal M, et al. Hypothalamic and pituitary c-Jun N-terminal kinase 1 signaling coordinately regulates glucose metabolism. Proc Natl Acad Sci U S A 107: 6028–6033.
20. Sabio G, Cavanagh-Kyros J, Barrett T, Jung DY, Ko HJ, et al. Role of the hypothalamic-pituitary-thyroid axis in metabolic regulation by JNK1. Genes Dev 24: 256–264.
21. Bruning JC, Michael MD, Winnay JN, Hayashi T, Horsch D, et al. (1998) A muscle-specific insulin receptor knockout exhibits features of the metabolic syndrome of NIDDM without altering glucose tolerance. Mol Cell 2: 559–569.
22. Plum L, Ma X, Hampel B, Balthasar N, Coppari R, et al. (2006) Enhanced PIP3 signaling in POMC neurons causes KATP channel activation and leads to diet-sensitive obesity. J Clin Invest 116: 1886–1901.
23. Fischer J, Koch L, Emmerling C, Vierkotten J, Peters T, et al. (2009) Inactivation of the Fto gene protects from obesity. Nature 458: 894–898.
24. Wunderlich FT, Luedde T, Singer S, Schmidt-Supprian M, Baumgartl J, et al. (2008) Hepatic NF-kappa B essential modulator deficiency prevents obesity-induced insulin resistance but synergizes with high-fat feeding in tumorigenesis. Proc Natl Acad Sci U S A 105: 1297–1302.
25. Whitmarsh AJ, Davis RJ (2001) Analyzing JNK and p38 mitogen-activated protein kinase activity. Methods Enzymol 332: 319–336.
26. Whitham M, Chan MH, Pal M, Matthews VB, Prelovsek O, et al. Contraction-induced IL-6 gene transcription in skeletal muscle is regulated by c-jun terminal kinase/Activator protein -1. J Biol Chem.
27. Chibalin AV, Leng Y, Vieira E, Krook A, Bjornholm M, et al. (2008) Downregulation of diacylglycerol kinase delta contributes to hyperglycemia-induced insulin resistance. Cell 132: 375–386.
28. Arkan MC, Hevener AL, Greten FR, Maeda S, Li ZW, et al. (2005) IKK-beta links inflammation to obesity-induced insulin resistance. Nat Med 11: 191–198.
29. Rohl M, Pasparakis M, Baudler S, Baumgartl J, Gautam D, et al. (2004) Conditional disruption of IkappaB kinase 2 fails to prevent obesity-induced insulin resistance. J Clin Invest 113: 474–481.
30. Farese RV, Sajan MP, Yang H, Li P, Mastorides S, et al. (2007) Muscle-specific knockout of PKC-lambda impairs glucose transport and induces metabolic and diabetic syndromes. J Clin Invest 117: 2289–2301.
31. Ueki K, Kondo T, Kahn CR (2004) Suppressor of cytokine signaling 1 (SOCS-1) and SOCS-3 cause insulin resistance through inhibition of tyrosine phosphorylation of insulin receptor substrate proteins by discrete mechanisms. Mol Cell Biol 24: 5434–5446.

32. Ueki K, Kondo T, Tseng YH, Kahn CR (2004) Central role of suppressors of cytokine signaling proteins in hepatic steatosis, insulin resistance, and the metabolic syndrome in the mouse. Proc Natl Acad Sci U S A 101: 10422–10427.

33. Bruning JC, Gautam D, Burks DJ, Gillette J, Schubert M, et al. (2000) Role of brain insulin receptor in control of body weight and reproduction. Science 289: 2122–2125.

34. Inoue H, Ogawa W, Asakawa A, Okamoto Y, Nishizawa A, et al. (2006) Role of hepatic STAT3 in brain-insulin action on hepatic glucose production. Cell Metab 3: 267–275.

35. Konner AC, Janoschek R, Plum L, Jordan SD, Rother E, et al. (2007) Insulin action in AgRP-expressing neurons is required for suppression of hepatic glucose production. Cell Metab 5: 438–449.

36. Wang Y, Su B, Sah VP, Brown JH, Han J, et al. (1998) Cardiac hypertrophy induced by mitogen-activated protein kinase kinase 7, a specific activator for c-Jun NH2-terminal kinase in ventricular muscle cells. J Biol Chem 273: 5423–5426.

37. Zheng C, Xiang J, Hunter T, Lin A (1999) The JNKK2-JNK1 fusion protein acts as a constitutively active c-Jun kinase that stimulates c-Jun transcription activity. J Biol Chem 274: 28966–28971.

38. Mao X, Fujiwara Y, Orkin SH (1999) Improved reporter strain for monitoring Cre recombinase-mediated DNA excisions in mice. Proc Natl Acad Sci U S A 96: 5037–5042.

Prenatal Exposure to Lipopolysaccharide Combined with Pre- and Postnatal High-Fat Diet Result in Lowered Blood Pressure and Insulin Resistance in Offspring Rats

Xue-Qin Hao[1], Jing-Xia Du[2], Yan Li[2], Meng Li[3], Shou-Yan Zhang[4]*

1 Department of Pharmacy, College of Animal Science and Technology, Henan University of Science and Technology, Luoyang, PR China, 2 Department of pharmacology, Medical College, Henan University of Science and Technology, Luoyang, PR China, 3 Luoyang Entry-Exit Inspection and Quarantine Bureau, Luoyang, PR China, 4 Department of Cardiology, Luoyang Central Hospital Affiliated to Zhengzhou University, Luoyang, PR China

Abstract

Background: Adult metabolic syndrome may in part have origins in fetal or early life. This study was designed to explore the effect of prenatal exposure to lipopolysaccharide and high-fat diet on metabolic syndrome in offspring rats.

Methods: 32 pregnant rats were randomly divided into four groups, including Control group; LPS group (pregnant rats were injected with LPS 0.4 mg/kg intraperitoneally on the 8th, 10th and 12th day of pregnancy); High-fat group (maternal rats had high-fat diet during pregnancy and lactation period, and their pups also had high-fat diet up to the third month of life); LPS + High-fat group (rats were exposed to the identical experimental scheme with LPS group and High-fat group).

Results: Blood pressure elevated in LPS group and High-fat group, reduced in LPS+High-fat group, accompanied by the increase of serum leptin level in LPS and High-fat group and increase of serum IL-6, TNF-a in High-fat group; both serum insulin and cholesterol increased in High-fat and LPS+High-fat group, as well as insulin in LPS group. HOMA-IR value increased in LPS, High-fat and LPS+High-fat group, and QUICKI decreased in these groups; H-E staining showed morphologically pathological changes in thoracic aorta and liver tissue in the three groups. Increased serum alanine and aspartate aminotransferase suggest impaired liver function in LPS+High-fat group.

Conclusion/Significance: Prenatal exposure to lipopolysaccharide combined with pre- and postnatal high-fat diet result in lowered blood pressure, insulin resistance and impaired liver function in three-month old offspring rats. The lowered blood pressure might benefit from the predictive adaptive response to prenatal inflammation.

Editor: Guillermo López Lluch, Universidad Pablo de Olavide, Centro Andaluz de Biología del Desarrollo-CSIC, Spain

Funding: This research was supported by Dr. Scientific Research Foundation of Henan University of Science and Technology (No 09001575) and Project of Henan Science and Technology (No 122300410234). The funders had no role in study design, data collection and analysis, decision to publish, or preparation of the manuscript.

Competing Interests: The authors have declared that no competing interests exist.

* E-mail: zsydoctor@163.com

Introduction

The pathophysiology of Type 2 diabetes (T2DM) is characterized by a low-grade chronic inflammation, with the release of inflammatory cytokines by innate immune cells (mainly macrophages and dendritic cells) that impair insulin action [1]. Accumulating evidence from animal studies suggest that chronic elevation of circulating lipopolysaccharide (LPS), a key component of gram negative bacteria cell walls, is considered to be a causative factor for insulin resistance [2]. Obese and T2DM subjects have elevated LPS concentrations in the circulation, and LPS directly inhibits insulin signaling and glucose transport in human muscle cells. Pharmacological and genetic inhibition of LPS-induced inflammation leads to enhanced insulin action [2]. It suggests that inflammation is a mechanism connected with the risk of type 2 diabetes [3].

A fat-enriched diet favors the development of gram negative bacteria in the intestine which is linked to the occurrence of T2DM. It was suggested that the intestinal microbiota contributes to the development of obesity and insulin-resistance. A switch from a normal diet towards a fat-enriched diet, where the daily amount of dietary fibers is reduced, was associated with a change in the ecology of the intestinal microbiota with an increase in gram-negative bacteria [1]. An increase in plasma LPS occurs in healthy individuals after a high-fat meal, whereas a chronic state of low-grade endotoxemia as measured by plasma LPS is evident in patients with obesity and insulin resistance [4].

A great deal of evidence have demonstrated the link between fetal and postnatal growth and development of adult cardiovascular risk factors including hypertension, dyslipidemia, obesity, altered vascular endothelial function and glucose homeostasis. It suggests that adult metabolic syndrome may in part have origins in fetal or early life [5]. Population-based studies suggest that fetal adaptive responses to maternal dietary imbalance confer survival benefit when the postnatal diet remains suboptimal but increase susceptibility to cardiovascular disease when postnatal nutrition is improved [6]. Predictive adaptive responses are also observed in adverse environmental conditions, for example, sweat gland density is determined in early postnatal life by environmental temperature, an adaptation that may determine the degree of tolerance to extremes of climate later in life [6,7]. In addition, fathers can also initiate intergenerational transmission of obesity/ metabolic diseases, induced indirectly or directly, such as through exposure to a high-fat diet [8].

The link between maternal high-fat diet and metabolic diseases has been well recognized [9-11], and previous studies have also showed that prenatal exposure to LPS (0.79 mg/kg) programs hypertension, obesity and insulin resistance in offspring rats [12–14]. But the influence of prenatal LPS exposure combined with pre- and early postnatal high-fat diet on metabolic diseases in offspring rats was not known. May they create a predictive additive effect due to the prenatal inflammation caused by both LPS treatment and high-fat diet, or chronic high-fat diet relative to acute LPS injection intraperitoneally may produce a benefit effect on offspring as a predictive adaptive response? This study was designed to explore the effect of prenatal LPS (0.4 mg/kg) exposure combined with pre- and early postnatal high-fat diet on metabolic syndrome in three-month old offspring rats.

Materials and Methods

Animals

Sixty Sprague-Dawley rats (40 females and 20 males) were purchased from Animal Center of Tongji Medical College, Huazhong University of Science and Technology (Wuhan, China). All animals had free access to standard laboratory rat chow and tap water in a room at constant temperature (24°C) and under a 12 h light-dark cycle. After acclimation for two weeks, the males were with the females for 15 hours, and day 0 of pregnancy was confirmed the next morning by the presence of a vaginal plug. After parturition, pups were raised with a lactating mother until 4 weeks of age, at which time they were removed to cages containing four rat pups. The present study was conducted in accordance with the principles outlined in the National Institutes of Health (NIH) *Guide for the Care and Use of Laboratory Animals* (http://grants1.nih.gov/grants/olaw/) and was approved by the local animal ethics committee at Henan University of Science and Technology.

Dams and litters

The pregnant rats were randomly divided into four groups (n = 8 in each): Control group, LPS group, High-fat group and LPS+High-fat group. The rats in Control group and LPS group had normal diet, and were intraperitoneally administered with vehicle, 0.40 mg/kg LPS (Sigma Chemical, St Louis, MO, USA) respectively on the 8th, 10th and 12th day of pregnancy. Rats in High-fat group were exposed to high-fat diet (based on the normal diet, added 10% lard oil, 5% cholesterin, 1.5% bile salt from pig, 10 egg yolks/kg, 0.14 kg milk powder/kg, some sugar and trace elements) during pregnancy and lactation period, and their pups also had High-fat diet up to the third month of life. Rats in LPS+High-fat group were exposed to the identical experimental scheme with LPS group and High-fat group.

Blood collection

Rats fasted for 12 h, were anesthetized with pentobarbital (40 mg/kg). Blood was taken from abdominal aorta and put at room temperature for 30 minutes, then was centrifuged at 3000 r/ min for 10 minutes. The supernatant serum was taken and stored at −20°C.

Measurement of serum IL-6, TNF-a and leptin concentration

Serum IL-6, TNF-a and leptin concentrations were measured with Enzyme-linked immunosorbent assay (Elisa) method using Rat IL-6, TNF-a and leptin ELISA kits (Shanghai Resun Biological Technology Co., Ltd., Shanghai, China) according to the instructions. The microplates were read using a SpectraMax M5 microplate reader (SpectraMax M5, US).

Systolic blood pressure measurement

Blood pressure was measured with Carotid Artery Intubation method using BL-420E Biological Signal Acquisition System (Chengdu Thai Union Electronics Co., Ltd., Chengdu, China) when offspring rats were three-month old. The offspring rats were anesthetized with pentobarbital (40 mg/kg) and put on the table; then carotid artery was exposed, intubated and connected to BL-420E Biological Signal Acquisition System. The average systolic blood pressure was recorded.

Measurement of serum glucose and insulin

Serum glucose was measured with Glucose Oxidase method using Glucose assay kit (Sichuan new biological technology Co., Ltd., Chengdu, China) and TBA-2000FR automatic biochemical analyzer (Toshiba Medical Systems Co., Ltd., Japan). Serum insulin was measured with Chemiluminescence method using Insulin determination kit (Tianjin Bo oasis Biological Technology Co., Ltd., Tianjin, China) and TBA-2000FR automatic biochemical analyzer (Toshiba Medical Systems Co., Ltd., Japan).

Measurement of serum triglyceride and cholesterol

Serum triglyceride and cholesterol were measured with Oxidase method using Triglyceride assay kit and Cholesterol assay kit (Intec Biotechnology Co., Ltd., Xiamen, China), respectively, and detected with TBA-2000FR automatic biochemical analyzer (Toshiba Medical Systems Co., Ltd., Japan).

Calculation of HOMA-IR and QUICKI

HOMA-IR was calculated according to the formulas below:

$$HOMA - IR =$$

$$[fasting\ glucose\ (mmol/L) \times fasting\ insulin\ (\mu IU/mL)/22.5]$$

Insulin sensitivity was estimated using the Quantitative Insulin Sensitivity Check Index (QUICKI) according to equation: QUICKI = $1/[(\log\ insulin\ (\mu IU/mL) + \log\ glucose\ (mg/dL)]$. Low QUICKI indicates low insulin sensitivity, while high QUICKI indicates high insulin sensitivity.

Evaluation of liver function

Liver function was evaluated by serum levels of alanine aminotransferase, aspartate aminotransferase, total bilirubin, total protein and albumin. Alanine aminotransferase and aspartate aminotransferase were determined with IFCC method using Alanine aminotransferase and Aspartate aminotransferase determination kits (Sichuan New Biological Technology Co., Ltd., Chengdu, China), respectively. Total bilirubin was measured with Vanadate Oxidation method using Total bilirubin assay kit (Sichuan New Biological Technology Co., Ltd., Chengdu, China). Total protein was determined with Biuret method using Total protein assay kit (Intec Biotechnology Co., Ltd., Xiamen, China); albumin was determined with Bromocresol Green Colorimetry

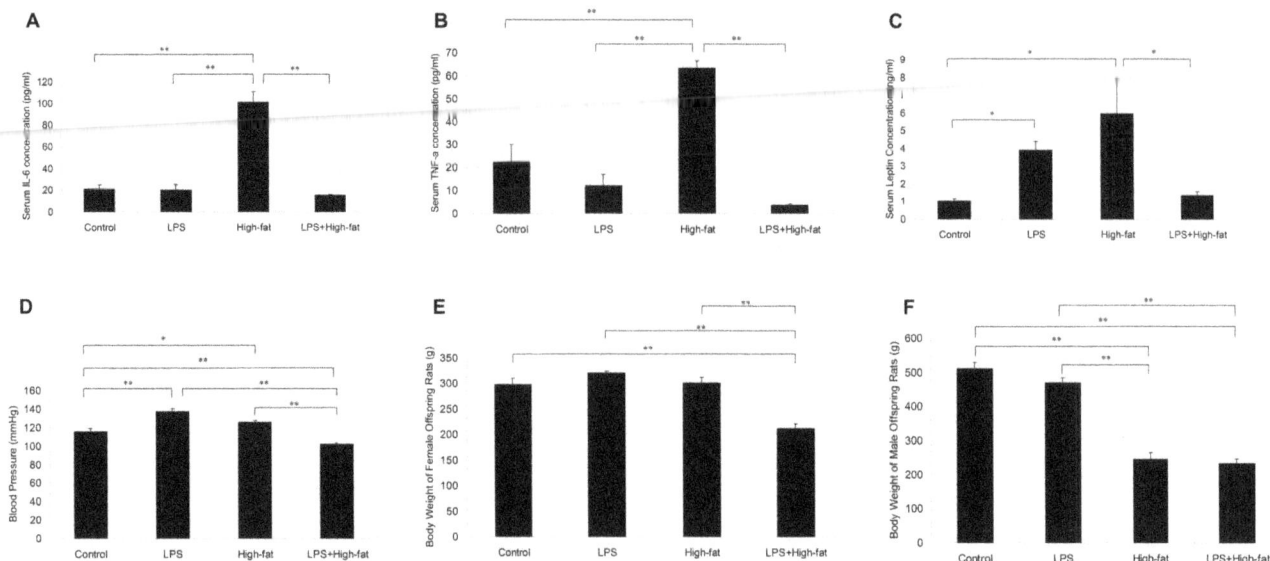

Figure 1. Effects of prenatal exposure to lipopolysaccharide combined with pre- and postnatal high-fat diet on serum IL-6 (A), TNF-a (B), leptin (C), blood pressure (D) and body weight (E, F) in three-month old offspring rats. Data are presented as the mean ± SEM (n = 8 in each group). ** P<0.01, * P<0.05 (one-way ANOVA).

method using Albumin assay kit (Intec Biotechnology Co., Ltd., Xiamen, China). All these indexes were detected with TBA-2000FR automatic biochemical analyzer (Toshiba Medical Systems Co., Ltd., Japan).

Evaluation of renal function

Renal function was evaluated by serum levels of urea nitrogen, creatinine and uric acid. Serum urea nitrogen was determined with UV-Glutamate Dehydrogenase method using Kit for determination of urea nitrogen; serum creatinine was determined with Sarcosine Oxidase method using Creatinine assay kit; serum uric acid was determined with Oxidase method using Uric acid assay kit. All these kits were purchased from Sichuan New Biological Technology Co., Ltd., Chengdu, China. These indexes were detected with TBA-2000FR automatic biochemical analyzer (Toshiba Medical Systems Co., Ltd., Japan).

Morphological changes of thoracic aorta and liver tissue

After perfusion with 0.9% Nacl and 4% paraformaldehyde, thoracic aorta and liver tissue were collected and incubated in 4% paraformaldehyde solution for 48 h, then dehydrated and embedded in paraffin wax; tissue was sliced into sections (4 µm) and HE staining was performed. Morphological changes of thoracic aorta and liver tissue were observed under light microscope.

Statistical analysis

Results are presented as means ± SEM. One-way ANOVA followed by Tukey's post hoc test was used to assess the statistical significance between groups. Two-way ANOVA followed by Bonferroni's post-test was used to assess the interaction between prenatal LPS exposure and high-fat diet on the values. P<0.05 was considered significant. All analyses were performed with SPSS 13.0 (SPSS Inc., Chicago, IL, USA).

Results

Delivery rate

Delivery rates for different groups are 10±2 puppies per litter in Control group and LPS group; 8±2 puppies per litter in High-fat group and LPS + High-fat group.

Food intake

Food intake of pregnant rats in Control group and LPS group was 46.3±4.2 g and 45.6±4.5 g per day; Food intake of pregnant rats in High-fat group and LPS+High-fat group was 29.3±3.5 g, 27.7±3.3 g per day, respectively.

Food intake of 3 month-old male offspring rats in Control group and LPS group was 34.7±3.4 g, 35.3±2.8 g per day, in female offspring rats was 26.6±1.3 g and 27.0±1.8 g, respectively. Food intake of 3 month-old male offspring rats in High-fat and LPS+High-fat group was 20.4±2.7 g, 19.0±2.5 g per day, in female offspring rats was 16.3±1.3 g and 15.5±1.5 g, respectively.

Serum IL-6, TNF-a and leptin concentration

Serum IL-6 and TNF-a concentration in High-fat group increased significantly compared with Control group, LPS group and LPS+High-fat group (p<0.01) (Figure 1A and 1B). There was no significant difference between Control group, LPS group and LPS+High-fat group. Serum leptin concentration in High-fat group increased significantly compared with Control group, LPS group and LPS+High-fat group (p<0.05) (Figure 1C). Significant interaction was found between prenatal LPS exposure and pre- and postnatal high-fat diet on serum IL-6 (F = 38.822, df = 1, p<0.01), TNF-a (F = 13.801, df = 1, p<0.01) and leptin concentration (F = 36.017, df = 1, p<0.01).

Systolic blood pressure

Systolic blood pressure in LPS group (p<0.01) and High-fat group (p<0.05) increased significantly compared with Control group, while systolic blood pressure in LPS+High-fat group decreased significantly compared with Control, LPS and High-fat groups ($p<0.01$). Significant interaction was found between prenatal LPS exposure and pre- and postnatal high-fat diet on systolic blood pressure (F = 22.686, df = 1, $p<0.01$) (Figure 1D).

Body weight

Body weight of female offspring rats in LPS+High-fat group decreased significantly compared with Control group, LPS group and High-fat group ($p<0.01$) (Figure 1E); body weight in male offspring rats in both High-fat group and LPS+High-fat group decreased significantly compared with Control group and LPS group ($p<0.01$) (Figure 1F). There existed significant interaction between prenatal LPS exposure and pre- and postnatal high-fat diet on body weight of female offspring rats (F = 33.624, df = 1, $p<0.01$).

Serum glucose and insulin concentration

Serum insulin in LPS, High-fat and LPS+High-fat groups increased significantly compared with Control group ($p<0.01$). Compared with LPS group, serum insulin in the LPS+High-fat group also increased significantly ($p<0.05$) (Figure 2A). No significant difference was found among all groups in serum glucose (Figure 2B).

Serum cholesterol and triglyceride concentration

Serum cholesterol concentration in High-fat group ($p<0.05$) and LPS+High-fat group ($p<0.01$) increased significantly compared with Control group and LPS group ($p<0.01$) (Figure 2C). There existed significant interaction between prenatal LPS exposure and pre- and postnatal high-fat diet on serum cholesterol concentration (F = 325.371, df = 1, $p<0.01$). There was no significant difference among all groups in serum triglyceride concentration (Figure 2D).

HOMA-IR and QUICKI

Compared with Control group, HOMA-IR in LPS, High-fat and LPS+High-fat groups increased significantly ($p<0.01$)

(Figure 2E). HOMA-IR in LPS+High-fat group also increased significantly compared with LPS group ($p<0.05$) (Figure 2E).

QUICKI in LPS group, High-fat group and LPS+High-fat group decreased significantly compared with Control group ($p<0.01$) (Figure 2F).

Liver and renal function evaluation

Serum alanine aminotransferase concentration increased significantly in LPS+High-fat group compared with Control group ($p<0.01$). Serum aspartate aminotransferase concentration increased significantly in High-fat group ($p<0.05$) and LPS+High-fat group ($p<0.01$). No significant difference was found among all groups in serum total bilirubin, total protein and albumin concentration (Table 1).

No significant difference was found among all groups in serum urea nitrogen, creatinine and uric acid (Table 1).

Morphological changes of thoracic aorta

Under light microscope, cells in thoracic aorta in Control group lined up in order without disruption, and the morphology structure of cells were normal, by contrast, the cells were disordered and loose, and with some deformed nucleus in LPS group and High-fat group (Figure 3A).

Morphological changes of liver

Under light microscope, liver tissue in Control group was normal without inflammation and hepatocytes disruption, whereas in LPS group, macrophages and lymphocytes infiltration was found around central vein. Lipid accumulates in most of the hepatocytes as vacuoles with many nucleus disappeared in High-fat group and LPS+High fat group (Figure 3B).

Discussion

The novel finding of this study was that prenatal exposure to LPS of 0.4 mg/kg resulted in hypertension and insulin resistance in offspring rats; prenatal exposure to LPS combined with pre- and postnatal high-fat diet resulted in lowered blood pressure, insulin

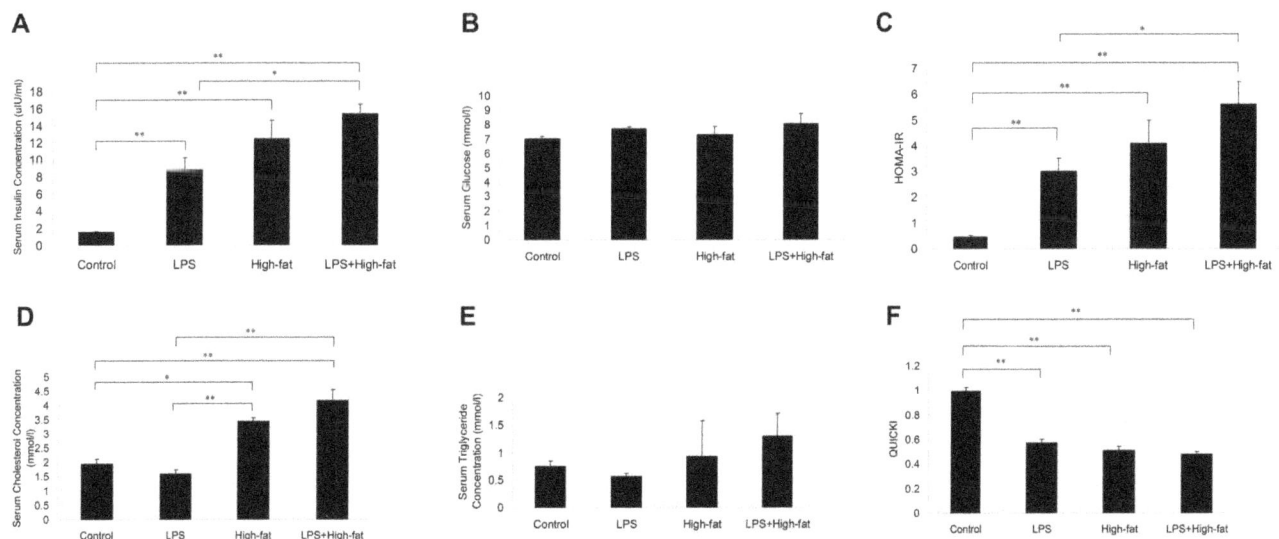

Figure 2. Effects of prenatal exposure to lipopolysaccharide combined with pre- and postnatal high-fat diet on serum insulin (A), glucose (B), HOMA-IR (C), serum cholesterol(D), serum triglyceride (E) and QUICKI (F) in three-month old offspring rats. Data are presented as the mean ± SEM (n = 8 in each group). ** $P<0.01$, * $P<0.05$ (one-way ANOVA).

Table 1. Effects of prenatal exposure to lipopolysaccharide combined with pre- and postnatal high-fat diet on liver and renal function in offspring rats.

	Control	LPS	High-fat	LPS+High-fat
Alanine aminotransferase (u/L)	29.88±3.74	29.75±2.89	39.00±6.00	74.75±22.32**
Aspartate aminotransferase (u/L)	87.00±7.93	94.75±6.35	211.50±32.50*#	228.75±49.56**##
Total bilirubin (umol/L)	0.55±0.11	0.34±0.11	0.35±0.25	0.13±0.06
Total protein (g/L)	75.38±3.42	69.25±0.79	71.00±1.00	73.00±1.63
Albumin (g/L)	41.13±1.30	39.50±0.60	42.00±1.00	36.75±1.38
Urea nitrogen (mmol/L)	5.85±0.48	5.93±0.49	8.65±1.15	4.30±0.45
Creatinine (mmol/L)	59.00±4.52	46.63±2.45	50.00±10.00	47.00±8.83
Uric acid (mmol/L)	34.25±5.77	44.63±5.14	96.50±6.50	53.50±13.38

*$p<0.05$ vs Control group; **$p<0.01$ vs Control group; # $p<0.05$ vs LPS group; ## $p<0.01$ vs LPS group.

resistance, lowered body weight and impaired liver function in offspring rats.

LPS acts as a non-specific immunostimulant to mimic the bacterial inflammatory response. It initiates a series of phosphorylation events by binding to Toll-like receptor 4 and promoting the translocation of nuclear transcription factor (NF)-κB into the nucleus, which promotes transcription of IL-6, IL-1β, and TNF-a, ultimately induces the inflammatory response [12]. Our previous study has showed that prenatal exposure to LPS (0.79 mg/kg) results in increased IL-6 and TNF-a concentration in amniotic fluid 12 h after intraperitoneal injection of LPS (mean value, LPS group vs control group, TNF-a concentration: 6.43 vs 3.10 fmol/ml; IL-6 concentration: 75 vs 50 pg/ml). We also found that prenatal LPS (0.79 mg/kg) exposure up-regulates IL-6 and TNF-a mRNA expression in fetus and causes hypertension in offspring rats [12,13].

According to my previous studies, prenatal exposure to LPS of 0.79 mg/kg can cause abortion at a rate of 10% to 15%, therefore, 0.4 mg/kg would be safer. In the present study, we found that prenatal exposure to LPS of 0.4 mg/kg resulted in hypertension in three-month old offspring rats. Besides, Serum IL-6 and TNF-a increased significantly in High-fat group, which suggests an apparent inflammatory state created by high-fat diet. These findings can be supported by the previous studies [6,12,14].

In Kohmura's study, the pregnant mice were injected intravenously with 0.05 or 0.1 mg of LPS on day 14 to 16 of gestation. I-labeled LPS were injected into mice. Considerable amounts of the radioactivity were accumulated in the placenta and also in fetuses. This indicates that LPS can pass through the placenta and into fetuses. However, it is well-established that many of the biologic effects of LPS are mediated through the action of proinflammatory mediators released by host cells in response to LPS. These mediators including TNF-a, IL-1 and nitric oxide are mainly produced by macrophages [15]. In Ning's study, pregnant mice were injected intraperitoneally with a single dose of LPS (0.5 mg/kg) on gestational day 17. TNF-a obviously increased in maternal serum and amniotic fluid in response to LPS. When the pregnant mice were pretreated with a low-dose LPS (0.01 mg/kg, i.p.) at 4, 12, 24 or 48 h before LPS (0.5 mg/kg, i.p.), LPS-evoked TNF-a in maternal serum and amniotic fluid was significantly inhibited. Importantly, low-dose LPS pretreatment also greatly attenuated LPS-induced increases in TNF-a protein in fetal liver and fetal brain. Taken together, these results indicate that perinatal exposure to low-dose LPS induces a reduced sensitivity to subsequent LPS challenge [16]. Xu also found that, pretreatment with a low-dose LPS (0.01 mg/kg, i.p.) 24 h before high-dose LPS (0.12 mg/kg, i.p.) reduced sensitivity to subsequent high-dose LPS-induced intra-uterine fetal death, TNF-a production and

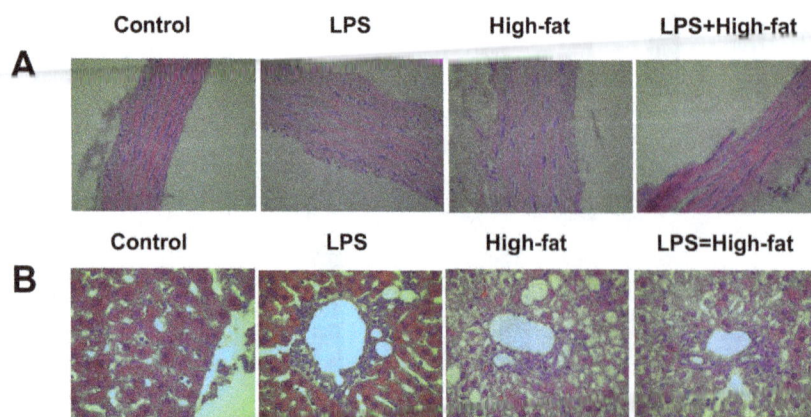

Figure 3. Prenatal exposure to lipopolysaccharide combined with pre- and postnatal high-fat diet result in morphological changes in thoracic aorta (A) and liver (B) tissue (H-E staining) in three-month old offspring rats.

oxidative stress in mice [17]. These can explain why prenatal exposure to LPS combined with high-fat diet result in normal level of serum TNF-a concentration in offspring rats.

Despite the hypertension or elevated blood pressure induced by prenatal exposure to LPS or high-fat diet, it was interesting to find that, a lowered blood pressure was found in LPS+High-fat group with lowered body weight both in male and female offspring rats. It seemed that prenatal LPS plus pre- and postnatal high-fat diet reversed hypertension caused by LPS. This phenomenon might due to the interaction between prenatal LPS treatment and high-fat diet. In the present study, the high-fat diet was given on the day when pregnancy was detected, that is, 8 days earlier than the intraperitoneal LPS injection during pregnancy. As has been demonstrated in Troseid's study that "An increase in plasma LPS occurs in healthy individuals after a high-fat meal" [4], therefore, we hypothesize that the reduced blood pressure in offspring rats of high-fat group might be the result of predictive adaptive response to inflammation caused by LPS and high-fat diet [6,7]. What in accordance with the lowered blood pressure was the normal level of serum IL-6 and TNF-a in LPS+High-fat group, which further convinced the beneficial effect of prenatal LPS exposure combined with pre- and early postnatal high-fat diet on blood pressure in offspring rats.

It was unexpected to find that body weight of male offspring in High-fat group was lower compared with Control and LPS group. It might because that the male fetuses are more vulnerable to prenatal adverse environment [8]. This result can be supported by previous study by Makarova who found that, leptin injections to C57Bl mice on day 17 of pregnancy decreased body weight in both male and female offspring but inhibited the food intake and diet-induced obesity only in male offspring. The maternal effect was more pronounced in male offspring. Their result showed that hyperleptinemia during pregnancy has gender-specific long-term effects on energy balance regulation in progeny and does not predispose offspring to developing obesity [18]. In Sánchez's study, offspring of dams supplemented with olive oil, butter, or margarine during late pregnancy and lactation were fed with normal fat diet until 4-month-old, and then with high fat diet until 6-month-old. In this model, the offspring displayed a lower body weight in both genders and lower body fat only in males, and the mechanism is also related to leptin [19]. Leptin suppresses food intake and increases energy expenditure by enhancing thermogenesis and metabolic rate [14]. It is associated with body mass index and body fat in non-obese and obese subjects and in patients

with T2DM [20]. In the present study, increased serum leptin level exhibited in high-fat group. Therefore, it is likely that, the reduction of body weight in male offspring in High-fat group might correlate with leptin level, while the reduction of body weight in LPS+High-fat group might result from the interaction between LPS and high-fat diet.

In addition, it was observed that a hyperinsulinemia, hypercholesterolemia, higher HOMA-IR and lower insulin sensitivity exhibited in offspring rats of LPS group, High-fat group and LPS+High-fat group, which suggest higher insulin resistance in these groups. Previous studies have demonstrated that maternal exposure to LPS of 0.79 mg/kg or high-fat diet results in insulin resistance in adult offspring rats [10,11,21]. If the lowered blood pressure in LPS+High-fat group is due to predictive adaptive response to prenatal inflammation, it seemed that it could not protect the offspring from insulin resistance. The possible mechanism need further study.

Serum levels of both alanine aminotransferase and aspartate aminotransferase evelated in LPS+High-fat group, and elevated aspartate aminotransferase was also found in High-fat group, which suggest impaired liver function [22]. The morphological changes in liver tissue also convinced this finding. In High-fat group and LPS+High-fat group, inflammation and serious liver steatosis was observed in the liver tissue. H-E staining of thoracic aorta also showed an impaired structure of thoracic aorta in LPS and High-fat group, but it seemed that it was less impaired in LPS+High-fat group. These morphological changes further convinced the findings in blood pressure and insulin resistance.

In conclusion, inflammation induced by prenatal exposure to LPS and pre- and postnatal high-fat diet might exert a predictive adaptive response which protects the offspring rats from hypertension; at the same time, the maternal metabolism might also be influenced, and in turn produced offspring with lowered body weight and insulin resistance. The further study will focus on whether prenatal exposure to LPS and High-fat diet cause change in maternal serum leptin level, and whether maternal exposure to LPS and high-fat diet only during pregnancy produce offspring without both hypertension and insulin resistance.

Author Contributions

Conceived and designed the experiments: XH. Performed the experiments: XH JD YL. Analyzed the data: XH. Contributed reagents/materials/analysis tools: ML SZ. Wrote the paper: XH.

References

1. Blasco-Baque V, Serino M, Vergnes JN, Riant E, Loubieres P, et al (2012) High-fat diet induces periodontitis in mice through lipopolysaccharides (LPS) receptor signaling: protective action of estrogens. PLoS One 7:e48220.

2. Liang H, Hussey SE, Sanchez-Avila A, Tantiwong P, Musi N (2013) Effect of lipopolysaccharide on inflammation and insulin action in human muscle. PLoS One 8:e63983.

3. Lappi J, Kolehmainen M, Mykkanen H, Poutanen K (2013) Do large intestinal events explain the protective effects of whole grain foods against type 2 diabetes? Crit Rev Food Sci Nutr 53:631–40.

4. Troseid M, Nestvold TK, Rudi K, Thoresen H, Nielsen EW, et al. (2013) Plasma lipopolysaccharide is closely associated with glycemic control and abdominal obesity: evidence from bariatric surgery. Diabetes Care. 2013 Jul 8. [Epub ahead of print].

5. Armitage JA, Lakasing L, Taylor PD, Balachandran AA, Jensen RI, et al. (2005) Developmental programming of aortic and renal structure in offspring of rats fed fat-rich diets in pregnancy. J Physiol 565:171–84.

6. Khan I, Dekou V, Hanson M, Poston L, Taylor P (2004) Predictive adaptive responses to maternal high-fat diet prevent endothelial dysfunction but not hypertension in adult rat offspring. Circulation 110:1097–102.

7. Rickard IJ, Lummaa V (2007) The predictive adaptive response and metabolic syndrome: challenges for the hypothesis. Trends Endocrinol Metab 18:94–9.

8. Ng SF, Lin RC, Laybutt DR, Barres R, Owens JA, et al. (2010) Chronic high-fat diet in fathers programs beta cell dysfunction in female rat offspring. Nature 467:963–6.

9. Guberman C, Jellyman JK, Han G, Ross MG, Desai M (2013) Maternal high-fat diet programs rat offspring hypertension and activates the adipose renin-angiotensin system. Am J Obstet Gynecol. 2013 Jun 4.[Epub ahead of print] .

10. Kruse M, Seki Y, Vuguin PM, Du XQ, Fiallo A, et al. (2013) High-fat intake during pregnancy and lactation exacerbates high-fat diet-induced complications in male offspring in mice. Endocrinology 154(10):3565–76.

11. Murabayashi N, Sugiyama T, Zhang L, Kamimoto Y, Umekawa T, et al. (2013) Maternal high-fat diets cause insulin resistance through inflammatory changes in fetal adipose tissue. Eur J Obstet Gynecol Reprod Biol 169:39–44.

12. Hao XQ, Zhang HG, Yuan ZB, Yang DL, Hao LY, et al. (2010) Prenatal exposure to lipopolysaccharide alters the intrarenal renin-angiotensin system and renal damage in offspring rats. Hypertens Res 33:76–82.

13. Hao XQ, Kong T, Zhang SY, Zhao ZS (2012) Alteration of embryonic AT_2-R and inflammatory cytokines gene expression induced by prenatal exposure to lipopolysaccharide affects renal development. Experimental and Toxicologic Pathology. 2012 Feb 17. [Epub ahead of print].

14. Liu X, Xue Y, Liu C, Lou Q, Wang J, et al. (2013) Eicosapentaenoic acid-enriched phospholipid ameliorates insulin resistance and lipid metabolism in diet-induced-obese mice. Lipids Health Dis 12:109.

15. Kohmura Y, Kirikae T, Kirikae F, Nakano M, Sato I (2000) Lipopolysaccharide (LPS)-induced intra-uterine fetal death (IUFD) in mice is principally due to maternal cause but not fetal sensitivity to LPS. Microbiol Immunol 44: 897–904.

16. Ning H, Wang H, Zhao L, Zhang C, Li XY, et al. (2008) Maternally-administered lipopolysaccharide (LPS) increases tumor necrosis factor alpha in fetal liver and fetal brain; its suppression by low-dose LPS pretreatment. Toxicol Lett 176. 13–19.

17. Xu DX, Wang H, Zhao L, Ning H, Chen YH, et al. (2007) Effects of low-dose lipopolysaccharide (LPS) pretreatment on LPS-induced intra-uterine fetal death and preterm labor. Toxicology 234: 167–175.

18. Makarova EN, Chepeleva EV, Panchenko PE, Bazhan NM (2013) The influence of abnormally high leptin levels during pregnancy on the metabolic phenotypes in progeny mice. Am J Physiol Regul Integr Comp Physiol 2013 Oct 2. [Epub ahead of print].

19. Sánchez J, Priego T, García AP, Llopis M, Palou M, et al. (2012) Maternal supplementation with an excess of different fat sources during pregnancy and lactation differentially affects feeding behavior in offspring: putative role of the leptin system. Mol Nutr Food Res 56:1715–28.

20. Muhammadnejadch O, Zargham N (2013) Serum leptin level is reduced in non-obese subjects with type 2 diabetes. Int J Endocrinol Metab 11:3–10.

21. Nilsson C, Larsson BM, Jennische E, Eriksson E, Bjorntorp P, et al. (2001) Maternal endotoxemia results in obesity and insulin resistance in adult male offspring. Endocrinology 142:2622–30.

22. de Luis DA, Aller R, Izaola O, Gonzalez Sagrado M, Conde R, et al. (2013) Role of insulin resistance and adipocytokines on serum alanine aminotransferase in obese patients with type 2 diabetes mellitus. Eur Rev Med Pharmacol Sci 17:2059–64.

3

Metabolic Syndrome and Fatal Outcomes in the Post-Stroke Event

Eric Vounsia Balti[1,2], André Pascal Kengne[2,3], Jean Valentin Fogha Fokouo[2], Brice Enid Nouthé[2,4], Eugene Sobngwi[2,5]*

1 Diabetes Research Center, Faculty of Medicine and Pharmacy, Brussels Free University, Brussels, Belgium, 2 National Obesity Center, Yaoundé Central Hospital and Faculty of Medicine and Biomedical Sciences, University of Yaoundé 1, Yaoundé, Cameroon, 3 NCRP for Cardiovascular and Metabolic Diseases, South African Medical Research Council and University of Cape Town, Cape Town, South Africa, 4 Department of Medicine, McGill University, Montreal, Quebec, Canada, 5 Institute of Health and Society, Newcastle University, Newcastle, United Kingdom

Abstract

Background and Purpose: Determinants of post-acute stroke outcomes in Africa have been less investigated. We assessed the association of metabolic syndrome (MetS) and insulin resistance with post-stroke mortality in patients with first ever-in-lifetime stroke in the capital city of Cameroon (sub-Saharan Africa).

Methods: Patients with an acute first-stroke event (n = 57) were recruited between May and October 2006, and followed for 5 years for mortality outcome. MetS definition was based on the Joint Interim Statement 2009, insulin sensitivity/resistance assessed via glucose-to-insulin ratio, quantitative insulin sensitivity check index and homeostatic model assessment.

Results: Overall, 24 (42%) patients deceased during follow-up. The prevalence of MetS was higher in patients who died after 28 days, 1 year and 5 years from any cause or cardiovascular-related causes (all $p \leq 0.040$). MetS was associated with an increased overall mortality both after 1 year (39% vs. 9%) and 5 years of follow-up (55% vs. 26%, $p = 0.022$). Similarly, fatal events due to cardiovascular-related conditions were more frequent in the presence of MetS both 1 year (37% vs. 9%) and 5 years after the first-ever-in-lifetime stroke (43% vs. 13%, $p = 0.017$). Unlike biochemical measures of insulin sensitivity and resistance (non-significant), in age- and sex-adjusted Cox models, MetS was associated with hazard ratio (95% CI) of 2.63 (1.03–6.73) and 3.54 (1.00–12.56) respectively for all-cause and cardiovascular mortality 5 years after stroke onset.

Conclusion: The Joint Interim Statement 2009 definition of MetS may aid the identification of a subgroup of black African stroke patients who may benefit from intensification of risk factor management.

Editor: Pierre-Marie Preux, Institute of Neuroepidemiology and Tropical Neurology, France

Funding: The authors have no support or funding to report.

Competing Interests: The authors have declared that no competing interests exist.

* E-mail: eugene.sobngwi@newcastle.ac.uk

Introduction

Metabolic syndrome (MetS) is a constellation of conditions which singly are associated with increased risk of cardiovascular diseases (CVD) [1,2]. Furthermore, the presence of MetS in an individual confers a risk of cardiovascular disease higher than that from each of the components of the syndrome [3,4]. Therefore, MetS has been intensively investigated over the recent years for a possible contribution to cardiovascular disease risk stratification and/or reduction.

The prevalence of MetS varies substantially across populations and settings, both as a result of background differences in the distribution of its components across populations, but also of the diversity of criteria for defining the condition. There have been recent efforts to harmonize the clinical definition of MetS by accounting for ethnic differences in the cutoff values of key components such as central obesity and atherogenic dyslipidemia [5,6]. How the harmonized definition reflects the risk of major outcomes has not been widely assessed. For instance, in the absence of cutoff values specific to populations of African ethnicity, those derived from Caucasians have been recommended in Africans, yet no evidence is available on the correlation of MetS based on those criteria and major incident health outcomes among black Africans [7–10]. Stroke is the most common cardiovascular outcome in sub-Saharan Africa and may serve this purpose.

We therefore sought to investigate the association of MetS with post-event survival in a cohort of patients following a first-ever-in-lifetime stroke from an urban area of Cameroon.

Methods

Study Setting and Participants

This study was conducted at Yaoundé Central Hospital, a major tertiary reference hospital in the capital city of Cameroon. The setting and the study population have been previously described [11]. Briefly, patients admitted for a first-ever-in-lifetime stroke were consecutively enrolled between May and October 2006. Diagnosis of stroke was based on WHO criteria [12] and stroke

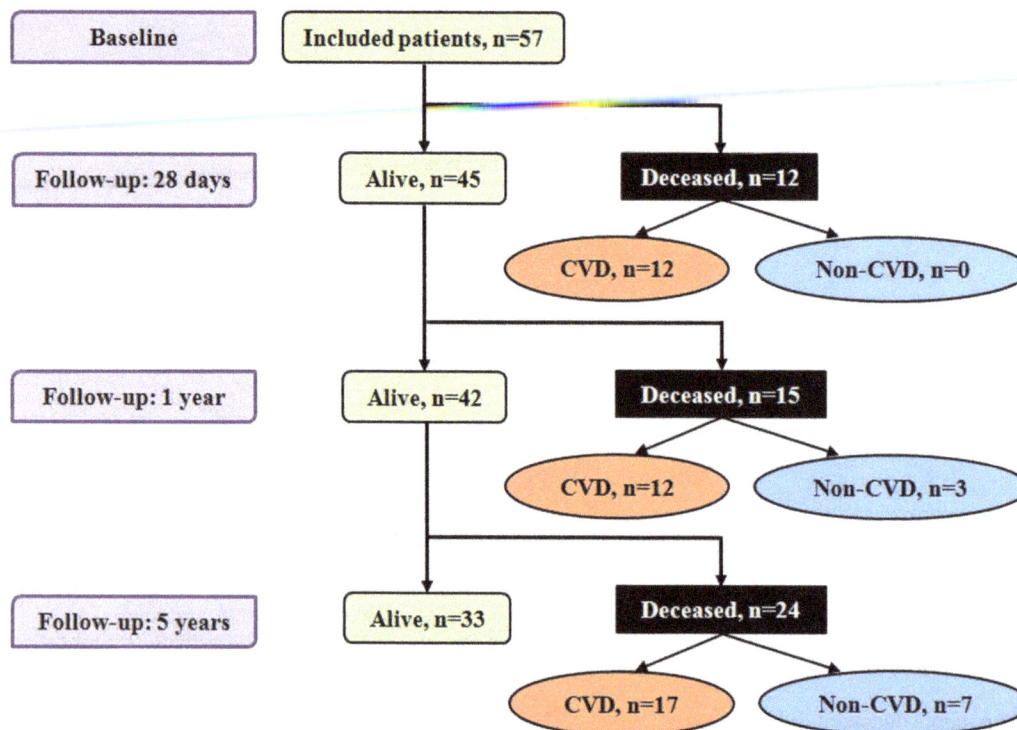

Figure 1. Flow chart of enrolled patients. Values are cumulative number of participants alive (green boxes) or who died (black boxes) at 28 days, 1 and 5 years of follow-up. The number of deaths at each time-point is further distinguished as cardiovascular disease (CVD) related (light-salmon ovals) or not (light-blue ovals).

was distinguished from transient ischemic attack by the duration of functional impairment or symptoms of more than 24 hours. Demographic, anthropometric and clinical data were collected at baseline using a standard questionnaire and blood samples were collected after an overnight fast for biological determinations. Waist circumference was measured in supine position since most patients were bedridden for major motor deficiency and could not assume the usual standing position required for such a measurement. Body mass index was calculated using the most recent measurement of height and weight in the last 12 months, in the absence of specific scale for measuring adult's weight in supine position. Follow-up contacts were established with patients, their relatives and/or their physicians 28 days, 1 year and 5 years from baseline for mortality outcome data collection (Figure 1). Mortality and causes of death were ascertained via hospital records or verbal autopsy and based on the 10th revision of the International Classification of Diseases (codes I 00–99) [13]. The study was approved by the Institutional Review Board of The Yaoundé Central Hospital (Cameroon). Patients, always in the presence of at least one relative, or two next of kin (for unconscious patients) provided the verbal informed consent to participate in the study. The purpose of the study was explained to participants/family in one of the official languages, or one of the national languages for illiterate patients, with the assistance of translators as appropriate. Informed verbal consent was deemed appropriate given the high illiteracy rate among patients with stroke and the nature of the disease with some patients presenting in unconscious or impotent states, and therefore unable to provide a written consent. The consent procedure was approved by the Institutional Review Board, and documented for each patient by a tick of boxes on the case report form, which was always presented to patients/families.

Definition of Metabolic Syndrome

MetS was defined based on the Joint Interim Statement (JIS) criteria [5]. Thus, positive diagnosis of the syndrome was established when at least three of the following were present: 1) fasting plasma glucose ≥100 mg/dL (or history of doctor-diagnosed diabetes), 2) systolic (and/or diastolic) blood pressure ≥130 (85) mmHg or treated hypertension, 3) serum triglycerides ≥150 mg/dL, 4) serum high-density lipoproteins (HDL) cholesterol <40 mg/dL in men and <50 mg/dL in women and 5) waist circumference of >80 cm in women and >94 cm in men. Blood pressure was measured on the left arm using a mercury sphygmomanometer with appropriate cuffs and the average of two measurements taken 5 minutes apart was used in the study.

Analytical Methods

Glucose was analyzed by the hexokinase method (Roche Diagnostics, Mannheim, Germany). Insulin levels were determined by radioimmunoassay (Linco Research; St. Charles, MO), while triglycerides (TG), total cholesterol (TC) and HDL cholesterol determinations used enzymatic colorimetric methods. A more detailed description of the analytical methods is available elsewhere [11]. Since none of the patients had a triglycerides level of 400 mg/dL or more, LDL cholesterol levels were calculated using Friedewald formula for all study participants [14]. Blood samples were collected between 72 hours and at most 1 week post-admission after an overnight fast of 12 hours.

Insulin sensitivity was assessed by both fasting glucose-to-insulin (Glu/Ins) ratio and quantitative insulin sensitivity check index (QUICKI) while insulin resistance was estimated by the Homeo-static model assessment of insulin resistance (HOMA-IR) three to seven days after admission [11].

Table 1. General characteristics of the study population at inclusion.

Characteristics	All patients (n = 57)	Men (n = 32)	Women (n = 25)	p
Age, years	61.9±12.9	63.1±10.4	60.4±15.6	0.439
Body mass index, kg/m^2	23.7±11.5	25.4±10.6	19.6±13.0	0.160
Waist girth, cm	90.5±14.0	92.1±15.5	88.3±11.5	0.318
Systolic blood pressure, mmHg	170±36	171±37	168±35	0.709
Diastolic blood pressure, mmHg	101±27	106±33	94±15	0.105
Total cholesterol, mg/dL	173±36	169±40	178±39	0.389
Triglycerides, mg/dL	129±56	135±57	122±55	0.411
LDL cholesterol, mg/dL	109±43	106±40	114±47	0.483
HDL cholesterol, mg/dL	37±21	36±14	39±28	0.528
Fasting blood glucose, g/l	1.33±0.79	1.20±0.51	1.47±1.03	0.205
Plasma insulin, mIU/L	5.86±5.37	5.2±3.3	6.7±7.4	0.316
Clinical type of stroke				
Hemorrhagic, n (%)	12 (21)	7 (22)	6 (24)	>0.99
Ischemic, n (%)	45 (79)	25 (78)	20 (80)	>0.99
Components of MetS				
High blood pressure, n (%)	37 (65)	22 (69)	15 (60)	0.684
Diabetes, n (%)	26 (47)	15 (50)	11 (44)	0.657
High waist girth, n (%)	30 (53)	12 (38)	18 (72)	0.010
Low HDL cholesterol, n (%)	38 (69)	19 (59)	19 (83)	0.123
High triglyceride, n (%)	22 (40)	14 (44)	8 (35)	0.696
Metabolic syndrome, n (%)	33 (59)	16 (50)	17 (71)	0.196
Number of components, n (%)				
1	8 (14)	5 (16)	3 (13)	>0.99
2	15 (27)	11 (34)	4 (17)	0.223
3	20 (36)	10 (31)	10 (42)	0.601
4 or 5	13 (24)	6 (19)	7 (30)	0.494

Statistical Analysis

Groups' comparison used Chi-square or Fisher's exact tests for categorical variables and student's t-test or Mann-Whitney U test for continuous variables. Results are expressed as counts (proportions), mean and standard deviation or median, inter-quartile range, minimum and maximum values. Early (28-day), one- and five-year mortality rates were derived with the use of the Kaplan-Meier estimator, with groups comparisons via Log-rank test. Cox proportional hazard regression models were then used to adjust for the effect of age and sex, with the non-violation of the proportional assumption confirmed via Schoenfeld residuals' plots. Follow-up duration was estimated from the day of hospital admission to death, lost to follow-up or maximum duration of 5 years, whichever came first. Because not all included patients (n = 31/57, 54%) could afford a CT-scan, we performed a sensitivity analysis and extrapolated our analysis to patients clinically diagnosed with ischemic stroke (n = 45). Clinical classification of stroke subtypes resulted in a 92% sensitivity and 60% specificity [11]. One participant was excluded from the survival analysis for missing data on MetS status. A p value <0.05 was used to characterize statistically significant results.

SPSS v20.0 for Windows (IBM statistics, Chicago, IL, USA) and GraphPad Prism v5.00 for Windows (San Diego, CA, USA) were used for statistical analysis.

Results

Baseline Profile of the Study Group

The general characteristics of the study population are shown in Table 1. Of the 57 participants included, 32 (56%) were men. With the exception of high waist circumference which was more frequent in women than in men (72% vs. 38%), there was no significant difference in the distribution of baseline characteristics between men and women (all p≥0.105, Table 1). Stroke was clinically classified as ischemic in 15 (79%) patients and as hemorrhagic in 12 (21%) patients (Table 1). Imaging studies (CT scan) were available for 31 patients (54%) among whom 26 (84%) had ischemic stroke and 5 (16%) had hemorrhagic stroke [11]. Low HDL cholesterol (69%) was the most frequent component of MetS followed by high blood pressure (65%) and high waist circumference 53%. The prevalence of MetS was 59% (n = 33) overall, 50% (n = 16) in men and 71% (n = 17) in women (p = 0.196, Table 1).

Fatal Outcomes

Of the 57 patients enrolled 33 (58%) were still alive after 5 years of follow-up. Table 2 summarizes the general characteristics of survivors and patients who died at all follow-up time-points. Men and women were equally distributed across all the study groups. Stroke survivors overall were mostly comparable to those who died with consideration to several baseline characteristics and at any

Table 2. Baseline characteristics of the study population according to mortality at different follow-up time-points.

Characteristics	Short term overall mortality			1-year overall mortality			5-year overall mortality			5-year cardiovascular-related mortality		
	Yes (n=12)	No (n=45)	p	Yes (n=15)	No (n=42)	p	Yes (n=24)	No (n=33)	p	Yes (n=17)	No (n=40)	p
Age, years	68±12	60±12	0.086	66±13	60±13	0.135	65±12	59±13	0.092	64.3±13.1	60.9±12.8	0.368
Sex ratio, men/women	5/7	27/18	0.255	7/8	25/17	0.389	13/11	19/14	0.798	8/9	24/16	0.542
Body mass index, kg/m²	25±13	23±11	0.718	27±12	23±11	0.353	26±13	23±11	0.477	26.9±11.0	22.7±11.7	0.348
Waist girth, cm	92±10	90±15	0.655	94±13	89±14	0.265	93±13	89±15	0.267	94.9±11.9	88.5±14.5	0.114
Systolic blood pressure, mmHg	159±37	173±36	0.246	159±36	174±36	0.185	163±35	174±36	0.242	164±35	172±37	0.488
Diastolic blood pressure, mmHg	90±15	104±29	0.130	91±16	104±30	0.127	94±15	106±33	0.094	94±15	104±31	0.212
Total cholesterol, mg/dL	185±36	169±40	0.229	173±41	172±39	0.941	170±39	175±41	0.664	171±37	173±41	0.893
Triglycerides, mg/dL	132±50	129±58	0.842	136±54	127±57	0.599	126±56	132±56	0.675	122±48	132±60	0.527
LDL cholesterol, mg/dL	125±41	105±43	0.171	113±45	108±43	0.714	112±43	107±44	0.714	112±41	108±44	0.765
HDL cholesterol, mg/dL	34±17	38±21	0.516	33±17	39±22	0.362	33±15	41±24	0.168	35±17	38±22	0.591
Fasting blood glucose, g/L	1.62±0.99	1.25±0.72	0.159	1.49±0.91	1.26±0.75	0.355	1.36±0.79	1.31±0.81	0.815	1.46±0.88	1.27±0.76	0.422
Plasma insulin, mIU/L	5.0±2.6	6.1±5.9	0.533	4.8±2.7	6.3±6.0	0.374	5.6±5.5	6.0±5.3	0.775	6.6±6.1	5.5±5.0	0.506
Components of MetS												
High blood pressure, n (%)	9 (75)	28 (62)	0.510	11 (73)	26 (62)	0.537	18 (75)	19 (56)	0.174	13 (77)	24 (60)	0.374
Diabetes, n (%)	8 (67)	18 (42)	0.128	9 (60)	17 (43)	0.247	13 (54)	13 (42)	0.368	10 (59)	16 (42)	0.392
High waist girth, n (%)	8 (67)	22 (49)	0.340	10 (67)	20 (48)	0.205	15 (62)	15 (45)	0.203	12 (71)	18 (45)	0.139
Low HDL cholesterol, n (%)	9 (75)	29 (67)	0.735	11 (73)	27 (67)	0.754	18 (75)	20 (64)	0.404	12 (32)	26 (68)	>0.99
High triglyceride, n (%)	5 (42)	17 (39)	0.894	6 (40)	16 (40)	1.00	8 (33)	14 (45)	0.375	5 (29)	17 (45)	0.439
Metabolic syndrome, n (%)	11 (92)	22 (50)	0.010	13 (87)	20 (49)	0.014	18 (75)	15 (47)	0.034	14 (82)	19 (49)	0.040
Number of components, n (%)												
1	1 (8)	7 (16)	0.672	1 (7)	7 (17)	0.428	3 (12)	5 (16)	1.00	2 (12)	6 (15)	>0.99
2	0 (0)	15 (34)	0.024	1 (7)	14 (34)	0.047	3 (12)	12 (37)	0.065	1 (6)	14 (36)	0.023
3	6 (50)	14 (31)	0.313	8 (53)	12 (29)	0.096	10 (42)	10 (31)	0.421	8 (47)	12 (31)	0.386
4 or 5	5 (42)	8 (19)	0.096	5 (33)	8 (20)	0.300	8 (33)	5 (16)	0.136	6 (35)	7 (18)	0.190

given time-point during follow-up. Although they tended to be younger, leaner, to have lower fasting blood glucose, insulin, triglycerides, HDL cholesterol and LDL cholesterol levels, and to display lower systolic and diastolic blood pressures than those who died, differences did not reach the conventional significance threshold (Table 2). Similar findings were observed in the subset of patients clinically diagnosed with ischemic stroke (Table S1).

Metabolic Syndrome and Insulin Resistance

The distribution of individual components of MetS was similar between survivors and deceased participants at any time-point. However, the prevalence of JIS-defined MetS was always higher among deceased patients. Prevalence figures (deceased vs. survivors) were 11/12 vs. 22/45 at 28 days, 13/15 vs. 20/42 at 1 year, 18/24 vs. 15/33 at 5 years for all-cause mortality, and 14/17 vs. 19/40 at 5 years for cardiovascular-related death (all $p \leq 0.04$, Table 2). No difference in the prevalence of individual components of MetS was observed although deceased patients from cardiovascular-related causes at 5-year among those with clinically diagnosed ischemic stroke had a higher waist circumference (Table S1).

As previously mentioned, HOMA-IR was used to evaluate insulin resistance while QUICKI and the Glu/Ins ratio were used as surrogates of sensitivity to insulin. Figure 2 shows that there was no significant difference between stroke survivors and those who

died with regard to the levels of those predictors of insulin response. Although deceased patients tended to be more insulin-resistant (and less insulin-sensitive) than their counterparts, overall, no significant difference was observed in insulin sensitivity (glucose-to-insulin ratio and QUICKI) and resistance indices (HOMA-IR) between the two groups.

Kaplan Meier and Cox Regression Analysis

Mortality rate from all causes and from cardiovascular-related causes in patients with first-ever-in-lifetime stroke was respectively 43% (95% CI, 30–56%) and 31% (95% CI, 18–43%) after 5 years. This and the stratification according to presence of MetS are illustrated in Figure 3. Overall mortality occurred more often in patients with MetS (Log-rank test, $p = 0.022$; Figure 3A). The latter group had a higher mortality rate both after 1 and 5 years follow-up (39% vs. 9% and 55% vs. 26% respectively). Survival analysis in patients who died from cardiovascular-related conditions suggests that 14/17 (82%) of deaths occurred within 12 months and the majority of deceased patients 14/17 (82%) had MetS. Mortality rates associated to MetS at 1 and 5 years were respectively 37% (20–53%) and 43% (26–60%). The 5-year mortality rate was significantly higher in the presence of MetS than in its absence ($p = 0.017$, Figure 3B). When patients with ischemic stroke were considered, 12/17 (71%) of deceased patients within 5 years had MetS which was associated with a 50%

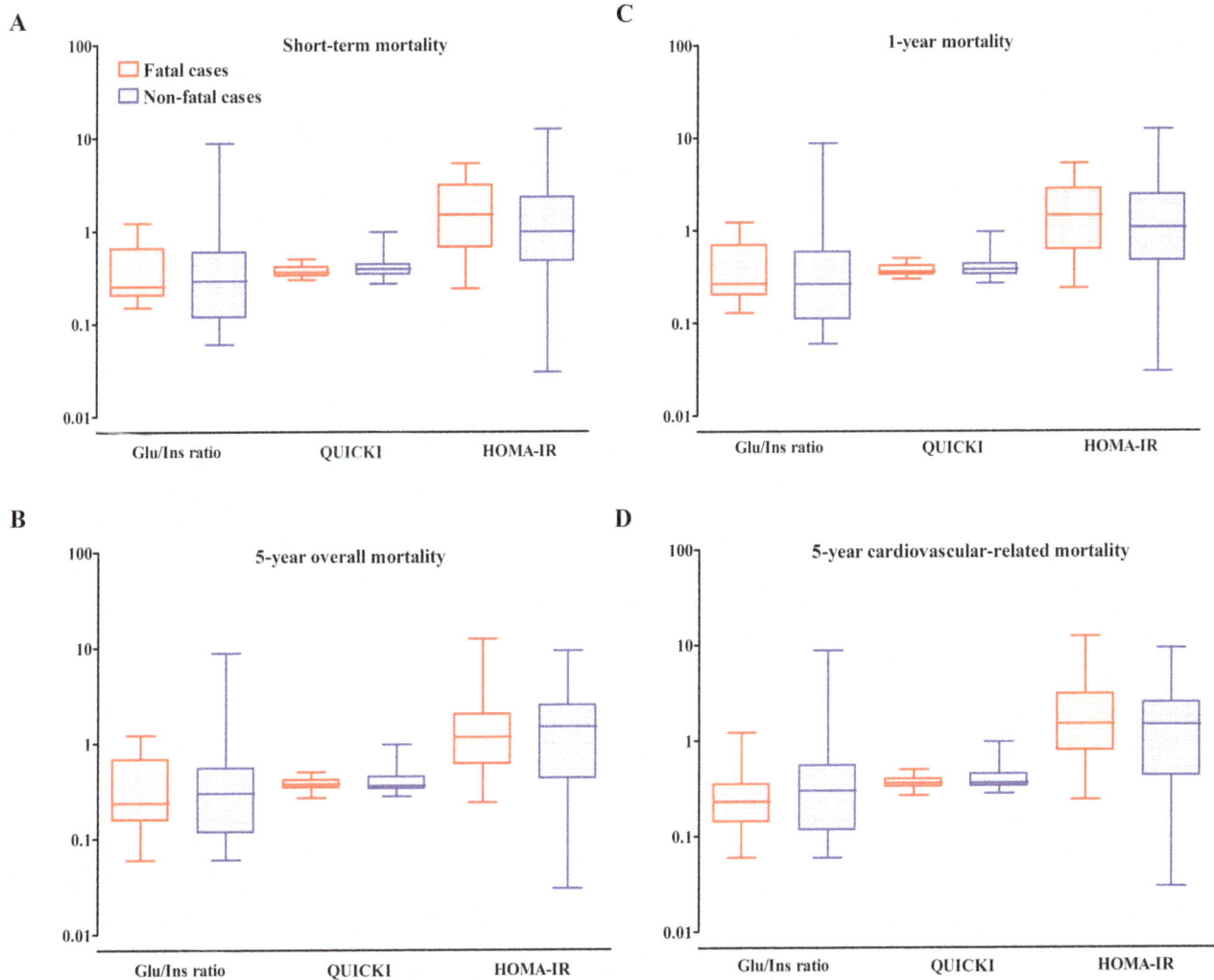

Figure 2. Insulin sensitivity and resistance according to outcome and cause of death during follow-up. Comparison of insulin resistance and sensitivity indices according to the vital status at 28 days (A), 1 year (B), 5 years from all-cause of death (C) and 5 years cardiovascular-related mortality (D). Data are expressed in a log scale. Boxes represent median (crossing horizontal bar) and interquartile range (lower and upper limits). The whiskers depict maximum and minimum values for each of the insulin resistance/sensitivity indices for deceased patients (red color) and those still alive (blue color) at the indicated follow-up time. For each insulin resistance/sensitivity index, and across figure panels, the boxes and whiskers for the deceased are always displayed on the right.

(95%CI, 30–70%; data not shown) all-cause mortality rate as opposed to 25% (95%CI, 6–44%; data not shown) among their counterparts without MetS ($p = 0.047$). In this subset of the study population, cardiovascular-related mortality occurred significantly earlier in the presence of MetS, 42 (95%CI, 22–62%; data not shown) vs. 10% (95%CI, 0–23%; data not shown), $p = 0.017$ (Figure S1).

In age- and sex-adjusted Cox regression analysis, the presence of MetS was associated with a hazard ratio (95% CI) of 2.63 (1.03–6.73), $p = 0.043$ and 3.54 (1.00–12.56), $p = 0.050$ respectively for all-cause and cardiovascular-related mortality after five years. Markers of insulin sensitivity or insulin resistance were not associated with 5-year mortality (all $p > 0.05$, Table 3). Similarly, none of the components of MetS taken separately was significantly associated with mortality risk (data not shown). In patients with ischemic stroke, none of the candidate markers reached statistical significance for the prediction of overall mortality (all $p > 0.05$) while MetS tended to be associated with 5-year mortality from cardiovascular-related conditions ($p = 0.048$, Table S2).

Discussion

We have investigated the relationship between post-stroke mortality and MetS using the recent definition criteria by the Joint Interim Statement for harmonization of MetS [5]. In our cohort, the prevalence of MetS but not its components was higher in stroke patients who died after 28 days, 1 and 5 years even after adjustment for age and gender. This was observed for both all-cause and cardiovascular-related mortality but with a less robust association with the latter.

Previous studies of MetS in sub-Saharan Africa used a variety of definitions including the ones proposed by the International Diabetes Federation, the World Health Organization (WHO) and the National Cholesterol Education Panel (NCEP) Adult Treatment Panel III [15]. The prevalence of MetS varies according to the criteria used for its definition in various ethnic groups and the JIS definition may result in a better estimate of the syndrome in sub-Saharan populations [5,16,17]. We found that hypertension and low HDL cholesterol were the most prevalent components of

A

5-year overall mortality

B

5-year cardiovascular-related mortality

MetS	0	13	15	16	17	18
no-MetS	0	2	2	3	5	6
All patients	0	15	17	18	22	24

1-year mortality rate % (95%CI)	5-year mortality rate % (95%CI)
- MetS: 39 (23-56)	- MetS: 55 (37-72)
- no-MetS: 9 (0-20)	- no-MetS: 26 (8-44)
- Overall: 26 (15-38)	- Overall: 42 (29-55)

MetS	0	12	14	14	14	14
no-MetS	0	2	2	2	3	3
All patients	0	14	14	14	17	17

1-year mortality rate % (95%CI)	5-year mortality rate % (95%CI)
- MetS: 37 (20-53)	- MetS: 43 (26-60)
- no-MetS: 9 (0-20)	- no-MetS: 13 (0-27)
- Overall: 25 (13-36)	- Overall: 30 (18-42)

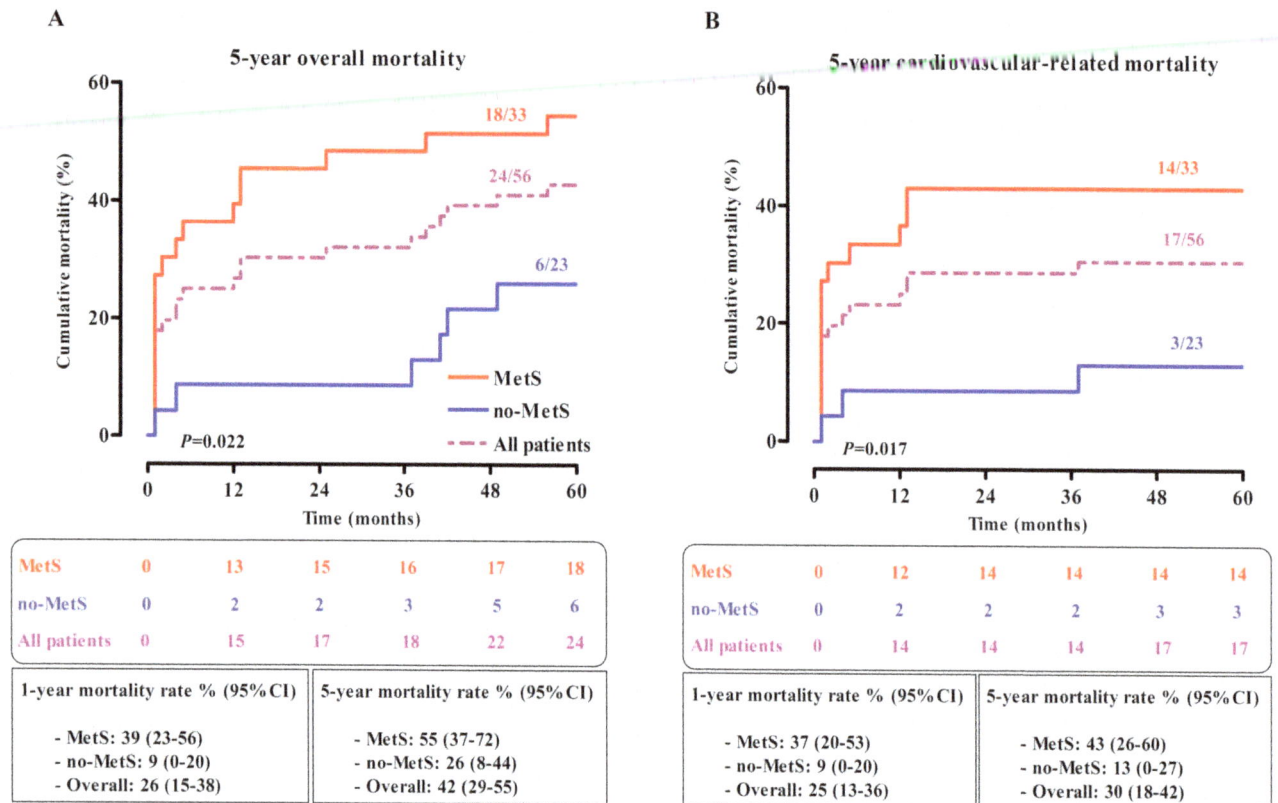

Figure 3. Kaplan-Meier curves in all included patients. Overall (A) and cardiovascular-related (B) mortalities according to the presence of metabolic syndrome. Comparisons were performed using Log-rank test. The total fraction of deceased patients during follow-up is indicated above each arm in the 2 panels. Cumulative number of deceased patients during follow-up and mortality rates (95%CI) after 1 and 5 years from overall and cardiovascular-related causes for all patients and in the presence or absence of MetS are indicated below the respective graphs.

MetS in both survivors and deceased patients without significant differences between the two groups for all components. Moreover, MetS was more prevalent among fatal stroke cases. This suggests that risk of stroke onset at baseline from the individual risk factors in all patients is the same but they tend to occur concomitantly and therefore increase mortality rate in deceased patients. Similar findings have been described in African-Caribbean population with stroke and coronary heart disease [18].

Unlike insulin resistance or sensitivity indices, in the presence of MetS, patients with ischemic stroke died significantly faster independently of the cause of death. Overall, MetS was associated with a higher mortality rate and was an independent predictor of 5-year post-stroke death independently of the cause. A similar trend was observed for deaths from cardiovascular-related conditions. This finding is consistent with previously reported data using other definitions of MetS. In a logistic regression analysis and using WHO criteria for diagnosis of MetS, Isomaa et al. reported a 1.81 relative risk of death from cardiovascular-related events over a follow-up duration of 6.9 years [19]. Other significant predictors in the study include hypertension and microalbuminuria. The latter has not been assessed in our study and the former is estimated by the WHO criteria using a higher

Table 3. Cox regression analysis of 5-year mortality in all study participants.

Covariates	5-year overall mortality			5-year cardiovascular-related mortality		
	HR*	95%CI	p	HR	95%CI	p
Glu/Ins ratio[†]	0.81	0.42-1.55	0.527	0.68	0.24-1.97	0.480
HOMA-IR[‡]	1.04	0.88-1.22	0.673	1.08	0.92-1.26	0.371
QUICKI[§]	0.06	0-16.88	0.331	0.10	0-10.36	0.171
Metabolic syndrome	2.63	1.03-6.73	0.043	3.54	1.00-12.56	0.050

All Cox models are adjusted for age and gender;
*hazard ratio;
[†]glucose-to-insulin ratio;
[‡]homeostatic model assessment of insulin resistance;
[§]quantitative insulin sensitivity check index.

cutoff for blood pressure. Similarly, other studies defining MetS according to the NCEP or WHO have shown an increased mortality associated with the condition [4,20,21]. More importantly, it is apparent from our results that cardiovascular mortality occurs more often few months after stroke onset in patients with MetS. This suggests that targeting MetS might be effective for prevention of early mortality associated to cerebrovascular events. However, it is worthwhile to notice that our observations are based on a model restricted to metabolic parameters. The interplay between MetS and other variables such as stroke severity or the stroke subtype might influence the resulting outcome.

Unlike the pathophysiology of cardiovascular events in individuals with MetS, the relationship between MetS and mortality following cardiovascular events in general and stroke in particular still needs to be clarified [22]. The differences in definition and heterogeneity in populations of interest in studies focusing on MetS make the findings difficult to pool together. For instance, in some reports, participants were enrolled based on diabetes status, gender or age and in others not [2,3,23–25]. Nevertheless, in recent meta-analysis, both Galassi et al. and Gami et al. have shown that independently of these differences, MetS is associated with an increased risk of death following a cardiovascular event [20,26]. Whether or not this excess mortality risk is due to the constellation of factors included in the definition of MetS is still unclear. Consistent with what has been described in other settings, our findings suggest that MetS is more prevalent and might predict poor outcome in patients with first-ever-in-lifetime stroke. However, no further inference about the relationship between the number of risk factors and mortality can be made due to the relatively small sample size.

The small sample size is the major limitation of this study. This may have affected our capacity for detecting some significant differences and precluded stratification according to stroke subtypes. Moreover, in the absence of systematic CT-Scan or magnetic resonance imaging studies, the definitive diagnosis of the subtypes of stroke was not available for all participants. Some patients with acute stroke would tend to die prior to hospital admission in this setting; therefore our use of hospital-based cohort would underestimate the true magnitude of early post-stroke mortality. We also lack data on medication prescription and adherence during follow-up, which could aid the understanding of some of the associations observed in this study. Lastly, waist girth was measured in supine position, and BMI calculated based on imputed weight using the most recent measurement in the last 12 months. Both approaches are imprecise, but are among the best alternatives for approximating those parameters in bedridden patients in our resources-limited setting. Our study also has major advantages including extensive baseline investigation, and a successful follow-up of a relatively large number of participants, which is rather uncommon in the African setting [8]. By demonstrating

a correlation between JIS-defined MetS and long-term outcome, we have provided evidence in support of the applicability of this definition, although larger studies will be needed to assess the validity of individual components of the syndrome based on JIS definition in this context.

In conclusion, JIS-defined MetS is associated with an increased cardiovascular-related and all-cause mortality in black African patients with first stroke event. MetS therefore appears as a useful tool for identifying a subgroup of patients with stroke whose long-term outcomes can potentially be improved by more intensive risk factor modifying therapies. However, our observations need to be confirmed in a bigger cohort and the process by which the combination of risk factors in MetS influences case fatality warrants further investigation. In such a cohort, further investigation of the relationship between MetS as defined by the JIS 2009 [5] criteria and stroke severity using currently available scores could also be addressed.

Supporting Information

Figure S1 Kaplan-Meier curves in the subgroup of patients clinically diagnosed with ischemic stroke. Overall (A) and cardiovascular-related (B) mortalities according to the presence of metabolic syndrome. Comparisons were performed using Log-rank test. The total fraction of deceased patients during follow-up is indicated above each arm in the 2 panels. Cumulative numbers of deceased patients during follow-up in the overall cohort of patients with ischemic stroke and in the presence or absence of MetS are mentioned below the panels.

Table S1 Baseline characteristics of study participants with ischemic stroke according to mortality at different follow-up time-points.

Table S2 Cox regression analysis for prediction of 5-year mortality in study participants with ischemic stroke.

Acknowledgments

We thank all patients and their families for volunteering to take part in this study.

Author Contributions

Conceived and designed the experiments: APK ES. Performed the experiments: EVB JVFF BEN. Analyzed the data: EVB APK. Contributed reagents/materials/analysis tools: EVB JVFF BEN. Wrote the paper: EVB APK JVFF BEN ES.

References

1. Grundy SM (2012) Pre-diabetes, metabolic syndrome, and cardiovascular risk. J Am Coll Cardiol 59: 635–643.
2. Wannamethee SG, Shaper AG, Lennon L, Morris RW (2005) Metabolic syndrome vs Framingham Risk Score for prediction of coronary heart disease, stroke, and type 2 diabetes mellitus. Arch Intern Med 165: 2644–2650.
3. Arnlov J, Ingelsson E, Sundstrom J, Lind L (2010) Impact of body mass index and the metabolic syndrome on the risk of cardiovascular disease and death in middle-aged men. Circulation 121: 230–236.
4. Gupta AK, Dahlof B, Sever PS, Poulter NR (2010) Metabolic syndrome, independent of its components, is a risk factor for stroke and death but not for coronary heart disease among hypertensive patients in the ASCOT-BPLA. Diabetes Care 33: 1647–1651.
5. Alberti KG, Eckel RH, Grundy SM, Zimmet PZ, Cleeman JI, et al. (2009) Harmonizing the metabolic syndrome: a joint interim statement of the International Diabetes Federation Task Force on Epidemiology and Prevention;

National Heart, Lung, and Blood Institute; American Heart Association; World Heart Federation; International Atherosclerosis Society; and International Association for the Study of Obesity. Circulation 120: 1640–1645.
6. Gaillard T, Schuster D, Osei K (2009) Metabolic syndrome in Black people of the African diaspora: the paradox of current classification, definition and criteria. Ethn Dis 19: S2–S7.
7. Kengne AP, Anderson CS (2006) The neglected burden of stroke in sub-Saharan Africa. Int J Stroke 1: 180–190.
8. Kengne AP, Ntyintyane LM, Mayosi BM (2012) A systematic overview of prospective cohort studies of cardiovascular disease in sub-Saharan Africa. Cardiovasc J Afr 23: 103–112.
9. Kolo PM, Jibrin YB, Sanya EO, Alkali M, Peter Kio IB, et al. (2012) Hypertension-Related Admissions and Outcome in a Tertiary Hospital in Northeast Nigeria. Int J Hypertens 2012: 960546.

10. O'Donnell MJ, Xavier D, Liu L, Zhang H, Chin SL, et al. (2010) Risk factors for ischaemic and intracerebral haemorrhagic stroke in 22 countries (the INTER-STROKE study): a case-control study. Lancet 376: 112–123.

11. Sobngwi E, Kengne AP, Balti EV, Fezeu L, Nouthe B, et al. (2012) Metabolic profile of sub-Saharan african patients presenting with first-ever ischemic stroke: association with Insulin Resistance. J Stroke Cerebrovasc Dis 21: 639–640.

12. Connor MD, Thorogood M, Modi G, Warlow CP (2007) The burden of stroke in Sub-Saharan Africa. Am J Prev Med 33: 172–173.

13. Setel PW, Sankoh O, Rao C, Velkoff VA, Mathers C, et al. (2005) Sample registration of vital events with verbal autopsy: a renewed commitment to measuring and monitoring vital statistics. Bull World Health Organ 83: 611–617.

14. Warnick GR, Knopp RH, Fitzpatrick V, Branson L (1990) Estimating low-density lipoprotein cholesterol by the Friedewald equation is adequate for classifying patients on the basis of nationally recommended cutpoints. Clin Chem 36: 15–19.

15. Okafor CI (2012) The metabolic syndrome in Africa: Current trends. Indian J Endocrinol Metab 16: 56–66.

16. Fezeu L, Balkau B, Kengne AP, Sobngwi E, Mbanya JC (2007) Metabolic syndrome in a sub-Saharan African setting: central obesity may be the key determinant. Atherosclerosis 193: 70–76.

17. Motala AA, Mbanya JC, Ramaiya KL (2009) Metabolic syndrome in sub-Saharan Africa. Ethn Dis 19: S2–10.

18. Tillin T, Forouhi NG, McKeigue PM, Chaturvedi N (2006) The role of diabetes and components of the metabolic syndrome in stroke and coronary heart disease mortality in U.K. white and African-Caribbean populations. Diabetes Care 29: 2127–2129.

19. Isomaa B, Almgren P, Tuomi T, Forsen B, Lahti K, et al. (2001) Cardiovascular morbidity and mortality associated with the metabolic syndrome. Diabetes Care 24: 683–689.

20. Galassi A, Reynolds K, He J (2006) Metabolic syndrome and risk of cardiovascular disease: a meta-analysis. Am J Med 119: 812–819.

21. Hunt KJ, Resendez RG, Williams K, Haffner SM, Stern MP (2004) National Cholesterol Education Program versus World Health Organization metabolic syndrome in relation to all-cause and cardiovascular mortality in the San Antonio Heart Study. Circulation 110: 1251–1257.

22. Miranda PJ, DeFronzo RA, Califf RM, Guyton JR (2005) Metabolic syndrome: definition, pathophysiology, and mechanisms. Am Heart J 149: 33–45.

23. Bruno G, Merletti F, Biggeri A, Bargero G, Ferrero S, et al. (2004) Metabolic syndrome as a predictor of all-cause and cardiovascular mortality in type 2 diabetes: the Casale Monferrato Study. Diabetes Care 27: 2689–2694.

24. Callahan A, Amarenco P, Goldstein LB, Sillesen H, Messig M, et al. (2011) Risk of stroke and cardiovascular events after ischemic stroke or transient ischemic attack in patients with type 2 diabetes or metabolic syndrome: secondary analysis of the Stroke Prevention by Aggressive Reduction in Cholesterol Levels (SPARCL) trial. Arch Neurol 68: 1245–1251.

25. Hu G, Qiao Q, Tuomilehto J, Balkau B, Borch-Johnsen K, et al. (2004) Prevalence of the metabolic syndrome and its relation to all-cause and cardiovascular mortality in nondiabetic European men and women. Arch Intern Med 164: 1066–1076.

26. Gami AS, Witt BJ, Howard DE, Erwin PJ, Gami LA, et al. (2007) Metabolic syndrome and risk of incident cardiovascular events and death: a systematic review and meta-analysis of longitudinal studies. J Am Coll Cardiol 49: 403–414.

4

Celastrol, an NF-κB Inhibitor, Improves Insulin Resistance and Attenuates Renal Injury in db/db Mice

Jung Eun Kim[1], Mi Hwa Lee[1], Deok Hwa Nam[1], Hye Kyoung Song[1], Young Sun Kang[1], Ji Eun Lee[2], Hyun Wook Kim[2], Jin Joo Cha[1], Young Youl Hyun[3], Sang Youb Han[4], Kum Hyun Han[4], Jee Young Han[5], Dae Ryong Cha[1]*

1 Department of Internal Medicine, Division of Nephrology, Korea University, Ansan City, Kyungki-Do, Korea, 2 Department of Internal Medicine, Division of Nephrology, Wonkwang University, Gunpo City, Kyungki-Do, Korea, 3 Department of Internal Medicine, Division of Nephrology, Sungkyunkwan University, Seoul, Korea, 4 Department of Internal Medicine, Division of Nephrology, Inje University, Goyang City, Kyungki-Do, Korea, 5 Department of Pathology, Inha University, Incheon City, Kyungki-Do, Korea

Abstract

The NF-κB pathway plays an important role in chronic inflammatory and autoimmune diseases. Recently, NF-κB has also been suggested as an important mechanism linking obesity, inflammation, and metabolic disorders. However, there is no current evidence regarding the mechanism of action of NF-κB inhibition in insulin resistance and diabetic nephropathy in type 2 diabetic animal models. We investigated the effects of the NF-κB inhibitor celastrol in db/db mice. The treatment with celastrol for 2 months significantly lowered fasting plasma glucose (FPG), HbA1C and homeostasis model assessment index (HOMA-IR) levels. Celastrol also exhibited significant decreases in body weight, kidney/body weight and adiposity. Celastrol reduced insulin resistance and lipid abnormalities and led to higher plasma adiponectin levels. Celastrol treatment also significantly mitigated lipid accumulation and oxidative stress in organs including the kidney, liver and adipose tissue. The treated group also exhibited significantly lower creatinine levels and urinary albumin excretion was markedly reduced. Celastrol treatment significantly lowered mesangial expansion and suppressed type IV collagen, PAI-1 and TGFβ1 expressions in renal tissues. Celastrol also improved abnormal lipid metabolism, oxidative stress and proinflammatory cytokine activity in the kidney. In cultured podocytes, celastrol treatment abolished saturated fatty acid-induced proinflammatory cytokine synthesis. Taken together, celastrol treatment not only improved insulin resistance, glycemic control and oxidative stress, but also improved renal functional and structural changes through both metabolic and anti-inflammatory effects in the kidney. These results suggest that targeted therapy for NF-κB may be a useful new therapeutic approach for the management of type II diabetes and diabetic nephropathy.

Editor: Pratibha V. Nerurkar, College of Tropical Agriculture and Human Resources, University of Hawaii, United States of America

Funding: This work was supported by the Korea Research Foundation Grant funded by the Korean Government (MOEHRD) as a Brain Korea 21 project (grant number KRF-2010-T1102051) and a special grant from Korea University (grant number R1003201). The funders had no role in study design, data collection and analysis, decision to publish, or preparation of the manuscript.

Competing Interests: The authors have declared that no competing interests exist.

* E-mail: cdragn@unitel.co.kr

Introduction

Type 2 diabetes mellitus is the leading cause of end-stage renal disease and is associated with morbidity and mortality due to cardiovascular disease. The increased mortality in type 2 diabetes mellitus is partially due to insulin resistance [1]. From a clinical perspective, insulin resistance is frequently combined with hyperinsulinemia, abnormal glucose metabolism, hypertension, atherosclerosis and dyslipidemia; collectively these conditions are referred to as metabolic syndrome [2,3].

Although the pathogenic mechanism of diabetic nephropathy is complex, inflammatory mechanisms may play important roles in the initiation and progression of diabetic nephropathy [4,5]. Macrophage infiltration, activation of inflammatory cytokines and adhesion molecules in the diabetic kidney have been reported in both human and animal diabetic models in a manner similar to other immunologic renal diseases [6,7,8].

NF-kappaB (NF-κB) is a ubiquitous and well-known transcription factor responsible for regulating the expressions of genes that are involved in inflammatory pathways such as proinflammatory cytokines, chemokines and adhesion molecules [9,10]. Since NF-κB plays a pivotal role in the inflammatory process, NF-κB has been an important and attractive therapeutic target for the management of many inflammatory diseases. Increasing evidence demonstrates that NF-κB is activated and contributes to macrophage infiltration in experimental models of diabetic kidney disease [11,12,13]. In addition, recent studies suggest that high glucose, mechanical stretching, angiotensin II and proteinuria contribute to NF-κB activation [13,14,15].

In terms of insulin resistance, NF-κB activation in adipose tissue has recently been implicated as an important mechanism in the development of insulin resistance [16]. Obesity is accompanied by the infiltration and activation of macrophages in adipose tissue, leading to chronic inflammation of adipose tissue [17]. Adipose tissue is an important organ in obesity-induced inflammation, since obesity induces phenotypic changes in adipocytes such as hypertrophy, and also induces an inflammatory response in adipocytes in an autocrine or paracrine fashion, resulting in impaired adipocyte function [18]. However, the roles of this pathway in diabetic nephropathy and insulin resistance have not been clearly delineated.

In this study we investigated the effect of celastrol, an NF-κB inhibitor, on insulin resistance and diabetic nephropathy under the hypothesis that inhibition of the NF-κB pathway may improve insulin resistance and renal function through the modulation of inflammatory processes in both adipose tissues and kidneys in db/db mice.

Materials and Methods

Animal experiments

Six-week-old male non-diabetic db/m and diabetic db/db mice (C57BLKS/J-lepr^{db}/lepr^{db}) were purchased from the Jackson Laboratory (Sacramento, CA, USA). The mice were given free access to food and tap water and were caged individually under controlled temperature ($23 \pm 2°C$) and humidity ($55 \pm 5\%$) with an artificial light cycle. At 8 weeks of age, mice were divided into 3 groups. Group 1 consisted of non-diabetic control db/m mice (n = 8), group 2 consisted of db/db mice as a control group (n = 8), and group 3 consisted of db/db mice that were treated via injection with 1 mg/kg/day of celastrol (Sigma. St. Louis, MO, USA) intraperitoneally for 2 months (n = 8). In addition, we performed another in vivo experiment to evaluate whether celastrol could potentially have significant effect on food intake and body weight in non-diabetic control db/m mice. Control non-diabetic db/m mice were divided into two groups with or without treatment with 1 mg/kg/day of celastrol for 2 weeks (n = 5 in each group), and compare the physical parameters after 2 weeks. During experiments, food intake, water intake, urine volume, body weight, fasting plasma glucose concentration, and HbA1c levels were measured monthly. Plasma glucose levels were measured by a glucose oxidase-based method and creatinine levels were determined using an HPLC method. Plasma insulin levels and plasma adiponectin levels were measured using an ELISA kit (Linco Research, St. Charles, MO, USA). Plasma triglyceride and cholesterol analyses were measured using a GPO-Trinder kit (Sigma, St. Louis, MO, USA). Plasma lipoprotein profiles were measured using a fast protein liquid chromatography (HPLC) system. The blood levels of hemoglobin A1c (HbA1c) were calculated by an IN2IT system (Bio-Rad, UK). The homeostasis model assessment index (HOMA-IR) was calculated by the following equation: fasting glucose (mmol/L) × fasting insulin (mU/L)/22.5. An insulin-tolerance test (ITT) was performed to assess the insulin resistance state. ITT was performed following 8-hour fasting and blood samples were collected through the tail vein. Mice received 0.75 units/kg of regular insulin by i.p. injection and blood sampling was done to measure blood glucose levels at 0, 30, 60, 90, and 120 min after insulin injection. To determine urinary microalbumin excretion, individual mice were placed in a metabolic cage and urine was collected for 24 h. The urinary microalbumin concentration was determined by a competitive enzyme-linked immunosorbent assay (Shibayagi, Shibukawa, Japan) and corrected by urinary creatinine concentration. Plasma and urinary levels of 8-isoprostane were measured using an ELISA kit (Cayman Chemical, Ann Arbor, MI, USA). Lipids from the hepatic, adipose, and renal cortical tissues were extracted as described by Bligh and Dyer [19]. Total cholesterol and triglyceride contents were measured using a commercial kit (Wako Chemicals, Richmond, VA, USA). The extent of peroxidative reaction in the hepatic, adipose, and kidney tissues was determined by directly measuring lipid hydroperoxides (LPOs) using redox reactions with ferrous ions from tissue homogenates and an LPO

assay kit (Cayman Chemical, Ann Arbor, MI, USA), as described previously [20]. At the end of the study period, systolic blood pressure was measured using tail-cuff plethysmography (LE 5001-Pressure Meter, Letica SA, Barcelona, Spain). Mice were sacrificed under anesthesia by i.p. injection of sodium pentobarbital (50 mg/kg). This study was carried out in strict accordance with the recommendations in the Guide for the Care and Use of Laboratory Animals of the National Institutes of Health. The protocol was approved by the Committee on the Ethics of Animal Experiments of the University of Korea (Permit Number: KUIACUC-20111001-1).

Analysis of gene expression by real-time quantitative PCR

Total RNA was extracted from experimental cells with Trizol reagent and further purified using an RNeasy Mini kit (Qiagen, Valencia, CA, USA). Primers were designed from the respective gene sequences using Primer 3 software and the secondary structures of templates were examined and excluded using the mfold software program. Table S1 shows the nucleotide sequences of the primers. Quantitative gene expression was performed on a Light Cycler 1.5 system (Roche Diagnostics Corporation, Indianapolis, IN, USA) using SYBR Green technology. Real-time reverse transcription-PCR was performed for 10 min at 50°C and 5 min at 95°C. Subsequently, 30–35 cycles were applied, consisting of denaturation for 10 s at 95°C and annealing with extension for 30 s at 60°C. At the end of the PCR cycle, samples were heated to 95°C to check that a single PCR product was obtained. The ratio of each gene and β-actin level (relative gene expression number) was calculated by subtracting the threshold cycle number (Ct) of the target gene from that of β -actin and raising 2 to the power of this difference.

Histopathological evaluation and immunohistochemistry

Cardiac, hepatic, and adipose tissues were fixed for 48 h with 10% paraformaldehyde at 4°C, dehydrated, embedded in paraffin, cut into 4 μm thick slices, and stained with periodic acid-Schiff (PAS), Masson's trichrome (MT), and hematoxylin and eosin. Glomerular mesangial expansion was scored semiquantitatively and the percentage of mesangial matrix occupying each glomerulus was rated from 0 to 4 as follows: 0, 0%; 1, <25%; 2, 25–50%; 3, 50–75%; and 4, >75%. For immunohistochemical staining, renal tissues were sliced into 4 μm sections. Slides were transferred to a 10 mmol/L citrate buffer solution at a pH of 6.0. Various staining conditions were then applied as follows: sections were microwaved for 10–20 min to retrieve antigens for TGF-β1 staining, transferred to Biogenex Retriever (pH 8.0) (ImmuGenex, San Ramon, CA, USA) for PAI-1 staining or treated with trypsin (Sigma, St Louis, MO, USA) for 30 min at 37°C for type IV collagen staining. After washing in water, 3.0% H_2O_2 in methanol was applied for 10 min in order to block endogenous peroxidase activity and the slides were incubated at room temperature for 40 min with normal goat serum (TGF-β1and type IV collagen) or 10% power block (PAI-1) to prevent nonspecific detection. Next, slides were incubated at 4°C overnight with a primary antibody including rabbit polyclonal anti-type IV collagen antibody (1:200; Santa Cruz Biotechnology, Santa Cruz, CA, USA), a rabbit polyclonal anti-TGF-β1 antibody (1:200; Santa Cruz Biotechnology) and a rabbit anti-PAI-1 antibody (1:50; American Diagnostica, Stanford, CT, USA). Slides were incubated in a secondary antibody for 30 min. For coloration, slides were incubated at room temperature with a mixture of 0.05% 3,3-diaminobenzidine containing 0.01% H_2O_2 and counterstained with Mayer's hematoxylin. Negative control sections were stained under identical conditions with the buffer solution substituting for the primary antibody. In order to evaluate the results of immunohistochemical staining, glomerular fields were graded semiquantitatively under a high-power field containing 50–60 glomeruli and an average score was calculated as described previously [21].

Western blot analysis

Nuclear and cytoplasmic proteins were extracted from renal cortical tissues and cells using a commercial nuclear extraction kit according to the manufacturer's instructions (Active Motif, Carlsbad, CA). Under denaturing conditions, 35 μg of protein were electrophoresed on a 10% SDS-PAGE mini-gel. Proteins were transferred onto a polyvinylidene difluoride membrane (Immobilon-P; Millipore, Bedford, MA, USA) for 60 min at 100 V. After incubation in blocking solution (Tris-buffered saline containing 150 mM NaCl, 50 nM Tris, 0.05% Tween-20 and 5% BSA, pH 7.5) for 1 h at room temperature, the membrane was hybridized in blocking buffer with goat polyclonal anti-TLR4 antibody (1:500, Santa Cruz Biotechnology, CA, USA), anti-NOX4 antibody (1:500, Novus Biologicals, USA), rabbit monoclonal anti- NF-κB p65 antibody(1:2000, Cell signaling, USA), rabbit monoclonal anti-α-tubulin antibody (1:1000,Cell Signaling Technology) or mouse monoclonal anti-β-actin antibody (1: 10000, Sigma Aldrich) overnight at 4°C with gentle shaking. Afterward, peroxidase conjugated secondary antibodies (1:5000) were applied for 1 h at room temperature, followed by reaction with chemiluminescence (ECL) reagent (Amersham, Buckinghamshire, UK).

Fatty acid analysis in hepatic and adipose tissues

Fatty acid compositions in hepatic and adipose tissue were analyzed at the end of study period by gas chromatography-flame ionization detection (GC-FID) method on a HP6890N GC-FID with a hydrogen flame ionization detector and an Supelco™ SP-2560 column (100 m×0.25 mm×0.20 μm). Helium served as the carrier gas, and 1 μl sample was loaded when the injection temperature was 260°C. Briefly, an extraction with chloroform was conducted. The dry extracts were dissolved in a few drops of chloroform and filled in thin liquid chromatography plates for separation of the lipids. The lipid esters were trans-methylated and the methyl esters were extracted. The FA methyl esters were separated by gas–liquid chromatography (GLC). The FAs were identified by comparison of the retention times of separation, controlled by SUPELCO™37 component FAME Mix (47885-U). Thirty seven fatty acids including saturated (SFA), monounsaturated (MUFA), and polyunsaturated (PUFA) fatty acids were identified and quantified.

Podocyte culture experiment

Since podocytes are the major target cells affected by high glucose and free fatty acid stimulation in the diabetic milieu, we used podocytes to further define the molecular mechanism of NF-κB inhibition on proinflammatory cytokine synthesis. A thermosensitive, SV 40-transfected immortalized mouse podocyte cell line that had been obtained as a generous gift from Peter Mundel (Albert Einstein college of medicine, N.Y.) was used for this study [22]. All cells were grown in a type I collagen coated dish (Iwaki, Tokyo, Japan) supplemented with RPMI media containing heat inactivated 10% fetal calf serum (Invitrogen, Carlsbad, CA), penicillin, and streptomycin. Differentiated podocytes were grown to subconfluence in the growth media and then cultured for 24 hours in a medium containing 5 mmol/L D-glucose and 1% FCS before being exposed to experimental conditions. The normal glucose group (NG group) used confluent cell monolayers cultured with 5 mmol/L of D-glucose, while the high glucose group (HG group) used 30 mmol/L of D-glucose. To evaluate the different effects of saturated (SFA), and monounsaturated (MUFA) fatty acids on proinflammatory cytokine synthesis, we treated some wells with palmitic acid (SFA) at a final concentration of 100 μM (Sigma, St. Louis, MO, USA) or oleic acid (PUFA) at a final concentration of 10 μM (Sigma, St. Louis, MO, USA) under either normal or high glucose conditions. To elucidate the effect of NF-κB inhibition, 1 μM of celastrol was added to the cells for 1 h before treatment with free fatty acid. All experimental groups were cultured in triplicate and harvested at 12 hours for extraction of the total RNA and secretory cytokine proteins. The secreted proinflammatory cytokines were measured in the culture supernatants using Millipore's MILLIPLEX™ Mouse Cytokine/Chemokine kit and the supernatant levels of cytokines were expressed relative to the total protein concentration. All experiments were performed in triplicate and cells were harvested at 12 hours to extract total RNA and protein.

Statistical analysis

A nonparametric analysis was used because of the relatively small number of samples. Results were expressed as mean ± standard error of the mean (SEM). Multiple comparisons were performed using the Kruskal-Wallis test with Bonferroni correction, followed by a Mann-Whitney U-test using a microcomputer-assisted program with SPSS for Windows 10.0 (SPSS, Chicago, IL, USA). $P<0.05$ was considered statistically significant.

Results

Effects of celastrol on biochemical and physical parameters in experimental animals

Table 1 shows biochemical results for each group. As expected, body weight, food intake, water intake, plasma insulin levels and fasting plasma glucose concentrations were significantly higher in diabetic *db/db* mice than those of non-diabetic *db/m* mice throughout the study period. Additionally, urine volume, organ mass of kidney, fat and liver was significantly higher in diabetic *db/db* mice compared with those of non-diabetic *db/m* mice. However, there were no significant differences in plasma levels of creatinine, adiponectin and 8-isoprostane, and systolic blood pressure between non-diabetic *db/m* mice and diabetic *db/db* mice. Interestingly, body weight was significantly lower in the celastrol-treated group due to decreases in food intake. In terms of organ mass change, celastrol treatment did not induce any significant changes in the weights of the liver or heart. Epididymal fat mass and kidney weight were significantly lower in the celastrol treatment group compared with the control group. However, there were no significant differences in systolic blood pressure or plasma levels of insulin or isoprostane between the two groups. Celastrol treatment induced a marked improvement in glycemic control. Even after only 4 weeks of treatment, fasting plasma glucose levels were significantly decreased; this hypoglycemia was persistently observed until the end of the study (Table 1). Furthermore, plasma adiponectin levels were significantly higher in the celastrol-treated group. In addition, we also performed another in vivo experiment in *db/m* mice to define celastrol also decrease food intake and body weight independent of diabetic status. As shown in Table S2, 2weeks treatment with celastrol also induced a significant decrease in food intake and body weight in *db/m* mice.

Table 1. Physical and biochemical parameters of experimental animals.

Parameters	week	db/m control	db/db + vehicle	db/db + celastrol
Body weight (g)	0	24.28±0.18	33.2±0.41***	33.4±0.81***
	4	29.14±0.40	45.7±1.29***	38.0±1.26***,‡
	8	29.00±0.53	46.5±1.94***	37.2±2.22***,†
Daily Food intake (g)	0	3.53±0.31	4.68±0.26	4.95±0.53
	4	3.14±0.09	4.93±0.08***	3.85±0.24**,‡
	8	2.97±0.17	5.06±0.18***	4.10±0.46**,†
Daily water intake (g)	0	5.35±0.25	7.87±0.22***	7.45±0.69**
	4	3.98±0.22	16.45±0.47***	4.45±0.43***,‡
	8	3.60±0.16	17.56±0.54***	8.14±0.62**,‡
Fasting plasma glucose (mmol/l)	0	9.3±0.5	18.2±1.9**	19.4±3.4**
	4	8.3±0.3	35.7±1.8***	17.2±4.2*,‡
	8	8.59±0.32	32.1±1.8***	16.2±3.1*,‡
UV (ml/day)	0	0.45±0.08	0.66±0.10	0.71±0.11
	4	0.39±0.08	0.75±0.12*	0.68±0.03*
	8	0.39±0.05	1.42±0.32**	0.76±0.14
Kidney/100 g BW	8	0.49±0.02	1.36±0.05***	0.52±0.03‡
Heart/100 g BW	8	0.36±0.02	0.38±0.02	0.35±0.02
Fat/100 g BW	8	1.15±0.08	6.08±0.41***	2.73±0.74*,‡
Liver/100 g BW	8	4.17±0.63	7.26±0.56**	7.58±1.13**
P-adiponectin (µg/ml)	8	2.89±0.20	2.51±0.05	29.1±2.44**,‡
P-8-isoprostane(pg/ml)	8	249±29.8	473±74.4	814±172
P-creatinine (µmol/l)	8	35.0±4.0	45.0±6.0	29.0±2.0†
P-insulin (ng/ml)	8	1.71±0.38	9.73±0.01***	8.80±2.41**
SBP (mmHg)	8	118±16	115±15	124±11

UV, urine volume; P, plasma. Values are expressed as means ± SEM. Statistical analysis was performed between groups at the same time periods; *P<0.05; **P<0.01; ***P<0.001 vs. db/m control; †P<0.05; ‡P<0.01 vs. db/db + vehicle.

Effects of celastrol on metabolic parameters in experimental animals

Celastrol treatment induced a marked improvement in insulin resistance. As shown in Figures 1A and 1B, levels of HOMA-IR and HbA1C were significantly decreased after celastrol treatment. The improvement in insulin resistance by celastrol treatment was further confirmed by intraperitoneal ITT (Figure 1C). In accordance with the improved insulin resistance, celastrol treatment significantly decreased plasma total cholesterol and triglyceride levels (Figure 1D).

Effects of celastrol on renal function and histological changes in experimental animals

Urinary albumin excretion was significantly higher in diabetic db/db mice than those of non-diabetic db/m mice throughout the study period (Figure 2). Celastrol treatment markedly decreased urinary albumin excretion after 4 weeks of treatment and this effect was persistently observed until the end of the study period (Figure 2). In terms of renal function, the celastrol group also showed significantly lower levels of plasma creatinine levels (Table 1). Consistent with marked attenuation of albuminuria, celastrol treatment significantly suppressed the expression of profibrotic and proinflammatory molecules in the kidney. Figures 3A–3L show representative renal pathology and immunostaining for TGFβ1, type IV collagen, and PAI-1. Consistent with marked attenuation of albuminuria, mesangial expansion was

more severe in diabetic db/db mice than non-diabetic db/m mice, and mesangial expansion was markedly improved in the celastrol treatment group (Figure 3A, 3E, 3I, Figure 4). Furthermore, the immunostaining scores for TGFβ1, type IV collagen and PAI-1, major fibrotic molecules in fibrotic glomeruli, also demonstrated dramatic improvement in the celastrol-treated group (Figure 3, 4).

Effects of celastrol on oxidative stress and inflammatory cytokines in experimental animals

Since celastrol treatment improved albuminuria and structural changes in diabetic kidneys and NF-κB inhibition can inhibit proinflammatory cytokine production, we next examined whether improvement in renal function was derived from the suppression of proinflammatory cytokines in the kidney. As shown in Figure 5, urinary excretion of inflammatory cytokines was markedly higher in diabetic db/db mice than non-diabetic db/m mice, and celastrol treatment markedly suppressed the urinary levels of these cytokines. Additionally, urinary levels of 8-isoprostane, an indicator of oxidative stress in the kidney, also profoundly decreased in celastrol-treated group (Figure 5). In addition, we performed western blot using renal cortical tissues for the NF-κB to elucidate whether the NF-κB is overexpressed in diabetic kidneys. As shown in Figure 6, diabetic mice showed significantly higher levels of activation in NF-κB compared with control db/m mice as determined by the nuclear expressions of the p65 subunit of NF-κB, toll-like receptor 4 (TLR4) and NADPH oxidase 4

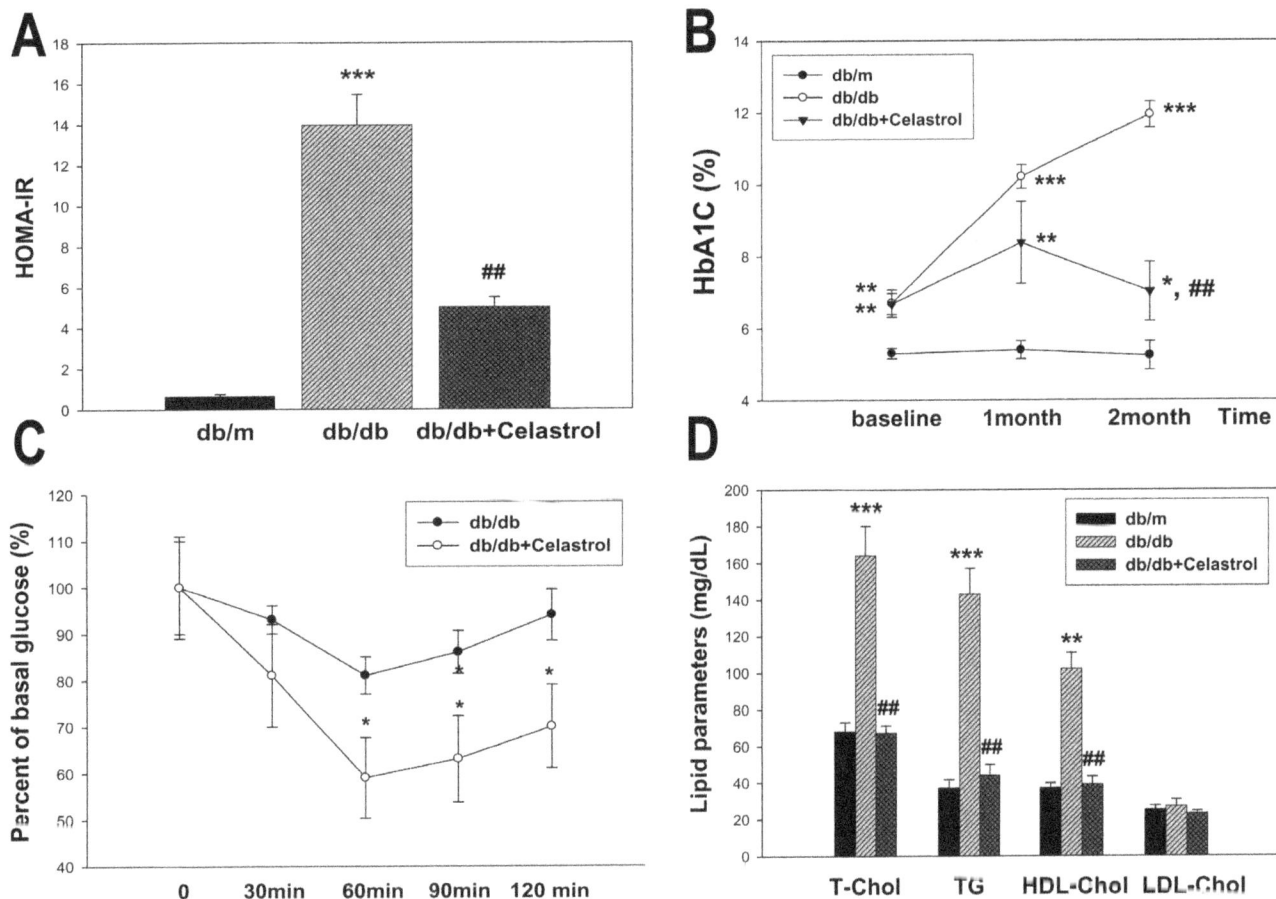

Figure 1. Effects of celastrol on HOMA-IR, HbA1C, insulin resistance and plasma lipid levels in experimental animals. Data are shown as the mean±SEM; *p<0.05, **p<0.01, ***p<0.001 vs. db/m group; ##p<0.01 vs. control db/db group.

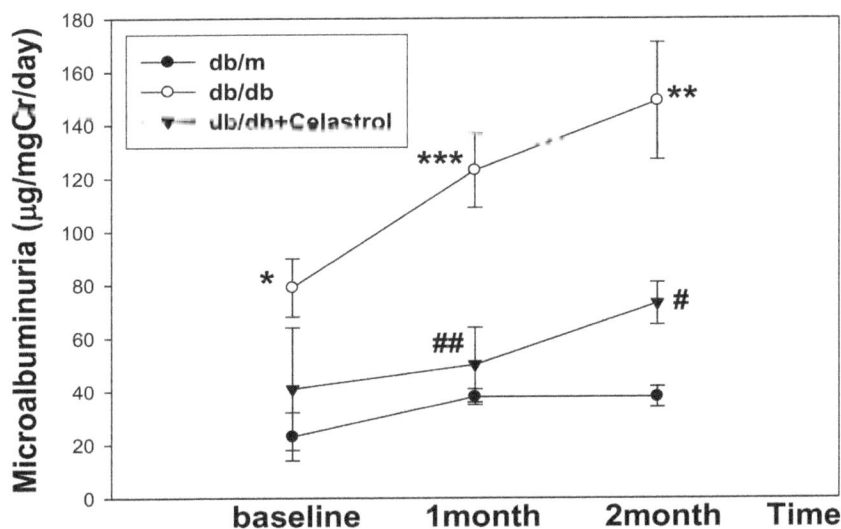

Figure 2. Effects of celastrol on urinary albumin excretion in experimental animals. Data are shown as the mean±SEM; *p<0.05, **p<0.01, ***p<0.001 vs. db/m group; #p<0.05; ##p<0.01 vs. control db/db group.

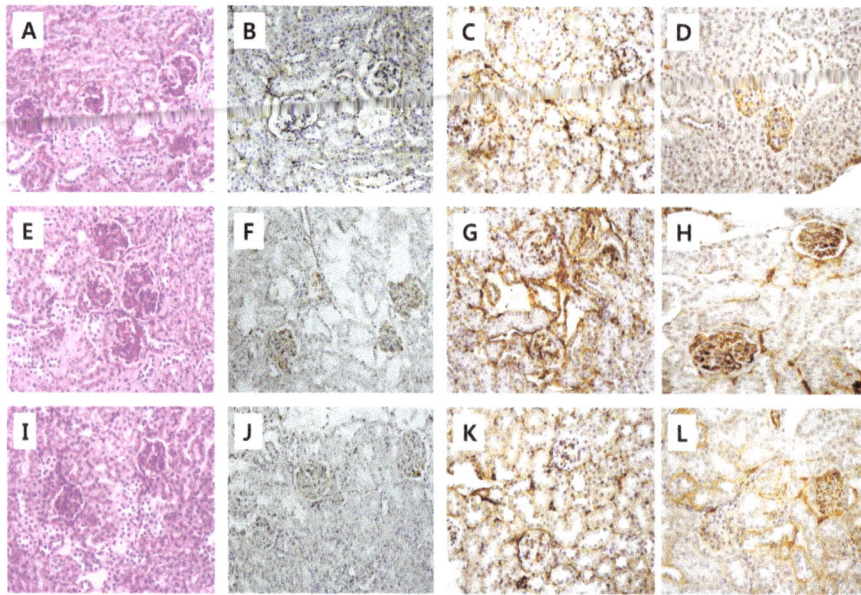

Figure 3. Representative renal histologic findings in experimental animals. (A, E, I) PAS, (B, F, J) TGFβ-1, (C, G, K) Type IV collagen, (D, H, L) PAI-1; A–D, *db/m*; E–H, *db/db*; I–L, *db/db*+celastrol. Original magnification X400.

(NOX4) in renal cortical tissues. Celastrol treatment significantly suppressed inflammatory molecules in diabetic kidney (Figure 6A, 6B)

Effects of celastrol on fatty acid composition in hepatic and adipose tissues in experimental animals

Table S3 shows the change in fatty acids composition in hepatic and adipose tissues after 2 months treatment with celastrol. In non-diabetic control *db/m* mice, most FAs were composed of n-6 PUFAs (42%), SFAs (35%) and MUFAs (22%) in fat, and n-6 PUFAs (72%), n-3 PUFAs (16%) and SFAs (11%) in liver. However, FAs composition in diabetic *db/db* mice showed significantly higher levels of SFAs and lower levels of n-6 PUFAs in fat and liver compared with those in control *db/m* mice. Interestingly, celastrol treated *db/db* mice showed significantly lower levels of SFAs, and higher levels of MUFAs in fat and liver compared with those in diabetic *db/db* mice (Table S3).

Effects of celastrol on histological changes in liver and adipose tissue

Figure S1 shows the representative adipose tissue and liver pathology in the experimental groups at the end of the study period. In accordance with improved plasma lipid abnormalities, celastrol treatment markedly decreased hepatic steatosis (Figure

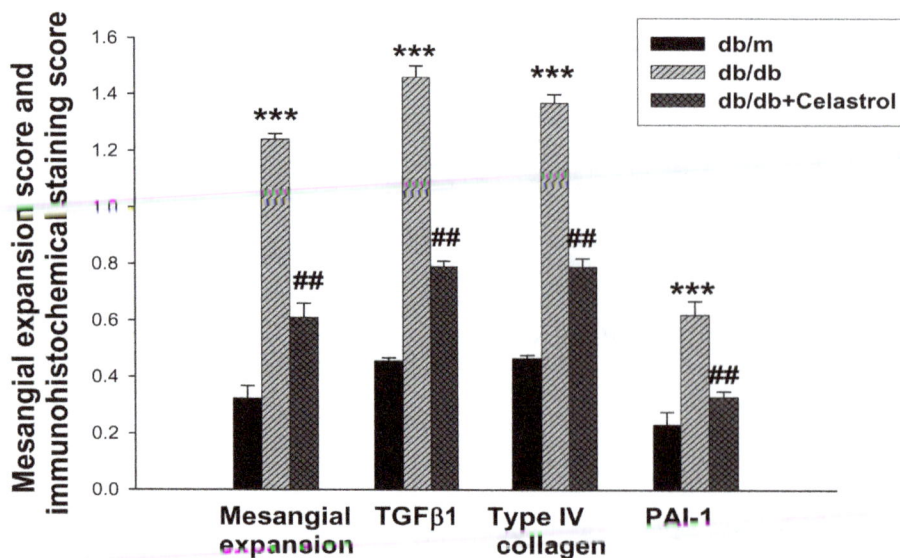

Figure 4. Glomerular mesangial expansion score and immunostaining score. Data are shown as the mean±SEM; ***p<0.001 vs. *db/m* group; ##p<0.01 vs. control *db/db* group.

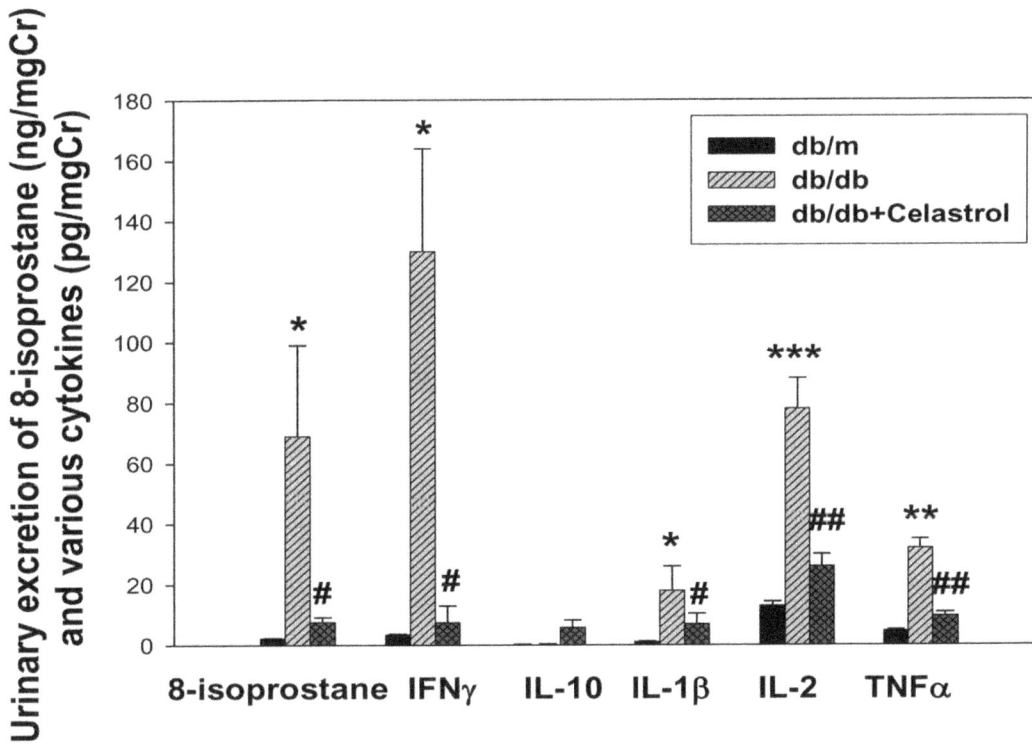

Figure 5. Effects of celastrol on urinary levels of cytokines in experimental animals. Data are shown as the mean±SEM; *p<0.05, **p<0.01, ***p<0.001 vs. *db/m* group; #p<0.05, ##p<0.01 vs. control *db/db* group.

A

B

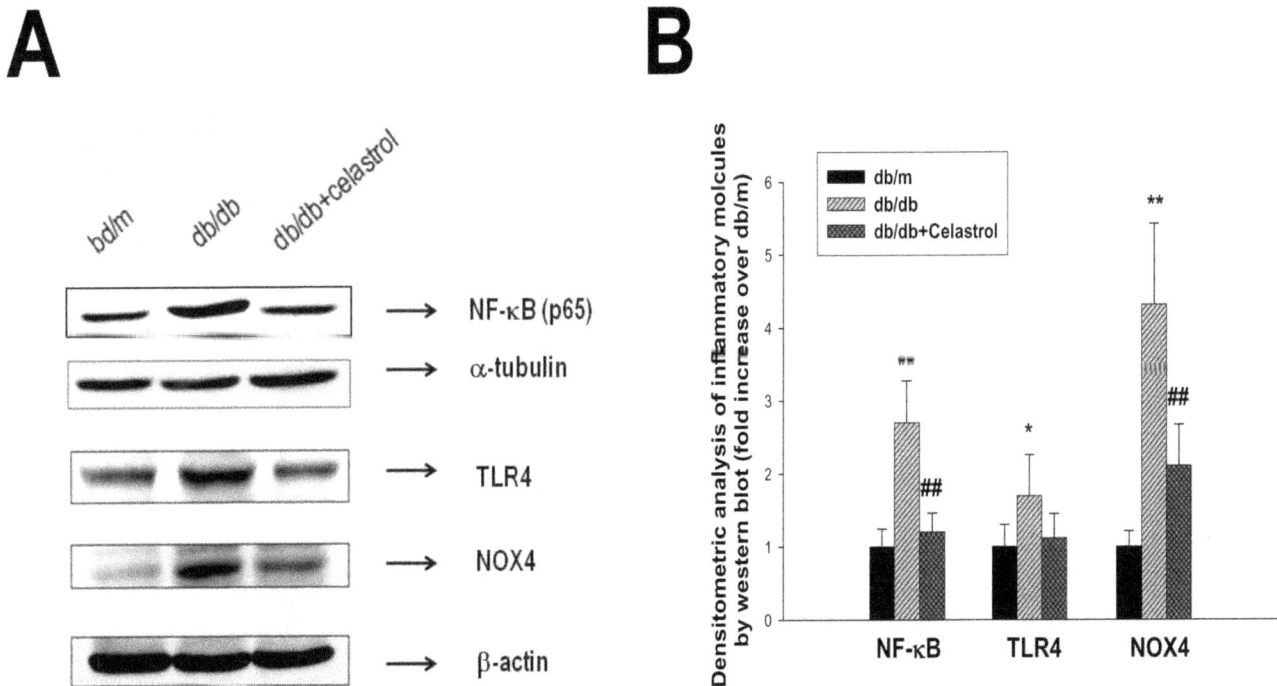

Figure 6. Effects of celastrol on inflammatory molecules in experimental animals. (A) Representative western blot for NF-κB p65, TLR4, and NOX4 protein in renal cortical tissues in experimental animals. (B) Densitometric analysis of western results. Data are shown as the mean±SEM; *p<0.05, **p<0.01, vs. *db/m* group; ##p<0.01 vs. control *db/db* group.

S1F). Interestingly, adipose tissue obtained from epididymal fat revealed that celastrol treatment induced phenotypic changes in adipocytes, causing differentiation into small adipocytes (Figure S1C). Further, this phenotypic change was consistent with the change in epididymal fat mass that was decreased by celastrol treatment.

Effects of celastrol on oxidative stress and lipid accumulation in experimental animals

Because celastrol administration improved microalbuminuria and insulin resistance and was related to improvements in metabolic dysfunction, we next investigated whether these improvements were related to a correction of lipotoxicity. As shown in Figure 7, cholesterol and triglyceride levels in renal and hepatic tissues were markedly increased in diabetic db/db mice than non-diabetic db/m mice, and significantly decreased by celastrol treatment, although these parameters did not show any significant differences in adipose tissue. Since oxidative stress in the diabetic condition induces the peroxidation of lipids and leads to cellular dysfunction, we also evaluated changes in LPO in tissues. LPO levels in the kidney, liver, and adipose tissues were significantly decreased by celastrol treatment (Figure 8).

Effects of celastrol on proinflammatory cytokine synthesis in cultured podocytes

Finally, we performed an *in vitro* experiment to further evaluate the direct effect of celastrol treatment in terms of anti-inflammatory effects in cultured podocytes. As shown in Figure 9A, stimulation with high glucose alone did not induce significant increases in the gene expression of inflammatory molecules including IFNγ, NOX4, TLR4, and TNFα, whereas stimulation with the palmitate (SFA) markedly up-regulated the expressions of these cytokine genes. Prior treatment with celastrol almost completely suppressed this SFA-induced cytokine molecule expression. However, oleic acid (MUFA) showed down-regulated

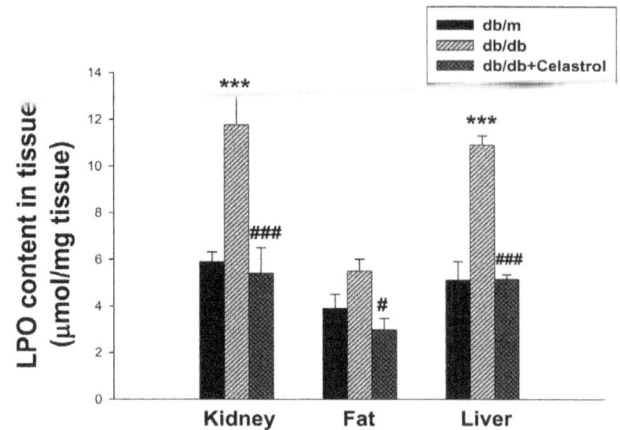

Figure 8. Effects of celastrol on lipid peroxidation in experimental animals. Data are shown as the mean±SEM; ***p<0.001 vs. db/m group; #p<0.05, ###p<0.001 vs. control db/db group.

tendency in inflammatory cytokine gene expression, although it did not reach statistical significance. However, there was no significant change in anti-inflammatory cytokines such as IL-10. In accordance with gene expression, inflammatory cytokine secretion was profoundly increased only after SFA stimulation and celastrol treatment completely abrogated fatty acid-induced inflammatory cytokine production (Figure 9B). In addition, NOX4 and TLR4 protein expression determined by western blot also showed similar changes (Figure 9C, 9D).

Discussion

In the present study, we demonstrated that celastrol treatment significantly improved insulin resistance, glycemic control and metabolic parameters in db/db mice. Celastrol treatment also

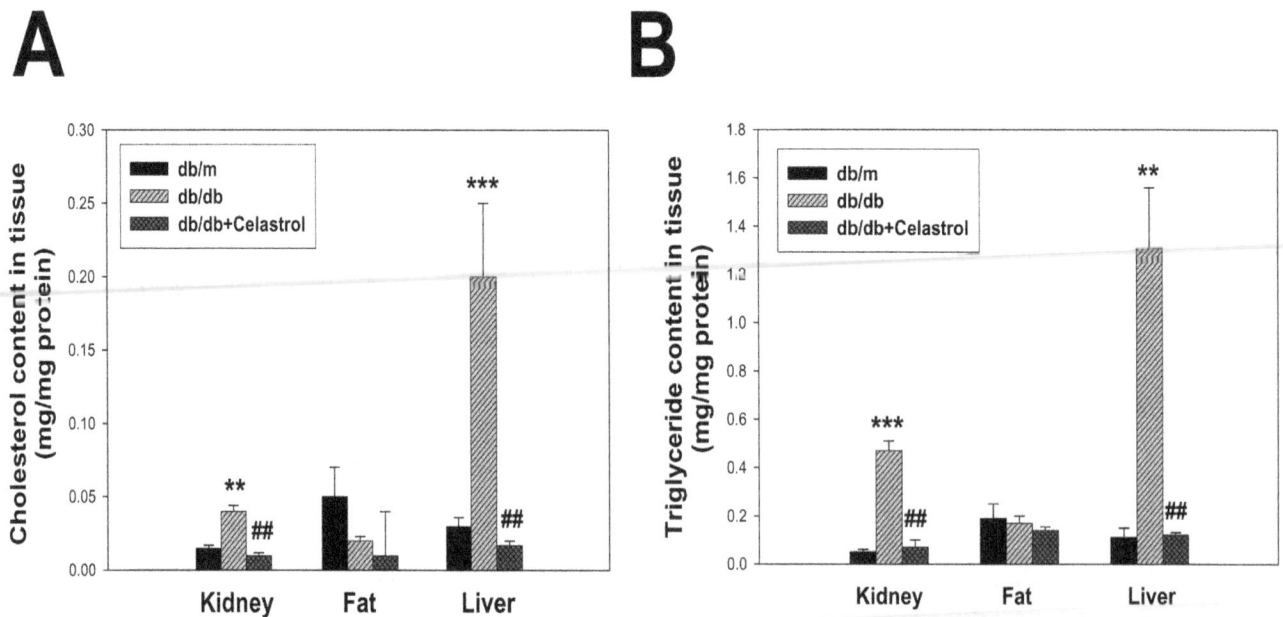

Figure 7. Effects of celastrol on tissue lipid accumulation in experimental animals. (A) Cholesterol contents in renal, adipose, and hepatic tissues. (B) Triglyceride contents in renal, adipose, and hepatic tissues. Data are shown as the mean±SEM; **p<0.01, ***p<0.001 vs. db/m group; ##p<0.01 vs. control db/db group.

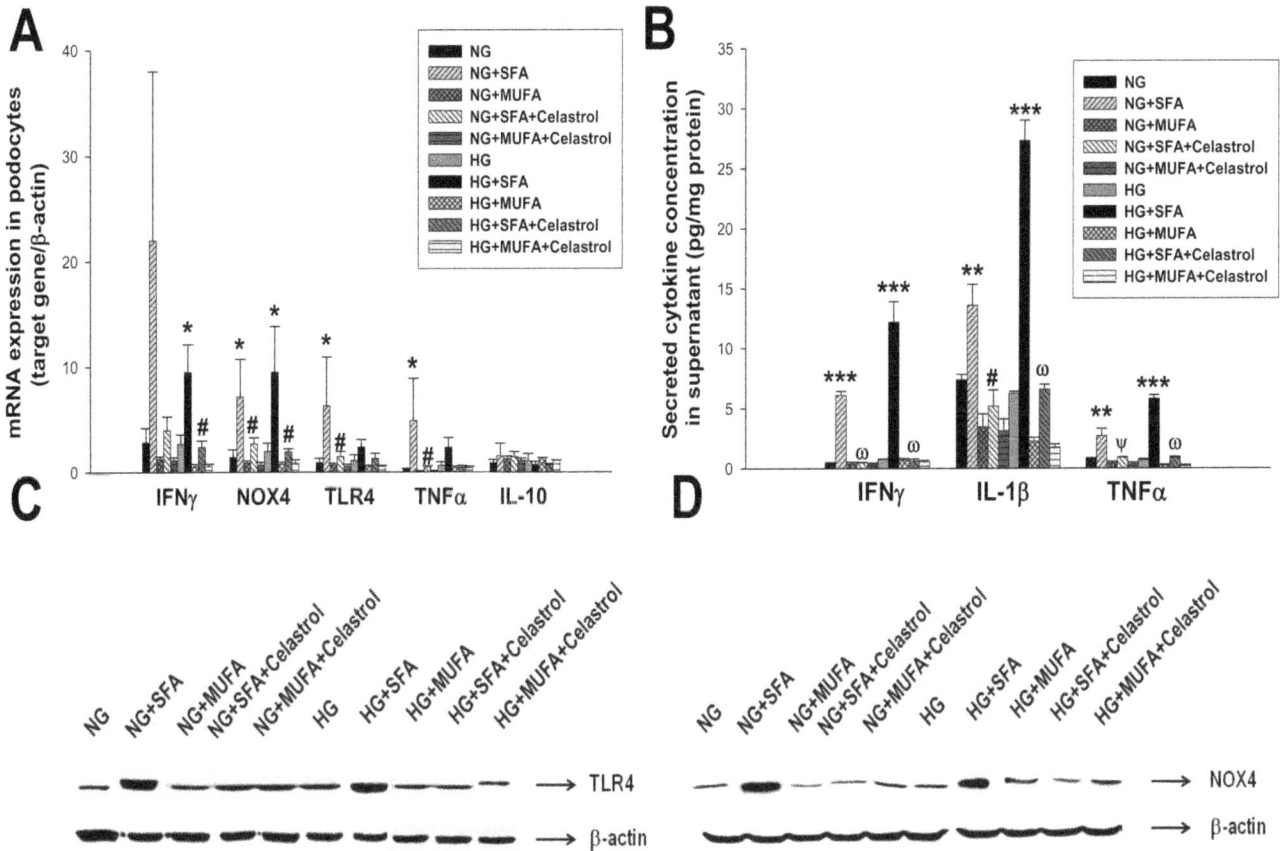

Figure 9. Effects of celastrol on inflammatory molecules in cultured podocytes. (A) mRNA expression in podocytes. (B) Secreted cytokine concentration in supernatant. Data are shown as the mean±SEM; (C) Representative western blot for TLR4 in podocytes. (D) Representative western blot for NOX4 in podocytes. SFA, saturated fatty acid; MUFA, monounsaturated fatty acids; *p<0.05, **p<0.01, ***p<0.001 vs. NG or HG; #p<0.05, Ψp<0.01, ω<0.0001 vs. SFA treated group.

significantly mitigated lipid accumulation and oxidative stress in various organs including the liver and adipose tissue. In addition, celastrol treatment exhibited renal protective effects through improvement in renal lipid accumulation, oxidative stress and proinflammatory cytokine activity in the kidney. We also provided evidence that celastrol treatment abolished free fatty acid-induced proinflammatory cytokine synthesis in cultured podocytes.

The NF-κB signaling pathway is a central axis in tissue inflammation because NF-κB controls the expression of genes including inflammatory cytokines, chemokines, and adhesion molecules, all of which play pivotal roles in controlling inflammation [9]. Due to this attractive characteristic, targeted therapy for the NF-κB pathway has been of interest in the treatment of many inflammatory diseases. Although a great deal of evidence suggests the indirect renoprotective effect of various drugs and drug targets such as RAS blockade, ROS inhibition, alpha-tocopherol, and PPARα and PPARγ agonists secondary to inhibition of the NF-κB pathway [11,13,23,24,25,26,27], there is little evidence suggesting that direct inhibition of the NF-κB pathway has a beneficial effect in diabetic nephropathy. Furthermore, increasing data suggest an important role of the NF-κB pathway in the development of insulin resistance associated with adipose tissue inflammation [9,28] and there is also some evidence regarding the effect of NF-κB inhibition on insulin resistance.

In the present study, we investigated the effects of celastrol, an NF-κB inhibitor, on insulin resistance and diabetic nephropathy in

type 2 diabetic mice that are a well-known animal model of insulin resistance and nephropathy. We found that celastrol treatment markedly improved glycemic control and reduced HbA1C levels and HOMA-IR index scores in these overtly diabetic insulin resistant mice. Improvements in insulin resistance were further confirmed by insulin tolerance test. Celastrol-treated animals exhibited much better lipid profiles, including decreases in total cholesterol and triglyceride levels associated with improvement in hepatic steatosis.

In agreement with these results, recent studies have explored potential mechanisms of the NF-κB pathway in the pathogenesis of insulin resistance. Women with polycystic ovarian syndrome demonstrate insulin resistance and increases in NF-κB activation in mononuclear cells [29]. NF-κB DNA-binding activity and IkBα protein levels were significantly more elevated in PBMCs from type 2 diabetic patients than in non-diabetic controls [30]. In addition, NF-κB binding was positively associated with both body mass index and the homeostasis model assessment of insulin resistance in type 2 diabetic patients [31]. Genetic polymorphism in the 3' region of the IkBα gene have been associated with insulin resistance in Hispanic Americans in the Insulin Resistance Atherosclerosis (IRAS) Family Study [32]. Taken together, this data suggests a possible link between NF-κB activation and insulin resistance.

Celastrol treatment significantly decreased body weight due to decreases in food consumption. These results contrast with those of a previous study in animal models of infection-associated anorexia and NF-κB transgenic mice [33,34]. Infection-related anorexia and weight loss are mediated via NF-κB activation in hypothalamic pro-opiomelanocortin (POMC) neurons. In addition, hypothalamic NF-κB was activated by leptin, an important anorexigenic hormone, and mediates leptin-stimulated POMC transcription [33]. Tang et al. reported that energy expenditure was elevated without a change in food intake in NF-κB transgenic mice [34]. Although it is not clear why the celastrol group showed lower body weight and decreased food intake, recent studies suggest that inhibition of NF-κB by celastrol in the hypothalamus may decrease levels of neuropeptide Y (NPY), which is an orexigenic hormone, resulting in decreased food intake and body weight. NPY is the most abundant neuropeptide within the central nervous system and its effects are mediated through the Y1 receptor, where it participates as an orexigenic hormone in the control of food intake [35]. Musso et al. reported that the Y1 receptor for NPY may represent one of the κB site-containing genes that is modulated by κB-related factors and acts as an enhancer element, inferring its potential role in regulating the expression of the Y1 receptor gene [36]. Furthermore, Zhang et al. also demonstrated that IKKβ/NF-κB remains inactive in hypo-thalamic neurons; however, overnutrition atypically activates hypothalamic IKKβ/NF-κB through elevated endoplasmic retic-ulum stress in the hypothalamus and activates hypothalamic AGRP neurons, leading to increased production of orexigenic hormones [37]. However, the potential adverse events such as decrease in food intake and body weight in healthy subjects should be considered before clinical application of celastrol as a new therapeutic strategy for treatment of diabetic nephropathy.

Obese adipose tissue has been proposed to be a pivotal organ in insulin resistance, whereby inflammatory processes such as infiltration of macrophages and increased cytokine synthesis occur, inducing systemic insulin resistance [17]. However, the physiologic action of NF-κB inhibition in adipose tissue remains uncertain.

In the present study, celastrol treatment significantly decreased epididymal fat masses and induced phenotypic changes to small differentiated adipocytes, which is a more insulin sensitive phenotype [38]. In addition, celastrol also markedly increased the adiponectin gene expression that is associated with increased plasma levels of adiponectin, all of which are related with improved insulin resistance. These results agree with those of a previous study that demonstrated that NF-κB levels were higher in mice treated with a high fat diet, and that inhibition of NF-κB restored the lipotoxicity of adipose tissue and decreased fat mass [39]. Furthermore, celastrol treatment significantly decreased the levels of SFAs, and increased the levels of MUFAs in hepatic and adipose tissue, that are more anti-inflammatory fatty acid composition. We also observed that adipose tissue lipid peroxida-tion was markedly decreased in the celastrol-treated group. Taken together, these results imply that NF-κB inhibition decreased inflammation and oxidative stress in adipose tissue and led to improved insulin resistance.

The most important finding of this study is that celastrol treatment decreased the urinary excretion of albumin and plasma creatinine levels. Additionally, celastrol decreased mesangial expansion in renal tissues, accompanied by suppression of the synthesis of profibrotic and proinflammatory molecules. We observed that NF-κB activation was increased in diabetic *db/db* mice compared with that in control db/m mice. Celastrol treatment decreased renal NF-κB activation in db/db mice. In addition, celastrol treatment markedly inhibited NOX4 expres-sion, a marker of oxidative stress in the kidney, and decreased the

urinary excretions of 8-isoprostane, a marker of oxidative stress, and inflammatory cytokines including TNFα and IL-2. Taken together, these results suggest that celastrol treatment inhibited oxidative stress and inflammatory processes in the kidney. These results agree with those of a previous report that concluded celastrol treatment attenuates hypertension-induced inflammation and oxidative stress in fructose-induced hypertensive rats [40].

Another interesting finding of this study is the improvement in renal lipid metabolism by celastrol treatment. In diabetic mice, mRNA expression levels of enzymes involved in cholesterol synthesis, such as HMG-CoA reductase and SREBP1c, were significantly increased in diabetic db/db mice compared with those in control *db/m* mice (data not shown). Celastrol treatment markedly decreased renal accumulation of cholesterol and triglyceride content in renal cortical tissues associated with the suppression of renal LPO content. This finding agrees with previous reports that suggest the role of abnormal renal lipid metabolism in the pathogenesis of diabetic nephropathy [41,42]. These results suggest that NF-κB inhibition in part improves renal function via improvements in renal lipid metabolic abnormalities.

In terms of decreased tissue levels of LPO, it may be possible that decreased tissue accumulation of lipid such as cholesterol and triglyceride may decrease the LPO contents in various organs instead of direct celastrol effects. To elucidate this point, we performed another in vivo experiment using *db/m mice*. As shown in Table S2, 2weeks treatment of celastrol significantly decreased tissue LPO contents in various organs without significant difference in tissue lipid accumulation. These results suggest that decreased tissue LPO contents are due to the direct effects of celastrol instead of lipotoxicity.

In the present study, we performed *in vitro* experiments to further elucidate the role of celastrol on diabetic nephropathy, and found that high glucose alone did not induce significant upregulation of inflammatory cytokines and oxidative stress markers, whereas free fatty acid treatment profoundly upregulated these molecules. We observed that celastrol abolished this free fatty acid-induced inflammatory and oxidative stress molecule synthesis. Considering the important role of free fatty acids on diabetic glomerular injury [43], these results suggest that decreased renal inflammation and oxidative stress by NF-κB inhibition resulted in improvement in renal lipid metabolism, leading to a partial contribution to the renoprotective effects of celastrol.

In conclusion, the NF-κB inhibitor celastrol provided a protective effect against target organ damage in type 2 diabetic mice through improved metabolic alterations as well as inhibition of profibrotic and proinflammatory processes in the target organs. These findings suggest that the NF-κB pathway may be a useful new therapeutic target in the treatment of type 2 diabetes mellitus and diabetic nephropathy.

Supporting Information

Figure S1 Effects of celastrol on histologic changes in adipose and hepatic tissues. (A, B, C) adipose tissue, (D, E, F) hepatic tissue, (A, D, *db/m*; B, E, *db/db*; C, F, *db/db*+celastrol. Original magnification X200.

Table S1 Primer sequences for real-time quantitative PCR.

Table S2 Physical and biochemical parameters of experimental animals.

Table S3   Fatty acid composition in various organs in experimental animals.

Acknowledgments

We thank Dr. Peter Mundel for the generous gift of podocytes [22] and obtaining permission for use of cell line, and Dr. In Ho Kim for design and discussion of this study.

References

1. Reaven GM (1998) Role of insulin resistance in human disease. Diabetes 37: 1495–1507.
2. Eckel RH, Alberti KG, Grundy SM, Zimmet PZ (2010) The metabolic syndrome. Lancet 375: 181–183.
3. Lakka HM, Laaksonen DE, Lakka TA, Niskanen LK, Kumpusalo E, et al. (2001) The metabolic syndrome and total and cardiovascular disease mortality in middle-aged men. JAMA 288: 2709–2716.
4. Galkina E, Ley K (2006) Leukocyte recruitment and vascular injury in diabetic nephropathy. J Am Soc Nephrol 17: 368–377.
5. Mora C, Navarro JF (2006) Inflammation and diabetic nephropathy. Curr Diab Rep 6: 463–468.
6. Furuta T, Saito T, Ootaka T, Soma J, Obara K, et al. (1993) The role of macrophages in diabetic glomerulosclerosis. Am J Kidney Dis 21: 480–485.
7. Sassy-Prigent C, Heudes D, Mandet C, Bélair MF, Michel O, et al. (2000) Early glomerular macrophage recruitment in streptozotocin-induced diabetic rats. Diabetes 49: 466–475.
8. Ruster C, Wolf G (2008) The role of chemokines and chemokine receptors in diabetic nephropathy. Front Biosci 13: 944–955.
9. Baker RG, Hayden MS, Ghosh S (2011) NF-kB, inflammation, and metabolic disease. Cell Metab 13: 11–22.
10. Barnes PJ, Karin M (1997) Nuclear factor-kB: A pivotal transcription factor in chronic inflammatory diseases. N Engl J Med 336: 1066–1071.
11. Chen L, Zhang J, Zhang Y, Wang Y, Wang B (2008) Improvement of inflammatory responses associated with NF-kappa B pathway in kidneys from diabetic rats. Inflamm Res 57: 199–204.
12. Mezzano S, Aros C, Droguett A, Burgos ME, Ardiles L, et al. (2004) NF-kappaB activation and overexpression of regulated genes in human diabetic nephropathy. Nephrol Dial Transplant 19: 2505–2512.
13. Lee FT, Cao Z, Long DM, Panagiotopoulos S, Jerums G, et al. (2004) Interactions between angiotensin II and NF-kappaB-dependent pathways in modulating macrophage infiltration in experimental diabetic nephropathy. J Am Soc Nephrol 15: 2139–2151.
14. Ha H, Yu MR, Choi YJ, Kitamura M, Lee HB (2002) Role of high glucose-induced nuclear factor-kappaB activation in monocyte chemoattractant protein-1 expression by mesangial cells. J Am Soc Nephrol 13: 894–902.
15. Gruden G, Setti G, Hayward A, Sugden D, Duggan S, et al. (2005) Mechanical stretch induces monocyte chemoattractant activity via an NF-kappaB-dependent monocyte chemoattractant protein-1-mediated pathway in human mesangial cells: inhibition by rosiglitazone. J Am Soc Nephrol 16: 688–696.
16. Zamboni M, Di Francesco V, Garbin U, Fratta Pasini A, Mazzali G, et al. (2007) Adiponectin gene expression and adipocyte NF-kappaB transcriptional activity in elderly overweight and obese women: inter-relationships with fat distribution, hs-CRP, leptin and insulin resistance. Int J Obes (Lond) 31: 1104–1109.
17. Ferrante AW Jr (2007) Obesity-induced inflammation: a metabolic dialogue in the language of inflammation. J Intern Med 262: 408–414.
18. Xu H, Barnes GT, Yang Q, Tan G, Yang D, et al (2003) Chronic inflammation in fat plays a crucial role in the development of obesity-related insulin resistance. J Clin Invest 112: 1821–1830.
19. Bligh EG, Dyer WJ (1959) A rapid method of total lipid extraction and purification. Can J Biochem Physiol 37: 911–917.
20. Lee MH, Song HK, Ko GJ, Kang YS, Han SY, et al. (2008) Angiotensin receptor blockers improve insulin resistance in type 2 diabetic rats by modulating adipose tissue. Kidney Int 74: 890–900.
21. Kang YS, Lee MH, Song HK, Ko GJ, Kwon OS, et al. (2010) CCR2 antagonism improves insulin resistance, lipid metabolism, and diabetic nephropathy in type 2 diabetic mice. Kidney Int 78: 883–894.
22. Mundel P, Reiser J, Zuniga Mejia Borja A, Pavenstadt H, Davidson GR, et al. (1997) Rearrangements of the cytoskeleton and cell contacts induce process formation during differentiation of conditionally immortalized mouse podocyte cell lines. Exp Cell Res 236: 248–258.
23. Liu W, Zhang X, Liu P, Shen X, Lan T, et al. (2010) Effects of berberine on matrix accumulation and NF-kappa B signal pathway in alloxan-induced diabetic mice with renal injury. Eur J Pharmacol 638: 150–155.
24. Lee WC, Chen HC, Wang CY, Lin PY, Ou TT, et al. (2010) Cilostazol ameliorates nephropathy in type 1 diabetic rats involving improvement in

oxidative stress and regulation of TGF-Beta and NF-kappaB. Biosci Biotechnol Biochem 74: 1355–1361.
25. Li L, Emmett N, Mann D, Zhao X (2010) Fenofibrate attenuates tubulointerstitial fibrosis and inflammation through suppression of nuclear factor-κB and transforming growth factor-β1/Smad3 in diabetic nephropathy. Exp Biol Med (Maywood) 235: 383–391.
26. Kuhad A, Chopra K (2009) Attenuation of diabetic nephropathy by tocotrienol: involvement of NFkB signaling pathway. Life Sci 84: 296–301.
27. Ohga S, Shikata K, Yozai K, Okada S, Ogawa D, et al. (2007) Thiazolidinedione ameliorates renal injury in experimental diabetic rats through anti-inflammatory effects mediated by inhibition of NF-kappaB activation. Am J Physiol Renal Physiol 292: F1141–F1150.
28. Donath MY, Shoelson SE (2011) Type 2 diabetes as an inflammatory disease. Nat Rev Immunol 11: 98–107.
29. González F, Rote NS, Minium J, Kirwan JP (2006) Increased activation of nuclear factor kappaB triggers inflammation and insulin resistance in polycystic ovary syndrome. J Clin Endocrinol Metab 91: 1508–1512.
30. Yang B, Hodgkinson A, Oates PJ, Millward BA, Demaine AG (2008) High glucose induction of DNA-binding activity of the transcription factor NFkappaB in patients with diabetic nephropathy. Biochim Biophys Acta 1782: 295–302.
31. He L, He M, Lv X, Pu D, Su P, et al. (2010) NF-kappaB binding activity and pro-inflammatory cytokines expression correlate with body mass index but not glycosylated hemoglobin in Chinese population. Diabetes Res Clin Pract 90: 73–80.
32. Miller MR, Zhang W, Sibbel SP, Langefeld CD, Bowden DW, et al. (2010) Variant in the 3' region of the IkappaBalpha gene associated with insulin resistance in Hispanic Americans: The IRAS Family Study. Obesity (Silver Spring) 18: 555–562.
33. Jang PG, Namkoong C, Gil Kang GM, Hur MW, Kim SW, et al. (2010) NF-kB Activation in Hypothalamic Pro-opiomelanocortin Neurons Is Essential in Illness- and Leptin-induced Anorexia. J Biol Chem 285: 9706–9715.
34. Tang T, Zhang J, Yin J, Staszkiewicz J, Gawronska-Kozak B, et al. (2010) Uncoupling of Inflammation and Insulin Resistance by NF-kB in Transgenic Mice through Elevated Energy Expenditure. J Biol Chem 285: 4637–4644.
35. Kalra SP, Sahu A, Kalra PS, Crowley WR (1990) Hypothalamic neuropeptide Y: a circuit in the regulation of gonadotropin and feeding behavior. Ann N Y.Acad Sci 611: 273–283.
36. Musso R, Grill M, Oberto A, Gamalero RS, Eva C (1997) Regulation of Mouse Neuropeptide Y Y1 Receptor Gene Transcription: A Potential Role for Nuclear Factor-kB/Rel Proteins. Mol Pharmacol 51: 327–357.
37. Zhang X, Zhang G, Zhang H, Karin M, Bail H, et al. (2008) Hypothalamic IKKβ/NF-κB and ER Stress Link Overnutrition to Energy Imbalance and Obesity. Cell 135: 61–73.
38. Marin P, Andersson B, Ottosson M, Olbe L, Chowdhury B, et al. (1992) The morphology and metabolism of intraabdominal adipose tissue in men. Metabolism 41: 1242–1248.
39. Melo AM, Bittencourt P, Nakutis FS, Silva AP, Cursino J, et al. (2011) Solidago chilensis Meyen hydroalcoholic extract reduces JNK/IκB pathway activation and ameliorates insulin resistance in diet-induced obesity mice. Exp Biol Med (Maywood) 236: 1147–1155.
40. Yu X, Tao W, Jiang F, Li C, Lin J, et al. (2010) Celastrol attenuates hypertension-induced inflammation and oxidative stress in vascular smooth muscle cells via induction of heme oxygenase-1. Am J Hypertens 23: 895–903.
41. Park CW, Kim HW, Ko SH, Lim JH, Ryu GR, et al. (2007) Long-term treatment of glucagon-like peptide-1 analog exendin-4 ameliorates diabetic nephropathy through improving metabolic anomalies in db/db mice. J Am Soc Nephrol 18: 1227–1238.
42. Proctor G, Jiang T, Iwahashi M, Wang Z, Li J, et al. (2006) Regulation of renal fatty acid and cholesterol metabolism, inflammation, and fibrosis in Akita and OVE26 mice with type 1 diabetes. Diabetes 55: 2502–2509.
43. Nosadini R, Tonolo G (2011) Role of oxidized low density lipoproteins and free fatty acids in the pathogenesis of glomerulopathy and tubulointerstitial lesions in type 2 diabetes. Nutr Metab Cardiovasc Dis 21: 79–85.

Author Contributions

Conceived and designed the experiments: JEK DRC. Performed the experiments: JEK MHL DHN HKS YSK SYH JEL. Analyzed the data: HWK JJC. Contributed reagents/materials/analysis tools: YYH KHH JYH. Wrote the paper: JEK.

Combined Impact of Cardiorespiratory Fitness and Visceral Adiposity on Metabolic Syndrome in Overweight and Obese Adults in Korea

Sue Kim[1], Ji-Young Kim[2], Duk-Chul Lee[1], Hye-Sun Lee[3], Ji-Won Lee[1]*, Justin Y. Jeon[2]*

1 Department of Family Medicine, Severance Hospital, Yonsei University College of Medicine, Seoul, Korea, 2 Department of Sport and Leisure Studies, Yonsei University, Seoul, Korea, 3 Biostatistics Collaboration Units, Department of Research Affairs, Yonsei University College of Medicine, Seoul, Korea

Abstract

Background: Obesity, especially visceral obesity, is known to be an important correlate for cardiovascular disease and increased mortality. On the other hand, high cardiorespiratory fitness is suggested to be an effective contributor for reducing this risk. This study was conducted to determine the combined impact of cardiorespiratory fitness and visceral adiposity, otherwise known as fitness and fatness, on metabolic syndrome in overweight and obese adults.

Methods: A total of 232 overweight and obese individuals were grouped into four subtypes according to their fitness level. This was measured by recovery heart rate from a step test in addition to visceral adiposity defined as the visceral adipose tissue area to subcutaneous adipose tissue area ratio (VAT/SAT ratio). Associations of fitness and visceral fatness were analyzed in comparison with the prevalence of metabolic syndrome.

Results: The high visceral fat and low fitness group had the highest prevalence of metabolic syndrome [Odds Ratio (OR) 5.02; 95% Confidence Interval (CI) 1.85–13.61] compared with the reference group, which was the low visceral adiposity and high fitness group, after adjustments for confounding factors. Viscerally lean but unfit subjects were associated with a higher prevalence of metabolic syndrome than more viscerally obese but fit subjects (OR 3.42; 95% CI 1.27–9.19, and OR 2.70; 95% CI 1.01–7.25, respectively).

Conclusions: Our study shows that visceral obesity and fitness levels are cumulatively associated with a higher prevalence of metabolic syndrome in healthy overweight and obese adults. This suggests that cardiorespiratory fitness is a significant modifier in the relation of visceral adiposity to adverse metabolic outcomes in overweight and obese individuals.

Editor: Reury F. P. Bacurau, University of Sao Paulo, Brazil

Funding: This work was supported by the Biomedical Technology Development Research Program through the National Research Foundation of Korea(NRF) funded by the Ministry of Science, ICT and Future Planning (NRF-2013M3A9B6046413). The funders had no role in study design, data collection and anlalysis, decision to publish, or preparation of the manuscript.

Competing Interests: The authors have declared that no competing interests exist.

* E-mail: indi5645@yuhs.ac (JWL); jjeon@yonsei.ac.kr (JYJ)

Introduction

Obesity is a major cause of metabolic dysregulation and leads to increased morbidity and mortality; therefore, it is a significant health concern worldwide [1,2]. Among obese characteristics, the accumulation of abdominal visceral adiposity has been shown to be strongly associated with a cluster of metabolic abnormalities and contributes to insulin resistance and metabolic syndrome [3,4]. Furthermore, visceral adiposity is an independent risk factor for cardiovascular diseases, such as hypertension and diabetes, irrespective of total body fat [5,6].

On the other hand, increased energy expenditure through physical activity prevents individuals from developing obesity and its related risks of metabolic abnormalities [7,8]. Cardiorespiratory fitness, or aerobic fitness, refers to the ability of circulatory and respiratory function to supply oxygen to muscles and other organs during sustained physical activity without tiring out [9]. Increased cardiorespiratory fitness is known to reduce the risk of cardiome-

tabolic diseases and can be estimated with recovery heart rate after exercise quantified as the indicator for physical fitness level [10,11]. Recent studies demonstrate that a greater level of measured recovery heart rate is associated with an increased risk for metabolic syndrome as well as cardiovascular diseases and all-cause mortality [12–14].

The effects of obesity and fitness as unfavorable and favorable contributors to the risk of developing cardiometabolic diseases have become of clinical interest. Indeed, some studies exploring the combination of fitness and fatness on metabolic disturbance and mortality have shown that fitness was a powerful modifier of this association [15,16]. Moreover, overweight but physically active individuals were shown to have an equivalent or even lower risk of death than lean but inactive individuals [17,18]. However, although central visceral adiposity is a critical determinant of metabolic profiles in obesity, little is known about visceral adiposity, cardiorespiratory fitness, and their combined impact on metabolic profiles in overweight and obese subjects.

We hypothesized that overweight and obese adults with high visceral adiposity and low fitness level would have high prevalence of metabolic syndrome, and furthermore, the combination of the two factors would be related to the magnitude of the association on the prevalence of metabolic syndrome. Therefore, this study was conducted to investigate the combined impact of visceral obesity and cardiorespiratory fitness on metabolic syndrome in overweight and obese adults as determined by abdominal computed tomography (CT) scan measurement and heart rate recovery after exercise.

Materials and Methods

Ethics Statement

All subjects participated in the study voluntarily, and written informed consent was obtained from each participant. The study complied with the Declaration of Helsinki and was approved by the Institutional Review Board of Severance Hospital.

Study participants

A total of 232 men and women participated in this substudy of the Korean Physical Activity and Obesity (K-POP) study, which is an ongoing study designed to examine physical fitness and metabolic markers of overweight and obese adults in Seoul, Korea. The participants were recruited from the visitors to the obesity clinic in the department of family medicine at Severance Hospital from January 2010 to March 2013.

Being overweight was defined as having a body mass index (BMI) $\geq$ 23 kg/m^2, and obesity was defined as having a BMI $\geq$ 25 kg/m^2, following Asian-pacific population specific BMI criteria by World Health Organization expert consultation [19]. Only healthy subjects aged 18 to 70 years without underlying medical conditions were included in this study, such that those with histories of hypertension, diabetes, dyslipidemia, chronic liver disease or other cardiovascular diseases were excluded. Those with medications that can affect cardiometabolic function, including anti-hypertensives, hypoglycemic agents, or anti-obesity drugs, were also excluded from the study. Participants who were not able to fulfill the cardiorespiratory fitness evaluation due to their physical or psychological conditions were likewise excluded.

Clinical and anthropometric evaluation

Data on past and current medical conditions and medications were collected from medical records. BMI was calculated as weight divided by height squared. Body weight was measured to the nearest 0.1 kg with an electronic scale, and height was measured to the nearest 0.1 cm with a stadiometer. Waist circumference was measured midway between the lowest rib and the iliac crest in the standing position. Blood pressure was measured two times by mercury sphygmomanometer after at least 10-min seated rest, and the average of the two measurements was recorded. Mean blood pressure was calculated based on this measurement. Lifestyle factors such as smoking status, alcohol consumption, and physical activity status were provided by participants through questionnaires. Smoking status was considered "yes" if the subjects reported themselves as a current smoker. Alcohol consumption was defined as a positive factor if alcohol consumption was 72 g or more per week. Physical activity status was analyzed from a participant's overall energy expenditure calculated in metabolic equivalents hour (MET-h) per week from information acquired through the Korean version of the International Physical Activity Questionnaire (IPAQ) [20].

Abdominal adipose tissue area was quantified by CT (Tomoscan 350; Philips, Mahwah, NJ, USA). Specifically, a 10-mm CT slice scan was acquired at the L4–L5 level with subjects in the supine position in order to measure the total abdominal tissue (TAT) and visceral adipose tissue (VAT) area. VAT was quantified by delineating the intra-abdominal cavity at the internal aspect of the abdominal and oblique muscle walls surrounding the cavity and the posterior aspect of the vertebral body. The subcutaneous adipose tissue (SAT) area was calculated by subtracting the VAT area from the TAT area. The coefficients of variation for inter- and intra-observer reproducibility for VAT were 1.4% and 0.5%, respectively.

Biochemical analyses

Biochemical analyses were performed on blood samples collected after overnight fasting (>12 hrs). Serum levels of fasting glucose, total cholesterol, triglycerides, high-density lipoprotein cholesterol, low-density lipoprotein cholesterol, and high-sensitivity C-reactive protein were measured with the Hitachi 7600 Automatic analyzer (High-Technologies Corporation, Hitachi, Tokyo, Japan). Fasting insulin was measured by electrochemiluminescence immunoassay using an Elecsys 2010 (Roche, Indianapolis, IN, USA), and insulin resistance was estimated using the homeostasis model assessment of insulin resistance (HOMA-IR) index [Insulin (mUl/L) $\times$ fasting glucose (mg/dl)/405] [21].

Metabolic syndrome was defined using the criteria proposed by the American Heart Association and the National Heart, Lung, and Blood Institute, with waist circumference criteria modification based on the following World Health Organization-Asian Pacific region criteria for abdominal obesity [19,22]: (1) a waist circumference $\geq$90 cm for men and $\geq$85 cm for women; (2) triglycerides $\geq$150 mg/dl; (3) serum HDL cholesterol <40 mg/dl for men and <50 mg/dl for women; (4) systolic blood pressure $\geq$130 mmHg, diastolic blood pressure $\geq$85 mmHg, or use of anti-hypertensive medication); and (5) fasting glucose $\geq$100 mg/dl, or insulin or hypoglycemic medication use.

Cardiorespiratory fitness

Cardiorespiratory fitness was evaluated using Tecumseh, a standardized 3-minute step test. Participants performed 24 steps per minute based on the protocol for the Tecumseh step test, maintaining a constant stepping rate on a 20.3 cm-high step for 3 minutes [10,23]. The participants were aided by an assistant's demonstration and a metronome cadence for proper stepping technique and constant step maintenance. Heart rates were measured and recorded by a heart rate monitor (Polar-FS3C, USA) attached on the anterior chest wall of the participant. Heart rates were recorded in a seating position 1 minute prior to exercise after at least 5 minutes of resting and 1 minute after the completion of the 3-minute step exercise (1 minute recovery heart rate). The expectation was that participants with greater cardiorespiratory fitness would have lower heart rates at 1 minute post-exercise than those with worse cardiorespiratory fitness [11].

Statistical analyses

To examine the joint impact of visceral fat and fitness level on the prevalence of metabolic syndrome, participants were divided into the following four groups according to the combination of their visceral obesity and fitness level: (1) low visceral fat and high level of fitness, (2) low visceral fat and low level of fitness, (3) high visceral adiposity and high level of fitness, and (4) high visceral adiposity and low level of fitness. Low visceral obesity was defined as having a VAT/SAT ratio measured by CT scan of less than 0.4, and high visceral obesity was defined as having a VAT/SAT ratio $\geq$ 0.4 [24]. Fitness level was divided into high or low according to the median value (50th percentile) of the distribution.

Data are expressed as means ± standard deviation (SD) or numbers (percentages). Normality of the variables was tested using the Kolmogorov-Smirnov test. The data between the groups were compared with analysis of variance for continuous data or chi-square test for categorical data. Bonferroni's post hoc tests were performed when significant differences were found to assess the magnitude of the differences.

To test the combined effect of visceral adiposity and fitness level, we tested their interactions with the interaction term for visceral adiposity*fitness level by logistic regression models for metabolic syndrome after adjusting for age and sex.

Multiple logistic regression analyses were performed to estimate the magnitude of the association of the four groups divided according to the combination of visceral adiposity and fitness level combined on the development of metabolic syndrome, after adjusting for age, sex, lifestyle factors (smoking, alcohol, and physical activity status), and BMI. The interaction between visceral adiposity and fitness level was tested at a significance level of 0.15 [25,26]. Hypothesis testing was two-sided at a significance level of 0.05. Statistical analyses were performed with SPSS (version 20.0; SPSS Inc., Chicago, IL, USA).

Results

Characteristics of the participants divided into the four groups according to visceral adiposity and fitness level are shown in Table 1. The VAT/SAT ratio was approximately 0.28 in the low adiposity groups and 0.65 in the high visceral adiposity groups, and was highest in the high visceral adiposity and low fitness level group. Recovery heart rate after exercise was approximately 81.1 beats per min (bpm) in the high fitness level groups and 105.8 bpm in the low fitness level groups, and was highest in the low visceral adiposity and low fitness level group. In comparison between the groups, the high visceral adiposity groups had a tendency to be older and the low visceral adiposity groups had more males in each of their groups. Notwithstanding having greater visceral adiposity, the high visceral adiposity and high fitness level group had lower parameters of insulin resistance, insulin, and HOMA-IR than did the low visceral adiposity and low fitness level group. There were no differences in lifestyle factors (smoking, alcohol, and physical activity status) between the groups.

Visceral adiposity and fitness level were seen to have a significant interaction for the prevalence of metabolic syndrome via the interaction term between the two factors, after adjusting for age and sex (p = 0.138).

Across the four groups in regards to the association with the prevalence of metabolic syndrome, and with the most favorable group defined by low visceral adiposity and high fitness as the reference, subjects with a high visceral fat and low fitness level were associated with the highest prevalence of metabolic syndrome among all other groups (OR: 5.02, 95% CI: 1.85–13.61), after adjustment for age, sex, smoking, alcohol, physical activity status, and BMI. Furthermore, low visceral adiposity but low fitness level had a significantly higher OR for the development of metabolic syndrome than did high visceral adiposity but high fitness level, after adjustment for the covariates (OR 3.42, 95% CI: 1.27–9.19 and OR 2.70, 95% CI: 1.01–7.25, respectively) (Figure 1).

Discussion

The objective of this study was to evaluate the joint impact of cardiorespiratory fitness and visceral adiposity on metabolic syndrome in overweight and obese adults. Our results showed that high visceral adiposity and low fitness level were cumulatively associated with metabolic syndrome. Furthermore, viscerally lean

but unfit subjects were found to have a greater odds for developing metabolic syndrome than visceral obese but highly fit individuals. These results indicate that the cardiorespiratory fitness level can alter the associations between visceral obesity and metabolic syndrome and is an important factor for reducing metabolic risk factors in overweight and obese adults.

Excessive visceral adipose tissue accumulation is one of the most important contributors to the clustering of adverse cardiometabolic profiles and metabolic syndrome that are associated with being overweight and obese [27]. Recent studies reveal that the characteristic of high visceral fat storage is a part of dysfunctional SAT expansion that leads to the functional loss of SAT as an energy deposit, resulting in ectopic fat deposition predominantly in abdominal visceral adipose tissue, liver, and skeletal muscle, and thus promoting insulin resistance [28,29]. The concept of the VAT/SAT ratio measurement has therefore been suggested to better represent visceral fat with metabolic abnormalities, reflecting relative distribution of abdominal adipose tissue [24,30,31]. Indeed, the VAT/SAT ratio has been reported to have associations with metabolic syndrome, hypertension, and diabetes independent of total visceral fat volume, and with glucose intolerance, insulin resistance, and dyslipidemia [31,32].

Cardiorespiratory fitness and metabolic syndrome may be related to the fact that unfit subjects are likely to have a high VAT [33]. Moreover, cardiorespiratory fitness is known to counteract the deleterious action of visceral adiposity [34]. In several studies, fitness level was shown to have an impact on modulating cardiovascular diseases such as diabetes as well as on mortality among overweight and obese individuals [35,36]. While visceral fat leads to greater release of deleterious cytokines and adipokines, improving fitness leads to a greater responsiveness to advantageous adipokines and cytokines, such as leptin, adiponectin, and interleukin (IL)-10 [37,38]. This adaptive change in sensitivity and metabolism concurrently decreases the release of unfavorable pro-inflammatory adipokines and cytokines, such as resistin, tumor necrosis factor-α, IL-6, retinol binding protein-4, etc [39]. Additionally, the increase in fat-free lean mass and decrease in resting cortisol levels through physical exercise are demonstrated to be associated with metabolic improvements [27,38]. As a result, fitness and fatness combine to define one's overall health status through fitness regulating metabolic adaptations and metabolic flexibility of the viscerally obese condition. In this study, fitness was demonstrated to be a modifier of the association between visceral obesity and the prevalence of metabolic syndrome.

Reduction in insulin resistance is known to be one of the primary metabolic adaptations of fitness, which leads to improvement in insulin sensitivity and glucose tolerance for skeletal muscle and throughout the body [34,40]. Increased expression of glucose transporter-4 protein and upregulation of glucose from enhanced skeletal muscle mitochondria enzyme activity may explain the link between cardiorespiratory fitness and improved insulin resistance [41,42]. Our results also demonstrate that fasting serum insulin levels and the insulin resistance marker HOMA-IR were lower in the high fitness group than the low fitness group despite the high fitness group having a higher visceral adiposity.

Only a few studies have explored the combined effect of visceral adiposity and cardiorespiratory fitness on metabolic outcomes or mortality. For instance, hypertensive patients with abdominal obesity (higher waist circumference) but a high degree of fitness were shown to have lower cardiovascular disease and all-cause death than were those with normal abdominal obesity but a low level of fitness [43]. In patients with cardiovascular disease, subjects with a high waist-to-hip ratio (WHR) and a high fitness level had a lower hazards ratio for mortality than those with a low

Table 1. Clinical characteristics according to visceral adiposity (VAT/SAT ratio) and fitness level (recovery heart rate).

	Low visceral adiposity High fitness level (n = 67)	Low visceral adiposity Low fitness level (n = 58)	High visceral adiposity High fitness level (n = 54)	High visceral adiposity Low fitness level (n = 53)	p-value[a]
Age (years)	31.63±8.90[‡§]	28.03±5.83[‡§]	38.06±9.52[*†]	37.70±9.78[*†]	<0.001
Male, n (%)	46 (68.7)[‡]	41 (70.7)[‡§]	21 (38.9)[*†]	25 (45.3)[†]	<0.001
BMI (kg/m²)	28.23±3.73[†]	30.80±5.03[*‡]	29.19±4.16[†]	29.38±4.22	0.002
Waist (cm)	94.11±9.37[†]	100.09±13.30[*]	98.92±11.43	98.58±11.58	0.008
Mean BP (mmHg)	89.68±10.58[†‡§]	97.09±15.10[*]	99.19±9.42[*]	99.00±9.44[*]	<0.001
Visceral fat (cm²)	80.00±27.44[‡§]	100.05±42.81[‡§]	148.92±71.91[*†§]	192.85±102.12[*†‡]	<0.001
Subcutaneous fat (cm²)	306.42±104.94[‡]	353.94±114.96[‡§]	238.72±77.28[*†]	286.08±108.91[†]	<0.001
VAT/SAT ratio	0.27±0.69[‡§]	0.29±0.68[‡§]	0.62±0.18[*†]	0.67±0.21[*†]	<0.001
Heart rate recovery	81.81±6.57[†§]	106.93±11.37[*‡]	80.35±8.06[†§]	104.62±12.30[‡]	<0.001
Alcohol, n (%)	20 (29.9)	16 (27.6)	15 (27.8)	18 (34.0)	0.878
Smoking, n (%)	9 (13.4)	10 (17.2)	13 (24.1)	16 (30.2)	0.227
Physical activity (MET-h/wk)	30.64±20.04	29.24±22.07	28.26±26.36	30.48±27.34	0.953
Cholesterol (mg/dl)	194.25±34.47	196.19±38.62	197.26±36.42	202.19±37.37	0.692
Triglyceride (mg/dl)	87.91±44.68[§]	122.74±67.81	127.81±49.54	165.15±183.78[*]	0.001
LDL (mg/dl)	121.01±32.86	123.16±36.33	123.13±35.74	121.92±34.00	0.983
HDL (mg/dl)	54.16±11.32[‡§]	50.72±11.82	48.20±10.06[*]	48.43±10.83[*]	0.010
Glucose (mg/dl)	88.76±8.11	108.43±119.52	88.76±11.23	93.36±15.36	0.247
Insulin (µU/ml)	10.02±9.27[†]	16.95±22.74[*‡]	9.50±4.54[†]	14.35±13.23	0.012
HOMA-IR	2.24±2.15[†]	4.19±5.98[*‡]	2.13±1.15[†]	3.03±2.61	0.005
hsCRP (mg/dL)	2.12±7.02	2.68±2.90	1.26±1.28	1.58±1.68	0.292

Abbreviations: VAT/SAT ratio, visceral adipose tissue area to subcutaneous adipose tissue area ratio; BMI, Body Mass Index; BP, Blood pressure; MET-h/wk, metabolic equivalents hour per week; LDL, low-density lipoprotein; HDL, high-density lipoprotein; HOMA-IR, Homeostasis model assessment of insulin resistance; hsCRP, high sensitive C-reactive protein.
[a]p-values are calculated by ANOVA with Bonferroni method.
*$p<0.05$ vs. Low visceral adiposity high fitness level; †$p<0.05$ vs. Low visceral adiposity low fitness level; ‡$p<0.05$ vs. High visceral adiposity high fitness level; §$p<0.05$ vs. High visceral adiposity low fitness level Variables are expressed as mean±SD for continuous variables or number (%) for categorical variables.

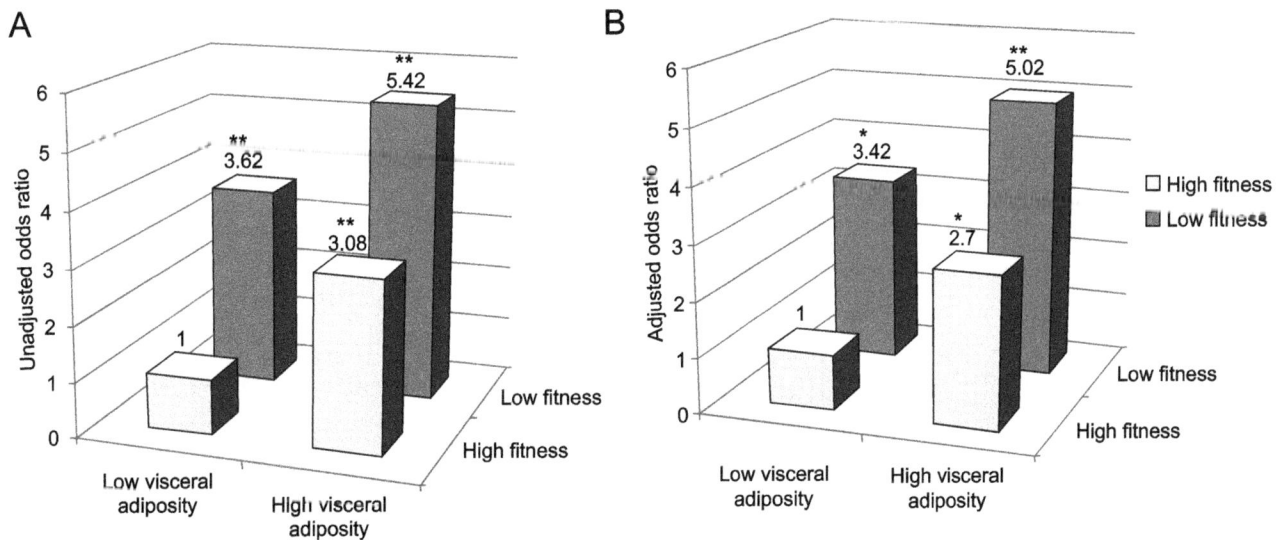

Figure 1. Odds ratio for metabolic syndrome according to visceral adiposity(VAT/SAT ratio) and fitness level(recovery heart rate).
Adjusted odds ratio: adjusted for age, sex, smoking, alcohol, physical activity status, and body mass index. *$p< 0.05$, **$p<0.01$, calculated by multiple logistic regression analyses.

WHR and a low fitness level [44]. Our study had results in accordance with these prior studies, but was strengthened by an accurate CT measurement of visceral adiposity and by using the criteria of VAT/SAT ratio. Additionally, Rheaume et al. suggested that changes in both visceral fat accumulation and cardiorespiratory fitness were associated with changes in metabolic syndrome components and that the two factors are both important for the maintenance of healthy cardiometabolic risk profiles, which is consistent with the results from our study [45]. Here, we compared these associations for individuals by stratifying their central adiposity by fitness level, permitting more rigorous analyses of combined subgroups than adjustment for either variable alone [43].

There were some limitations to our study. The directionality and causality of the results of cross-sectional analyses could not be determined with certainty. The 3-minute step test was used to measure fitness level instead of a direct measure of maximal oxygen uptake (VO_2 max). However, the correlation between the 3-minute step test results and VO_2 max has been validated in many studies so far, and the 3 minute step test is known to be a relatively quick and easy method used in clinical settings and in epidemiologic studies since the early 20th century [46,47]. Also, the HOMA-IR index was used instead of direct measurement for the representation of insulin resistance. Nonetheless, HOMA-IR has been validated as a reliable and clinically useful marker for assessing beta-cell function and insulin resistance [48]. Finally, as the sample was composed of more young to middle-aged adults, it may be difficult to generalize the data and results to older populations with a greater tendency toward higher visceral adiposity accumulation. Further studies are warranted to clearly identify the combined effect of fitness and visceral fatness to metabolic characteristics in an older and larger population.

Conclusions

In conclusion, visceral obesity and fitness level are cumulatively associated with the prevalence of metabolic syndrome in healthy overweight and obese adults. This suggests that cardiorespiratory fitness is a significant modifier of the relation between visceral adiposity and adverse metabolic outcomes, and the effects of improvement in fitness can be an important target for maintenance of the overall healthy metabolic characteristics in overweight and obese individuals.

Author Contributions

Conceived and designed the experiments: SK JYK JWL JYJ. Performed the experiments: SK JYK JWL JYJ. Analyzed the data: SK DCL HSL. Contributed reagents/materials/analysis tools: DCL JWL JYJ. Wrote the paper: SK JYK.

References

1. Pischon T, Boeing H, Hoffmann K, Bergmann M, Schulze MB, et al. (2008) General and abdominal adiposity and risk of death in Europe. N Engl J Med 359: 2105–2120.
2. Mokdad AH, Ford ES, Bowman BA, Dietz WH, Vinicor F, et al. (2003) Prevalence of obesity, diabetes, and obesity-related health risk factors, 2001. JAMA 289: 76–79.
3. Bjorntorp P (1997) Body fat distribution, insulin resistance, and metabolic diseases. Nutrition 13: 795–803.
4. Despres JP (2006) Is visceral obesity the cause of the metabolic syndrome? Ann Med 38: 52–63.
5. Mathieu P, Poirier P, Pibarot P, Lemieux I, Despres JP (2009) Visceral obesity: the link among inflammation, hypertension, and cardiovascular disease. Hypertension 53: 577–584.
6. Liu J, Fox CS, Hickson DA, May WD, Hairston KG, et al. (2010) Impact of abdominal visceral and subcutaneous adipose tissue on cardiometabolic risk factors: the Jackson Heart Study. J Clin Endocrinol Metab 95: 5419–5426.
7. Katzmarzyk PT, Church TS, Blair SN (2004) Cardiorespiratory fitness attenuates the effects of the metabolic syndrome on all-cause and cardiovascular disease mortality in men. Arch Intern Med 164: 1092–1097.
8. LaMonte MJ, Barlow CE, Jurca R, Kampert JB, Church TS, et al. (2005) Cardiorespiratory fitness is inversely associated with the incidence of metabolic syndrome: a prospective study of men and women. Circulation 112: 505–512.
9. Steele RM, Brage S, Corder K, Wareham NJ, Ekelund U (2008) Physical activity, cardiorespiratory fitness, and the metabolic syndrome in youth. J Appl Physiol 105: 342–351.
10. McArdle WD (2000) Essentials of Exercise Physiology. USA: Lipincott Williams and Wilkins.
11. Siconolfi SF, Garber CE, Lasater TM, Carleton RA (1985) A simple, valid step test for estimating maximal oxygen uptake in epidemiologic studies. Am J Epidemiol 121: 382–390.
12. Nilsson G, Hedberg P, Jonason T, Lonnberg I, Ohrvik J (2007) Heart rate recovery is more strongly associated with the metabolic syndrome, waist circumference, and insulin sensitivity in women than in men among the elderly in the general population. Am Heart J 154: 460 e461–467.
13. Morshedi-Meibodi A, Larson MG, Levy D, O'Donnell CJ, Vasan RS (2002) Heart rate recovery after treadmill exercise testing and risk of cardiovascular disease events (The Framingham Heart Study). Am J Cardiol 90: 848–852.
14. Shishehbor MH, Litaker D, Pothier CE, Lauer MS (2006) Association of socioeconomic status with functional capacity, heart rate recovery, and all-cause mortality. JAMA 295: 784–792.
15. Sui X, LaMonte MJ, Laditka JN, Hardin JW, Chase N, et al. (2007) Cardiorespiratory fitness and adiposity as mortality predictors in older adults. JAMA 298: 2507–2516.
16. Stevens J, Evenson KR, Thomas O, Cai J, Thomas R (2004) Associations of fitness and fatness with mortality in Russian and American men in the lipids research clinics study. Int J Obes Relat Metab Disord 28: 1463–1470.
17. Lee CD, Blair SN, Jackson AS (1999) Cardiorespiratory fitness, body composition, and all-cause and cardiovascular disease mortality in men. Am J Clin Nutr 69: 373–380.
18. Lee DC, Sui X, Artero EG, Lee IM, Church TS, et al. (2011) Long-term effects of changes in cardiorespiratory fitness and body mass index on all-cause and cardiovascular disease mortality in men: the Aerobics Center Longitudinal Study. Circulation 124: 2483–2490.
19. Consultation WHOE (2004) Appropriate body-mass index for Asian populations and its implications for policy and intervention strategies. Lancet 363: 157–163.
20. Hagstromer M, Oja P, Sjostrom M (2006) The International Physical Activity Questionnaire (IPAQ): a study of concurrent and construct validity. Public Health Nutr 9: 755–762.
21. Matthews DR, Hosker JP, Rudenski AS, Naylor BA, Treacher DF, et al. (1985) Homeostasis model assessment: insulin resistance and beta-cell function from fasting plasma glucose and insulin concentrations in man. Diabetologia 28: 412–419.
22. Grundy SM, Cleeman JI, Daniels SR, Donato KA, Eckel RH, et al. (2005) Diagnosis and management of the metabolic syndrome: an American Heart Association/National Heart, Lung, and Blood Institute Scientific Statement. Circulation 112: 2735–2752.
23. Jekal Y, Lee MK, Park S, Lee SH, Kim JY, et al. (2010) Association between Obesity and Physical Fitness, and Hemoglobin A1c Level and Metabolic Syndrome in Korean Adults. Korean Diabetes J 34: 182–190.
24. Fujioka S, Matsuzawa Y, Tokunaga K, Tarui S (1987) Contribution of intra-abdominal fat accumulation to the impairment of glucose and lipid metabolism in human obesity. Metabolism 36: 54–59.
25. Lentner C (ed) (1982) Geigy Scientific Tables. Basel: Ciba-Geigy Limited.
26. Lai CL, Gane E, Liaw YF, Hsu CW, Thongsawat S, et al. (2007) Telbivudine versus Lamivudine in Patients with Chronic Hepatitis B. N Engl J Med 357:2576–88.
27. Tchernof A, Despres JP (2013) Pathophysiology of human visceral obesity: an update. Physiol Rev 93: 359–404.
28. Heilbronn L, Smith SR, Ravussin E (2004) Failure of fat cell proliferation, mitochondrial function and fat oxidation results in ectopic fat storage, insulin resistance and type II diabetes mellitus. Int J Obes Relat Metab Disord 28 Suppl 4: S12–21.
29. Despres JP, Lemieux I (2006) Abdominal obesity and metabolic syndrome. Nature 444: 881–887.
30. Lee JW, Lee HR, Shim JY, Im JA, Kim SH, et al. (2007) Viscerally obese women with normal body weight have greater brachial-ankle pulse wave velocity than nonviscerally obese women with excessive body weight. Clin Endocrinol (Oxf) 66: 572–578.
31. Kaess BM, Pedley A, Massaro JM, Murabito J, Hoffmann U, et al. (2012) The ratio of visceral to subcutaneous fat, a metric of body fat distribution, is a unique correlate of cardiometabolic risk. Diabetologia 55: 2622–2630.
32. Miyazaki Y, DeFronzo RA (2009) Visceral fat dominant distribution in male type 2 diabetic patients is closely related to hepatic insulin resistance, irrespective of body type. Cardiovasc Diabetol 8: 44.

33. Arsenault BJ, Lachance D, Lemieux I, Almeras N, Tremblay A, et al. (2007) Visceral adipose tissue accumulation, cardiorespiratory fitness, and features of the metabolic syndrome. Arch Intern Med 167: 1518–1525.

34. Clark JE (2012) An overview of the contribution of fatness and fitness factors, and the role of exercise, in the formation of health status for individuals who are overweight. J Diabetes Metab Disord 11: 19.

35. McAuley PA, Smith NS, Emerson BT, Myers JN (2012) The obesity paradox and cardiorespiratory fitness. J Obes 2012: 951582.

36. Kelley DE, Goodpaster BH (1999) Effects of physical activity on insulin action and glucose tolerance in obesity. Med Sci Sports Exerc 31: S619–623.

37. Nannipieri M, Bonotti A, Anselmino M, Cecchetti F, Madec S, et al. (2007) Pattern of expression of adiponectin receptors in human adipose tissue depots and its relation to the metabolic state. Int J Obes (Lond) 31: 1843–1848.

38. Izquierdo M, Ibanez J, Calbet JA, Navarro-Amezqueta I, Gonzalez-Izal M, et al. (2009) Cytokine and hormone responses to resistance training. Eur J Appl Physiol 107: 397–409.

39. Jones TE, Basilio JL, Brophy PM, McCammon MR, Hickner RC (2009) Long-term exercise training in overweight adolescents improves plasma peptide YY and resistin. Obesity (Silver Spring) 17: 1189–1195.

40. Sieverdes JC, Sui X, Lee DC, Church TS, McClain A, et al. (2010) Physical activity, cardiorespiratory fitness and the incidence of type 2 diabetes in a prospective study of men. Br J Sports Med 44: 238–244.

41. Houmard JA, Shinebarger MH, Dolan PL, Leggett-Frazier N, Bruner RK, et al. (1993) Exercise training increases GLUT-4 protein concentration in previously sedentary middle-aged men. Am J Physiol 264: E896–901.

42. Horowitz JF, Klein S (2000) Lipid metabolism during endurance exercise. Am J Clin Nutr 72: 558S–563S.

43. McAuley PA, Sui X, Church TS, Hardin JW, Myers JN, et al. (2009) The joint effects of cardiorespiratory fitness and adiposity on mortality risk in men with hypertension. Am J Hypertens 22: 1062–1069.

44. Goel K, Thomas RJ, Squires RW, Coutinho T, Trejo-Gutierrez JF, et al. (2011) Combined effect of cardiorespiratory fitness and adiposity on mortality in patients with coronary artery disease. Am Heart J 161: 590–597.

45. Rheaume C, Arsenault BJ, Dumas MP, Perusse L, Tremblay A, et al. (2011) Contributions of cardiorespiratory fitness and visceral adiposity to six-year changes in cardiometabolic risk markers in apparently healthy men and women. J Clin Endocrinol Metab 96: 1462–1468.

46. Wener J, Sandberg AA, Scherlis L, Dvordin J, Master AM (1953) The electrocardiographic response to the standard 2-step exercise test. Can Med Assoc J 68: 368–374.

47. Santo AS, Golding LA (2003) Predicting maximum oxygen uptake from a modified 3-minute step test. Res Q Exerc Sport 74: 110–115.

48. Yokoyama H, Emoto M, Fujiwara S, Motoyama K, Morioka T, et al. (2004) Quantitative insulin sensitivity check index and the reciprocal index of homeostasis model assessment are useful indexes of insulin resistance in type 2 diabetic patients with wide range of fasting plasma glucose. J Clin Endocrinol Metab 89: 1481–1484.

An Extract of *Artemisia dracunculus* L. Inhibits Ubiquitin-Proteasome Activity and Preserves Skeletal Muscle Mass in a Murine Model of Diabetes

Heather Kirk-Ballard[1], Zhong Q. Wang[2], Priyanka Acharya[1,2], Xian H. Zhang[2], Yongmei Yu[2], Gail Kilroy[1], David Ribnicky[3], William T. Cefalu[2], Z. Elizabeth Floyd[1]*

1 Ubiquitin Biology Laboratory, Pennington Biomedical Research Center, Baton Rouge, Louisiana, United States of America, 2 Diabetes and Nutrition Laboratory, Pennington Biomedical Research Center, Baton Rouge, Louisiana, United States of America, 3 Department of Plant Biology and Pathology, Rutgers University, New Brunswick, New Jersey, United States of America

Abstract

Impaired insulin signaling is a key feature of type 2 diabetes and is associated with increased ubiquitin-proteasome-dependent protein degradation in skeletal muscle. An extract of *Artemisia dracunculus* L. (termed PMI5011) improves insulin action by increasing insulin signaling in skeletal muscle. We sought to determine if the effect of PMI5011 on insulin signaling extends to regulation of the ubiquitin-proteasome system. C2C12 myotubes and the KK-A^y murine model of type 2 diabetes were used to evaluate the effect of PMI5011 on steady-state levels of ubiquitylation, proteasome activity and expression of Atrogin-1 and MuRF-1, muscle-specific ubiquitin ligases that are upregulated with impaired insulin signaling. Our results show that PMI5011 inhibits proteasome activity and steady-state ubiquitylation levels *in vitro* and *in vivo*. The effect of PMI5011 is mediated by PI3K/Akt signaling and correlates with decreased expression of Atrogin-1 and MuRF-1. Under *in vitro* conditions of hormonal or fatty acid-induced insulin resistance, PMI5011 improves insulin signaling and reduces Atrogin-1 and MuRF-1 protein levels. In the KK-A^y murine model of type 2 diabetes, skeletal muscle ubiquitylation and proteasome activity is inhibited and Atrogin-1 and MuRF-1 expression is decreased by PMI5011. PMI5011-mediated changes in the ubiquitin-proteasome system *in vivo* correlate with increased phosphorylation of Akt and FoxO3a and increased myofiber size. The changes in Atrogin-1 and MuRF-1 expression, ubiquitin-proteasome activity and myofiber size modulated by PMI5011 in the presence of insulin resistance indicate the botanical extract PMI5011 may have therapeutic potential in the preservation of muscle mass in type 2 diabetes.

Editor: Cedric Moro, INSERM/UMR 1048, France

Funding: This study was supported by pilot funding (ZEF and ZQW) from the Botanical Research Center of Pennington Biomedical Research Center and The Biotech Center of Rutgers University, which is funded by the National Center for Complementary and Alternative Medicine and the Office of Dietary Supplements P50AT002776-01, and the American Diabetes Association (grant 1-10-BS-55, awarded to ZEF). This project used Genomics Core and Cell Biology and Imaging Core facilities that are supported in part by Centers of Biomedical Research Excellence (NIH P20-RR021945) and Nutrition Obesity Research Centers (NIH P30-DK072476) center grants from the National Institutes of Health. The funders had no role in study design, data collection and analysis, decision to publish, or preparation of the manuscript.

Competing Interests: The authors have declared that no competing interests exist.

* E-mail: elizabeth.floyd@pbrc.edu

Introduction

Insulin resistance in clinical states of metabolic syndrome and type 2 diabetes involves multiple tissues, including liver, adipose tissue and skeletal muscle. Specifically, skeletal muscle is the largest contributor to whole-body glucose disposal, making defective insulin signaling in skeletal muscle a primary feature of type 2 diabetes. Along with its role as the primary site of glucose uptake, skeletal muscle is also the main protein reservoir in the body. Protein levels in skeletal muscle are determined by insulin-mediated dual regulation of protein synthesis and protein degradation [1]. Impairment of insulin-stimulated phosphoinositol 3-kinase/Akt signaling is suggested to tilt the balance between protein synthesis and degradation toward protein degradation in skeletal muscle [2], generating amino acids that are released from skeletal muscle to meet whole body energy needs under catabolic conditions. If prolonged, the accelerated protein degradation associated with insulin resistance can lead to loss of skeletal muscle mass and function [3]. A relationship between type 2 diabetes and loss of skeletal muscle mass has been clearly demonstrated in older adults, particularly in women with type 2 diabetes [4] and in sarcopenic muscle loss [5]. Preservation of skeletal muscle mass and strength in this high risk population may depend on strategies designed to diminish the skeletal muscle protein degradation associated with type 2 diabetes.

Protein degradation in skeletal muscle is carried out primarily by the ubiquitin-proteasome system, a complex network of enzymes through which multiple ubiquitin molecules are covalently attached to a protein substrate, leading to degradation of the substrate by the 26S proteasome [6]. Various models of skeletal muscle atrophy show striking increases in components of the ubiquitin proteasome system, particularly the muscle-specific ubiquitin ligases Muscle Atrophy F-box protein (MAFBx, also called Atrogin-1) and Muscle Ring Finger-1 (MuRF-1) [7].

Expression of Atrogin-1 and MuRF-1 [8,9] as well as proteasome activity [10] is regulated by insulin in skeletal muscle via the PI3Kinase/Akt signaling pathway. The essential role of Atrogin-1 and MuRF-1 in maintaining skeletal muscle mass [11,12,13] makes these two muscle-specific ubiquitin ligases attractive targets for pharmacological intervention in insulin resistance and type 2 diabetes.

Botanical extracts have historically been an important source of medically beneficial compounds [14]. Metformin, one of the most commonly used agents in the treatment of type 2 diabetes, was synthesized based on the antihyperglycemic properties of the French Lilac [15].

In this regard, recent studies show that an ethanolic extract of *Artemisia dracunculus* L. (Russian tarragon), termed PMI5011, improves carbohydrate metabolism in animal models of type 2 diabetes [16]. The changes in whole body glucose levels mediated by PMI5011 correlate with increased insulin sensitivity in primary human skeletal muscle cells [17] and in rodent models of type 2 diabetes [18]. PMI5011 enhanced insulin signaling in skeletal muscle is associated with increased phosphatidylinositol 3-kinase activity and Akt phosphorylation along with increased protein content [18]. These results suggest that the effect of PMI5011 in skeletal muscle extends to regulation of ubiquitin-proteasome activity. If so, PMI5011 may be therapeutically useful in the preservation of skeletal muscle mass in insulin resistance and type 2 diabetes.

The aim of this study was to further evaluate the mechanism of action of PMI5011 by determining the effect of PMI5011 on the ubiquitin-proteasome system in skeletal muscle. In particular, we focused on the effect of PMI5011 on ubiquitin-proteasome activity and the expression of Atrogin-1 and MuRF-1 *in vitro* and *in vivo*.

Materials and Methods

Ethics statement

This study was carried out in strict adherence to the recommendations in the Guide for the Care and Use of Laboratory Animals of the National Institutes of Health. The animal studies were approved by the Institutional Animal Care and Use Committee of Pennington Biomedical Research Center (protocol number 695).

Materials

Dulbecco's Modified Eagle's Media (DMEM) was purchased from MediaTech (Manassas, Va). Fetal bovine (FBS) and horse serums were from Hyclone (Logan, UT). The AKT and phospho-AKT (Ser473) antibodies were purchased from Cell Signaling (Danvers, MA), FoxO3a antibody from Millipore (Billerica, MA) and the Atrogin-1 antibody was obtained from ECM Biosciences (Versailles, KY). The MuRF-1 and phospho-FoxO3a antibodies were obtained from Abcam (Cambridge, MA). The IRS-1, PI3K, and 19SRPN2 antibodies were purchased from Upstate (Lake Placid, NY); the ubiquitin antibody from BD Pharmingen (San Diego, CA). All TaqMan primer/probes pairs were obtained from Applied Biosystems (Carlsbad, CA). The 20S Proteasome Activity Assay kit was purchased from Millipore (Billerica, MA) and proteasome substrates were purchased from Boston Biochem (Cambridge, MA) and Bachem (Torrance, CA). Wortmannin, dexamethasone and palmitic acid were obtained from Sigma Aldrich (St. Louis, MO). The Ultra-Sensitive Mouse Insulin ELISA kit was obtained from Crystal Chem (Downers Grove, IL) and the glucose assay kit was from Cayman Chemical (Ann Arbor, MI)

Sourcing and characterization of PMI5011 extract

The PMI5011 botanical extract from *Artemisia dracunculus* L. was provided by the Botanical Research Center at Pennington Biomedical Research Center. Detailed information about quality control, preparation and biochemical characterization of PMI5011 has been previously reported [14,16,17,18,19,20,21]. PMI5011 was obtained from plants grown hydroponically in greenhouses under uniform and strictly controlled conditions, thereby standardizing the plants for their phytochemical content. The PMI5011 extract was dissolved in DMSO for the *in vitro* experiments.

Cell culture

Murine C2C12 myoblasts (American Type Culture Collection; Manassas, VA) were cultured in DMEM, high glucose (25 mM) with 10% fetal bovine serum (FBS), 2 mM glutamine, and antibiotics (100 units/ml penicillin G and 100 μg/ml streptomycin). While the myoblasts grew optimally in 25 mM glucose, the glucose concentration was lowered to 5 mM prior to differentiation to minimize any effect of the hyperglycemic conditions on insulin sensitivity of the myotubes. To obtain fully differentiated myotubes, the media was exchanged for DMEM, low glucose (5 mM) with 2% horse serum, glutamine, and penicillin G/streptomycin when the myoblasts reached confluence. The media was replaced every 48 hours and the cells were maintained in this medium. The myotubes were fully formed by the fourth day post-induction.

Wortmannin treatment

C2C12 myotubes were preincubated with PMI5011 (10 μg/ml) for 16 hours prior to the addition of wortmannin (200 nM). After a 1 hour preincubation in the absence or presence of wortmannin, insulin (100 nM) was added. Whole cell extracts were harvested two hours thereafter for isolation of whole cell extracts. Inhibition of PI3K/Akt signaling by wortmannin was confirmed by loss of Akt phosphorylation.

Free fatty acid treatment

Palmitic acid was diluted in ethanol (100 mM) and further diluted to a 6 mM working solution in 2% fatty acid free Bovine Serum Albumin (BSA) in DMEM. The 6 mM solution was sonicated and incubated at 55°C until a clear solution was observed. The resulting solution was diluted to the final concentration and filter-sterilized. C2C12 myotubes were incubated in the absence or presence of palmitic acid (200 μM) and PMI5011 (10 μg/ml) for 16 hours in the induction media. Thereafter, the media was exchanged for DMEM containing 0.3% fatty acid free BSA for 6 hours prior to insulin stimulation (100 nM insulin). Two hours after adding insulin, the cells were harvested for isolation of RNA and whole cell extracts.

Dexamethasone treatment

C2C12 myotubes were incubated in the absence or presence of dexamethasone (1 μM) and PMI5011 (10 μg/ml). When added, PMI5011 was present for 4 hours prior to adding dexamethasone. The cells were harvested for isolation of RNA and whole cell extracts 24 hours after adding dexamethasone.

Animal studies

KK-A^y mice are a murine model of obesity-induced insulin resistance and diabetes causes by mutation of the yellow obese gene A^y [22] that was previously used to establish PMI5011 regulates insulin receptor signaling in skeletal muscle [18]. Six-

A

B

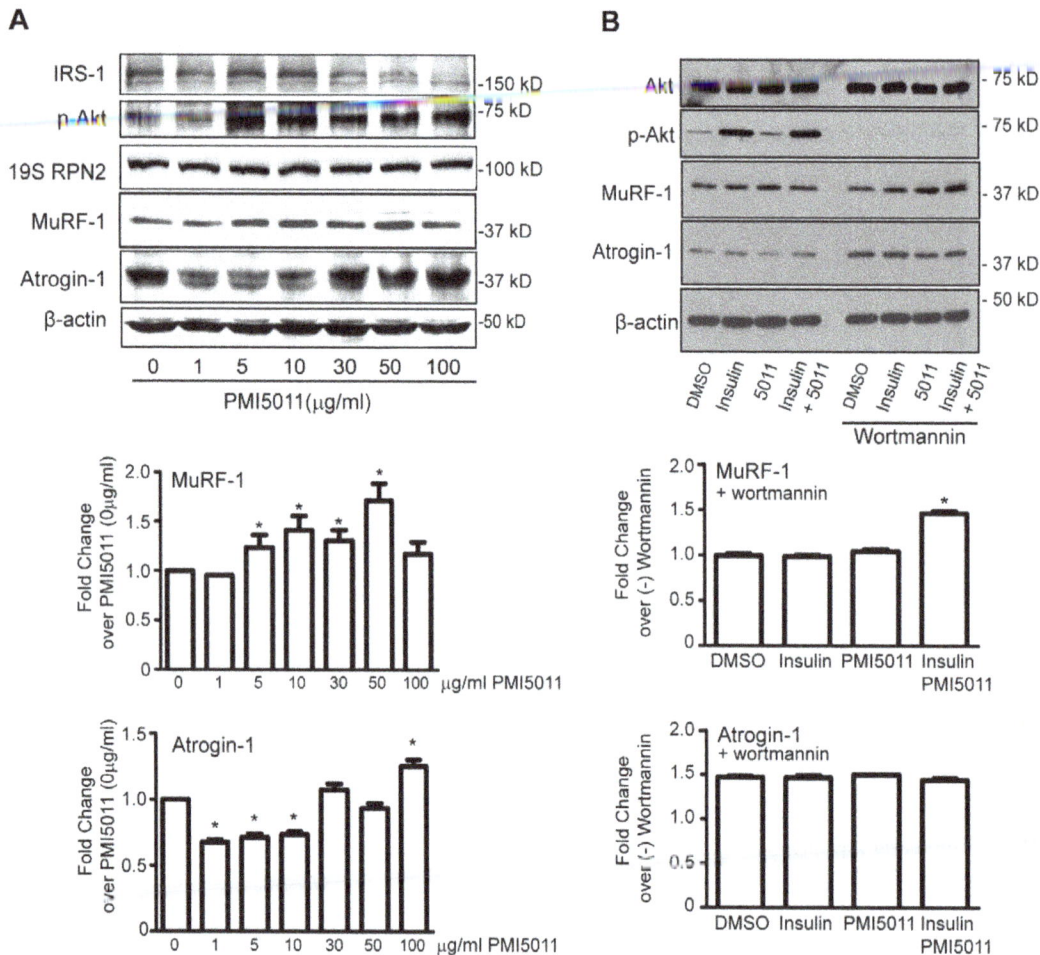

Figure 1. PMI5011 regulates expression of Atrogin-1 and MuRF-1 in skeletal muscle in a PI3K/Akt dependent manner. (A) C2C12 myotubes were incubated with the indicated concentrations of PMI5011 and whole cell extracts were harvested 16 hours thereafter. The levels of IRS-1, pAkt, 19S proteasome subunit RPN2, Atrogin-1 and MuRF-1 were assayed by western blot analysis. The fold change in Atrogin-1 and MuRF-1 expression was analyzed from three separate experiments. The fold change in Atrogin-1 and MuRF-1 protein expression compared to expression in the absence of PMI5011 was analyzed from three independent experiments. (B) C2C12 myotubes were preincubated with PMI5011 (10 μg/ml) for 16 hours as indicated prior to the addition of wortmannin (200 nM). After a 1 hour preincubation with wortmannin, insulin (100 nM) was added as indicated. Whole cell extracts were harvested two hours thereafter and subjected to SDS-PAGE followed by western blot analysis. Inhibition of PI3K/Akt signaling by wortmannin was confirmed by loss of Akt phosphorylation. The fold change in Atrogin-1 and MuRF-1 protein expression in the presence of Wortmannin relative to the corresponding (−) wortmannin conditions was analyzed from three independent experiments. * $p < 0.05$.

week-old male KK-Ay mice (n = 16) (Jackson Laboratory; Bar Harbor, ME) were single housed in animal rooms maintained at 25°C with a 12-h light dark cycle. The mice were fed a low-fat diet containing 16.4 kcal% protein, 10.5 kcal% fat, and 71.3 kcal% carbohydrate (D12329; Research Diets, Inc.; New Brunswick, NJ). At 10 weeks of age, the mice were randomly divided into a control group (n = 8) and a PMI5011-treated group (n = 8). The control group was fed the low fat diet *ad libitum* and the PMI5011 treatment group was fed *ad libitum* the low-fat diet containing 1% (w/w) PMI5011. Body weight was recorded weekly and food intake was monitored daily. Fasting glucose and insulin levels were measured at 0, 4, and 8 weeks on the diets.

Blood glucose and insulin measurements

Serum glucose levels were measured by a colorimetric hexokinase glucose assay and serum insulin levels were assayed via ELISA, according to the manufacturers' instructions. Skeletal muscle (gastrocnemius) was harvested from mice that were fasted for 4 hours prior to euthanasia. Human insulin (Humulin, Eli

Lilly, Indianapolis, IN) was administered to a subgroup of the control and PMI5011 mice at a dose of 1.5 U/kg and tissue was harvested after 90 minutes in order to assay potential changes in gene expression while maintaining skeletal muscle in an insulin-stimulated state.

Histological analysis of skeletal muscle

A portion of the skeletal muscle was fixed in 10% formalin and subjected to standard Hematoxylin and Eosin (H&E) staining. The H&E stained myofibers were scanned (NanoZoomer Digital Pathology, Hamamatsu Corp., Bridgewater, NJ) and the cross-sectional area of the myofibers was calculated from a minimum of fifty myofibers/animal using ImageJ (Research Services Branch, NIH, rsbweb.nih.gov/ij/) software.

Proteasome activity assay

Proteasome activity in C2C12 cells and skeletal muscle was measured according to the manufacturer's instructions (28)

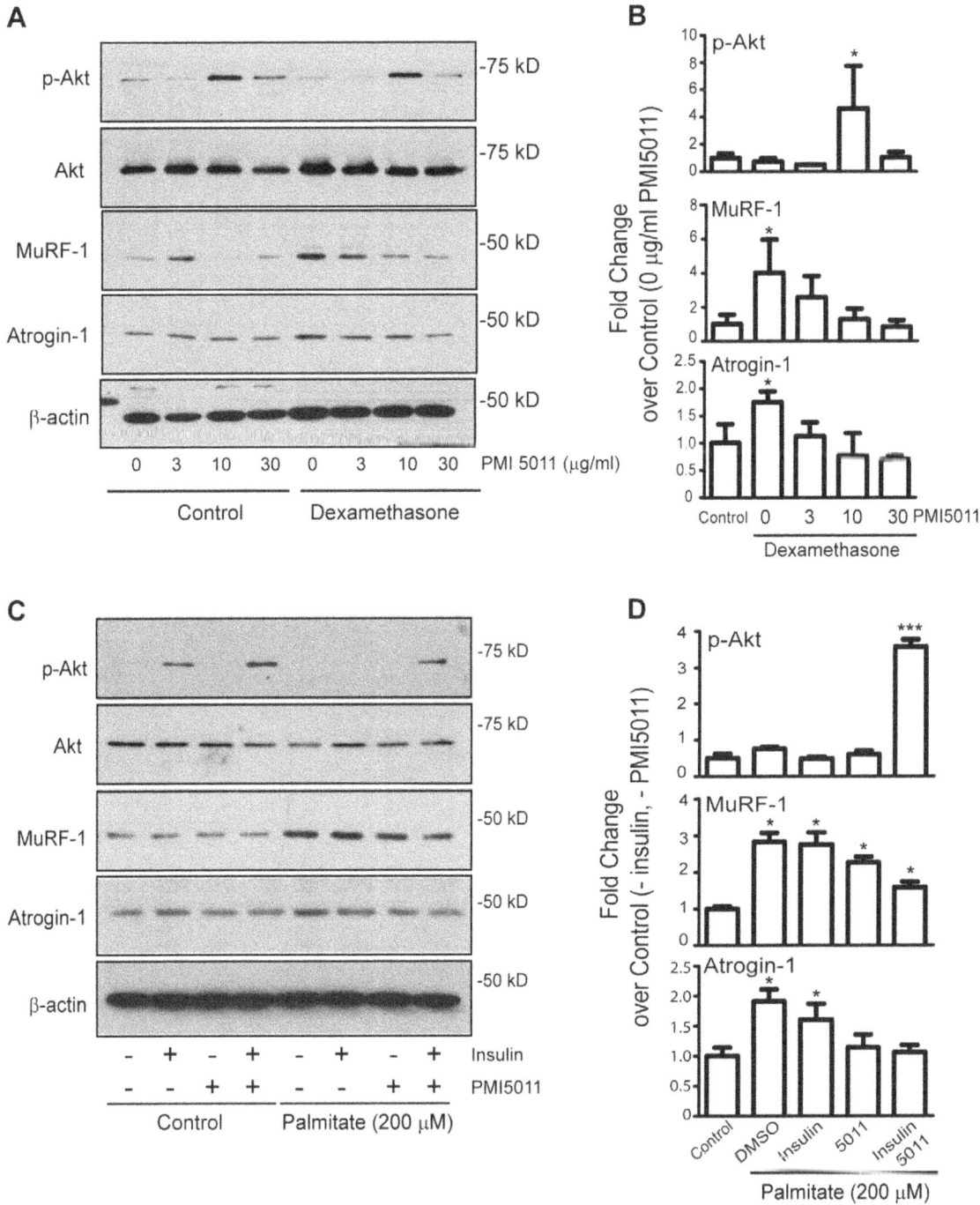

Figure 2. PMI5011 regulates expression of Atrogin-1 and MuRF-1 in two models of insulin resistance *in vitro*. (A) C2C12 myotubes were incubated in the absence (DMSO) or presence of PMI5011 at the indicated concentrations for 16 hours prior to the addition of dexamethasone (1 μM). Twenty-four hour after adding dexamethasone, whole cell extracts were harvested and subjected to SDS-PAGE followed by western blot analysis to determine phospho-Akt, total Akt, Atrogin-1 and MuRF-1 protein levels. β-actin is included as a loading control. (B) The fold change over control for phospho-Akt, MuRF-1 and Atrogin-1 protein levels was analyzed from three independent experiments. * $p < 0.05$ compared to control. (C) The C2C12 myotubes were incubated in the absence (DMSO) or PMI5011 (10 μg/ml) for 16 hours prior to adding palmitic acid (200 μM) as indicated. Twenty-four hours later, the cells were serum-deprived for 4 hours prior to insulin-stimulation (100 nM insulin) for 2 hours. Whole cell extracts were harvested and subjected to SDS-PAGE followed by western blot analysis of phospho-Akt, total Akt, Atrogin-1 and MuRF-1 protein levels. (D) The fold change over control for phospho-Akt, MuRF-1 and Atrogin-1 protein levels was analyzed from three independent experiments. * $p < 0.05$,*** $p < 0.001$ compared to control.

Millipore (Billerica, MA). Briefly, the cell lysates were harvested in 50 mM Tris-Cl, pH 7.4 with 25 mM KCl, 2 mM MgCl$_2$, 0.1% Triton X-100, 2 mM ATP, 2 mM PMSF. MgATP is included in the lysis buffer to maintain 26S proteasome activity. Proteasome activity was measured by incubating 20 μg of protein per sample of each lysate at 37°C for 60 min. Chymotrypsin-like activity was assayed with the 7-Amino-4-methylcoumarin (AMC) labeled peptide substrate Suc-Leu-Leu-Val-Tyr-AMC, tryspin-like activity was assayed using Ac-Arg-Leu-Arg-AMC and caspase-like activity using Ac-Nle-Pro-Nle-Asp-AMC. The free AMC released by proteasome activity was quantified using a 380/460 nm filter set (Molecular Devices, Sunnyvale, CA). Protcasome activity is reported as Relative Fluorescence Units (RFU)/µg protein/hr. Each sample was measured in triplicate both in the presence and in the absence of epoxomicin (20 µM, Boston Biochem), a highly specific 26S proteasome inhibitor, to account for any non-proteasomal degradation of the substrate. Non-proteasomal proteolysis is reported as the protease activity occurring in the presence of epoxomicin.

Analysis of protein expression

Skeletal muscle tissue lysates were prepared by dissecting the muscle free of adipose tissue and homogenizing in 25 mM HEPES, pH 7.4, 1% Igepal CA630, 137 mM NaCl, 1 mM PMSF, 10 µg/ml aprotinin, 1 µg/ml pepstatin, 5 µg/ml leupeptin using a PRO 200 homogenizer (PRO Scientific, Inc., Oxford, CT). The samples were centrifuged at $14,000 \times g$ for 20 min at 4°C. Whole cell extracts were harvested from the C2C12 myotubes in 50 mM Tris-Cl, pH 7.4 with 150 mM NaCl, 1 mM EDTA, 1% Igepal CA 630, 0.5% Na-deoxycholate, 0.1% SDS, 10 mM N-EM and protease inhibitors, and lysed via sonication. Protein concentrations were determined using a BCA assay (Thermo Fisher Scientific, Rockford, IL) according to the manufacturer's instructions. The tissue supernatants (50 µg) and C2C12 whole cell extracts (50 µg) were resolved by SDS-PAGE and subjected to immunoblotting using chemiluminescence detection (Thermo Fisher Scientific, Rockford, IL) and quantified as described [23].

Analysis of gene expression

Total RNA was purified from the skeletal muscle tissue using an RNeasy Fibrous Tissue Minikit (Qiagen, Valencia, CA). In each case, RNA (200 ng) was reverse transcribed using Multiscribe Reverse Transcriptase (Applied Biosystems, Carlsbad, CA) with random primers at 37°C for 2 hour. Real-time PCR was performed with TaqMan chemistry using the 7900 Real-Time PCR system and universal cycling conditions (50°C for 2 minutes; 95°C for 10 minutes; 40 cycles of 95°C for 15 seconds and 60°C for 1 minute; followed by 95°C for 15 seconds, 60°C for 15 seconds and 95°C for 15 seconds). The results were normalized to *Cyclophilin B* mRNA or 18S rRNA levels.

Statistical analysis

Normal distribution of the data for glucose and insulin levels, food intake and body weight was determined using the D'Agostino-Pearson omnibus K2 normality test. Statistical significance for body weight, glucose and insulin levels was determined using two-way mixed model ANOVA with post hoc Bonferroni correction. Statistical significance for all other data was determined using a two-tailed t test. All statistical analysis was carried out using GraphPad Prism 5 software (GraphPad Software, La Jolla, CA). Variability is expressed as the mean −/+ standard deviation.

Results

PMI5011 regulates expression of Atrogin-1 and MuRF-1 in C2C12 myotubes

To determine if the effect of PMI5011 on insulin signaling [18] involves regulating the expression of the Atrogin-1 and MuRF-1

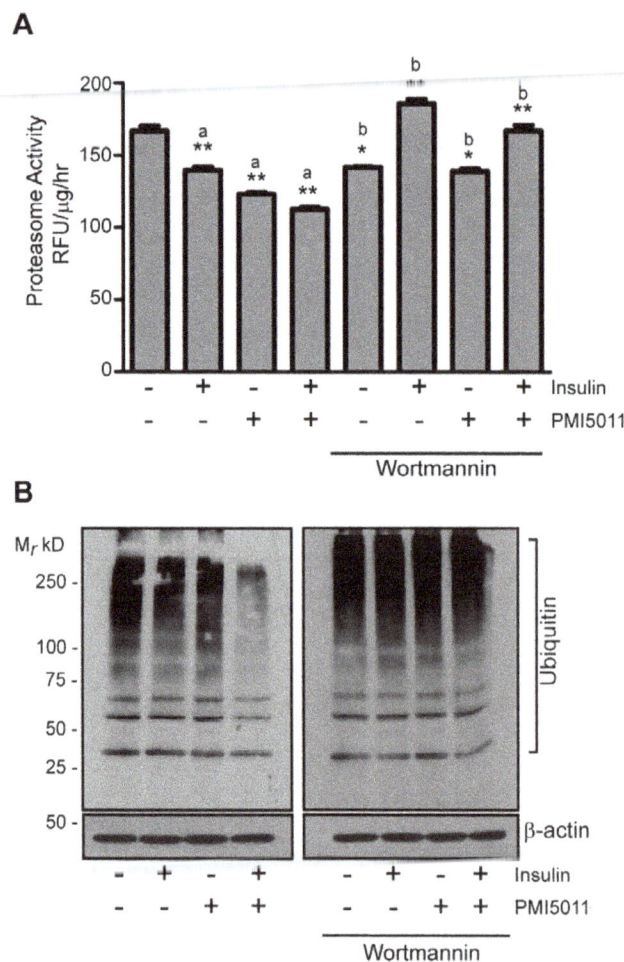

Figure 3. PMI5011 enhances the effect of insulin on proteasome activity and inhibits ubiquitylation in skeletal muscle. C2C12 myotubes were incubated with 10 µg/ml PMI5011 for 16 hours. The cells were subsequently incubated with wortmannin (200 nM) for 1 hour prior to the addition of insulin (100 nM) for 2 hours as indicated. (A) The cells were harvested and assayed for the chymotrysin-like protease activity of the proteasome. Proteasome activity is reported as Relative Fluorescence Units (RFU) RFU/µg protein/hr. The data are reported as the mean −/+ standard deviation from triplicate measurements and are representative of three independent experiments. a = compared to control; b = compared to related treatment (−) wortmannin; *$p<0.05$, **$p<0.01$ (B) Whole cell extracts were also subjected to SDS-PAGE followed by western blot analysis using an anti ubiquitin antibody to assay steady-state ubiquitylation levels. The data are representative of three independent experiments.

ubiquitin ligases, we assayed Atrogin-1 and MuRF-1 protein expression with increasing amounts of PMI5011 in C2C12 myotubes. As shown in **Figure 1A**, Atrogin-1 protein levels are decreased at concentrations of PMI5011 corresponding to maximal stimulation of Akt phosphorylation while MuRF-1 protein levels show a slight, but significant increase in the presence of PMI5011. Atrogin-1 levels are significantly increased and IRS-1 expression reduced at 100 µg/ml PMI5011, suggesting the beneficial effects of PMI5011 on insulin signaling are limited to 5–10 µg/ml PMI5011 *in vitro*. In contrast, PMI5011 has no effect on the expression of RPN2, a proteasome subunit that is required for funneling substrates into the 20S catalytic core of the 26S proteasome [24].

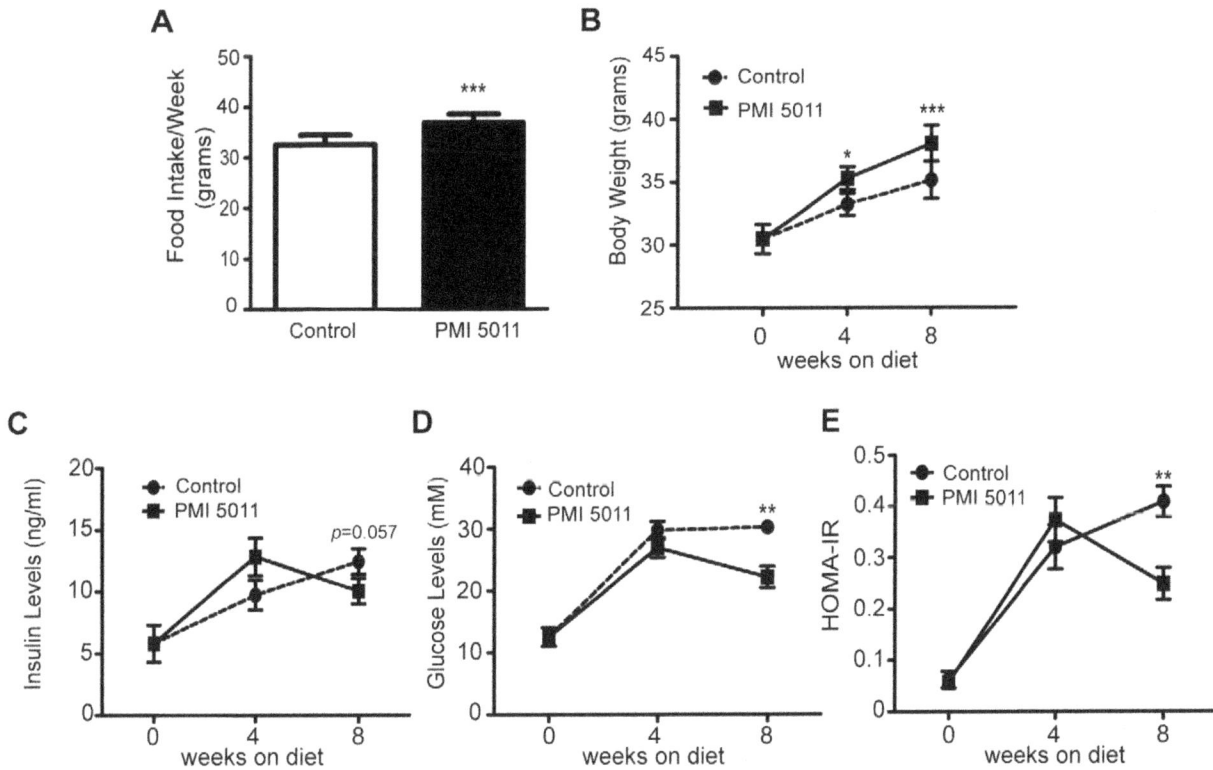

Figure 4. PMI5011 supplementation improves insulin sensitivity *in vivo.* KK-A^y mice were singly housed and maintained on a low fat diet (control, N = 8) or a low fat diet containing 1% PMI5011 (w/w) (PMI5011, N = 8) for two months. (A) Food intake was measured daily and (B) body weight has measured each week. (C) Plasma insulin and (D) glucose levels were determined at baseline, 4 and 8 weeks. (E) The index of homeostasis model assessment of insulin resistance [HOMA-IR; insulin (mU/L) x glucose (mM)/22.5] was calculated from fasting glucose and insulin levels.

The effect of PMI5011 on Atrogin-1 and MuRF-1 expression is mediated by phosphatidylinositol 3-kinase (PI3K) activity

The PI3K/Akt signaling pathway regulates expression of Atrogin-1 and MuRF-1 in skeletal muscle [25,26]. To determine if PMI5011 regulates Atrogin-1 and MuRF-1 expression via PI3K signaling, a set of experiments was carried out using wortmannin-mediated inhibition of PI3K activity. Inhibition of PI3K activity and Akt phosphorylation increased Atrogin-1 expression in the presence of insulin, PMI5011 or insulin and PMI5011 combined (**Figure 1B**). In contrast, inhibition of PI3K increased MuRF-1 expression only in the presence of insulin and PMI5011 combined when the wortmannin treated MuRF-1 levels were compared to the corresponding untreated samples.

PMI5011 regulates Atrogin-1 and MuRF-1 expression in hormone-induced insulin resistance

Treatment of C2C12 myotubes with the synthetic glucocorticoid dexamethasone (Dex) induces *atrogin-1* mRNA expression along with other markers of muscle atrophy [27,28,29] and inhibits Akt phosphorylation [27], providing an *in vitro* model of hormone-induced insulin resistance and muscle atrophy to assess the effects of PMI5011 in skeletal muscle with impaired insulin signaling. Dex treatment increases Atrogin-1 and MuRF-1 protein levels in the absence of PMI5011 (Figure 2A, see Dexamethasone, 0 μg/ml PMI5011) when compared to the level of each protein in the absence of Dex or PMI5011 (control, 0 μg/ml PMI5011) (**Figure 2 A, B**). However, the Dex-mediated increase in Atrogin-1 and MuRF-1 protein expression is inhibited by PMI5011

(**Figure 2A, B**) with the maximal effect of PMI5011 observed at 10–30 μg/ml. The PMI5011-mediated reduction in Atrogin-1 and MuRF-1 levels coincides with PMI5011 stimulation of Akt phosphorylation in the Dex-treated myotubes (**Figure 2A, B**).

PMI5011 enhances the effect of insulin on Atrogin-1 and MuRF-1 expression in fatty acid-induced insulin resistance

To determine if PMI5011 regulates Atrogin-1 and MuRF-1 expression in a different *in vitro* model of skeletal muscle insulin resistance, we assayed the effect of PMI5011 on Atrogin-1 and MuRF-1 expression in the presence of palmitic acid, a fatty acid that inhibits insulin signaling in C2C12 myotubes [30], modeling fatty acid induced insulin resistance. To confirm inhibition of insulin signaling by palmitic acid, we assayed the effect of palmitic acid on phosphorylation of Akt (**Figure 2C, D**). As expected, Akt is phosphorylated in response to insulin and the extent of Akt phosphorylation is increased by PMI5011. Palmitic acid inhibits insulin-dependent Akt phosphorylation, but this effect is reversed in the presence of insulin and PMI5011 combined, but not PMI5011 alone. Insulin resistance induced by palmitic acid also modestly increased Atrogin-1 protein expression, but this increase was reversed by the addition of insulin and PMI5011 (**Figure 2C, D**). MuRF-1 protein levels were substantially increased by palmitic acid under all conditions. The palmitic acid-mediated increase in MuRF-1 protein was significantly inhibited when both insulin and PMI5011 were present, but not with the addition of insulin alone (**Figure 2C, D**). Consistent with the results obtained with Dex treatment, the increase in Atrogin-1 and MuRF-1 levels in the

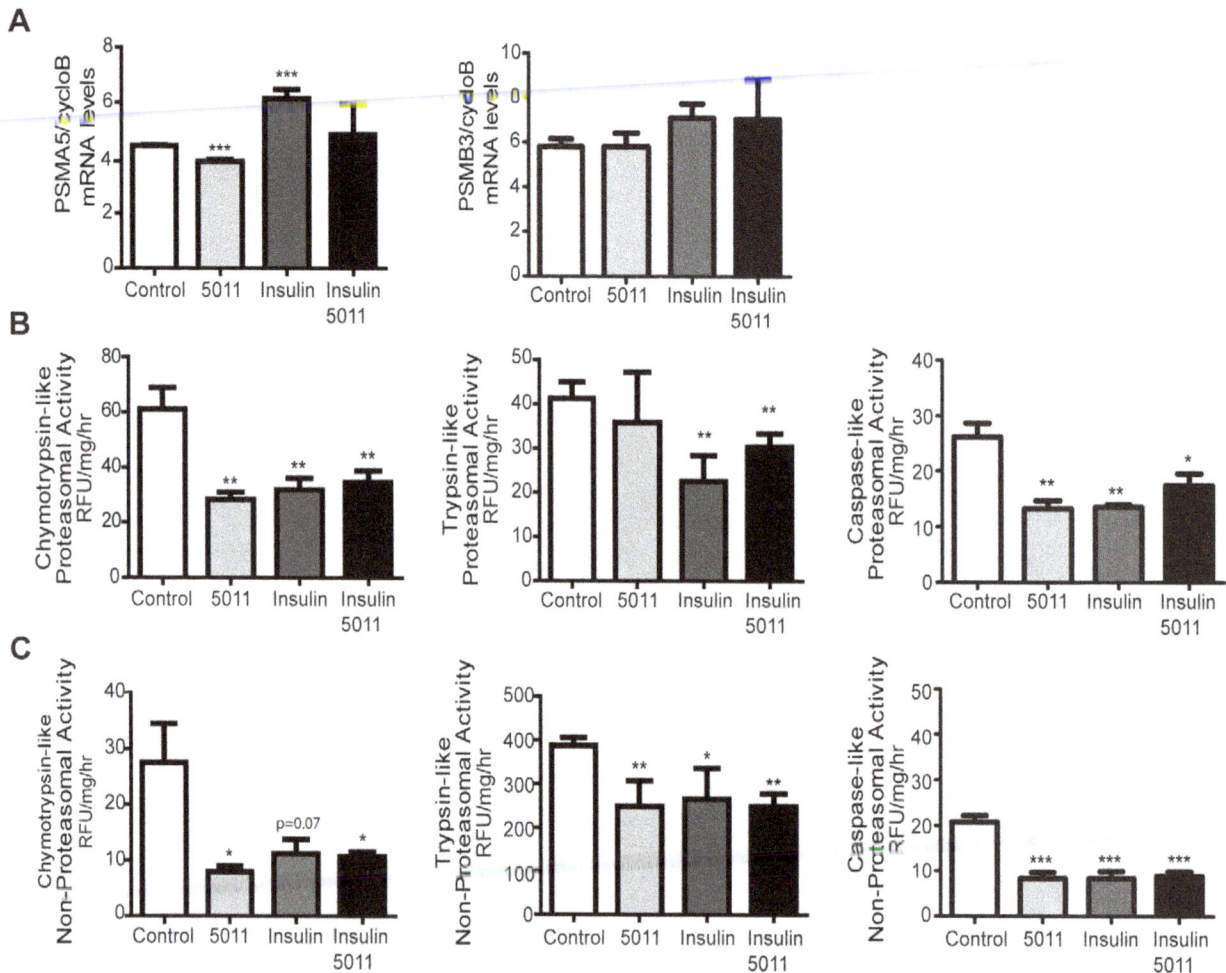

Figure 5. PMI5011 regulates proteasome and non-proteasome protease activity in skeletal muscle. At the end of the study, the KK-A^y mice were fasted for 4 hours and insulin (1.5 U/kg) or an equal volume of sterile PBS was administered by intraperitoneal injection to a subgroup (N = 4) of the control or PMI5011 supplemented (N = 4) mice. Skeletal muscle tissue (gastrocnemious) was harvested 90 minutes thereafter. (A) Gene expression of two proteasome subunits, PSMA5 and PSMB3, was analyzed by realtime RT-PCR. (B) The chymotrypin-like, trypsin-like and caspase-like 26S proteasome activities were assayed in a buffer containing MgATP to maintain the 26S proteasome structure. (C) Non-proteasomal protease activity was assayed as the chymotrypsin-like, trypsin-like or caspase-like activity measured in the presence of epoxomicin (20 μM), a highly specific proteasome inhibitor. Proteasome and nonproteasome activities are reported as RFU/μg protein/hr. The data are reported as the mean −/+ standard deviation (4 animals/group). Statistical significance is compared to control. *$p < 0.05$, ** $p < 0.01$, ***$p < 0.001$.

presence of palmitate over the levels of each protein in the absence of palmitate (control -insulin, - PMI5011) (Figure 2C,D) is reduced by PMI5011 (Figure 2C,D). Maximal reductions in Atrogin-1 and MuRF-1 expression in the presence of palmitate coincide with an increase in Akt phosphorylation that is mediated by insulin and PMI5011 combined (Figure 2C, D).

PMI5011 enhances the effect of insulin on proteasome activity and ubiquitylation in C2C12 myotubes

We next asked if PMI5011 altered the effect of insulin on proteasome activity and steady-state levels of ubiquitylated proteins *in vitro*. As shown in **Figure 3A**, 26S proteasome activity is significantly decreased in C2C12 myotubes in the presence of insulin or PMI5011 and insulin-mediated modulation of proteasome activity is enhanced by PMI5011. Inhibition of PI3K signaling is associated with increased proteasome activity in the presence of insulin or insulin and PMI5011 combined, indicating PMI5011-mediated enhancement of the effect of insulin on proteasome activity depends on PI3K activity.

We anticipated the decrease in proteasome activity would correlate with an increase in ubiquitylated proteins since the degradation of ubiquitin-modified proteins would be impaired and insulin-mediated changes in proteasome activity are accompanied by accumulation of ubiquitin-conjugated proteins [10]. However, we observed that steady-state levels of ubiquitylation are substantially inhibited in the presence of insulin and PMI5011 combined, but not with PMI5011 alone or in the presence of insulin alone (**Figure 3B**). The effects on ubiquitylation are abrogated in the presence of wortmannin, indicating the changes in steady-state levels of ubiquitylation observed in the presence of insulin and PMI5011 require activation of PI3K.

PMI5011 regulates ubiquitin-proteasome activity and non-proteasomal protein degradation in skeletal muscle in vivo

To determine if our results from the *in vitro* model of fatty acid-induced insulin resistance can be reproduced in an *in vivo* model of insulin resistance, we carried out experiments using the KK-A^y

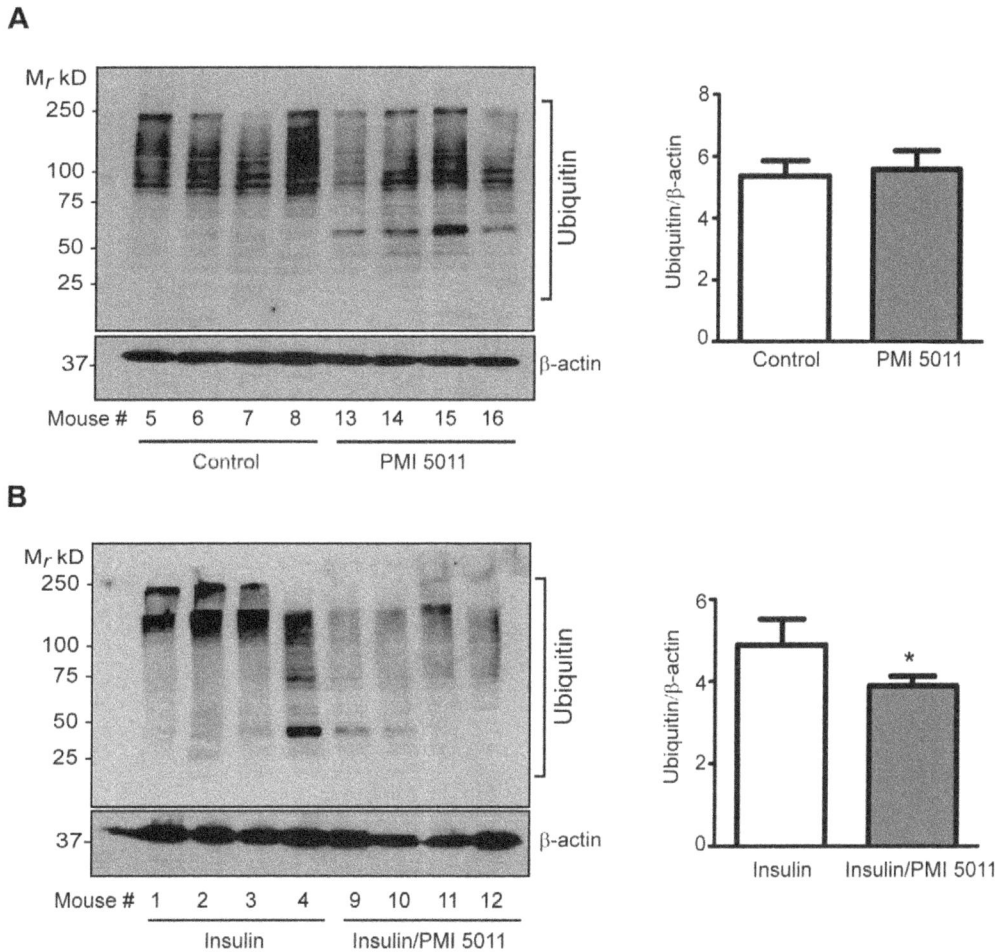

Figure 6. PMI5011 alters ubiquitin conjugation patterns in skeletal muscle. Steady-state ubiquitylation were measured in (A) control (N = 4) and PMI5011 supplemented (N = 4) KK-A^y mice or (B) control (N = 4) and PMI5011 supplemented (N = 4) KK-A^y mice administered insulin (1.5 U/kg IP) at the end of the study with tissue harvested 90 minutes thereafter. Whole cell extracts were subjected to SDS-PAGE followed by western blot analysis using an anti-ubiquitin antibody. β-actin is included as a loading control. Statistical significance is compared to insulin-treated animals in (B). *p<0.05.

model of obesity-related type 2 diabetes. Characterized by severe hyperinsulinemia, hyperglycemia, and hypertriglyceridemia [22], the KK-A^y mouse is one of several murine models that show obesity is linked to the development of insulin resistance [22,31]. Obesity is also associated with an increase in free fatty acids that leads to skeletal muscle insulin resistance [32] and recent evidence indicates that diet-induced obesity leads to skeletal muscle atrophy [33]. To determine if the changes in skeletal muscle protein content reported in the KK-A^y murine model of diabetes [18] are accompanied by changes in ubiquitin-proteasome system activity, male KK-A^y mice were randomized to PMI5011 dietary supplementation (N = 8 each group) and skeletal muscle was obtained after twelve weeks. The animals treated with PMI5011 had a small, but significant increase in food intake that corresponded with a slight, but significant increase in body weight (**Figure 4A, B**). At the end of eight weeks, serum glucose levels for the PMI5011-fed animals were significantly lower than the control animals and serum insulin levels trended downward (**Figure 4C, D**). These changes indicate improved glucose disposal and are reflected in an improved Homeostatis Model of Assessment of Insulin Resistance (HOMA-IR) (**Figure 4E**), a measure of insulin sensitivity based on the glucose and insulin levels [34].

Loss of muscle protein in a rat model of diabetes (streptozotocin-induced) is associated with increased expression of genes involved in ubiquitin-proteasome-dependent degradation, including subunits of the 26S proteasome and Atrogin-1 and MuRF-1 [7]. We assayed the effect of PMI5011 on the mRNA levels of two of the 26S proteasome subunits that are strongly upregulated with muscle loss, the 20S proteasome subunits alpha 5 (PSMA5) and beta 3 (PSMB3) [7]. As shown in **Figure 5A**, dietary supplementation with PMI5011 leads to a small, but significant decrease in the gene expression of PSMA5, but not PSMB3. Although decreased expression of PSMA5, with no change in PSMB3 expression suggests specificity in the effect of PMI5011 on proteasome subunit gene expression, PMI5011 had no effect on the gene expression of either proteasomal subunit in the insulin-stimulated muscle. Moreover, the changes in the gene expression of each subunit with acute insulin stimulation do not parallel the changes in proteasome activity, suggesting insulin-mediated regulation of the gene expression of these proteasome subunits does not influence proteasome activity. To determine the effect of PMI5011 on proteasome activity, we assayed the three types of protease activity that constitute proteasome activity (**Figure 5B**): chymotrypsin-like, trypsin-like, and caspase-like activity. PMI5011

A

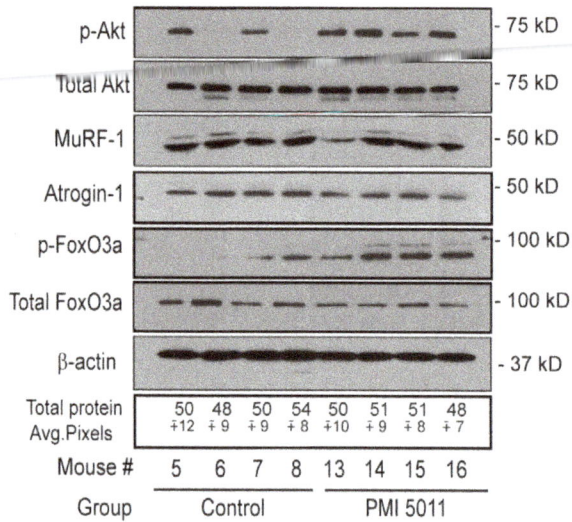

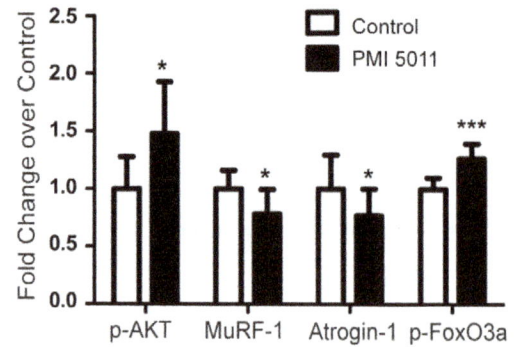

B

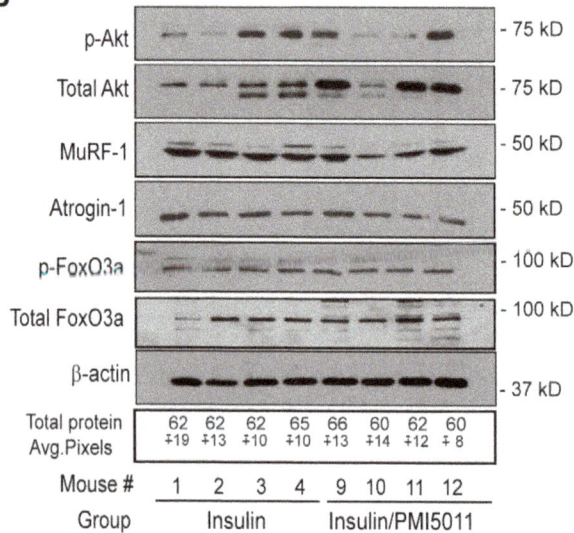

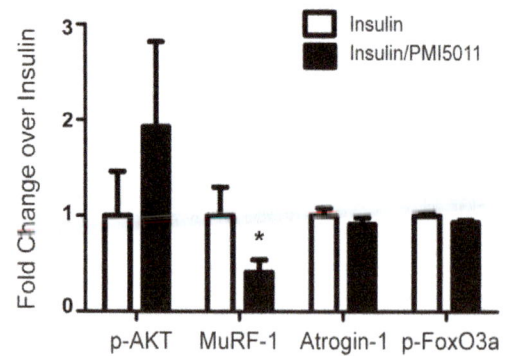

C

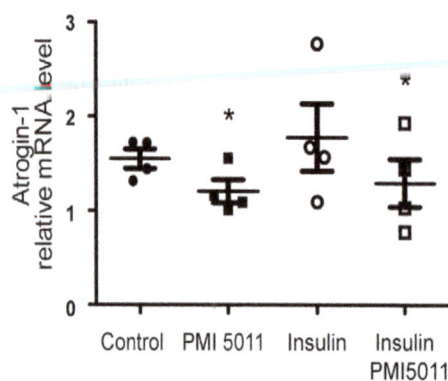

D

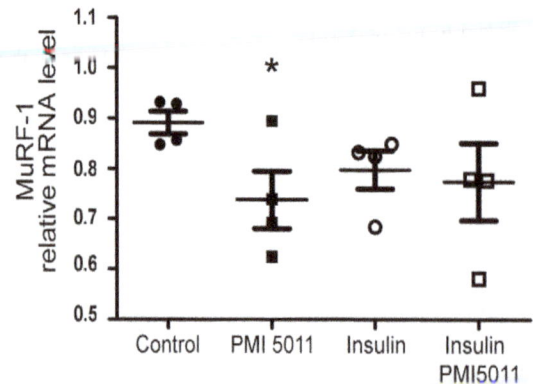

Figure 7. PMI5011 regulates Atrogin-1 and MuRF-1 gene and protein expression in skeletal muscle. (A, B) Skeletal muscle from KK-Ay mice was processed for whole cells extracts and analyzed using SDS-PAGE followed by western blot analysis of phospho-Akt, total Akt, MuRF-1, Atrogin-1, phospho-FoxO3a and total FoxO3a. β-actin and quantitation of the total protein loaded via MemCode staining are included as loading controls. Fold change for phospho-Akt/total Akt, phospho-FoxO3a/total FoxO3a, MuRF-1/total protein and Atrogin-1/total protein is reported for PMI5011 relative to control (A) or PMI5011 combined with insulin relative to insulin alone (B). (C, D) Atrogin-1 and MuRF-1 gene expression was determined using realtime RT-PCR. Results are reported as the mean −/+ standard deviation (N = 4/group). * $p < 0.05$, *** $p < 0.001$. Significance is reported relative to control in (C, D).

substantially reduces chymotrypsin-like and caspase-like protea-some activity without affecting trypsin-like activity. Acute exposure to insulin reduces all three activities, but is not more effective than dietary supplementation with PMI5011 in reducing chymotrypin and caspase-like proteasome activity. PMI5011-mediated changes in non-proteasomal protein degradation mirror the changes observed with chymotrypin and caspase-like proteasome activity (**Figure 5C**). In addition, PMI5011 inhibits the trypsin-like activity of non-proteasome proteases.

Although proteasome activity is decreased, steady-state levels of high molecular weight ubiquitin conjugates (>75 kD) are signif-icantly (p = 0.031) lower with PMI5011 supplementation com-pared to the untreated animals while ubiquitin conjugates near 50 kD accumulate with PMI5011, suggesting PMI5011 alters the specificity of proteins modified by ubiquitin without changing the overall level of ubiquitylation (**Figure 6A**). The overall levels of ubiquitylation are lowered by PMI5011 dietary supplementation when compared to insulin, and the pattern of ubiquitin conjugate accumulation also changes (**Figure 6B**), further supporting the notion that PMI5011 alters the specificity of ubiquitin conjugation in skeletal muscle.

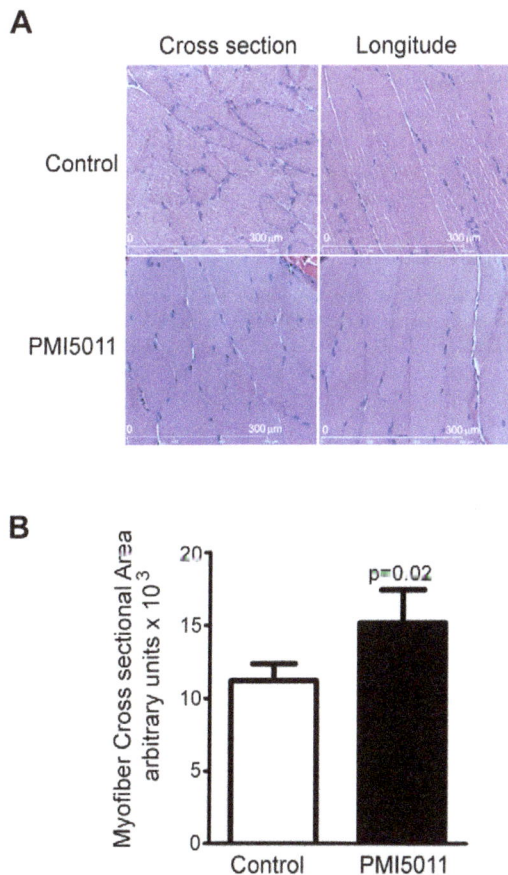

A

B

Figure 8. Skeletal muscle myofiber size is larger with dietary intake of PMI5011. (A) H&E staining of cross-section and longitudinal section of gastrocnemious skeletal muscle from control and PMI5011 supplemented KK-Ay mice. (B) The cross-sectional area of fifty myofibers/animal in each group was determined using ImageJ software. The statistical significance is reported as the mean −/+ standard deviation, p = 0.02.

PMI5011 decreases Atrogin-1 and MuRF-1 expression in skeletal muscle in vivo

PMI5011 supplementation improves insulin signaling in skeletal muscle when assayed as increased phosphorylation of Akt (**Figure 7A**). In addition, PMI5011 enhances insulin-stimulated Akt phosphorylation (**Figure 7B**). The changes in Akt phosphor-ylation with PMI5011 supplementation correlate with reduced expression of Atrogin-1 and MuRF-1 proteins (**Figure 7A**) while MuRF-1 protein levels are also reduced by PMI5011 when compared to insulin (**Figure 7B**).

The FoxO1 and FoxO3a members of the FoxO class of forkhead transcription factors are downstream targets of Akt that regulate the gene expression of *atrogin-1* and *MuRF-1* [25,27]. To determine if the effect of PMI5011 on atrogin-1 and MuRF-1 protein expression is related to regulation of FoxO phosphoryla-tion, we measured the levels of FoxO3a and phosphorylated FoxO3a (serine 253) in the skeletal muscle. Dietary intake of PMI5011 significantly increases phosphorylation of FoxO3a while the total amount of FoxO3a is decreased compared to the untreated animals (**Figure 7A**). The PMI5011-mediated increase in FoxO3a phosphorylation corresponds to decreased *atrogin-1* and *MuRF-1* expression (**Figure 7C**) when compared to the control animals, consistent with a role for FoxO3a in the effect of PMI5011 on atrogin-1 and MuRF-1 protein levels. Acute insulin treatment does not increase FoxO3a phosphorylation or signifi-cantly decrease *atrogin-1* and *MuRF-1* expression in skeletal muscle (**Figure 7B, D**) over that observed with PMI5011 supplementa-tion, although MuRF-1 protein levels are decreased by PMI5011 in the insulin-stimulated muscle (**Figure 7B**).

Skeletal muscle myofiber size is larger in PMI5011 supplemented animals

Consistent with inhibition of ubiquitylation and proteasome and non-proteasome activity, the cross-sectional area of myofibers from the PMI5011 treated animals was significantly larger than the myofibers from the control animal (**Figure 8A, B**), indicating muscle mass is conserved in the presence of PMI5011.

Discussion

PMI5011 is a well-characterized botanical extract from *A. dracunculus* L., whose effects on carbohydrate metabolism are comparable to the ability of known antidiabetic drugs (troglitazone and metformin) to lower glucose and insulin levels in murine models of diabetes and insulin resistance [16]. Studies exploring the mechanisms underlying the insulin sensitizing effects of PMI5011 show that PMI5011 enhances insulin signaling in skeletal muscle as demonstrated by increased PI3K activity, increased Akt phosphorylation, and decreased activity of protein tyrosine phosphatase 1B (PTP-1B), which serves as a negative regulator of insulin signaling [18]. The current study provides additional insight into the mechanism of action of PMI5011 in skeletal muscle by demonstrating PMI5011-mediated regulation of the ubiquitin-proteasome system.

Herein, we show PMI5011-enhanced insulin signaling specifi-cally inhibits chymotrypsin-like and caspase-like proteasome activity and all three non-proteasome protease activities, reduces steady-state ubiquitylation levels, regulates expression of the ubiquitin ligases, Atrogin-1 and MuRF-1 and enhances myofiber size in insulin resistant skeletal muscle. In contrast to PMI5011-mediated reductions in Atrogin-1 levels *in vitro* in the absence of insulin resistance (Figure 1A), MuRF-1 levels are increased by PMI5011. PMI5011-mediated decreases in MuRF-1 expression are apparent only in the *in vitro* models of insulin resistance. The

PMI5011-mediated change in MuRF-1 expression *in vivo* is comparable to the effect of insulin on MuRF-1 expression. Together, these results suggest MuRF-1 is the more relevant PMI5011 target in the presence of insulin resistance.

PI3K/Akt signaling regulates Atrogin-1 and MuRF-1 protein levels by inhibiting FoxO transcription factor-mediated induction of *atrogin-1* and *MuRF-1* gene expression [25,26,27]. Akt-dependent phosphorylation of FoxO1 or FoxO3a excludes the FoxO proteins from the nucleus, either via binding of the phosphorylated FoxO protein to 14-3-3 proteins in the cytoplasm or degradation of the phosphorylated FoxO protein by the proteasome [reviewed in [35]]. The PMI5011-mediated increase in Akt phosphorylation and FoxO3a phosphorylation, coupled with reduced atrogin-1 and MuRF-1 gene expression, suggests PMI5011 mediated reductions in Atrogin-1 and MuRF-1 protein expression are linked to enhanced Akt-dependent regulation of FoxO3a transcriptional activity.

The effects of PMI5011 on Atrogin-1 and MuRF-1 expression are not as pronounced as the PMI5011-mediated inhibition of proteasome and non-proteasome protease activity. As the major site of protein breakdown, proteasome activity is upregulated in muscle loss associated with insulin resistance [2,3,7]. PMI5011 substantially reduces the chymotrypsin and caspase-like protease activities in the absence or presence of insulin stimulation. This indicates PMI5011 action has the potential to broadly inhibit protein degradation in insulin resistant skeletal muscle since the proteasomal chymotrypsin-like activity is required for generalized protein degradation, in conjunction with either the trypsin-like or caspase-like activities [36]. However, the proteasome does not degrade intact myofibrillar proteins, the primary group of proteins targeted for breakdown in skeletal muscle atrophy [37,38]. Although the myofibrillar proteins are ultimately degraded by the proteasome, the filament proteins must be dissociated from the myofibrillar structure for recognition by the proteasome [39]. This task is most likely accomplished by the calpains, calcium-dependent proteases that interact with the ubiquitin-proteasome system [38,40], although initial cleavage of the filament components may also be carried out by caspases [41]. PMI5011-mediated inhibition of non-proteasome chymotrypsin-like and caspase activities is consistent with an effect of PMI5011 on

calpain and caspase proteases activities, suggesting PMI5011 acts to reduce degradation of the myofibrillar proteins by regulating the activity of several classes of proteases.

A potential role for PMI5011 in preventing degradation of the myofibrillar proteins in insulin resistance is further supported by our results showing PMI5011 regulates expression of MuRF-1 in the presence of insulin resistance *in vitro* and *in vivo*. MuRF-1 dependent ubiquitylation of skeletal muscle proteins accounts for the majority of ubiquitin modification in muscle atrophy and MuRF-1 directly interacts with and regulates the ubiquitylation of several myofibrillar proteins [42].

A role for MuRF-1 is well established in muscle loss due to insulin resistance associated with fasting or catabolic disease states. But insulin resistance also exacerbates muscle loss associated with aging, termed sarcopenia [43,44,45,46]. In contrast to the rapid muscle atrophy associated with fasting or catabolic diseases, sarcopenic muscle loss occurs gradually and is worsened by obesity [5]. Insulin resistance associated with obesity accelerates sarcopenia by suppressing protein synthesis and stimulating skeletal muscle protein degradation [46], even in the absence of type 2 diabetes [47]. In turn, the loss of muscle mass in sarcopenic obesity increases the risk of developing type 2 diabetes due to decreased glucose disposal in skeletal muscle. There are indications that sarcopenic muscle loss is mechanistically different from rapid muscle loss [48,49], but enhanced proteasome activity remains a common factor in both forms of muscle loss related to insulin resistance [49]. PMI5011-mediated enhanced insulin signaling, coupled with decreased MuRF-1 expression, decreased 26S proteasome activity and larger myofiber size in the obesity-related insulin resistant animals indicates PMI5011 has therapeutic potential for preserving muscle mass in insulin resistant skeletal muscle, including treatment of muscle loss due to sarcopenia.

Author Contributions

Conceived and designed the experiments: HKB ZQW WTC ZEF. Performed the experiments: HKB ZQW PA XHZ YY GK DR ZEF. Analyzed the data: HKB ZQW PA GK DR WTC ZEF. Contributed reagents/materials/analysis tools: ZQW DR WTC ZEF. Wrote the paper: HKB ZQW WTC ZEF.

References

1. Bassel-Duby R, Olson EN (2006) Signaling pathways in skeletal muscle remodeling. Annu Rev Biochem 75: 19–37.
2. Wang X, Hu Z, Hu J, Du J, Mitch WE (2006) Insulin resistance accelerates muscle protein degradation: Activation of the ubiquitin-proteasome pathway by defects in muscle cell signaling. Endocrinology 147: 4160–4168.
3. Mitch WE, Goldberg AL (1996) Mechanisms of muscle wasting. The role of the ubiquitin-proteasome pathway. N Engl J Med 335: 1897–1905.
4. Park SW, Goodpaster BH, Lee JS, Kuller LH, Boudreau R, et al. (2009) Excessive loss of skeletal muscle mass in older adults with type 2 diabetes. Diabetes Care 32: 1993–1997.
5. Srikanthan P, Hevener AL, Karlamangla AS (2010) Sarcopenia Exacerbates Obesity-Associated Insulin Resistance and Dysglycemia: Findings from the National Health and Nutrition Examination Survey III. PLoS One 5: e10805.
6. Aaron Ciechanover AO, Schwartz AL (2000) Ubiquitin-mediated proteolysis: biological regulation via destruction. BioEssays 22: 442–451.
7. Lecker SH, Jagoe RT, Gilbert A, Gomes M, Baracos V, et al. (2004) Multiple types of skeletal muscle atrophy involve a common program of changes in gene expression. FASEB J 18: 39–51.
8. Kettelhut IC, Pepato MT, Migliorini RH, Medina R, Goldberg AL (1994) Regulation of different proteolytic pathways in skeletal muscle in fasting and diabetes mellitus. Braz J Med Biol Res 27: 981–993.
9. Sacheck JM, Ohtsuka A, McLary SC, Goldberg AL (2004) IGF-I stimulates muscle growth by suppressing protein breakdown and expression of atrophy-related ubiquitin ligases, atrogin-1 and MuRF1. Am J Physiol Endocrinol Metab 287: E591–601.
10. Bennett RG, Hamel FG, Duckworth WC (2000) Insulin inhibits the ubiquitin-dependent degrading activity of the 26S proteasome. Endocrinology 141: 2508–2517.
11. Gomes MD, Lecker SH, Jagoe RT, Navon A, Goldberg AL (2001) Atrogin-1, a muscle-specific F-box protein highly expressed during muscle atrophy. Proc Natl Acad Sci U S A 98: 14440–14445.
12. Koyama S, Hata S, Witt CC, Ono Y, Lerche S, et al. (2008) Muscle RING-finger protein-1 (MuRF1) as a connector of muscle energy metabolism and protein synthesis. J Mol Biol 376: 1224–1236.
13. Bodine SC, Latres E, Baumhueter S, Lai VK, Nunez L, et al. (2001) Identification of ubiquitin ligases required for skeletal muscle atrophy. Science 294: 1704–1708.
14. Schmidt B, Ribnicky DM, Poulev A, Logendra S, Cefalu WT, et al. (2008) A natural history of botanical therapeutics. Metabolism 57: S3–9.
15. Witters LA (2001) The blooming of the French lilac. J Clin Invest 108: 1105–1107.
16. Ribnicky DM, Poulev A, Watford M, Cefalu WT, Raskin I (2006) Antihyperglycemic activity of Tarralin, an ethanolic extract of Artemisia dracunculus L. Phytomedicine 13: 550–557.
17. Wang ZQ, Ribnicky D, Zhang XH, Raskin I, Yu Y, et al. (2008) Bioactives of Artemisia dracunculus L enhance cellular insulin signaling in primary human skeletal muscle culture. Metabolism 57: S58–64.
18. Wang ZQ, Ribnicky D, Zhang XH, Zuberi A, Raskin I, et al. (2011) An extract of Artemisia dracunculus L. enhances insulin receptor signaling and modulates gene expression in skeletal muscle in KK-A(y) mice. J Nutr Biochem 22: 71–78.
19. Ribnicky DM, Kuhn P, Poulev A, Logendra S, Zuberi A, et al. (2009) Improved absorption and bioactivity of active compounds from an anti-diabetic extract of Artemisia dracunculus L. Int J Pharm 370: 87–92.
20. Zuberi AR (2008) Strategies for assessment of botanical action on metabolic syndrome in the mouse and evidence for a genotype-specific effect of Russian tarragon in the regulation of insulin sensitivity. Metabolism 57: S10–15.

21. Logendra S, Ribnicky DM, Yang H, Poulev A, Ma J, et al. (2006) Bioassay-guided isolation of aldose reductase inhibitors from Artemisia dracunculus. Phytochemistry 67: 1539–1546.
22. Ikeda H (1994) KK mouse. Diabetes Res Clin Pract 24 Suppl: S313–316.
23. Wang ZQ, Floyd ZE, Qin J, Liu X, Yu Y, et al. (2009) Modulation of skeletal muscle insulin signaling with chronic caloric restriction in cynomolgus monkeys. Diabetes 58: 1488–1498.
24. Rosenzweig R, Osmulski PA, Gaczynska M, Glickman MH (2008) The central unit within the 19S regulatory particle of the proteasome. Nature structural & molecular biology 15: 573–580.
25. Stitt TN, Drujan D, Clarke BA, Panaro F, Timofeyva Y, et al. (2004) The IGF-1/PI3K/Akt pathway prevents expression of muscle atrophy-induced ubiquitin ligases by inhibiting FOXO transcription factors. Mol Cell 14: 395–403.
26. Glass DJ (2010) PI3 kinase regulation of skeletal muscle hypertrophy and atrophy. Curr Top Microbiol Immunol 346: 267–278.
27. Sandri M, Sandri C, Gilbert A, Skurk C, Calabria E, et al. (2004) Foxo transcription factors induce the atrophy-related ubiquitin ligase atrogin-1 and cause skeletal muscle atrophy. Cell 117: 399–412.
28. Sultan KR, Henkel B, Terlou M, Haagsman HP (2006) Quantification of hormone-induced atrophy of large myotubes from C2C12 and L6 cells: atrophy-inducible and atrophy-resistant C2C12 myotubes. American Journal of Physiology - Cell Physiology 290: C650–C659.
29. Carballo-Jane E, Pandit S, Santoro JC, Freund C, Luell S, et al. (2004) Skeletal muscle: a dual system to measure glucocorticoid-dependent transactivation and transrepression of gene regulation. The Journal of Steroid Biochemistry and Molecular Biology 88: 191–201.
30. Chavez JA, Holland WL, Bar J, Sandhoff K, Summers SA (2005) Acid ceramidase overexpression prevents the inhibitory effects of saturated fatty acids on insulin signaling. The Journal of biological chemistry 280: 20148–20153.
31. Winzell MS, Ahrén B (2004) The High-Fat Diet–Fed Mouse. Diabetes 53: S215–S219.
32. Boden G (2011) Obesity, insulin resistance and free fatty acids. Current opinion in endocrinology, diabetes, and obesity 18: 139–143.
33. Sishi B, Loos B, Ellis B, Smith W, du Toit EF, et al. (2010) Diet-induced obesity alters signalling pathways and induces atrophy and apoptosis in skeletal muscle in a prediabetic rat model. Exp Physiol.
34. Matthews DR, Hosker JP, Rudenski AS, Naylor BA, Treacher DF, et al. (1985) Homeostasis model assessment: insulin resistance and beta-cell function from fasting plasma glucose and insulin concentrations in man. Diabetologia 28; 412–419.
35. Huang H, Tindall DJ (2007) Dynamic FoxO transcription factors. Journal of cell science 120: 2479–2487.
36. Kisselev AF, Callard A, Goldberg AL (2006) Importance of the Different Proteolytic Sites of the Proteasome and the Efficacy of Inhibitors Varies with the Protein Substrate. Journal of Biological Chemistry 281: 8582–8590.
37. Munoz KA, Satarug S, Tischler ME (1993) Time course of the response of myofibrillar and sarcoplasmic protein metabolism to unweighting of the soleus muscle. Metabolism: clinical and experimental 42: 1006–1012.
38. Goll DE, Neti G, Mares SW, Thompson VF (2008) Myofibrillar protein turnover: the proteasome and the calpains. Journal of animal science 86: E19–35.
39. Hasselgren PO, Fischer JE (2001) Muscle cachexia: current concepts of intracellular mechanisms and molecular regulation. Ann Surg 233: 9–17.
40. Wing SS, Lecker SH, Jagoe RT (2011) Proteolysis in illness-associated skeletal muscle atrophy: from pathways to networks. Critical reviews in clinical laboratory sciences 48: 49–70.
41. Du J, Wang X, Miereles C, Bailey JL, Debigare R, et al. (2004) Activation of caspase-3 is an initial step triggering accelerated muscle proteolysis in catabolic conditions. J Clin Invest 113: 115–123.
42. Cohen S, Brault JJ, Gygi SP, Glass DJ, Valenzuela DM, et al. (2009) During muscle atrophy, thick, but not thin, filament components are degraded by MuRF1-dependent ubiquitylation. The Journal of Cell Biology 185: 1083–1095.
43. Kim TN, Park MS, Lim KI, Choi HY, Yang SJ, et al. (2012) Relationships between Sarcopenic Obesity and Insulin Resistance, Inflammation, and Vitamin D Status:The Korean Sarcopenic Obesity Study (KSOS). Clinical endocrinology.
44. Fielding RA, Vellas B, Evans WJ, Bhasin S, Morley JE, et al. (2011) Sarcopenia: an undiagnosed condition in older adults. Current consensus definition: prevalence, etiology, and consequences. International working group on sarcopenia. Journal of the American Medical Directors Association 12: 249–256.
45. Levine ME, Crimmins EM (2012) The Impact of Insulin Resistance and Inflammation on the Association Between Sarcopenic Obesity and Physical Functioning. Obesity.
46. Abbatecola AM, Paolisso G, Fattoretti P, Evans WJ, Fiore V, et al. (2011) Discovering pathways of sarcopenia in older adults: a role for insulin resistance on mitochondria dysfunction. The journal of nutrition, health & aging 15: 890–895.
47. Lee CG, Boyko EJ, Strotmeyer ES, Lewis CE, Cawthon PM, et al. (2011) Association between insulin resistance and lean mass loss and fat mass gain in older men without diabetes mellitus. Journal of the American Geriatrics Society 59: 1217–1224.
48. Edstrom E, Altun M, Hagglund M, Ulfhake B (2006) Atrogin-1/MAFbx and MuRF1 are downregulated in aging-related loss of skeletal muscle. The journals of gerontology Series A, Biological sciences and medical sciences 61: 663–674.
49. Altun M, Besche HC, Overkleeft HS, Picchillo R, Edelmann MJ, et al. (2010) Muscle Wasting in Aged, Sarcopenic Rats Is Associated with Enhanced Activity of the Ubiquitin Proteasome Pathway. Journal of Biological Chemistry 285: 39597–39608.

Midkine, a Potential Link between Obesity and Insulin Resistance

Nengguang Fan[1,2], Haiyan Sun[1], Yifei Wang[1], Lijuan Zhang[2], Zhenhua Xia[2], Liang Peng[3], Yanqiang Hou[3], Weiqin Shen[3], Rui Liu[1], Yongde Peng[1]*

1 Department of Endocrinology, Shanghai First People's Hospital, Shanghai Jiao Tong University, Shanghai, China, 2 Department of Endocrinology, Shanghai Songjiang Center Hospital, Shanghai, China, 3 Department of Laboratory Medicine, Shanghai Songjiang Center Hospital, Shanghai, China

Abstract

Obesity is associated with increased production of inflammatory mediators in adipose tissue, which contributes to chronic inflammation and insulin resistance. Midkine (MK) is a heparin-binding growth factor with potent proinflammatory activities. We aimed to test whether MK is associated with obesity and has a role in insulin resistance. It was found that MK was expressed in adipocytes and regulated by inflammatory modulators (TNF-α and rosiglitazone). In addition, a significant increase in MK levels was observed in adipose tissue of obese ob/ob mice as well as in serum of overweight/obese subjects when compared with their respective controls. *In vitro* studies further revealed that MK impaired insulin signaling in 3T3-L1 adipocytes, as indicated by reduced phosphorylation of Akt and IRS-1 and decreased translocation of glucose transporter 4 (GLUT4) to the plasma membrane in response to insulin stimulation. Moreover, MK activated the STAT3-suppressor of cytokine signaling 3 (SOCS3) pathway in adipocytes. Thus, MK is a novel adipocyte-secreted factor associated with obesity and inhibition of insulin signaling in adipocytes. It may provide a potential link between obesity and insulin resistance.

Editor: Guillermo López Lluch, Universidad Pablo de Olavide, Centro Andaluz de Biología del Desarrollo-CSIC, Spain

Funding: This study was supported by the National Natural Science Foundation of China (Grant No. 81370904, 81070682 and 30800562). The funders had no role in study design, data collection and analysis, decision to publish, or preparation of the manuscript.

Competing Interests: The authors have declared that no competing interests exist.

* E-mail: pengyongde0908@126.com

Introduction

Obesity has become a global epidemic that is closely associated with the development of insulin resistance, type 2 diabetes and cardiovascular diseases [1,2]. Initially viewed as a major site for energy storage, adipose tissue has recently been identified as an important endocrine and immune organ [3,4]. It secretes a variety of bioactive molecules, including adiponectin, leptin, and various inflammatory mediators (e.g., TNF-α, IL-6 and MCP-1), which are collectively termed as adipokines [3,4]. Obesity leads to a dramatically changed secretory profile of adipose tissue, characterized by increased production of proinflammatory cytokines, such as TNF-α, IL-1β and IL-6 [5,6]. These cytokines exert direct actions on adipocytes and other insulin target cells, inducing chronic inflammation and insulin resistance [5,6]. To date, many novel adipokines with proinflammatory properties have been identified and linked to obesity-induced inflammation and insulin resistance [7].

Midkine (MK), also known as neurite growth-promoting factor 2, is a 13-kDa heparin-binding growth factor with pleiotropic activities [8]. It was originally identified as a retinoic acid-inducible molecule in mouse embryonic carcinoma cells, and is expressed in mouse embryos at mid-gestation [9]. Structurally, MK shares 50% sequence identity with pleiotrophin, both of which are composed of two domains (N- and C-domain) [9,10]. It has been shown that MK promotes cell proliferation, differentiation, survival and migration, and is involved in a variety of biological processes, including neuronal development, angiogenesis and oncogenesis

[10–13]. In addition, growing evidence has indicated a key role of MK in inflammation [14]. It promotes chemotaxis of neutrophils and macrophages and suppresses expansion of regulatory T cells [15–17]. Accordingly, MK-deficient mice were protected against antibody-induced rheumatoid arthritis, neointima formation after vascular injury, and experimental autoimmune encephalomyelitis, associated with decreased inflammatory cell infiltration and enhanced regulatory T cell expansion [16–18]. Clinically, patients with inflammatory diseases including rheumatoid arthritis, ulcerative colitis and Crohn's disease had increased blood MK compared with control subjects [18–20]. Together, MK appears to be a mediator implicated in many inflammatory processes and diseases. However, the relationship between MK and obesity, a state of chronic inflammation, is unclear.

Indeed, MK is synthesized and secreted by adipocytes [21]. During in vitro adipogenesis of 3T3-L1 preadipocytes, MK expression was markedly increased after initiation of differentiation. It exerted an essential role in the mitotic clonal expansion of 3T3-L1 preadipocytes [21], in line with its mitogenic effects on other cell types [22,23]. These in vitro findings seem to have their clinical relevance. Compared with control subjects, obese and diabetic children and adolescents had significantly higher levels of serum MK [24]. However, the relationship between MK and obesity and the role of MK in mature adipocytes remain to be further determined.

In the present study, we initially assessed MK expression levels in 3T3-L1 adipocytes and its regulation by inflammatory modulators. Then, we investigated the association between MK and obesity by examining MK levels in adipose tissue of mice and in serum of humans. Furthermore, in vitro experiments were performed to investigate the impact of MK on insulin signaling and GLUT4 translocation in 3T3-L1 adipocytes. Finally, the proinflammatory effects of MK on adipocytes were determined.

Materials and Methods

Ethics Statement

All research involving human participants was approved by the Institutional Review Board of Shanghai First People's Hospital affiliated to Shanghai Jiao Tong University School of Medicine, and performed in accordance with the principle of the Helsinki Declaration II. Written informed consent was obtained from all subjects. Animal procedures were approved by the Committee on the Ethics of Animal Experiments of Shanghai Jiao Tong University and were carried out in strict accordance with the recommendations in the Guide for the Care and Use of Laboratory Animals of Shanghai Jiao Tong University. All operations were performed under sodium pentobarbital anesthesia, and all efforts were made to minimize suffering.

Chemicals and Reagents

Dulbecco's modified Eagle's medium (DMEM) was purchased from Hyclone (Beijing, China). Fetal bovine serum (FBS) and penicillin-streptomycin were from Gibco (Carlsbad, CA). Isobutylmethylxanthine, dexamethasone, insulin and rosiglitazone were from Sigma (St. Louis, MO). Recombinant mouse MK was obtained from Pepro Tech (Rocky Hill, NJ) and the endotoxin level was below 1.0 EU per 1 μg of the protein by the LAL method. Human TNF-α was also from Pepro Tech (Rocky Hill, NJ). Specific antibodies against STAT3, phospho-STAT3 (Tyr705), phospho-p65 (Ser536), Akt, phospho-Akt (Ser473), GLUT4 and GAPDH were purchased from Cell signaling Technology (Beverly, MA). Antibody against MK was from Santa Cruz Biotechnology (Santa Cruz, CA). Phospho-IRS1 (Tyr612) antibody was from Abcam (Cambridge, MA). Na/K ATPase α-1 antibody was obtained from Novus Biologicals (Littleton, CO). Horseradish peroxidase-conjugated antibodies against rabbit or goat IgG were from Jackson Laboratories (West Grove, PA).

Subjects

A total of 206 individuals who consecutively visited the Medical Examination Center of Shanghai First People's Hospital for routine health check-ups were invited and 165 individuals agreed to attend our study. After excluding 30 ineligible subjects with diabetes, acute or chronic infectious diseases, autoimmune diseases, heart failure, hepatic or renal diseases, 135 individuals were included in our final analysis. Based on body mass index (BMI), the subjects were divided into two groups: normal weight

Table 1. Primer sequences for real-time PCR.

Genes	Sense	Anti-sense
Midkine	TGGAGCCGACTGCAAATACAA	GGCTTAGTCACGCGGATGG
SOCS3	ATGGTCACCCACAGCAAGTTT	TCCAGTAGAATCCGCTCTCCT
IL-6	GAGGATACCACTCCCAACAGACC	AAGTGCATCATCGTTGTTCATACA
MCP-1	CTTCTGGGCCTGCTGTTCA	CCAGCCTACTCATTGGGATCA
β-actin	GGCTGTATTCCCCTCCATCG	CCAGTTGGTAACAATGCCATGT

(NW; BMI <25 kg/m^2, n = 84) and overweight/obese subjects (OW/OB; BMI ≥ 25 kg/m^2, n = 51).

Anthropometric and Biochemical Measurements

All subjects were assessed after overnight fasting for at least 10 h. Body weight, height, systolic blood pressure (SBP) and diastolic blood pressure (DBP) were measured by an experienced physician. BMI was calculated as body weight in kilograms divided by body height squared in meters. Two 5-ml blood samples were collected from the cubital vein by one experienced nurse. Fasting blood glucose (FBG), triglycerides (TG), total cholesterol (TC), low-density lipoprotein cholesterol (LDL-C), and high-density lipoprotein cholesterol (HDL-C) were measured using an autoanalyzer (Beckman, Palo Alto, CA). Serum MK levels were determined with a commercially available enzyme-linked immunosorbent assay (ELISA) kit (DuoSet, R&D Systems, Minneapolis, MN). The linear range of the assay was 78.1–5000 pg/ml.

Animals

Male C57BL/6J leptin-deficient (ob/ob) mice and their lean littermates (6 weeks of age; n = 4 per group) were purchased from the Model Animal Research Center of Nanjing University (Nanjing, China). Mice were housed in a pathogen-free barrier facility with a 12 h light/12 h dark cycle, and given free access to water and standard chow diet (Slaccss, Shanghai) containing 20% protein and 5% fat (w/w). At 16 weeks of age, all mice were sacrificed under sodium pentobarbital anesthesia. Then, epididymal adipose tissues of the mice were immediately desected and fixed in 4% paraformaldehyde at 4°C, or snap-frozen in liquid nitrogen and stored at −80°C until use.

Cell Culture and Treatment

3T3-L1 preadipocytes and RAW264.7 macrophages were obtained from American Type Culture Collection (Rockville, MD) and maintained in DMEM supplemented with 10% FBS, 100 U/ml penicillin and 100 μg/ml streptomycin in a 5% CO2 humidified atmosphere at 37°C. Differentiation of 3T3-L1 preadipocytes was performed as described previously [25]. Briefly, 2 days postconfluence (defined as D0), cells were exposed to differentiation medium containing 0.5 mM isobutylmethylxanthine, 1 μM dexamethasone, 1.67 μM insulin (MDI) and 10% FBS. After 48 h of incubation (D2), the medium was replaced with DMEM containing 10% FBS and 1.67 μM insulin. On D4, the cells were switched to DMEM containing 10% FBS and refed every other day for the following 4–6 days until the cells were fully differentiated. Typically, more than 90% of the 3T3-L1 cells showed accumulation of multiple lipid droplets as determined by staining with Oil Red O. Before each treatment, fully differentiated 3T3-L1 adipocytes were serum starved in DMEM containing 0.25% FBS for 16 h.

To explore the effects of TNF-α and rosiglitazone on the expression of MK, serum-starved 3T3-L1 adipocytes were treated with or without TNF-α (20 ng/ml) in the presence or absence of rosiglitazone (1 μM) for 24 h. RNA and protein were extracted to evaluate the relative expression of MK mRNA by RT-PCR, and protein by western blot. To examine the role of MK on insulin signaling, serum-starved 3T3-L1 adipocytes were exposed to recombinant mouse MK (100 and 200 ng/ml) or vehicle for 24 h, followed by stimulation with 100 nM insulin for 10 min. Subsequently, phosphorylation of Akt (Ser473) and IRS-1 (Tyr612) were assessed by western blot analysis. When assessing the impact of MK on GLUT4 translocation, 3T3-L1 adipocytes were treated with MK (200 ng/ml) for 24 h, followed by insulin (100 nM) stimulation for 30 min. Plasma membrane proteins were

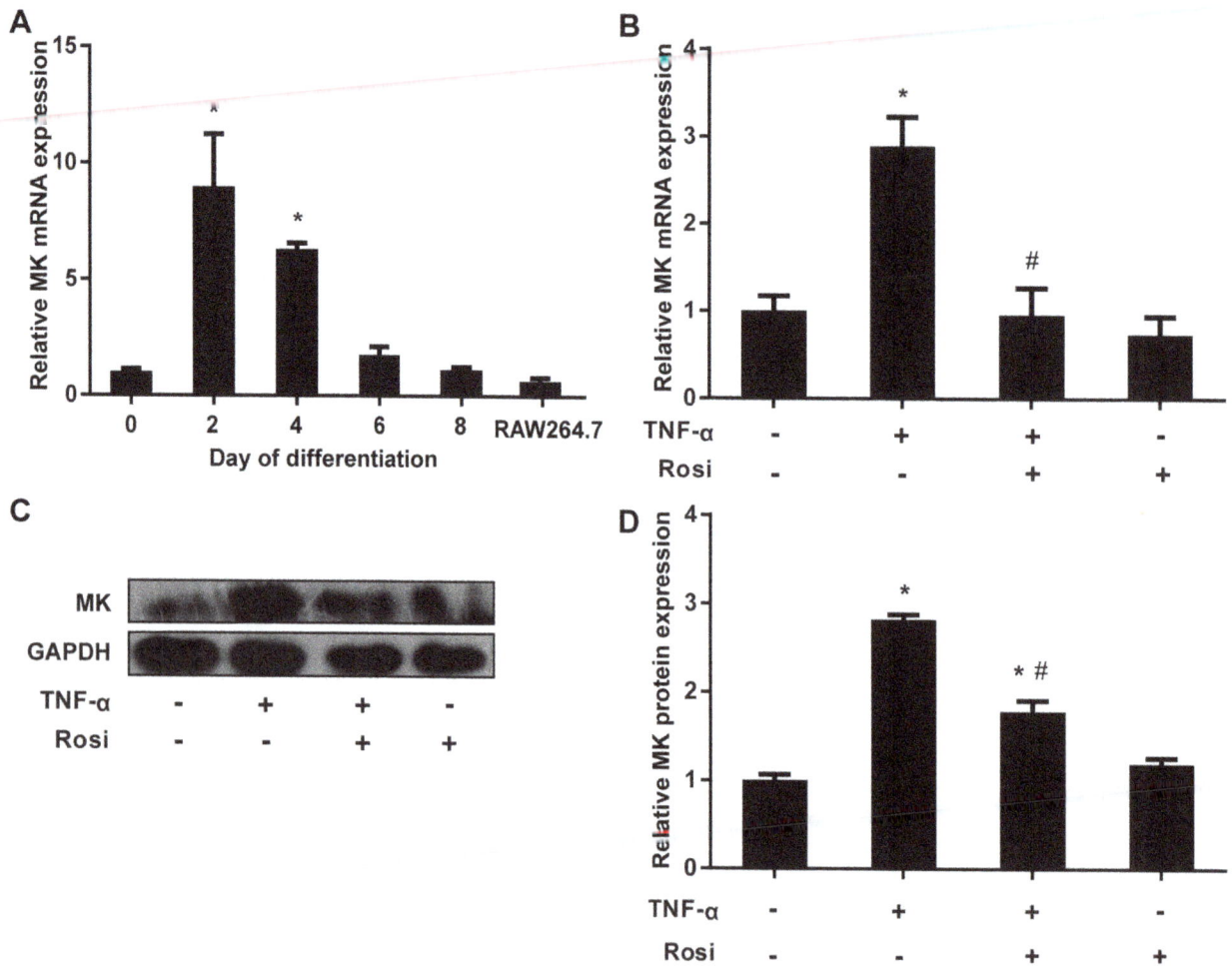

Figure 1. MK expression during preadipocyte differentiation and its regulation by inflammatory modulators in mature adipocytes.
A. 3T3-L1 preadipocytes were exposed to differentiation medium and MK mRNA expression was evaluated by quantitative RT-PCR at the indicated time points. Additionally, MK expression in RAW264.7 macrophages was also examined. Relative MK mRNA expression was expressed as fold of the D0 value. **B, C.** Differentiated 3T3-L1 adipocytes were incubated with or without TNF-α for 24 h in the presence or not of rosiglitazone (Rosi). MK expression was evaluated by quantitative RT-PCR (B) or western blot (C), and was expressed as fold of controls. D, Intensity of bands was quantified by densitometry. MK levels were normalized to GAPDH and expressed as fold of controls. Data are mean ± SE; n = 3. *P<0.05 versus control cells, #P<0.05 versus cells only treated with TNF-α.

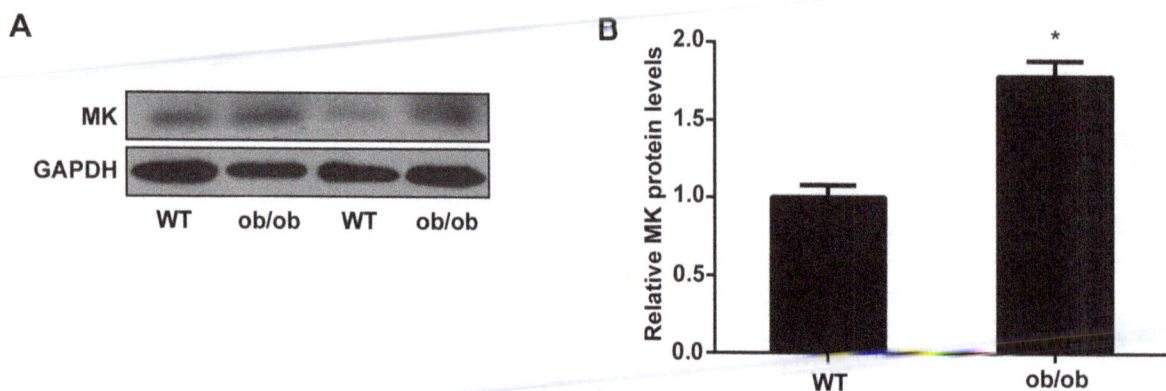

Figure 2. MK expression is increased in epididymal adipose tissue of obese ob/ob mice. A. Western blot analysis of MK protein levels in epididymal adipose tissue of leptin deficiency mice (ob/ob) and their wild-type littermate controls (WT) (n = 4 per group). Representative results are shown. **B.** Intensity of bands was quantified by densitometry. MK protein levels were normalized to GAPDH protein levels and expressed as fold of controls. Data are mean ± SE. *P<0.05 versus controls.

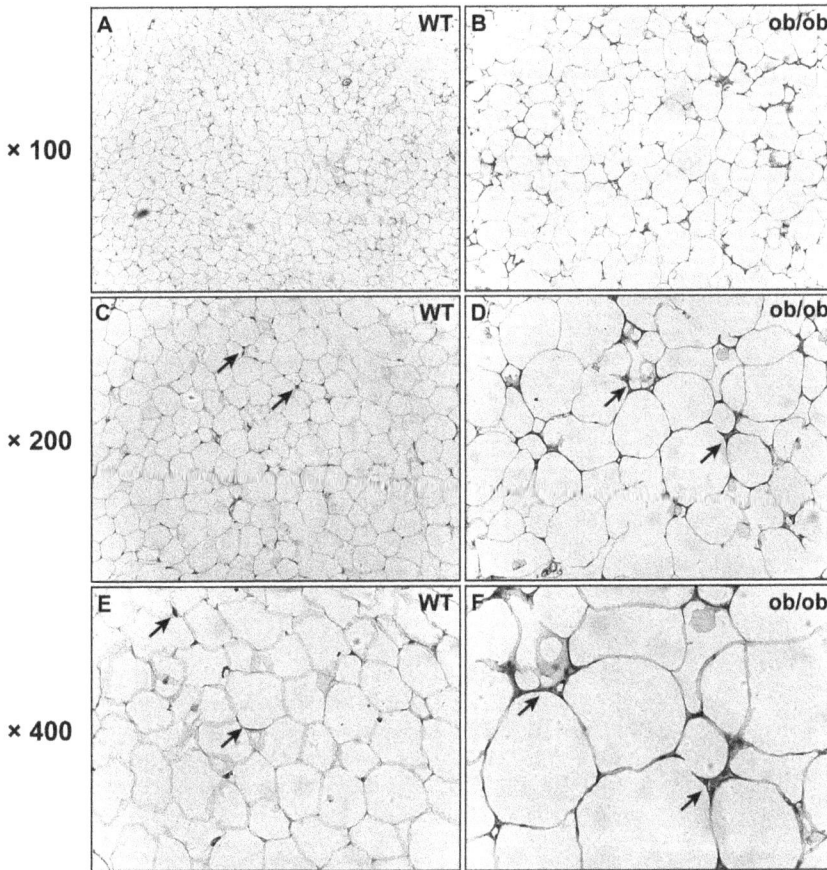

Figure 3. Immunohistochemical analysis of MK expression in epididymal adipose tissue of mice. MK expression was analyzed by immunohistochemistry in epididymal adipose tissue of leptin deficiency mice (ob/ob) (B, D, F) and their wild-type littermate controls (WT) (A, C, E) (n = 4 per group). Representative results are shown. Arrow, positive staining.

isolated and subjected to western blot. To further determine the potential mechanisms underlying the effects of MK on insulin signaling, differentiated 3T3-L1 adipocytes were treated with recombinant MK (100 ng/ml) for various time periods. Phos-

phorylated (Tyr705) and total STAT3 protein levels were assessed by western blot analysis. Moreover, SOCS3 mRNA expression was evaluated in 3T3-L1 adipocytes treated with increasing dose

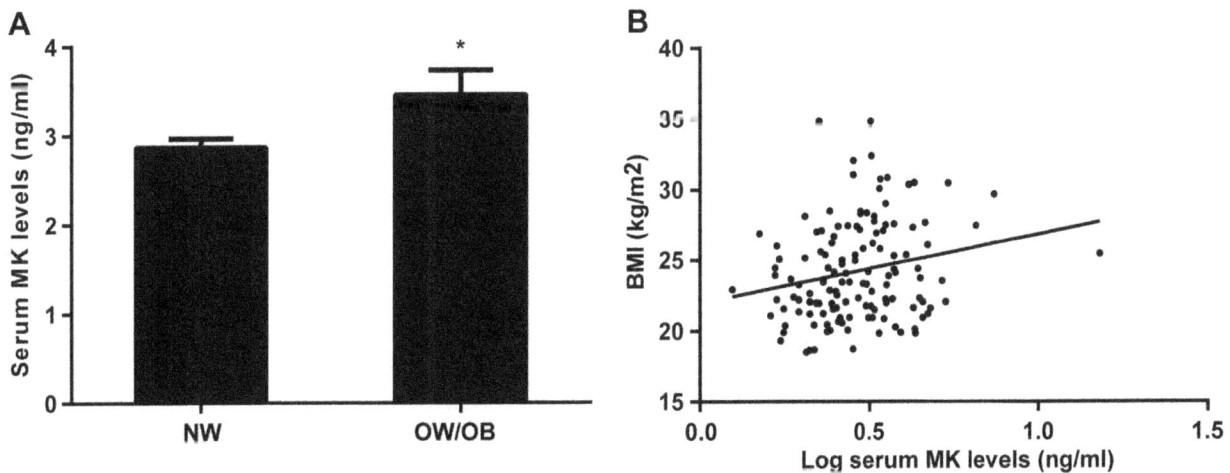

Figure 4. Serum levels of MK are associated with obesity in humans. A. Serum levels of MK in normal weight (n = 84) and overweight/obese subjects (n = 51). Data are means ± SE. NW, normal weight; OW/OB, overweight/obese. **B.** Correlation between serum levels of MK (Log transformed) and BMI. *$P < 0.05$ versus normal weight subjects.

Table 2. Clinical and biochemical characteristics of the study subjects.

Characteristics	Normal Weight	Overweight/ obese	P Value
Number of Subjects	84	51	
Age (years)	51.1±1.6	49.4±1.8	0.093
Male, n (%)	32 (38)	27 (53)	0.092
BMI (kg/m²)	22.0±0.2	27.9±0.3	<0.001
SBP (mmHg)	119.6±1.9	127.8±2.3	0.007
DBP (mmHg)	74.7±0.9	80.0±1.2	0.001
FBG (mmol/L)	4.74±0.04	4.94±0.05	0.004
TG (mmol/L)	1.31±0.08	1.86±0.12	<0.001
TC (mmol/L)	4.92±0.09	5.03±0.14	0.495
LDL-C (mmol/L)	3.14±0.09	3.29±0.13	0.338
HDL-C (mmol/L)	1.50±0.04	1.30±0.05	0.001

Data are presented as number (percentage) for categorical data, mean ± SE for continuous data. BMI, body mass index; SBP, systolic blood pressure; DBP, diastolic blood pressure; FBG, fasting blood glucose; TG, triglycerides; TC, total cholesterol; LDL-C; low-density lipoprotein cholesterol; HDL-C; high-density lipoprotein cholesterol.

of recombinant mouse MK (0, 50, 100 and 200 ng/ml) for 16 h. The cellular experiments were repeated at least 3 times.

RNA Preparation and Quantitative Real-time PCR Analysis

Total RNA was extracted from adipose tissues or cells with TRIzol Reagent (Invitrogen, Carlsbad, CA) according to the manufacturer's instructions. Next, 1 µg of total RNA was reverse-transcribed into first-strand cDNA using the Reverse Transcription system (Promega, Madison, WI). Quantitative real-time PCR was then performed in duplicate using the SYBR premix Ex Taq kit (TaKaRa, Dalian, China) on a DNA Engine Opticon 2 Real-Time PCR Detection System (Bio-Rad, Hercules, CA). Reaction conditions were 95°C for 2 min, and then 40 cycles of 95°C for 15 s/60°C for 30 s. The primer sequences are listed in Table 1. Gene expression was normalized to β-actin using the ΔΔct method.

Western Blot Analysis

For whole cell protein extraction, adipose tissues or cells were lysed in RIPA buffer (50 mM Tris·HCl, pH 7.4, 150 mM NaCl, 1% NP-40, 0.5% sodium deoxycholate, 0.1% SDS) containing protease and phosphatase inhibitors (5 mM EDTA, 1 mM PMSF, 1 mM sodium orthovanadate) for 30 min on ice. After centrifugation, the supernatants were collected and protein concentrations were determined by the BCA protein assay (Pierce, Rockford, IL). For plasma membrane protein isolation, the Pierce Cell Surface Protein Isolation Kit was used according to the manufacturer's instructions (Pierce, Rockford, IL). Equal amounts of protein from each sample were electrophoresed on 12% SDS-PAGE gels and then transferred to polyvinylidene difluoride membranes (Millipore, Bedford, MA). The membranes were blocked with 5% skim milk in TBS containing 0.1% Tween-20 for 1 h at room temperature, and then incubated with different primary antibodies overnight at 4°C. After washing and incubating with HRP-conjugated secondary antibodies for 1 h at room temperature, immunoreactive proteins were visualized using SuperSignal Pico ECL reagent (Pierce, Rockford, IL) and exposed to film. To

reprobe with different antibodies, the membranes were stripped in stripping buffer containing 62.5 mM Tris·HCl, PH 6.8, 2% SDS, and 100 mM β-mercaptoethanol at 50°C for 20–30 min with shaking.

Immunohistochemical Analysis

Adipose tissues fixed in 4% paraformaldehyde were embedded in paraffin and sectioned to a thickness of 5 µm. The sections were then deparaffinized in xylene and endogenous peroxidase activity was depleted with 0.3% hydrogen peroxide for 30 min at room temperature. For immunostaining of MK, the sections were first blocked with phosphate-buffered saline (PBS) containing 5% normal goat serum for 60 min at room temperature, followed by incubation with goat anti-MK antibody overnight at 4°C. The sections were washed three times with PBS and then incubated with HRP-conjugated rabbit anti-goat secondary antibody for 1 h at room temperature. After three washes with PBS, the sections were incubated with 0.1% diaminobenzidine (DAB) solution for 5–10 min. The nuclei were counterstained with hematoxylin for 5 min. Finally, images were acquired on a Zeiss microscope fitted with an Axiocam MRc camera and using Axiovision software (Carl Zeiss, Thornwood, NY).

Statistical Analysis

Data are presented as means ± SE unless otherwise stated. Non-normally distributed data were logarithmically transformed before analysis. Comparisons between groups were carried out using unpaired Student's t-test (for comparisons between two groups) or one-way ANOVA with Bonferroni post hoc test (for multiple group comparisons). MK expression at different time points during preadipocyte differentiation was compared using repeated measures of ANOVA. Pearson's test was used for the correlation analyses in the clinical study. All statistical analyses were performed with SPSS 13.0 (Chicago, IL). $P<0.05$ was considered statistically significant.

Results

MK Expression is Dynamically Regulated during Preadipocyte Differentiation

To explore the role of MK in adipocytes, we first assessed the expression pattern of MK upon 3T3-L1 preadipocyte differentiation. As previously reported [21], MK mRNA expression increased dramatically after differentiation and reached a peak on D2 (9-fold relative to D0, $P<0.05$) (Figure 1A). Thereafter, the expression of MK gradually decreased and returned to the D0 levels on D8 (Figure 1A), consistent with its mitogenic effect on preadipocytes after initiation of differentiation [21]. Additionally, MK mRNA expression levels in differentiated 3T3-L1 adipocytes on D8 were comparable to those in RAW264.7 macrophages (Figure 1A).

TNF-α and Rosiglitazone Regulate MK Expression in Adipocytes

It has been reported that MK is upregulated by inflammatory stimuli (e.g., TNF-α and IL-1β) in several cell types [26,27]. To determine whether MK expression in adipocytes is also modulated by inflammatory modulators, we treated 3T3-L1 adipocytes with TNF-α and/or rosiglitazone, which are well known to promote and attenuate inflammation in adipocytes, respectively [28,29]. As shown in Figure 1B, TNF-α treatment led to a marked increase in MK mRNA expression in 3T3-L1 adipocytes. Of note, this increase was completely abrogated by rosiglitazone (Figure 1B).

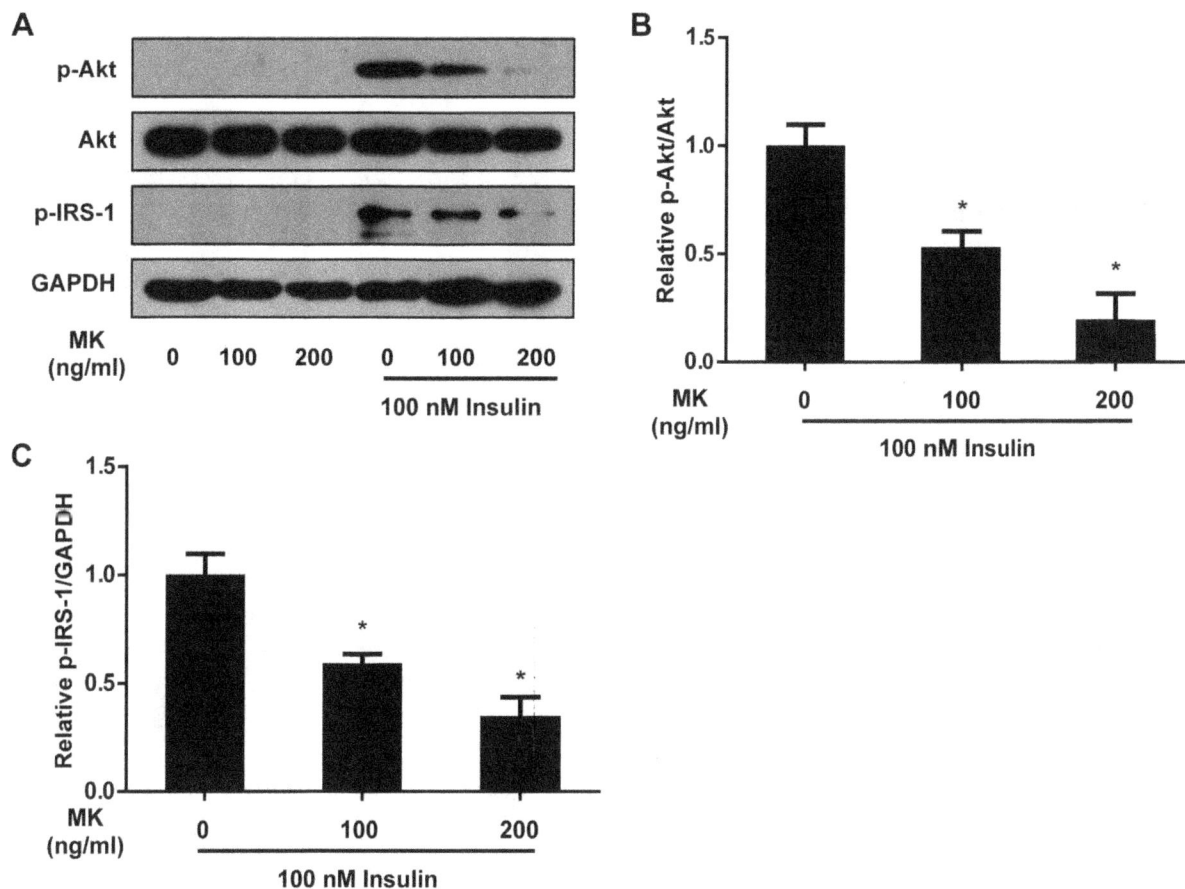

Figure 5. MK inhibits insulin signaling in 3T3-L1 adipocytes. A. Differentiated 3T3-L1 adipocytes were treated with recombinant mouse MK or vehicle for 24 h, and subsequently stimulated with insulin for 10 min. Phosphorylation of Akt (Ser473) and IRS-1 (Tyr612) were assessed by western blot analysis and representative results are shown. B, C. Intensity of bands was quantified by densitometry. Phosphorylated protein levels were normalized to total protein or GAPDH and expressed as fold of insulin-stimulated controls. Data are mean ± SE; n = 3. *P<0.05 versus control cells stimulated with insulin.

Consistent with the mRNA results, TNF-α induced MK protein expression in adipocytes, which was significantly attenuated by rosiglitazone (Figure 1C and D). Together, MK expression in adipocytes seems to be regulated by inflammatory modulators.

MK Expression is Increased in Adipose Tissue of Obese ob/ob Mice

To probe the role of MK in vivo, we then examined its expression levels in epididymal adipose tissue of ob/ob mice, a

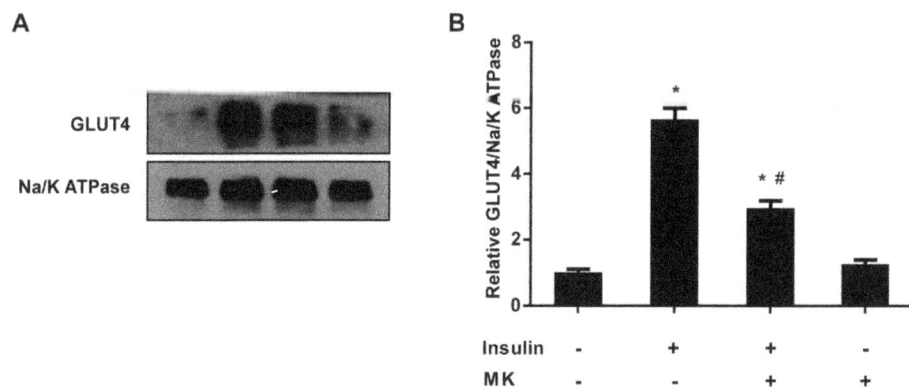

Figure 6. MK inhibits insulin-stimulated GLUT4 translocation in 3T3-L1 adipocytes. A. Differentiated 3T3-L1 adipocytes were treated with recombinant mouse MK or vehicle for 24 h, and subsequently stimulated with insulin for 30 min. Plasma membrane proteins were isolated and GLUT4 was assessed by western blot analysis. Representative results are shown. B. Intensity of bands was quantified by densitometry. GLUT4 protein levels were normalized to Na/K ATPase and expressed as fold of controls. Data are mean ± SE; n = 3. *P<0.05 versus control cells. #P<0.05 versus cells only treated with insulin.

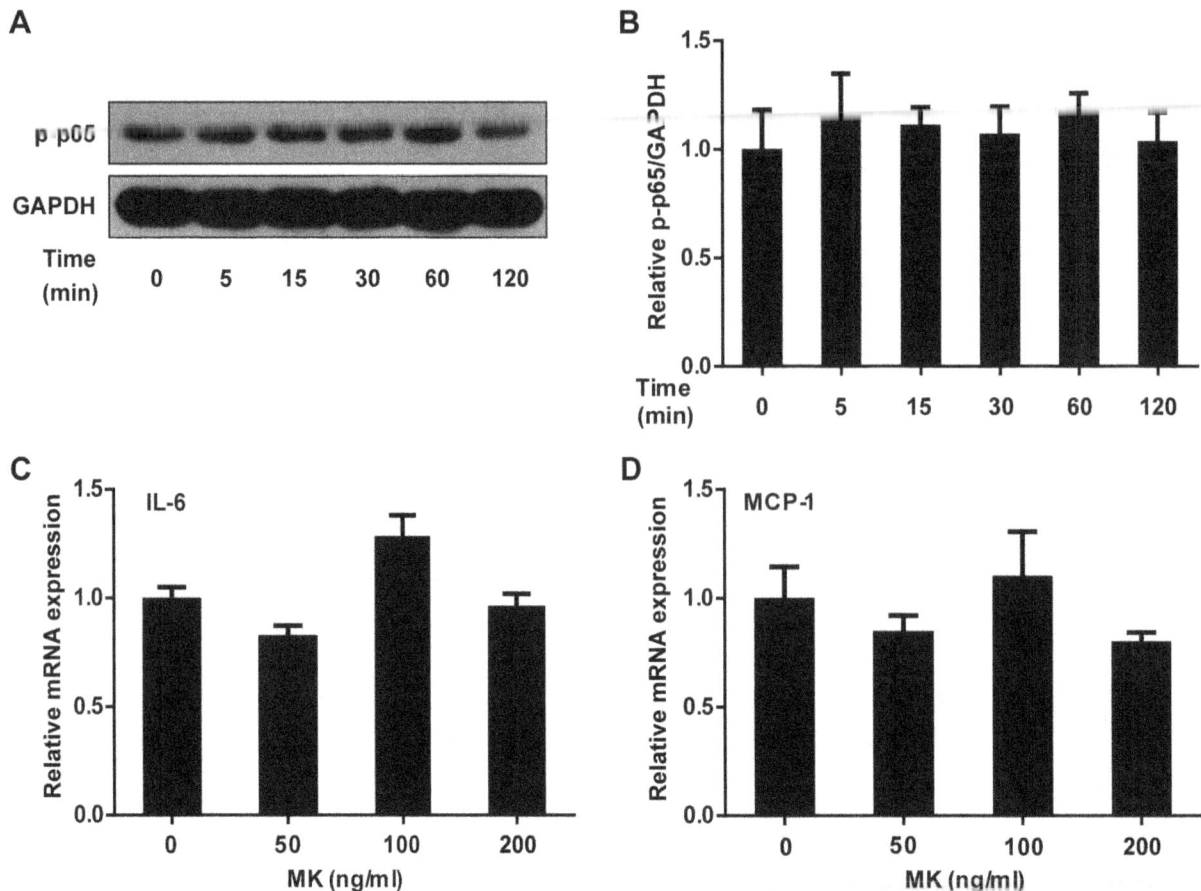

Figure 7. MK does not activate NFκB signaling in 3T3-L1 adipocytes. A. Differentiated 3T3-L1 adipocytes were treated with recombinant MK for the indicated time periods. Phosphorylation of p65/NFκB (Ser536) was assessed by western blot analysis and representative results are shown. **B.** Intensity of bands was quantified by densitometry. Phosphorylated p65/NFκB levels were normalized to GAPDH and expressed as fold of controls. **C, D.** Differentiated 3T3-L1 adipocytes were treated with increasing dose of recombinant MK for 16 h. IL-6 (C) and MCP-1 (D) mRNA expression were evaluated by quantitative RT-PCR. Relative gene expression was expressed as fold of controls. Data are mean ± SE; n = 3. *$P < 0.05$ versus controls.

well-characterized model of severe genetic obesity and insulin resistance due to leptin deficiency [30]. As assessed by western blot analysis, MK protein expression was significantly increased in epididymal adipose tissue of ob/ob mice when compared with their lean littermate controls (Figure 2). In addition, we performed immunohistochemical analysis of adipose tissue from mice. As shown in Figure 3, MK was detected in both adipocytes and stromal cells of adipose tissue. Moreover, MK expression was increased in epididymal adipose tissue of ob/ob mice relative to controls (Figure 3). Together, these results indicate an association between MK and obesity in vivo.

Serum MK Levels are Associated with Obesity in Humans

In light of the above in vitro and animal results, we further assessed the clinical relevance of MK in humans by determining its serum levels in overweight/obese subjects. Clinical and biochemical characteristics of the study subjects are shown in Table 2. Serum MK levels were significantly higher in overweight/obese subjects than in control subjects, [3.46±0.28 ng/ml versus 2.07±0.10 ng/ml, $P = 0.022$] (Figure 4A). After adjustment for age and sex by covariance analysis, the difference remained significant [3.50±0.20 ng/ml versus 2.84±0.16 ng/ml,

$P = 0.012$]. Furthermore, there was a positive correlation between serum MK levels and BMI ($r = 0.214$, $P = 0.013$, Figure 4B), and the correlation remained significant after adjusting for age and sex by partial correlation analysis ($r = 0.234$, $P = 0.007$). Together, our results show that MK is associated with obesity in humans.

MK Impairs Insulin Signaling in 3T3-L1 Adipocytes

We next sought to explore the pathophysiological significance of increased MK expression in obesity. Given its proinflammatory properties, we determined whether MK could attenuate insulin signaling in adipocytes, just like other inflammatory mediators [7]. Fully differentiated 3T3-L1 adipocytes were exposed to recombinant MK for 24 h and insulin signal transduction was then examined. As shown in Figure 5A and B, insulin-stimulated phosphorylation of Akt on Ser473, a commonly used marker of insulin signaling [31], was markedly reduced by MK treatment. Additionally, insulin signaling event upstream of Akt was also assessed. Consistently, MK decreased specific tyrosine phosphorylation of insulin receptor substrate 1 (IRS-1) on Tyr612 in response to insulin stimulation (Figure 5A and C). Taken together, our results show that MK impairs insulin signaling in 3T3-L1 adipocytes.

A

p-STAT3

STAT3

Time (min) 0 5 15 30 60 120

B

C

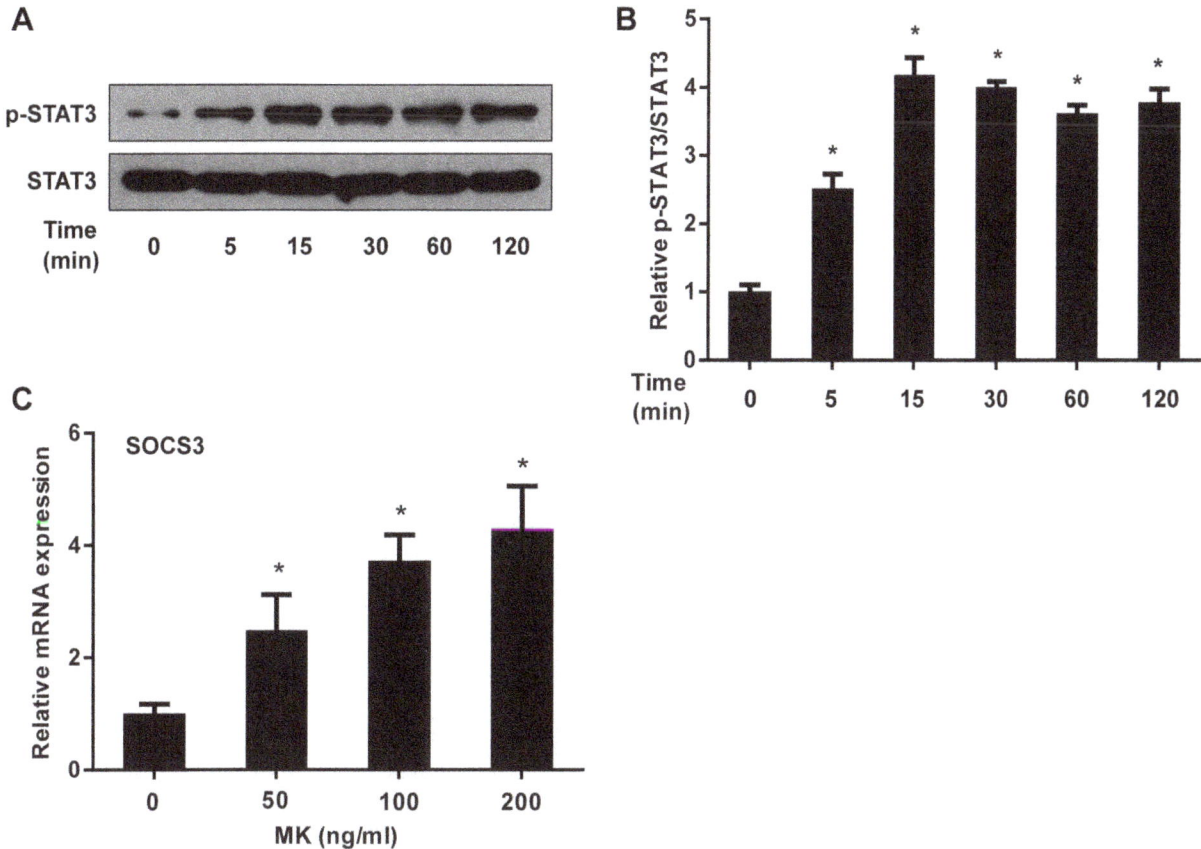

Figure 8. MK activates the STAT3-SOCS3 pathway in 3T3-L1 adipocytes. A. Differentiated 3T3-L1 adipocytes were treated with recombinant MK for the indicated time periods. Phosphorylated (Tyr705) and total STAT3 protein were assessed by western blot analysis and representative results are shown. **B.** Intensity of bands was quantified by densitometry. Phosphorylated STAT3 levels were normalized to total STAT3 and expressed as fold of controls. **C.** Differentiated 3T3-L1 adipocytes were treated with increasing dose of recombinant mouse MK for 16 h. SOCS3 mRNA expression was evaluated by quantitative RT-PCR. Relative gene expression was expressed as fold of controls. Data are mean ± SE; n = 3. *$P<0.05$ versus controls.

MK Reduces Insulin-stimulated GLUT4 Translocation in 3T3-L1 Adipocytes

Insulin-stimulated translocation of the glucose transporter GLUT4 to the cell surface in adipocytes is the basis for insulin-stimulated glucose uptake. In light of the inhibitory effects of MK on insulin signaling, we tested whether MK could reduce insulin-stimulated translocation of GLUT4. After 24 h treatment with MK, 3T3-L1 adipocytes were stimulated with 100 nM insulin for 30 min and plasma membrane GLUT4 protein was evaluated by western blot analysis. As shown in Figure 6, MK significantly reduced insulin-stimulated translocation of GLUT4 to the plasma membrane, consistent with its inhibitory effects on insulin signaling in adipocytes.

MK Does Not Activate NFκB Signaling in Adipocytes

The possible mechanisms underlying the suppressive effects of MK on insulin signaling were further investigated. As NFκB signaling plays a central role in insulin resistance and can be activated by MK in other cell types [32,33], we examined the actions of MK on this pathway in adipocytes. 3T3-L1 adipocytes were treated with recombinant MK, and the phosphorylaion of NFκB as well as the expression of inflammatory mediators was assessed. As shown in Figure 7A and B, MK did not induce the phosphorylation of p65/NFκB. Accordingly, IL-6 and MCP-1 mRNA expression in adipocytes were unchanged by MK

(Figure 7C and D). Thus, MK does not activate NFκB signaling in adipocytes.

MK Activates the STAT3-SOCS3 Pathway in Adipocytes

In addition to NFκB signaling, the STAT3-SOCS3 pathway is critical in cytokine-induced insulin resistance [34–36]. Of note, MK has been reported to activate STAT3 in 3T3-L1 preadipocytes, which prompted us to test whether MK also stimulates this signaling pathway in mature adipocytes. As shown in Figure 8A and B, as early as 5 min after MK treatment, significantly increased phosphorylation of STAT3 on Tyr705 was observed. This increase sustained up to 120 min. Moreover, the expression of SOCS3, a downstream target of STAT3, was also induced by MK in a dose-dependent manner (Figure 8C). These findings indicate that MK is a potent activator of the STAT3-SOCS3 pathway in mature adipocytes.

Discussion

As a novel endocrine and immune organ, adipose tissue secretes a variety of adipokines that are directly involved in inflammation and insulin resistance. In this study, we investigated the association of MK with obesity and its actions on adipocytes. MK was found to be expressed in adipocytes and regulated by inflammatory modulators. Notably, MK levels were increased in adipose tissue of obese mice and in serum of overweight/obese subjects as

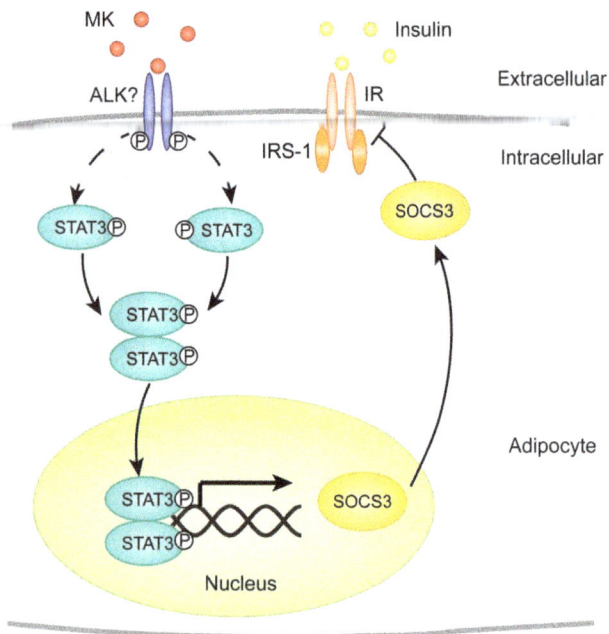

Figure 9. Schematic diagram of mechanisms of MK actions in adipocytes. Probably through anaplastic lymphoma kinase (ALK), a transmembrane receptor, MK induces tyrosine phosphorylation and dimeration of STAT3, which translocates to the nucleus and stimulates the transcription of SOCS3. Subsequently, SOCS3 inhibits insulin signaling by interacting with insulin receptor and IRS-1.

compared with their controls. In vitro experiments further revealed inhibitory effects of MK on insulin signaling in 3T3-L1 adipocytes, with activation of the STAT3-SOCS3 pathway. Our findings suggest a potential role of MK in obesity-induced insulin resistance.

MK is expressed in multiple cell types, including various immune and cancer cells [37,38]. Here, we found MK expression in both 3T3-L1 preadipocytes and mature adipocytes. In preadipocytes, MK expression increased immediately after differentiation and then declined progressively to the beginning levels, consistent with its essential role in promoting the mitotic clonal expansion of preadipocytes [21]. In mature adipocytes, MK was regulated by inflammatory modulators. TNF-α treatment led to a marked increase in MK expression, which was completely abolished by rosiglitazone, a potent PPARγ agonist with antiinflammatory actions. Thus, in line with its inflammatory properties, MK seems closely associated with the inflammatory state of mature adipocytes.

In addition to the adipocyte cell line in vitro, MK is also expressed in adipose tissue of mice. Importantly, MK expression was upregulated in epididymal adipose tissue of obese mice. Furthermore, overweight/obese humans had significantly increased serum MK levels compared with control subjects, with a positive correlation between serum MK and BMI. Collectively, MK is associated with obesity in both mice and humans. The mechanisms for MK upregulation in obese adipose tissue may be multiple and remain to be elucidated. TNF-α, which is increased in obesity [39], induces MK expression in adipocytes, and is therefore a potential candidate for the upregulation of MK. As MK is also expressed by macrophages, which are recruited into adipose tissue in obesity, they may be another source of MK in adipose tissue. In fact, we observed increased expression of MK in stromal cells, which are largely composed of macrophages, in

adipose tissue of ob/ob mice compared with controls. Nevertheless, the relative contribution of adipocytes and macrophages to the elevated expression of MK in obese adipose tissue remains to be determined. In addition, as a secreted protein by adipose tissue, MK serum concentration in mice and its relationship with obesity warrant future study.

Adipose tissue produces a range of adipokines that are directly involved in insulin resistance [7]. Herein, we showed that MK suppressed insulin signaling in adipocytes, as indicated by reduced phosphorylation of Akt and IRS-1 in response to insulin stimulation. These findings provide the first evidence that MK may be a novel inducer of insulin resistance. Since MK expression was increased in adipose tissue of obese mice, it warrants further investigation whether MK induces insulin resistance in vivo. Moreover, as serum MK levels were significantly elevated in obese subjects and correlated with BMI, further analysis of its relationship with insulin sensitivity will provide additional evidence for its actions on insulin resistance in humans. In addition, given the chemotactic activities of MK towards macrophages [16], which play a central role in obesity-induced inflammation and insulin resistance [40], future studies will also investigate the involvement of MK in macrophage recruitment into adipose tissue during obesity.

Though MK attenuates insulin signaling in adipocytes, the signal events by which MK interacts with insulin signal transduction remain to be clarified. The STAT3-SOCS3 pathway has been demonstrated to play a critical role in insulin resistance [34,41]. On activation, STAT3 dimerizes and translocates to the nucleus, inducing the expression of SOCS3, which in turn inhibits insulin signaling by direct interaction with the insulin receptor and by preventing the coupling of IRS-1 with the insulin receptor [42,43]. To date, a range of adipokines (e.g., IL-6, TNF-α and resistin) have been reported to promote insulin resistance in adipocytes through the STAT3-SOCS3 pathway [34–36]. In this study, we observed that MK also activated the STAT3-SOCS3 pathway in 3T3-L1 adipocytes, consistent with previous studies showing stimulative effects of MK on STAT3 in preadipocytes and keratinocytes [21,44]. Thus, MK is a potent activator of the STAT3-SOCS3 signaling cascade, which may mediate the inhibitory effects of MK on insulin signaling in adipocytes.

Another question not addressed is how MK activates the STAT3-SOCS3 pathway in adipocytes. Previous studies have proposed multiple molecules as the receptor of MK, including anaplastic lymphoma kinase (ALK), protein-tyrosine phosphatase ζ (PTPζ), low density lipoprotein receptor-related protein (LRP) and integrin [8,45–47]. Among them, ALK is a transmembrane receptor tyrosine kinase that has been shown to activate STAT3 [48]. Additionally, we detected ALK expression in adipocytes (data not shown). Thus, it may be through ALK that MK activates the STAT3-SOCS3 pathway in adipocytes, which further impairs insulin signal transduction, as illustrated in Figure 9.

In summary, we show here that MK is expressed in adipocytes and is associated with obesity in both mice and humans. Moreover, as revealed by reduced phosphorylation of Akt and IRS-1 and decreased GLUT4 translocation in response to insulin stimulation, MK suppresses insulin signaling in adipocytes, associated with activation of the STAT3-SOCS3 signaling pathway. Therefore, MK is a potential link between obesity and insulin resistance, and may offer a new target to treat insulin resistance and other obesity-associated diseases.

Acknowledgments

We thank Dr. Jiqiu Wang, Dr. Maopei Chen, Dr. Yinkai Sun, and Dr Minglan Liu for technical assistance.

Author Contributions

Conceived and designed the experiments: NGF YDP. Performed the experiments: NGF HYS YFW. Analyzed the data: NGF LJZ RL.

Contributed reagents/materials/analysis tools: ZHX LP YQH WQS. Wrote the paper: NGF.

References

1. Franks PW, Hanson RL, Knowler WC, Sievers ML, Bennett PH, et al. (2010) Childhood obesity, other cardiovascular risk factors, and premature death. N Engl J Med 362: 485–493.
2. Shang X, Li J, Tao Q, Li J, Li X, et al. (2013) Educational Level, Obesity and Incidence of Diabetes among Chinese Adult Men and Women Aged 18–59 Years Old: An 11-Year Follow-Up Study. PLoS One 8: e66479.
3. Waki H, Tontonoz P (2007) Endocrine functions of adipose tissue. Annu Rev Pathol 2: 31–56.
4. Galic S, Oakhill JS, Steinberg GR (2010) Adipose tissue as an endocrine organ. Mol Cell Endocrinol 316: 129–139.
5. Maury E, Brichard SM (2010) Adipokine dysregulation, adipose tissue inflammation and metabolic syndrome. Mol Cell Endocrinol 314: 1–16.
6. Tilg H, Moschen AR (2006) Adipocytokines: mediators linking adipose tissue, inflammation and immunity. Nat Rev Immunol 6: 772–783.
7. Ouchi N, Parker JL, Lugus JJ, Walsh K (2011) Adipokines in inflammation and metabolic disease. Nat Rev Immunol 11: 85–97.
8. Kadomatsu K, Kishida S, Tsubota S (2013) The heparin-binding growth factor midkine: the biological activities and candidate receptors. J Biochem 153: 511–521.
9. Kadomatsu K, Tomomura M, Muramatsu T (1988) cDNA cloning and sequencing of a new gene intensely expressed in early differentiation stages of embryonal carcinoma cells and in mid-gestation period of mouse embryogenesis. Biochem Biophys Res Commun 151: 1312–1318.
10. Muramatsu T (1993) Midkine (MK), the product of a retinoic acid responsive gene, and pleiotrophin constitute a new protein family regulating growth and differentiation. Int J Dev Biol 37: 183–188.
11. Weckbach LT, Groesser L, Borgolte J, Pagel JI, Pogoda F, et al. (2012) Midkine acts as proangiogenic cytokine in hypoxia-induced angiogenesis. Am J Physiol Heart Circ Physiol 303: H429–438.
12. Sueyoshi T, Jono H, Shinriki S, Ota K, Ota T, et al. (2012) Therapeutic approaches targeting midkine suppress tumor growth and lung metastasis in osteosarcoma. Cancer Lett 316: 23–30.
13. Michikawa M, Kikuchi S, Muramatsu H, Muramatsu T, Kim SU (1993) Retinoic acid responsive gene product, midkine, has neurotrophic functions for mouse spinal cord and dorsal root ganglion neurons in culture. J Neurosci Res 35: 530–539.
14. Weckbach LT, Muramatsu T, Walzog B (2011) Midkine in inflammation. ScientificWorldJournal 11: 2491–2505.
15. Takada T, Toriyama K, Muramatsu H, Song XJ, Torii S, et al. (1997) Midkine, a retinoic acid-inducible heparin-binding cytokine in inflammatory responses: chemotactic activity to neutrophils and association with inflammatory synovitis. J Biochem 122: 453–458.
16. Horiba M, Kadomatsu K, Nakamura E, Muramatsu H, Ikematsu S, et al. (2000) Neointima formation in a restenosis model is suppressed in midkine-deficient mice. J Clin Invest 105: 489–495.
17. Wang J, Takeuchi H, Sonobe Y, Jin S, Mizuno T, et al. (2008) Inhibition of midkine alleviates experimental autoimmune encephalomyelitis through the expansion of regulatory T cell population. Proc Natl Acad Sci U S A 105: 3915–3920.
18. Maruyama K, Muramatsu H, Ishiguro N, Muramatsu T (2004) Midkine, a heparin-binding growth factor, is fundamentally involved in the pathogenesis of rheumatoid arthritis. Arthritis Rheum 50: 1420–1429.
19. Krzystek-Korpacka M, Neubauer K, Matusiewicz M (2010) Circulating midkine in Crohn's disease: clinical implications. Inflamm Bowel Dis 16: 208–215.
20. Krzystek-Korpacka M, Neubauer K, Matusiewicz M (2009) Clinical relevance of circulating midkine in ulcerative colitis. Clin Chem Lab Med 47: 1085–1090.
21. Cernkovich ER, Deng J, Hua K, Harp JB (2007) Midkine is an autocrine activator of signal transducer and activator of transcription 3 in 3T3-L1 cells. Endocrinology 148: 1598–1604.
22. Ratovitski EA, Kotzbauer PT, Milbrandt J, Lowenstein CJ, Burrow CR (1998) Midkine induces tumor cell proliferation and binds to a high affinity signaling receptor associated with JAK tyrosine kinases. J Biol Chem 273: 3654–3660.
23. Kadomatsu K, Hagihara M, Akhter S, Fan QW, Muramatsu H, et al. (1997) Midkine induces the transformation of NIH3T3 cells. Br J Cancer 75: 354–359.
24. Lucas S Fau - Henze G, Henze G Fau - Schnabel D, Schnabel D Fau - Barthlen W, Barthlen W Fau - Sakuma S, Sakuma S Fau - Kurtz A, et al. (2010) Serum levels of Midkine in children and adolescents without malignant disease.
25. Student AK, Hsu RY, Lane MD (1980) Induction of fatty acid synthetase synthesis in differentiating 3T3-L1 preadipocytes. J Biol Chem 255: 4745–4750.
26. You Z, Dong Y, Kong X, Beckett LA, Gandour-Edwards R, et al. (2008) Midkine is a NF-kappaB-inducible gene that supports prostate cancer cell survival. BMC Med Genomics 1: 6.
27. Yazihan N, Karakurt O, Ataoglu H (2008) Erythropoietin reduces lipopolysaccharide-induced cell Damage and midkine secretion in U937 human histiocytic lymphoma cells. Adv Ther 25: 502–514.
28. Hotamisligil GS, Peraldi P, Budavari A, Ellis R, White MF, et al. (1996) IRS-1-mediated inhibition of insulin receptor tyrosine kinase activity in TNF-alpha- and obesity-induced insulin resistance. Science 271: 665–668.
29. Delerive P, Fruchart JC, Staels B (2001) Peroxisome proliferator-activated receptors in inflammation control. J Endocrinol 169: 453–459.
30. Friedman JM, Halaas JL (1998) Leptin and the regulation of body weight in mammals. Nature 395: 763–770.
31. Stienstra R, Joosten LA, Koenen T, van Tits B, van Diepen JA, et al. (2010) The inflammasome-mediated caspase-1 activation controls adipocyte differentiation and insulin sensitivity. Cell Metab 12: 593–605.
32. Kuo AH, Stoica GE, Riegel AT, Wellstein A (2007) Recruitment of insulin receptor substrate-1 and activation of NF-kappaB essential for midkine growth signaling through anaplastic lymphoma kinase. Oncogene 26: 859–869.
33. Baker RG, Hayden MS, Ghosh S (2011) NF-kappaB, inflammation, and metabolic disease. Cell Metab 13: 11–22.
34. Serrano-Marco L, Rodriguez-Calvo R, El Kochairi I, Palomer X, Michalik L, et al. (2011) Activation of peroxisome proliferator-activated receptor-beta/−delta (PPAR-beta/−delta) ameliorates insulin signaling and reduces SOCS3 levels by inhibiting STAT3 in interleukin-6-stimulated adipocytes. Diabetes 60: 1990–1999.
35. Steppan CM, Wang J, Whiteman EL, Birnbaum MJ, Lazar MA (2005) Activation of SOCS-3 by resistin. Mol Cell Biol 25: 1569–1575.
36. Ishizuka K, Usui I, Kanatani Y, Bukhari A, He J, et al. (2007) Chronic tumor necrosis factor-alpha treatment causes insulin resistance via insulin receptor substrate-1 serine phosphorylation and suppressor of cytokine signaling-3 induction in 3T3-L1 adipocytes. Endocrinology 148: 2994–3003.
37. Narita H Fau - Chen S, Chen S Fau - Komori K, Komori K Fau - Kadomatsu K, Kadomatsu K (2008) Midkine is expressed by infiltrating macrophages in in-stent restenosis in hypercholesterolemic rabbits.
38. Dai LC, Yao X, Wang X, Niu SQ, Zhou LF, et al. (2009) In vitro and in vivo suppression of hepatocellular carcinoma growth by midkine-antisense oligonucleotide-loaded nanoparticles. World J Gastroenterol 15: 1966–1972.
39. Hotamisligil GS, Shargill NS, Spiegelman BM (1993) Adipose expression of tumor necrosis factor-alpha: direct role in obesity-linked insulin resistance. Science 259: 87–91.
40. Olefsky JM, Glass CK (2010) Macrophages, inflammation, and insulin resistance. Annu Rev Physiol 72: 219–246.
41. Palanivel R, Fullerton MD, Galic S, Honeyman J, Hewitt KA, et al. (2012) Reduced Socs3 expression in adipose tissue protects female mice against obesity-induced insulin resistance. Diabetologia 55: 3083–3093.
42. Emanuelli B, Peraldi P, Filloux C, Chavey C, Freidinger K, et al. (2001) SOCS-3 inhibits insulin signaling and is up-regulated in response to tumor necrosis factor-alpha in the adipose tissue of obese mice. J Biol Chem 276: 47944–47949.
43. Emanuelli B, Peraldi P, Filloux C, Sawka-Verhelle D, Hilton D, et al. (2000) SOCS-3 is an insulin-induced negative regulator of insulin signaling. J Biol Chem 275: 15985–15991.
44. Huang Y, Hoque MO, Wu F, Trink B, Sidransky D, et al. (2008) Midkine induces epithelial-mesenchymal transition through Notch2/Jak2-Stat3 signaling in human keratinocytes. Cell Cycle 7: 1613 1622.
45. Stoica GE, Kuo A, Powers C, Bowden ET, Sale EB, et al. (2002) Midkine binds to anaplastic lymphoma kinase (ALK) and acts as a growth factor for different cell types. J Biol Chem 277: 35990–35998.
46. Maeda N, Ichihara-Tanaka K, Kimura T, Kadomatsu K, Muramatsu T, et al. (1999) A receptor-like protein-tyrosine phosphatase PTPzeta/RPTPbeta binds a heparin-binding growth factor midkine. Involvement of arginine 78 of midkine in the high affinity binding to PTPzeta. J Biol Chem 274: 12474–12479.
47. Muramatsu H, Zou P, Suzuki H, Oda Y, Chen GY, et al. (2004) alpha4beta1- and alpha6beta1-integrins are functional receptors for midkine, a heparin-binding growth factor. J Cell Sci 117: 5405–5415.
48. Chiarle R, Simmons WJ, Cai H, Dhall G, Zamo A, et al. (2005) Stat3 is required for ALK-mediated lymphomagenesis and provides a possible therapeutic target. Nat Med 11: 623–629.

PPAR Agonist-Induced Reduction of Mcp1 in Atherosclerotic Plaques of Obese, Insulin-Resistant Mice Depends on Adiponectin-Induced Irak3 Expression

Maarten Hulsmans[1,◐], Benjamine Geeraert[1,◐], Thierry Arnould[2], Christos Tsatsanis[3], Paul Holvoet[1]*

1 Atherosclerosis and Metabolism Unit, Department of Cardiovascular Sciences, KU Leuven, Leuven, Belgium, **2** Laboratory of Biochemistry and Cell Biology (URBC), NAmur Research Institute for LIfe Sciences (NARILIS), University of Namur (FUNDP), Namur, Belgium, **3** Department of Clinical Chemistry, School of Medicine, University of Crete, Heraklion, Greece

Abstract

Synthetic peroxisome proliferator-activated receptor (PPAR) agonists are used to treat dyslipidemia and insulin resistance. In this study, we examined molecular mechanisms that explain differential effects of a PPARα agonist (fenofibrate) and a PPARγ agonist (rosiglitazone) on macrophages during obesity-induced atherogenesis. Twelve-week-old mice with combined leptin and LDL-receptor deficiency (DKO) were treated with fenofibrate, rosiglitazone or placebo for 12 weeks. Only rosiglitazone improved adipocyte function, restored insulin sensitivity, and inhibited atherosclerosis by decreasing lipid-loaded macrophages. In addition, it increased *interleukin-1 receptor-associated kinase-3* (*Irak3*) and decreased *monocyte chemoattractant protein-1* (*Mcp1*) expressions, indicative of a switch from M1 to M2 macrophages. The differences between fenofibrate and rosiglitazone were independent of *Pparγ* expression. In bone marrow-derived macrophages (BMDM), we identified the rosiglitazone-associated increase in adiponectin as cause of the increase in Irak3. Interestingly, the deletion of Irak3 in BMDM (IRAK3$^{-/-}$ BMDM) resulted in activation of the canonical NFκB signaling pathway and increased Mcp1 protein secretion. Rosiglitazone could not decrease the elevated Mcp1 secretion in IRAK3$^{-/-}$ BMDM directly and fenofibrate even increased the secretion, possibly due to increased mitochondrial reactive oxygen species production. Furthermore, aortic extracts of high-fat insulin-resistant LDL-receptor deficient mice, with lower *adiponectin* and *Irak3* and higher *Mcp1*, showed accelerated atherosclerosis. In aggregate, our results emphasize an interaction between PPAR agonist-mediated increase in adiponectin and macrophage-associated Irak3 in the protection against atherosclerosis by PPAR agonists.

Editor: Andrea Cignarella, University of Padova, Italy

Funding: Funding was provided by the Fonds voor Wetenschappelijk Onderzoek-Vlaanderen (G.0548.08, G0846.11, and Vascular Biology Network), and by Interdisciplinair Ontwikkelingsfonds - Kennisplatform (KP/12/009). M. Hulsmans is a postdoctoral fellow of the Fonds voor Wetenschappelijk Onderzoek-Vlaanderen. The funders had no role in study design, data collection and analysis, decision to publish, or preparation of the manuscript.

Competing Interests: The authors have declared that no competing interests exist.

* E-mail: paul.holvoet@med.kuleuven.be

◐ These authors contributed equally to this work.

Introduction

Low-grade chronic inflammation is associated with obesity and obesity-induced metabolic disorders such as insulin resistance, type 2 diabetes, the metabolic syndrome and atherosclerosis [1,2]. The recruitment of monocytes and differentiation and polarization to classically activated pro-inflammatory M1 macrophages instead of anti-inflammatory M2 macrophages, have been causally linked to the development of adipose tissue dysfunction, the metabolic syndrome and atherosclerosis [3]. The monocyte chemoattractant protein-1 (Mcp1, also known as chemokine (C-C motif) ligand-2, Ccl2), a marker of M1 macrophages, increases macrophage infiltration, inflammation and insulin resistance in transgenic mice. Conversely, disruption of Mcp1 or its receptor Ccr2 impairs migration of macrophages thereby lowering adipose tissue inflammation and improving insulin sensitivity [4]. It is also recognized that maladaptive production of various adipocytokines (e.g. adiponectin, resistin, visfatin, and leptin) and pro-inflammatory cytokines, such as tumor necrosis factor-α (TNFα) and interleukin (IL)-6, are implicated in the development of obesity-

related systemic inflammation and insulin resistance. In particular, the blood levels of adiponectin are significantly lower in obese individuals and have been associated with metabolic inflammation, insulin resistance and the development of cardiovascular disease [5]. The protective effect of adiponectin has mainly been attributed to its anti-inflammatory action [6]. Interestingly, interleukin-1 receptor-associated kinase-3 (IRAK3; also referred to as IRAK-M), a kinase deficient member of the IRAK family and an important negative regulator of toll-like receptor/nuclear factor κB (NFκB) signaling [7,8], is a major mediator of globular adiponectin-induced endotoxin tolerance in macrophages [9]. Recently, we showed that decreased expression of *IRAK3* in monocytes of obese patients is associated with a high prevalence of metabolic syndrome; weight loss results in an increase in *IRAK3* that is associated with decreased systemic inflammation [10].

Several clinical trials support the use of peroxisome proliferator-activated receptor (PPAR) agonists to treat dyslipidemia and insulin resistance in obesity and type 2 diabetes. PPARα agonists such as fenofibrate regulate lipoprotein metabolism [11]. PPARγ agonists such as rosiglitazone reduce blood glucose levels in patients with type 2 diabetes [12]. Recent data also suggest critical roles of PPAR agonists in inhibiting vascular inflammation and atherosclerosis [13–15]. However, it remains to be determined if molecular mechanisms that confer their vascular protection are identical for PPARα and PPARγ agonists.

In the present study, we aimed to analyze the consequences of PPARα and PPARγ agonist treatment on macrophage activation in relation to atherogenesis using mice with combined leptin (Ob/Ob) and LDL-receptor deficiency (double knockout [DKO] mice). These mice are characterized by morbid obesity, dyslipidemia, glucose intolerance and insulin resistance, and accelerated atherosclerosis [16,17]. Atherosclerotic lesions cover 20% of total area of the thoracic abdominal aorta in double-mutant mice compared with 3.5% in LDL-receptor deficient mice. Ob/Ob mice have no detectable lesions. Higher macrophage homing is detected prior to increase in plaque volumes in the aortic root of DKO mice [16]. In intra-abdominal adipose tissues of DKO mice, Pparγ expression is lower than in LDL-receptor deficient and Ob/Ob mice, and Pparα expression is lower than in LDL-receptor deficient mice. Weight loss increases Pparα and Pparγ, associated with a decrease in atherosclerosis [17]. Because DKO mice, in contrast to single KO mice, are characterized by decreases in Pparα and Pparγ and accelerated atherosclerosis, we selected DKO mice to investigate the effect of fenofibrate and rosiglitazone. We found that rosiglitazone treatment in contrast to fenofibrate increases systemic adiponectin levels and *Irak3* expression, resulting in decreased expression of *Mcp1* in atherosclerotic plaques. Moreover, the presence of Irak3 in macrophages is necessary for the indirect Mcp1-reducing effects of PPAR agonists. Because defective leptin signaling was found to modulate inflammation and atherosclerosis [18], we also studied the relation between low *adiponectin* (*Adipoq*) and *Irak3* expression in aortic extracts of high-fat and insulin resistant LDL-receptor deficient mice characterized by high plasma leptin levels.

Materials and Methods

Experimental Protocol of Animal Studies

Animal experiments conformed to the Guide for the Care and Use of Laboratory Animals published by the US National Institutes of Health. They were approved by the Institutional Animal Care and Research Advisory Committee of the KU Leuven (Permit Number: P087/2007). Breeding and genotyping of DKO mice, on the C57BL/6 J background, were performed as previously described [16,17]. Figure 1 shows a schematic diagram of the experimental protocol. For comparison, age- and gender-matched lean C57BL/6 J mice (n = 12) were used. Fenofibrate and rosiglitazone (Avandia) were purchased from Sigma-Aldrich and GlaxoSmithKline. DKO mice were treated with fenofibrate (n = 14), rosiglitazone (n = 13) or placebo (n = 26) for 12 weeks starting at the age of 12 weeks. Fenofibrate (50 mg kg^{-1} day^{-1}) and rosiglitazone (10 mg kg^{-1} day^{-1}) were added to standard diet (SD) containing 4% fat (Ssniff), placebo-treated mice received the grinded chow only. Food and water were available *ad libitum*. Food intake of the DKO mice was ≈5.7 g/day and was not affected by the treatments. LDL-receptor deficient mice, on the C57BL/6 J background, were fed *ad libitum* for a period of 12 weeks starting at the age of 12 weeks with SD (n = 32) or with a high-fat diet (HFD) containing 45% fat (n = 9). Food intake was 50% of that of DKO mice, and was not different between SD- and HFD-fed mice. All mice were sacrificed by Nembutal overdose at the age of 24 weeks.

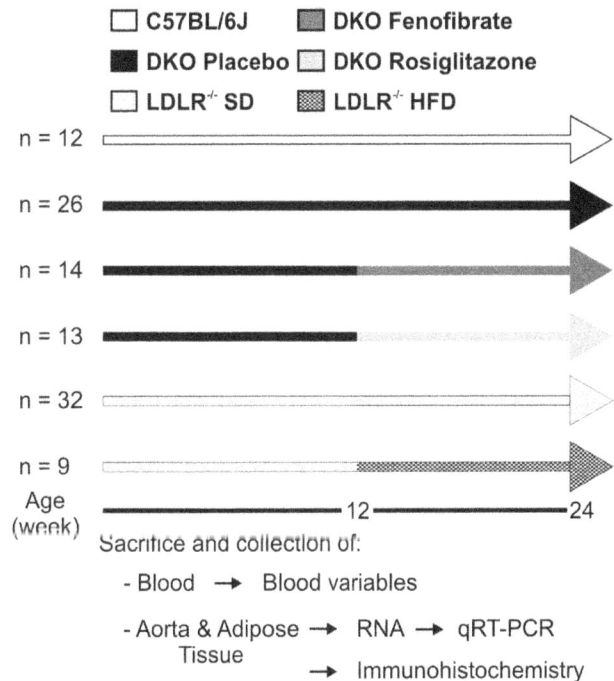

Figure 1. Experimental protocol. Twelve-week old DKO mice were treated for 12 weeks with fenofibrate (50 mg kg^{-1} day^{-1}) or with rosiglitazone (10 mg kg^{-1} day^{-1}) and were compared with placebo-treated DKO and C57BL/6 J background mice. LDL-receptor deficient (LDLR$^{-/-}$) mice, on the C57BL/6 J background, were fed for a period of 12 weeks with standard diet (SD) or with a high-fat diet (HFD). The mice were sacrificed at 24 weeks and total blood, the aortic arch, the abdominal aorta, and visceral adipose tissue were collected.

Blood Values

After an overnight fast, blood was collected by puncturing the *vena cava*. Plasma was obtained by centrifugation. Total cholesterol and triglycerides were measured using standard enzymatic colorimetric assays (Boehringer Mannheim). Glucose was measured with a glucometer (Menarini Diagnostics) and plasma insulin with a mouse insulin enzyme-linked immunosorbent assay (ELISA) (Mercodia). To convert from mg/dL to mM, we divided glucose by 18 (= molecular weight), triglycerides by 89 and total cholesterol by 39. Insulin resistance was calculated by a homeostasis model assessment of insulin resistance (HOMA-IR) = fasting plasma insulin (mU/L) x fasting blood glucose (mM)/22.5. To determine glucose tolerance, glucose was measured in samples obtained by tail bleeding before and 15, 30, 60, 120 and 240 minutes after intraperitoneal administration of glucose (20% glucose solution; 2 g/kg). Plasma adiponectin, TNFα and IL6 were measured with specific mouse ELISAs (R&D Systems) [19,20].

Histological Analysis of Visceral Adipose Tissue and Atherosclerosis

Ten μm-thick paraffin sections of adipose tissue were stained for macrophages with an antibody against mouse Mac-3 antigen (Pharmingen). Blinded analysis was performed on 12 fields of 3 sections from different levels (every 0.1 mm) of the visceral adipose depot for each individual mouse with the Quantimet600 image analyzer (Leica) and a light microscope with 20× magnification. Adipocyte size was determined as the mean adipocyte area calculated by dividing the total adipocyte area by the total number

Table 1. Primers used for qRT-PCR analysis.

Gene symbol	Forward primer	Reverse primer
Adipoq	5′-CTCCTCATTTCTGTCTGTACGATTG-3′	5′-ACAGTAGCATCCTGAGCCCTTT-3′
β-actin	5′-ACGGCCAGGTCATCACTATTG-3′	5′-CACAGGATTCCATACCCAAGAAG-3′
IL6	5′-CTGTTGGGGAGTGGTATCCTCTGT-3′	5′-CCACGGCCTTCCCTACTTC-3′
Irak3 or Irak-m	5′-TTTGCTAGGTTTTGGTTGTCAGAA-3′	5′-TGAGAAGCTAAACTGGAGCCAAT-3′
Mcp1 or Ccl2	5′-GCAGTTAACGCCCCACTCA-3′	5′-CAGCCTACTCATTGGGATCATCTT-3′
Pparα	5′-TCAGGGTACCACTACGGAGTTCA-3′	5′-CCGAATAGTTCGCCGAAAGA-3′
Pparγ	5′-GCAGCTACTGCATGTGATCAAGA-3′	5′-GTCAGCGGGTGGGACTTTC-3′
Tnfα	5′-GGGAGGCCATTTGGGAACT-3′	5′-GCCACCACGCTCTTCTGTCTA-3′

of adipocytes for each mouse. The number of nuclei of Mac-3-positive cells was averaged over 12 different fields, which were most enriched with macrophages, and expressed as ratio to the number of adipocytes. Dead/dying adipocytes were identified by the presence of crown-like structures (CLS). CLS density was

obtained by counting the number of CLS in each section and expressed as ratio to the number of adipocytes. Preparation of sections of the aortic valves, determination of the extent of atherosclerosis, and lipid (oil red O) and macrophage (Mac-3

Table 2. Blood, adipose tissue and plaque variables.

	C57BL/6 J	DKO Placebo	Fenofibrate	Rosiglitazone	ANOVA
A. Weight and blood variables					
Weight (g)	28.1±1.0	61.8±0.8***	58.7±1.1***/§	54.9±1.0***/§§§/£	P<0.001
Total cholesterol (mM)	1.1±0.1	13.4±0.8***	13.7±1.0***	16.6±1.2***/§	P<0.001
Triglycerides (mM)	0.30±0.24	3.1±0.3***	2.4±0.3***	1.9±0.3***/§	P<0.001
Glucose (mM)	4.2±0.2	8.2±0.5***	7.0±0.5***	4.9±0.3*/§§§/££	P<0.001
Insulin (mU/L)	74.3±4.4	213.3±24.7***	106.3±5.9***/§§§	67.1±16.3§§§	P<0.001
HOMA-IR	14.2±1.0	90.1±15.1***	31.2±2.2***/§§	15.8±4.5§§§/£	P<0.001
AUC of IPGTT	35.1±0.4	87.6±4.9***	74.8±4.2***	50.8±1.2***/§§§/£££	P<0.001
TNFα (pg/mL)	22.4±1.2	29.7±1.9**	29.6±1.0***	24.7±1.3§/££	P<0.01
IL6 (pg/mL)	17.9±0.6	29.3±2.4***	21.1±2.3§	14.6±1.7§§§/£	P<0.001
Adiponectin (mg/mL)	5.4±0.6	2.9±0.4**	1.1±0.2***/§§§	16.2±0.7***/§§§/£££	P<0.001
B. Adipose tissue variables					
Adipocyte size (x 10³ μm³)	2.1±0.2	7.9±0.2***	8.1±0.2***	6.4±0.4***/§§/££	P<0.001
Macrophages/adipocyte	2.8±0.5	219.7±10.8***	122.5±15.3***/§§§	49.9±3.0***/§§§/£££	P<0.001
CLS (%)	0.08±0.03	10.9±1.1***	5.9±1.3***/§§	1.3±0.2***/§§§/££	P<0.001
C. Plaque variables					
Plaque volume (x 10⁻³ μm³)	ND	93.9±5.4	114.6±10.1	60.3±14.2§/££	P<0.01
Plaque macrophages (% of plaque area)	ND	28.5±2.2	22.5±1.3§	11.6±1.2§§§/£££	P<0.001
Plaque lipids (% of plaque area)	ND	30.3±1.4	28.4±1.2	24.3±1.2§§/£	P<0.05

Data are means ± SEM.
*P<0.05,
**P<0.01 and
***P<0.001 DKO compared with C57BL/6 J mice;
§P<0.05,
§§P<0.01 and
§§§P<0.001 PPAR agonist-treated compared with placebo-treated DKO mice;
£P<0.05,
££P<0.01 and
£££P<0.001 rosiglitazone-treated compared with fenofibrate-treated DKO mice.
Abbreviations: CLS, crown-like structures; ND, not detectable.

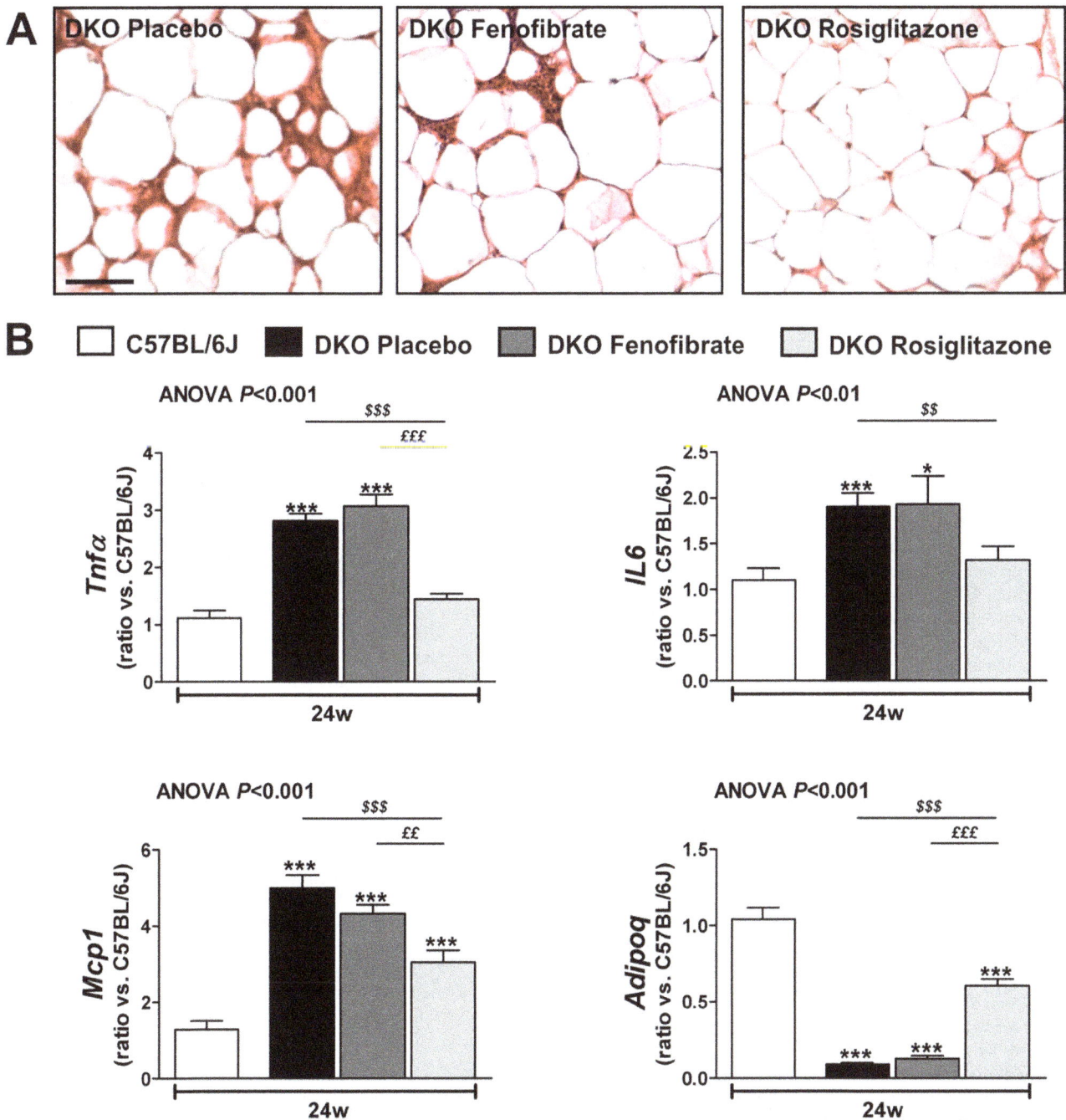

Figure 2. Rosiglitazone and not fenofibrate treatment reduces macrophage accumulation and improves adiponectin expression in visceral adipose tissue. (**A**) Representative Mac-3 staining of visceral adipose tissue of placebo-, fenofibrate- and rosiglitazone-treated DKO mice at 24 weeks. (**B**) Relative *RNA* levels of *Tnfα, IL6, Mcp1* and *Adipoq* as determined by qRT-PCR. Data are means $\pm$ SEM. Scale bar = 100 μm. *$P<0.05$ and ***$P<0.001$ DKO compared with C57BL/6 J mice; $^{\$\$}P<0.01$ and $^{\$\$\$}P<0.001$ PPAR agonist-treated compared with placebo-treated DKO mice; $^{££}P<0.01$ and $^{£££}P<0.001$ rosiglitazone-treated compared with fenofibrate-treated DKO mice.

antibody) stainings were performed according to previously described protocols [19,20].

Cell Culture

Bone marrow cells were isolated from 24-weeks-old C57BL/6 J, DKO and IRAK3$^{-/-}$ mice. IRAK3$^{-/-}$ mice were kindly provided by Dr. Flavell (Yale University) [8]. After euthanasia, the mice were sprayed with 70% ethanol and the femurs were

dissected. Muscles connected to the bone were removed using clean gauze, and the femurs were placed into a Petri dish containing sterile PBS on ice. Both epiphyses were removed using sterile scissors and the bones were flushed with a syringe with DMEM containing 10% FBS (Gibco) to extrude bone marrow. Single cell suspensions were prepared by passing the cells through a 70-μm cell strainer. Cells were washed and incubated in erythrocyte-lysis buffer (Miltenyi) for 10 minutes, according to the

Table 3. *Pparα* and *Pparγ* expressions in visceral adipose and aortic tissues of PPAR agonist-treated DKO mice.

	DKO			ANOVA
	Placebo	Fenofibrate	Rosiglitazone	
A. Visceral adipose tissue				
Pparα	0.23±0.02***	0.37±0.04***/^{SS}	1.83±0.17***/^{SSS}/$^{£££}$	P<0.001
Pparγ	0.21±0.01***	0.33±0.03***/^{SS}	0.43±0.02***/^{SSS}/$^{£}$	P<0.001
B. Abdominal aorta				
Pparα	0.58±0.05*	0.57±0.05*	3.33±0.39***/^{SSS}/$^{£££}$	P<0.001
Pparγ	0.67±0.07*	1.00±0.05^{SSS}	1.11±0.09^{SSS}	P<0.001

Data are means ± SEM.
*P<0.05 and
***P<0.001 DKO compared with C57BL/6 J mice;
^{SS}P<0.01 and
^{SSS}P<0.001 PPAR agonist-treated compared with placebo-treated DKO mice;
$^{£}$P<0.05 and
$^{£££}$P<0.001 rosiglitazone-treated compared with fenofibrate-treated DKO mice.

manufacturer's instructions. These fresh bone marrow cells were differentiated to bone marrow-derived macrophages (BMDM) [21], using L929 cell conditioned medium (LCCM) as a source of granulocyte/macrophage colony stimulating factor [22]. The cells derived from one femur were resuspended in 25 mL bone marrow differentiation media, which is DMEM supplemented with 20% FBS, 30% LCCM, 100 U/mL penicillin, 100 mg/mL streptomycin, and 2 mM L-glutamine (Gibco). Cells were seeded in non-tissue culture-treated 150 mm Petri dishes and incubated at 37°C in a 5% CO_2 atmosphere. Six days after seeding the cells, the attached cells were washed and incubated overnight under normal growth conditions. Then, cells were incubated with 50 μM fenofibrate, 10 μM rosiglitazone, 5 μM GW9662 (Sigma-Aldrich) and 1 or 10 μg/mL murine globular adiponectin (PeproTech) for 24 hours. Cell viability, as determined by trypan blue exclusion, was >80%.

RNA Extraction and Gene Expression Analysis

Total *RNA* was extracted with TRIzol reagent (Invitrogen) and purified on RNeasy Mini kit columns (Qiagen). First-strand cDNA was generated from total *RNA* with the SuperScript VILO cDNA synthesis kit (Invitrogen). Quantitative real-time PCR (qRT-PCR) was performed using Fast SYBRGreen master mix according to the supplier's protocol (Applied Biosystems). Oligonucleotides (Invitrogen) used as forward and reverse primers were designed using the Primer Express software (Applied Biosystems) and are summarized in Table 1. Data were normalized to the housekeeping gene *β-actin* as previously described [20].

Western Blotting

Western blot analysis was performed with 20 μg of total protein. Protein was electrophoresed through a 10–20% SDS-polyacrylamide gel (Bio-Rad) and transferred to a polyvinylidene difluoride membrane (Millipore). Membranes were processed according to standard Western blotting procedures. To detect protein levels, membranes were incubated with primary antibodies against β-actin (Cell Signaling Technology) and Irak3 (Rockland Immunochemicals). The membranes were then incubated with horseradish peroxidase-coupled secondary antibody (Santa Cruz Biotechnology) and developed with SuperSignal chemiluminescent substrate

(Pierce). A PC-based image analysis program was used to quantify the intensity of each band (Bio-1D).

Soluble Mcp1 Cytokine Levels

Conditioned medium was harvested after treatment of BMDM and stored at −80°C. Soluble Mcp1 protein levels in the conditioned medium were determined by ELISA according to the manufacturer's instructions (R&D Systems).

NFκB p50 DNA Binding Activity

NFκB p50 DNA binding activity was assessed on isolated nuclear extracts of BMDM by ELISA using the TransAM NFκB p50 transcription factor assay kit according to the manufacturer's protocol (Active Motif). Briefly, 10 μg of nuclear extract diluted in complete lysis buffer was used in the p50 binding assay. The samples were shaken for 1 hour at room temperature in 30 μL binding buffer. After washing, anti-p50 antibody diluted 1:1000 was applied to the wells for 1 hour at room temperature. Specific binding was estimated by spectrophotometry after incubation with a horseradish peroxidaseconjugated antibody (1 hour at room temperature, 1:1000 diluted) at 450 nm wave length.

Mitochondrial Reactive Oxygen Species Detection

To detect mitochondrial reactive oxygen species (mROS) formation in treated BMDM, measurements of MitoSOX Red (Invitrogen) fluorescence were performed by flow cytometry (Becton, Dickinson and Company). Cells were incubated with PBS containing 5 μM MitoSOX for 10 minutes at 37°C and 5% CO_2. The labeled cells were washed twice with PBS and then suspended in warm PBS for analysis by flow cytometry.

Statistical Analysis

The Kruskal-Wallis nonparametric one-way ANOVA, followed by the Dunn's multiple comparisons test was used to compare more than two independent samples. The unpaired t-test with Welch's correction test was used for the two-sample comparisons (Graph Pad Prism version 5). Correlations were calculated using the nonparametric Spearman's correlation coefficient (r_s). Non-parametric tests were used because Gaussian distribution cannot be expected in small sample size studies as performed in this article. The area under the curve of the intraperitoneal glucose tolerance test (AUC of IPGTT) was calculated in Graph Pad Prism version 5. A probability value of P<0.05 was considered statistically significant.

Results

Rosiglitazone in Contrast to Fenofibrate Decreases Systemic Inflammation and Restores Insulin Sensitivity

Body weight, plasma total cholesterol and triglycerides were significantly higher in placebo-treated DKO mice compared with lean C57BL/6 J background mice. Glucose and insulin levels, and thus the HOMA-IR index were similarly elevated. Glucose tolerance as measured by AUC of IPGTT was increased. The higher levels of TNFα and IL6, and the lower adiponectin levels indicated systemic inflammation (Table 2A). Both fenofibrate and rosiglitazone decreased weight and insulin levels. Interestingly, only rosiglitazone treatment reduced glucose levels resulting in a decrease in HOMA-IR and a partial normalization of glucose tolerance. Systemic inflammation was only decreased after rosiglitazone treatment evidenced by lower levels of TNFα and IL6 and increased adiponectin levels. Both treatments had almost no effect on total cholesterol and triglycerides (Table 2A).

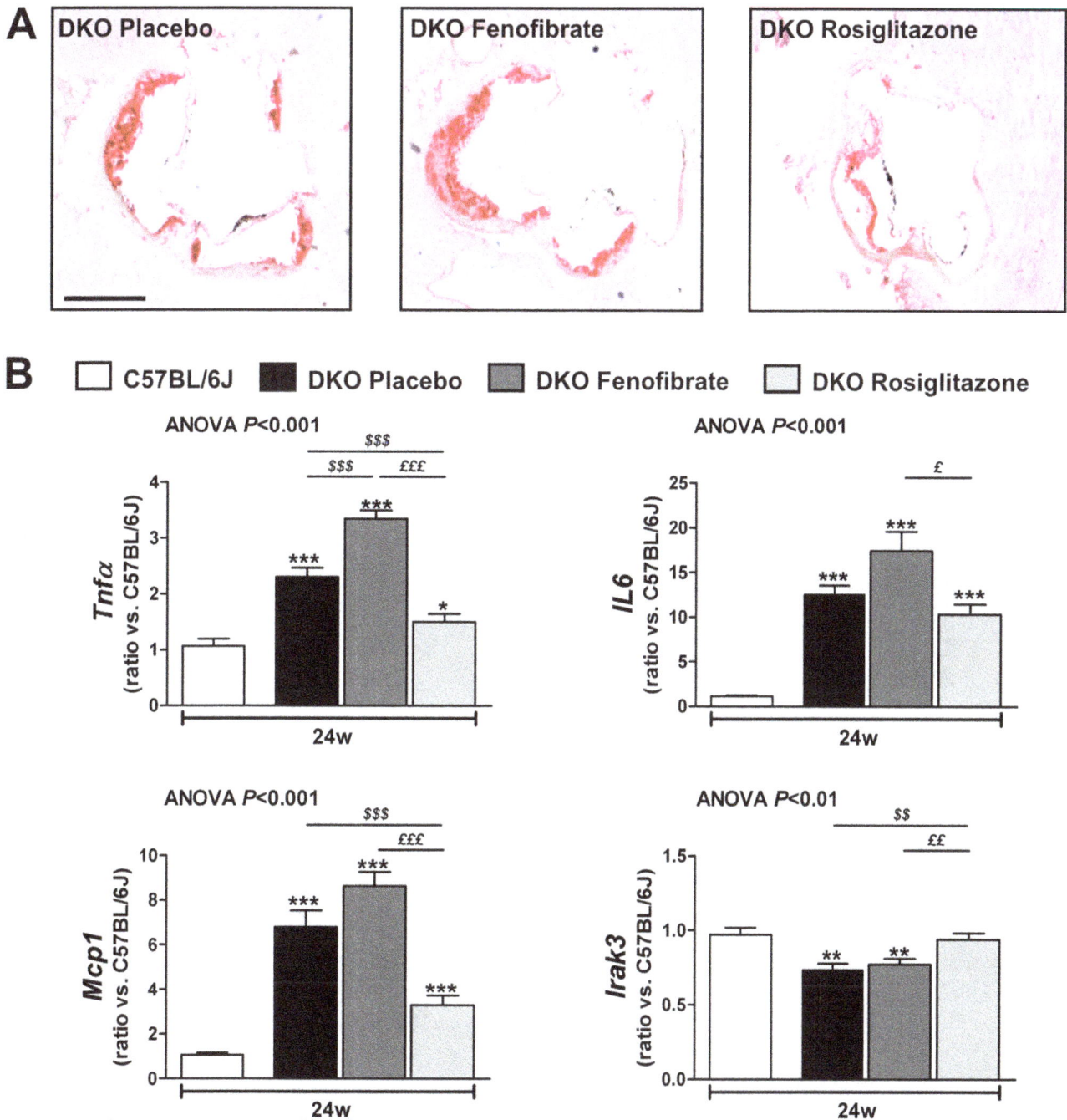

Figure 3. Rosiglitazone and not fenofibrate treatment decreases atherogenesis in obese, insulin resistant mice. (**A**) Representative Mac-3 staining of aortic sinus plaques of placebo-, fenofibrate- and rosiglitazone-treated DKO mice at 24 weeks. (**B**) Gene expression in the aorta was analyzed by measuring relative *RNA* levels using qRT-PCR for *Tnfα, IL6, Mcp1* and *Irak3*. Data are means ± SEM. Scale bar = 500 μm. *$P<0.05$, **$P<0.01$ and ***$P<0.001$ DKO compared with C57BL/6 J mice; $^{$$}P<0.01$ and $^{$$$}P<0.001$ PPAR agonist-treated compared with placebo-treated DKO mice; $^{£}P<0.05$, $^{££}P<0.01$ and $^{£££}P<0.001$ rosiglitazone-treated compared with fenofibrate-treated DKO mice.

Rosiglitazone and not Fenofibrate Improves Adipocyte Function by Decreasing Macrophage Accumulation

Figure 2A shows representative sections of visceral adipose tissue stained for macrophages of placebo-, fenofibrate-, and rosiglitazone-treated DKO mice. The adipocyte size, number of macrophages and CLS, which indicates necrotic adipocytes surrounded by phagocytes, were increased in DKO mice compared with lean C57BL/6 J mice (Table 2B). Only rosiglita-

zone decreased the adipocyte size. Both treatments, but rosiglitazone more than fenofibrate, reduced the number of macrophages and CLS in adipose tissue of DKO mice (Table 2B and Figure 2A). Furthermore, rosiglitazone decreased *Tnfα, IL6* and *Mcp1* expressions, and increased the expression of *Adipoq* (Figure 2B). Rosiglitazone treatment also resulted in a greater increase in *Pparα* than fenofibrate treatment; differences in *Pparγ* were less pronounced (Table 3A).

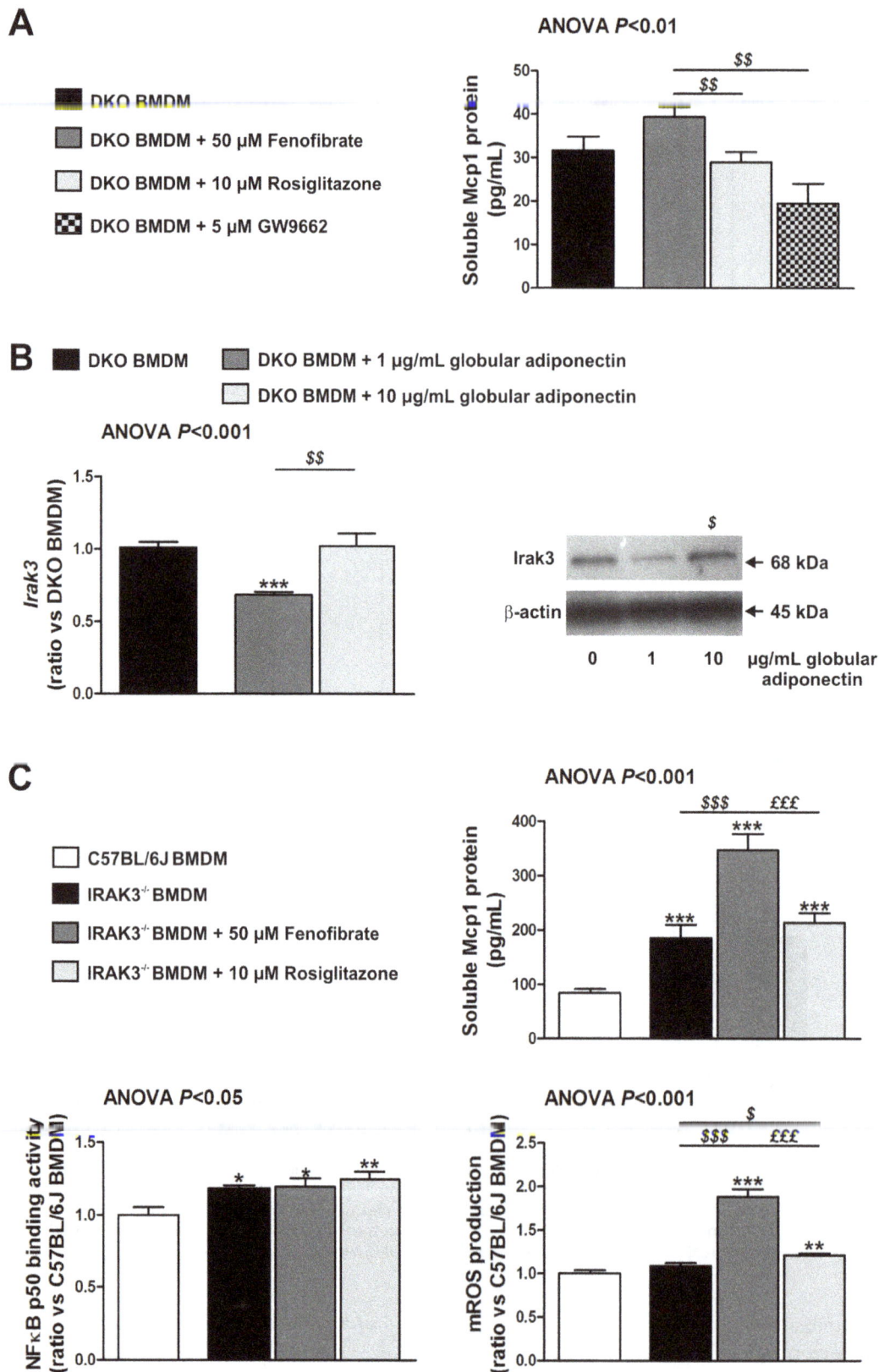

Figure 4. Adiponectin-induced Irak3 plays an important role in rosiglitazone-mediated decrease of Mcp1. (A) Soluble Mcp1 protein levels in DKO BMDM exposed to 50 μM fenofibrate, 10 μM rosiglitazone or 5 μM GW9662 for 24 hours as determined by LLISA. Data are means ± SEM; n = 16 from three different mice. $^{\$\$}P<0.01$ compared with fenofibrate-treated BMDM. **(B)** Irak3 *RNA* and protein levels of DKO BMDM exposed to 1 or 10 μg/mL globular adiponectin for 24 hours as determined by qRT-PCR and Western blotting. Data are means ± SEM; n = 6. $^{***}P<0.001$ compared with DKO BMDM; $^{\$}P<0.05$ and $^{\$\$}P<0.01$ compared with DKO BMDM exposed to 1 μg/mL globular adiponectin. **(C)** Soluble Mcp1 protein

levels (n = 18 from three different mice), NFκB p50 DNA binding activity (n = 8 from two different mice) and mROS production (n = 6) in IRAK3$^{-/-}$ BMDM exposed to 50 μM fenofibrate or 10 μM rosiglitazone for 24 hours as determined by ELISA and flow cytometry. Data are means ± SEM. *P<0.05, **P<0.01 and ***P<0.001 compared with C57BL/6 J BMDM; $^{$}P$<0.05 and $^{$$$}P$<0.001 compared with IRAK3$^{-/-}$ BMDM; $^{£££}P$<0.001 compared with fenofibrate-treated BMDM. Abbreviations: BMDM, bone marrow-derived macrophages; mROS, mitochondrial reactive oxygen species.

Rosiglitazone and not Fenofibrate Reduces Atherosclerotic Plaque Volume and Macrophage Content by Decreasing Macrophage Accumulation

Figure 3A shows representative sections of atherosclerotic lesions stained for macrophages of placebo-, fenofibrate-, and rosiglitazone-treated DKO mice. Fenofibrate had no effect on overall plaque volume. In contrast, rosiglitazone decreased plaque volume by inhibiting macrophage and lipid deposition (Table 2C). In addition, rosiglitazone treatment decreased *Tnfα*, *IL6* and *Mcp1* expressions in extracts of abdominal aorta. Furthermore, *Irak3* expression was increased after rosiglitazone treatment (Figure 3B). *Irak3* in the aorta correlated positively with circulating adiponectin levels (r_s = 0.41, P<0.01) and negatively with *Tnfα* (r_s = −0.43, P<0.01), *IL6* (r_s = −0.35, P<0.05) and *Mcp1* (r_s = −0.46, P<0.001). The expression of *Adipoq* in aortic extracts, 2.1-fold decreased in DKO compared with C57BL/6 J mice (P<0.01), increased more after rosiglitazone treatment (1.8-fold *vs*. DKO,

P<0.01; 1.4-fold *vs*. fenofibrate treatment, P<0.05) than fenofibrate treatment (1.2-fold *vs*. DKO, P<0.05). Rosiglitazone treatment also resulted in a greater increase in *Pparα* than fenofibrate treatment; differences in *Pparγ* were not significant (Table 3B).

Irak3 Induction Dependent on High Adiponectin is Required for the Decreased Expression of Mcp1 after Rosiglitazone Treatment

We investigated the direct effect of fenofibrate, rosiglitazone, and PPARγ antagonist (GW9662) treatment on BMDM from DKO mice to elucidate the observed differences between PPAR treatments. Fenofibrate tended to increase Mcp1 protein. Rosiglitazone did not decrease Mcp1 protein and addition of the PPARγ antagonist did not increase Mcp1 protein. In aggregate, we did not observe a direct inhibitory effect of PPAR agonists on

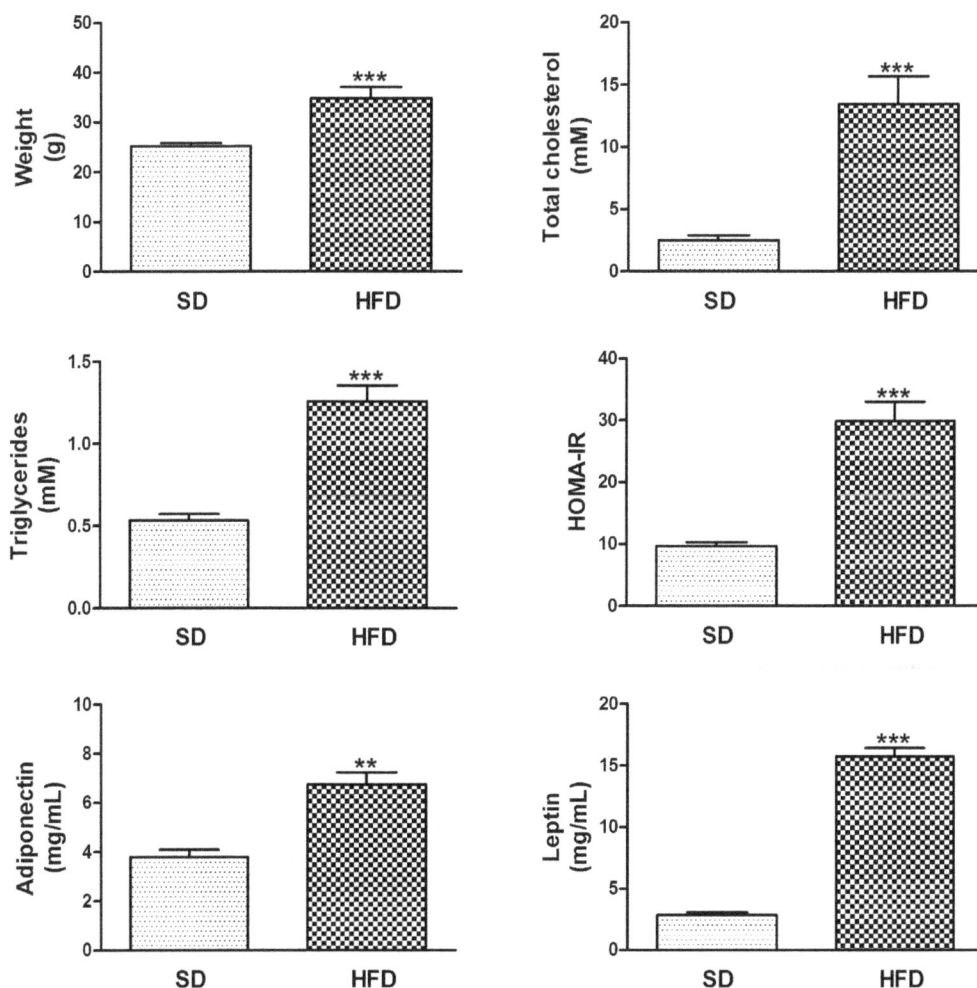

Figure 5. HFD-induced weight gain is associated with dyslipidemia, insulin resistance and hyperleptinemia in the presence of high blood adiponectin. Data are means ± SEM. **P<0.01 and ***P<0.001 HFD-fed compared with SD-fed LDL-receptor deficient mice. Abbreviations: HFD, high fat diet; SD, standard diet.

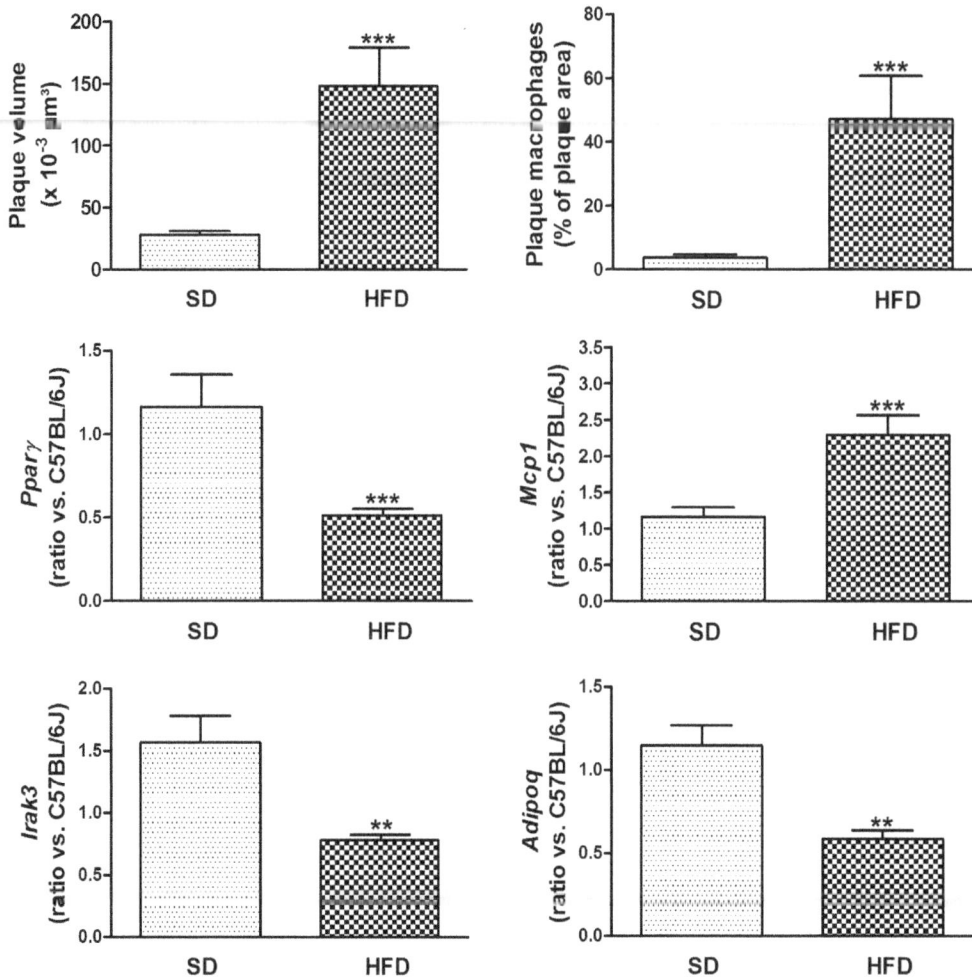

Figure 6. HFD increases atherogenesis in insulin resistant mice. Plaque volume was determined by measuring lipid (oil red O)-stained surfaces in subsequent sections; macrophages were stained with anti-Mac-3 antibody. Gene expression in the aorta was analyzed by measuring relative *RNA* levels using qRT-PCR for *Pparγ*, *Mcp1*, *Irak3* and *Adipoq*. Data are means ± SEM. **$P < 0.01$ and ***$P < 0.001$ HFD-fed compared with SD-fed LDL-receptor deficient mice. Abbreviations: HFD, high fat diet; SD, standard diet.

Mcp1 protein secretion (average Mcp1 concentration in DKO BMDM: 31.8 ± 1.6 pg/mL) (Figure 4A).

However, we have previously shown that there is a causal relation between variable globular adiponectin levels and IRAK3 expression in blood monocytes of obese patients [10]. Because we found that rosiglitazone increased adiponectin more than fenofibrate, we determined the effect of low (as in untreated and fenofibrate-treated DKO mice) and high (as in rosiglitazone-treated DKO mice) globular adiponectin concentrations on the Irak3 expression in BMDM. Indeed, exposure to 10 μg/mL globular adiponectin increased the Irak3 expression (*RNA* and protein) in comparison with exposure to 1 μg/mL globular adiponectin (Figure 4B).

Then, we investigated if Irak3 deletion had an effect on Mcp1 expression. The deletion of Irak3 in BMDM (IRAK3$^{-/-}$ BMDM) was characterized by activation of the canonical NFκB signaling pathway as determined by NFκB p50 DNA binding activity. This resulted in a 2.2-fold increase in Mcp1 protein secretion compared with control cells (185.5 ± 24.5 *vs.* 84.5 ± 7.3 pg/mL, $P < 0.001$). Rosiglitazone treatment did not decrease the elevated Mcp1 secretion in IRAK3$^{-/-}$ BMDM and fenofibrate even increased the production of Mcp1, independently from NFκB p50 DNA

binding activity. However, the observed increase in Mcp1 after fenofibrate treatment was associated with increased mROS production (Figure 4C).

Lower Adipoq and Irak3 Expressions are Associated with M1 Macrophages and Accelerated Atherosclerosis in High-fat Insulin Resistant Mice

Body weight, plasma total cholesterol and triglycerides were significantly higher in HFD-fed LDL-receptor deficient mice compared with SD-fed mice, with C57BL/6 J background. Glucose tolerance, as measured by AUC of IPGTT and HOMA-IR index was elevated. In contrast to DKO, HFD-fed LDL-receptor deficient mice had increased blood levels of adiponectin. In addition, their leptin levels were elevated (Figure 5).

Figure 6 shows accelerated atherosclerosis in aortic arch of high-fat insulin resistant mice, due to increased macrophage content. Aortic *Pparγ*, *Adipoq* and *Irak3* expressions were decreased, whereas *Mcp1* expression was increased. *Pparα* expression was not significantly decreased in aorta of HFD-fed mice (data not shown). Increased aortic inflammation in HFD-fed mice was further evidenced by a 1.6-fold increase in *Tnfα* ($P < 0.01$) and a 7.2-fold increase in *IL6* ($P < 0.001$).

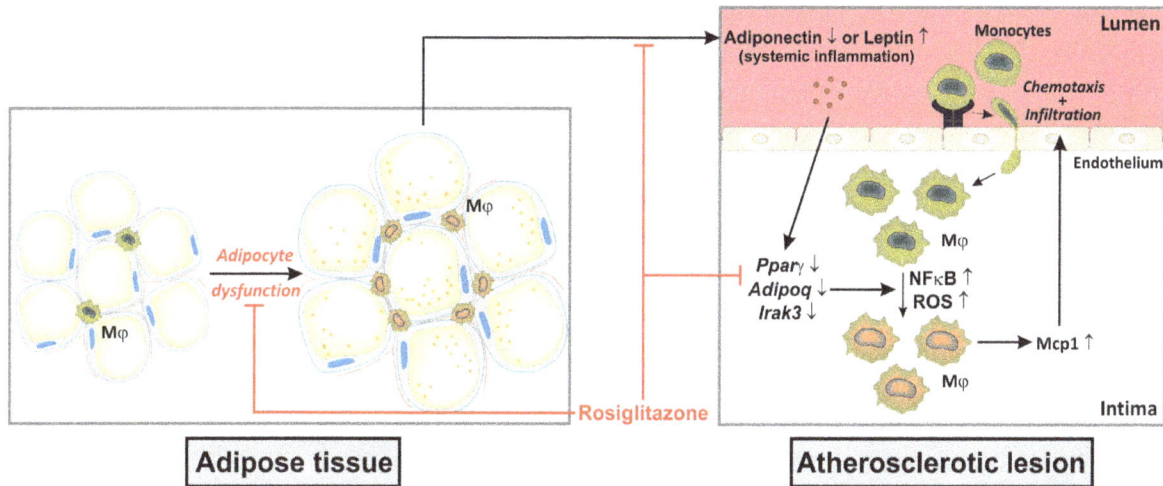

Figure 7. Adiponectin and macrophage-associated Irak3 are indispensable molecules in the anti-atherosclerotic properties of PPAR agonists. The schematic draw demonstrates the anti-atherosclerotic properties of the PPARγ agonist rosiglitazone. Treatment with rosiglitazone improves the adipocyte function characterized by a decrease in adipocyte size, a reduction in adipose tissue macrophages and an increased expression of anti-inflammatory adiponectin. The increase in blood adiponectin and *de novo* adiponectin production in atherosclerotic lesions is necessary for the upregulation of Irak3 in plaque macrophages, which is crucial for the indirect rosiglitazone-mediated decrease in Mcp1 secretion. Abbreviations: Mφ, macrophages; ROS, reactive oxygen species.

Discussion

Previous studies have shown that treatment with PPAR agonists could prevent vascular inflammation, atherosclerosis and the development of cardiovascular disease [23–25]. In the present study, we showed that rosiglitazone, a PPARγ agonist, could reduce obesity-induced systemic inflammation, insulin resistance, macrophage accumulation and atherosclerotic plaque formation. In contrast, treatment with fenofibrate, a PPARα agonist, did not reduce systemic inflammation or plaque formation.

PPARγ agonists not only increase peripheral insulin sensitivity but also cause dramatic decreases in systemic inflammation. In obese diabetic patients, rosiglitazone has been shown to decrease circulating C-reactive protein and IL6 levels [26,27]. Rosiglitazone, but not fenofibrate, also increased adiponectin in our DKO mice. Previously, we demonstrated a relation between adiponectin and Pparγ in the heart, insulin sensitivity, and cardiac function, independent of cholesterol and triglycerides [28]. PPARγ increases adiponectin through a PPAR-responsive element in the adiponectin promoter in adipocytes [29,30]. The increase in adiponectin may explain the more pronounced increase in *Pparα* expression in adipose and aortic tissues [31,32]. Our study also confirmed that adiponectin is essential for the indirect vascular protective effect of rosiglitazone [33–35] at least partially through upregulation of Irak3 in plaque macrophages. Indeed, we observed that high levels of adiponectin increases the expression of Irak3 in BMDM, which at its turn is necessary for the indirect vascular protective effect of rosiglitazone on macrophages as evidenced by the elevated Mcp1 protein secretion in IRAK3$^{-/-}$ BMDM *in vitro*. Several recent studies have demonstrated that IRAK3 regulates critical aspects of innate immunity, including the development of endotoxin tolerance after adiponectin exposure. Adiponectin induces IRAK3 expression through ERK1/2 and PI3K/Akt signaling cascades [9]. Furthermore, IRAK3 is an important regulator by which tumor-associated macrophages mimic the phenotype of alternatively activated (M2) macrophages [36]. IRAK3 also attenuates post-infarction remodeling by protecting the heart from uncontrolled inflammation and excessive

matrix degradation [37]. A surprising finding was that aortic expression of *Irak3* in HFD-fed insulin resistant mice was observed in association with increased blood levels of adiponectin. But aortic *Adipoq* expression was decreased in association with lower *Pparγ* expression, suggesting that local expression in macrophages is more relevant than systemic expression by adipose tissues. This is in agreement with the observation that rosiglitazone inhibited monocyte/macrophage adhesion through *de novo* adiponectin production in human monocytes [38]. Also, HFD-fed mice had elevated levels of leptin that together with high insulin induces inflammation [39,40]. Previously, it has been suggested that PPARγ guarantees a balanced and adequate production of secretion from adipose tissue of adipocytokines such as adiponectin and leptin, which are important mediators of insulin action in peripheral tissues [41]. Our data in HFD-fed mice indicate that imbalanced production does not necessarily imply high leptin and low adiponectin. Elevated leptin, even in presence of high adiponectin, is sufficient to generate an inflammatory response.

Similar to PPARγ agonists, PPARα agonists, like fenofibrate, have also demonstrated anti-inflammatory properties in addition to their other beneficial effects on metabolism [15,42]. However, in our study, fenofibrate treatment had no effect on systemic inflammatory markers, and did not increase adiponectin levels and *Irak3* expression and did not decrease the expression of *Mcp1*. In addition, exposure of IRAK3$^{-/-}$ BMDM to fenofibrate resulted in an increased secretion of Mcp1 protein *in vitro*. The different Mcp1 secretion after rosiglitazone and fenofibrate treatment is independent of activation of the canonical NFκB signaling pathway but is possibly due to the increased ROS production observed after fenofibrate treatment. Indeed, it has been suggested that ROS production is involved in the regulation of *Mcp1* expression [43]. However, we have to take into account that a mouse model is not the best model to evaluate PPARα selective compounds for their anti-atherosclerotic efficacy because in humans fenofibrate also influences lipid metabolism through modulation of cholesteryl ester transfer protein [44]. In diet-fed hamsters, the anti-atherosclerotic efficacy of fenofibrate occurred primarily *via* reductions in pro-atherogenic lipoproteins. However, these hamsters were not obese and did not display insulin resistance [45]. Furthermore, the dosages of fenofibrate and rosiglitazone were approximately 2 and 6 times higher than the maximum recommended daily dose in humans. However, in this study, fenofibrate and rosiglitazone were used as experimental tools to identify underlying mechanisms that could apply to patients treated with the drug. Finally, our data are in agreement with previous data of Duez *et al.* showing that fenofibrate did not reduce atherosclerotic lesion area in the aortic sinus of ApoE deficient mice [46]. However, they found a reduction of cholesterol content in descending aortas of treated mice, an effect that was more pronounced in older mice exhibiting more advanced lesions. Unfortunately, in our study we did not measure cholesterol levels in the descending aorta. Interestingly, fenofibrate reduced lesions in the aortic sinus of ApoE deficient mice overexpressing human apolipoprotein-A1 [46].

Conclusions

In summary, we found that rosiglitazone in contrast to fenofibrate improves insulin sensitivity and adiponectin levels

and inhibits inflammation and atherosclerotic plaque formation by reducing M1 macrophage accumulation in the vascular wall. In addition, the adiponectin-dependent upregulation of Irak3 in macrophages is necessary for the reduction in Mcp1 secretion, and thus switch from M1 to M2. HFD-induced increase in leptin causes inflammation associated with decreased *Irak3* expression in association with accelerated atherosclerosis, even in presence of high blood levels of adiponectin but decreased plaque expression of *Adipoq*. In summary, we showed that Irak3 as an inhibitor of NFκB and ROS production is required for the protective action of particularly the PPARγ agonist (Figure 7).

Acknowledgments

We thank Roxane Menten for excellent technical assistance.

Author Contributions

Conceived and designed the experiments: MH BG PH. Performed the experiments: MH BG. Analyzed the data: MH BG PH. Contributed reagents/materials/analysis tools: TA CT. Wrote the paper: MH BG PH.

References

1. Hotamisligil GS (2006) Inflammation and metabolic disorders. Nature 444: 860–867.
2. Hulsmans M, Holvoet P (2010) The vicious circle between oxidative stress and inflammation in atherosclerosis. J.Cell Mol.Med. 14: 70–78.
3. Weisberg SP, McCann D, Desai M, Rosenbaum M, Leibel RL, et al. (2003) Obesity is associated with macrophage accumulation in adipose tissue. J.Clin.Invest 112: 1796–1808.
4. Odegaard JI, Ricardo-Gonzalez RR, Goforth MH, Morel CR, Subramanian V, et al. (2007) Macrophage-specific PPARgamma controls alternative activation and improves insulin resistance. Nature 447: 1116–1120.
5. Kadowaki T, Yamauchi T, Kubota N, Hara K, Ueki K, et al. (2006) Adiponectin and adiponectin receptors in insulin resistance, diabetes, and the metabolic syndrome. J.Clin.Invest 116: 1784–1792.
6. Yang WS, Lee WJ, Funahashi T, Tanaka S, Matsuzawa Y, et al. (2001) Weight reduction increases plasma levels of an adipose-derived anti-inflammatory protein, adiponectin. J.Clin.Endocrinol.Metab 86: 3815–3819.
7. Wesche H, Gao X, Li X, Kirschning CJ, Stark GR, et al. (1999) IRAK-M is a novel member of the Pelle/interleukin-1 receptor-associated kinase (IRAK) family. Journal of Biological Chemistry 274: 19403–19410.
8. Kobayashi K, Hernandez LD, Galan JE, Janeway CA Jr, Medzhitov R, et al. (2002) IRAK-M is a negative regulator of Toll-like receptor signaling. Cell 110: 191–202.
9. Zacharioudaki V, Androulidaki A, Arranz A, Vrentzos G, Margioris AN, et al. (2009) Adiponectin promotes endotoxin tolerance in macrophages by inducing IRAK-M expression. Journal of Immunology 182: 6444–6451.
10. Hulsmans M, Geeraert B, De Keyzer D, Mertens A, Lannoo M, et al. (2012) Interleukin-1 receptor-associated kinase-3 is a key inhibitor of inflammation in obesity and metabolic syndrome. PLoS.ONE. 7: e30414.
11. Staels B, Dallongeville J, Auwerx J, Schoonjans K, Leitersdorf E, et al. (1998) Mechanism of action of fibrates on lipid and lipoprotein metabolism. Circulation 98: 2088–2093.
12. Phillips LS, Grunberger G, Miller E, Patwardhan R, Rappaport EB, et al. (2001) Once- and twice-daily dosing with rosiglitazone improves glycemic control in patients with type 2 diabetes. Diabetes Care 24: 308–315.
13. Zhang LL, Gao CY, Fang CQ, Wang YJ, Gao D, et al. (2011) PPAR{gamma} attenuates intimal hyperplasia through inhibiting TLR4-mediated inflammation in vascular smooth muscle cells. Cardiovascular Research 92: 484–493.
14. Kadoglou NP, Iliadis F, Angelopoulou N, Perrea D, Liapis CD, et al. (2008) Beneficial effects of rosiglitazone on novel cardiovascular risk factors in patients with Type 2 diabetes mellitus. Diabetic Medicine 25: 333–340.
15. Delerive P, Martin-Nizard F, Chinetti G, Trottein F, Fruchart JC, et al. (1999) Peroxisome proliferator-activated receptor activators inhibit thrombin-induced endothelin-1 production in human vascular endothelial cells by inhibiting the activator protein-1 signaling pathway. Circ.Res. 85: 394–402.
16. Mertens A, Verhamme P, Bielicki JK, Phillips MC, Quarck R, et al. (2003) Increased low-density lipoprotein oxidation and impaired high-density lipoprotein antioxidant defense are associated with increased macrophage homing and atherosclerosis in dyslipidemic obese mice: LCAT gene transfer decreases atherosclerosis. Circulation 107: 1640–1646.
17. Verreth W, De Keyzer D, Pelat M, Verhamme P, Ganame J, et al. (2004) Weight-loss-associated induction of peroxisome proliferator-activated receptor-alpha and peroxisome proliferator-activated receptor-gamma correlate with reduced atherosclerosis and improved cardiovascular function in obese insulin-resistant mice. Circulation 110: 3259–3269.

18. Taleb S, Herbin O, Ait-Oufella H, Verreth W, Gourdy P, et al. (2007) Defective leptin/leptin receptor signaling improves regulatory T cell immune response and protects mice from atherosclerosis. Arteriosclerosis, Thrombosis, and Vascular Biology 27: 2691–2698.
19. Verreth W, De Keyzer D, Davey PC, Geeraert B, Mertens A, et al. (2007) Rosuvastatin restores superoxide dismutase expression and inhibits accumulation of oxidized LDL in the aortic arch of obese dyslipidemic mice. British Journal of Pharmacology 151: 347–355.
20. Geeraert B, Crombe F, Hulsmans M, Benhabiles N, Geuns JM, et al. (2010) Stevioside inhibits atherosclerosis by improving insulin signaling and antioxidant defense in obese insulin-resistant mice. Int.J.Obes.(Lond) 34: 569–577.
21. Zamboni DS, Rabinovitch M (2003) Nitric oxide partially controls Coxiella burnetii phase II infection in mouse primary macrophages. Infect.Immun. 71: 1225–1233.
22. Englen MD, Valdez YE, Lehnert NM, Lehnert BE (1995) Granulocyte/macrophage colony-stimulating factor is expressed and secreted in cultures of murine L929 cells. J.Immunol.Methods 184: 281–283.
23. Bouhlel MA, Derudas B, Rigamonti E, Dievart R, Brozek J, et al. (2007) PPARgamma activation primes human monocytes into alternative M2 macrophages with anti-inflammatory properties. Cell Metab 6: 137–143.
24. Wayman NS, Hattori Y, McDonald MC, Mota-Filipe H, Cuzzocrea S, et al. (2002) Ligands of the peroxisome proliferator-activated receptors (PPAR-gamma and PPAR-alpha) reduce myocardial infarct size. FASEB Journal 16: 1027–1040.
25. Calkin AC, Forbes JM, Smith CM, Lassila M, Cooper ME, et al. (2005) Rosiglitazone attenuates atherosclerosis in a model of insulin insufficiency independent of its metabolic effects. Arteriosclerosis, Thrombosis, and Vascular Biology 25: 1903–1909.
26. Haffner SM, Greenberg AS, Weston WM, Chen H, Williams K, et al. (2002) Effect of rosiglitazone treatment on nontraditional markers of cardiovascular disease in patients with type 2 diabetes mellitus. Circulation 106: 679–684.
27. Chu NV, Kong AP, Kim DD, Armstrong D, Baxi S, et al. (2002) Differential effects of metformin and troglitazone on cardiovascular risk factors in patients with type 2 diabetes. Diabetes Care 25: 542–549.
28. Verreth W, Ganame J, Mertens A, Bernar H, Herregods MC, et al. (2006) Peroxisome proliferator-activated receptor-alpha,gamma-agonist improves insulin sensitivity and prevents loss of left ventricular function in obese dyslipidemic mice. Arteriosclerosis, Thrombosis, and Vascular Biology 26: 922–928.
29. Combs TP, Wagner JA, Berger J, Doebber T, Wang WJ, et al. (2002) Induction of adipocyte complement-related protein of 30 kilodaltons by PPARgamma agonists: a potential mechanism of insulin sensitization. Endocrinology 143: 998–1007.
30. Iwaki M, Matsuda M, Maeda N, Funahashi T, Matsuzawa Y, et al. (2003) Induction of adiponectin, a fat-derived antidiabetic and antiatherogenic factor, by nuclear receptors. Diabetes 52: 1655–1663.
31. Padmalayam I, Suto M (2013) Role of Adiponectin in the metabolic syndrome: current perspectives on its modulation as a treatment strategy. Curr Pharm Des doi:CPD-EPUB-20130220-9.
32. Hu D, Fukuhara A, Miyata Y, Yokoyama C, Otsuki M, et al. (2013) Adiponectin Regulates Vascular Endothelial Growth Factor-C Expression in Macrophages via Syk-ERK Pathway. PLoS.ONE. 8: e56071.

33. Tao L, Wang Y, Gao E, Zhang H, Yuan Y, et al. (2010) Adiponectin: an indispensable molecule in rosiglitazone cardioprotection following myocardial infarction. Circulation Research 106: 409–417.

34. Wong WT, Tian XY, Xu A, Yu J, Lau CW, et al. (2011) Adiponectin is required for PPARgamma-mediated improvement of endothelial function in diabetic mice. Cell Metab 14: 104–115.

35. Bahia L, Aguiar LG, Villela N, Bottino D, Godoy-Matos AF, et al. (2007) Adiponectin is associated with improvement of endothelial function after rosiglitazone treatment in non-diabetic individuals with metabolic syndrome. Atherosclerosis 195: 138–146.

36. Standiford TJ, Kuick R, Bhan U, Chen J, Newstead M, et al. (2011) TGF-beta-induced IRAK-M expression in tumor-associated macrophages regulates lung tumor growth. Oncogene 30: 2475–2484.

37. Chen W, Saxena A, Li N, Sun J, Gupta A, et al. (2012) Endogenous IRAK-M Attenuates Postinfarction Remodeling Through Effects on Macrophages and Fibroblasts. Arteriosclerosis, Thrombosis, and Vascular Biology 32: 2598–2608.

38. Tsai JS, Chen CY, Chen YL, Chuang LM (2010) Rosiglitazone inhibits monocyte/macrophage adhesion through de novo adiponectin production in human monocytes. J.Cell Biochem. 110: 1410–1419.

39. Burgos-Ramos E, Sackmann-Sala L, Baquedano E, Cruz-Topete D, Barrios V, et al. (2012) Central leptin and insulin administration modulates serum cytokine- and lipoprotein-related markers. Metabolism 61: 1646–1657.

40. de Heredia FP, Gomez-Martinez S, Marcos A (2012) Obesity, inflammation and the immune system. Proceedings of the Nutrition Society 71: 332–338.

41. Kintscher U, Law RE (2005) PPARgamma-mediated insulin sensitization: the importance of fat versus muscle. Am.J.Physiol Endocrinol.Metab 288: E287–E291.

42. Madej A, Okopien B, Kowalski J, Zielinski M, Wysocki J, et al. (1998) Effects of fenofibrate on plasma cytokine concentrations in patients with atherosclerosis and hyperlipoproteinemia IIb. Int.J Clin.Pharmacol.Ther. 36: 345–349.

43. Chakrabarti S, Blair P, Freedman JE (2007) CD40–40L signaling in vascular inflammation. Journal of Biological Chemistry 282: 18307–18317.

44. van der Hoogt CC, de Haan W, Westerterp M, Hoekstra M, Dallinga-Thie GM, et al. (2007) Fenofibrate increases HDL-cholesterol by reducing cholesteryl ester transfer protein expression. Journal of Lipid Research 48: 1763–1771.

45. Srivastava RA (2011) Evaluation of anti-atherosclerotic activities of PPAR-alpha, PPAR-gamma, and LXR agonists in hyperlipidemic atherosclerosis-susceptible F(1)B hamsters. Atherosclerosis 214: 86–93.

46. Duez H, Chao YS, Hernandez M, Torpier G, Poulain P, et al. (2002) Reduction of atherosclerosis by the peroxisome proliferator-activated receptor alpha agonist fenofibrate in mice. Journal of Biological Chemistry 277: 48051–48057.

Effects of Green Tea Extract on Insulin Resistance and Glucagon-Like Peptide 1 in Patients with Type 2 Diabetes and Lipid Abnormalities

Chia-Yu Liu[1,2], Chien-Jung Huang[3], Lin-Huang Huang[1], I-Ju Chen[1,2], Jung-Peng Chiu[1,2], Chung-Hua Hsu[1,2]*

1 Institute of Traditional Medicine, School of Medicine, National Yang-Ming University, Taipei, Taiwan, 2 Department of Chinese Medicine, Branch of Linsen and Chinese Medicine, Taipei City Hospital, Taipei, Taiwan, 3 Department of Metabolism, Branch of Linsen and Chinese Medicine, Taipei City Hospital, Taipei, Taiwan

Abstract

The aim of this study is to investigate the effect of green tea extract on patients with type 2 diabetes mellitus and lipid abnormalities on glycemic and lipid profiles, and hormone peptides by a double-blinded, randomized and placebo-controlled clinical trial. This trial enrolled 92 subjects with type 2 diabetes mellitus and lipid abnormalities randomized into 2 arms, each arm comprising 46 participants. Of the participants, 39 in therapeutic arm took 500 mg green tea extract, three times a day, while 38 in control arm took cellulose with the same dose and frequency to complete the 16-week study. Anthropometrics measurements, glycemic and lipid profiles, safety parameters, and obesity-related hormone peptides were analyzed at screening and after 16-week course. Within-group comparisons showed that green tea extract caused a significant decrease in triglyceride and homeostasis model assessment of insulin resistance index after 16 weeks. Green tea extract also increased significantly high density lipoprotein cholesterol. The HOMA-IR index decreased from 5.4±3.9 to 3.5±2.0 in therapeutic arm only. Adiponectin, apolipoprotein A1, and apolipoprotein B100 increased significantly in both arms, but only glucagon-like peptide 1 increased in the therapeutic arm. However, only decreasing trend in triglyceride was found in between-group comparison. Our study suggested that green tea extract significantly improved insulin resistance and increased glucagon-like peptide 1 only in within-group comparison. The potential effects of green tea extract on insulin resistance and glucagon-like peptide 1 warrant further investigation.

Trial Registration: ClinicalTrials.gov NCT01360567

Editor: Stephen L. Atkin, Postgraduate Medical Institute & Hull York Medical School, University of Hull, United Kingdom

Funding: This study was supported financially by the National Science Council, Taiwan, under Grant No. 101-2320-B-010-075. The funders had no role in study design, data collection and analysis, decision to publish, or preparation of the manuscript.

Competing Interests: The authors have declared that no competing interests exist.

* E-mail: owlherbs@yahoo.com.tw

Introduction

Both type 2 diabetes mellitus (T2DM) and dyslipidemia are individually associated with a cluster of risk factors of atherosclerosis. Lipoprotein abnormalities also increase the thrombotic risk of diabetic patients [1]. Common risk factors for coronary artery disease explain only 25–50% of increased atherosclerotic risk in diabetes mellitus. Other obvious risk factors are hyperglycemia and dyslipidemia. However, hyperglycemia is a very late stage in the sequence of events from insulin resistance to frank diabetes, whereas lipoprotein abnormalities are manifested during the largely asymptomatic diabetic prodrome and contribute to the increased risk of macrovascular disease [2]. Combining medication with lifestyle modification is a logical approach to reduce cardiovascular risk in individuals with dyslipidemia and T2DM [3].

Tea, derived from the plant Camellia sinensis is consumed in the world as green, black or Oolong tea. Among them, green tea has the most significant effects on cardiovascular protection, and the effects of green tea are mainly attributed to its flavonoid-like polyphenols, such as catechins. Catechins concluded mainly epigallocatechin gallate (EGCG), epigallocatechin, epicatechin gallate, and epicatechin, which are the most common green tea extracts (GTE). EGCG is the major catechin in tea and may account for 50–80% of the total catechins in tea [4]. Although several studies implied that EGCG may have the potential to improve the glycemic and lipid profiles in patients with diabetes and dyslipidemia [5–8], the effect of GTE on glucose and lipid control was inconsistent, and the underlying mechanism was still unclear. Therefore, this study aims to investigate the effects of decaffeinated GTE on anthropometric measurements, glycemic and lipid profile, as well as hormone levels by a randomized, double-blinded, and placebo-controlled clinical trial.

Subjects and Methods

This clinical trial was conducted from April 2011 to March 2012 at Taipei City Hospital in Taiwan. Among 236 registered patients with T2DM, whose glycemic hemoglobin higher than 6.5% within 3 months, screened at our outpatient clinic, 102 subjects met the following criteria were enrolled: (1) age between 20 and 65 years, (2) diagnosis of type 2 diabetes for more than one year, (3) body mass index (BMI) ≥ 18 kg/m2 and ≤30 kg/m2, (4) fasting triglyceride ≥ 150 mg/dl or fasting low-density-lipoprotein cholesterol (LDL) ≥100 mg/dl and (5) willing to participate in and fill out questionnaires for this trial. The exclusion criteria include (1) serum alanine transaminase >80 U/L, (2) serum creatinine >1.8 mg/dl, (3) breast feeding or pregnancy, (4) heart failure, acute myocardial infarction, stroke, heavy injury, and (5) any other conditions not suitable for trial as evaluated by the physician. Letters explaining the purpose of the study were sent to all the patients inviting their participation. Finally, with a written informed consent, 102 subjects were enrolled in this study. The protocol was approved by the Human Ethics Committee of Taipei City Hospital. This trial (NCT01360567) was registered with the ClinicalTrials.gov Registry on 20 May 2011 and followed the CONSORT 2010 statements. The protocol for this trial and supporting CONSORT checklist are available as supporting information; see Checklist S1 and Protocol S1.

Subjects were randomly allocated to receive a decaffeinated GTE EGCG (Group A) or a placebo (cellulose; Group B) for 16 weeks (Figure 1). Both experimental and placebo treatments were contained in the same opaque capsules, which were administered by a blinded research assistant. Subjects were instructed to maintain an isocaloric diet and to continue their previous eating habits during the study period. Every four weeks, subjects returned to our clinics and reported to the study center for adverse events and compliance assessment. Subjects were free to withdraw at any time. Throughout the study period, subjects were directed to continue taking the same dose of any prescribed hypoglycemic agents unless hypoglycemia or severe complications occurred, in which case they were directed to reduce their dose immediately.

Preparation of samples and treatment

Decaffeinated GTE was obtained from the Tea Research and Extension Station, Taoyuan County, Taiwan. It was extracted from dried leaves of green tea according to pre-set standard procedures. The decaffeinated GTE used in this study was standardized for several tea catechins in addition to EGCG (Table 1). The placebo comprised pure microcrystalline cellulose. Capsules contained either 500 mg decaffeinated GTE extract or cellulose. Subjects were asked to take one capsule 30 minutes after meals three times daily for 16 weeks. Table 1 lists the total daily dose of GTE compounds received by the active group.

Analysis of obesity-related hormone peptides

The levels of obesity-related hormone peptides, including leptin, insulin, ghrelin, adiponectin, apolipoprotein (apo) A1, apolipoprotein B100, and glucagon-like peptide 1 (GLP-1) (7–36) were measured in the morning after 8–9 hours of fasting. Whole blood sample was drawn and centrifuged at 4°C, with 1 ml aliquot of serum rapidly frozen at −80°C for the subsequent radioimmunoassay concentration analysis. Leptin was detected by the Millipore Human Leptin assay (Millipore, St. Charles, MO, USA) using I125-labled human leptin antiserum with a sensitivity of 0.5 ng/ml for a 100-μL sample. Ghrelin and adiponectin were detected by Millipore Ghrelin RIA Kits (Millipore, St. Charles) and Millipore Adiponectin RIA kits (Millipore, St. Charles) with a sensitivity of 93 pg/ml and 1 ng/ml, respectively. We used the same process as

that for leptin detection only with different I125-labled antibodies specific for ghrelin or adiponectin. BioSource INS-IRMA Kits (BioSource Europe S.A., Nivelles, Belgium) were employed to determine the level of insulin in serum as previously reported [9,10]. The intra- and inter-assay coefficients of variation were 3.1% and 4.9%, respectively. The limit of sensitivity is 0.5 ng/ml. Sampling would be reported if a difference exceeding 10% coefficients of variation was found between duplicated results of the sample. The level of insulin resistance was evaluated by the homeostasis model assessment of insulin resistance index (HOMA-IR), which was calculated with the following model: HOMA-IR = insulin [mIU/L] × glucose [mmol/L]/22.5, and values exceeding 2.25 would denote insulin resistance [11]. Circulating level of GLP-1 (7–36) was determined by the Millipore Human glucagon-like peptide-1 RIA kits (Millipore, St. Charles) with a sensitivity of 3 pmol for a 300-μL extracted sample. [12,13] Apo AI and apo B-100 were detected by immunoturbidimetric assay (K-assay, Kamiya Biomedical Company, Seattle, USA).

Quality of life

To measure the health-related quality of life (HRQOL) among our subjects, we used the self-administered life-quality questionnaires, world health organization quality of life-BREF (WHO-QOL-BREF), Taiwan version which was well validated with consistency coefficients ranging from 0.70 to 0.77 [14]. The WHOQOL-BREF questionnaire evaluated quality of life in physical, psychological, social and environmental domains, with scores ranging from 0 to 100. Higher scores in this questionnaire represent better health condition. Previous study showed that body weight loss could improve HRQOL; hence we use WHOQOL-BREF questionnaire to assess the effects of green tea extracts on quality of life [15].

Assessment

The single primary outcome was defined as the change of triglyceride (TG) level. The secondary outcomes were evaluated by anthropometric measurements in terms of body weight, height, BMI, waist circumference, and hip circumference. Biochemical characteristics of blood sample including fasting blood sugar, hemoglobin A1c (HbA1c), total cholesterol, low density lipoprotein (LDL)-cholesterol, high density lipoprotein (HDL)-cholesterol levels, high sensitivity C-reactive protein (hsCRP), obesity-related hormone peptides, and HRQOL scores on the WHOQOL-BREF were also assessed. The safety parameters included serum alanine transaminase, creatinine, estimated glomerular filtration rate (eGFR), and adverse event reports. All measurements of biochemical characteristics and obesity-related hormone peptides of blood sample were made at 0800–0900 after an overnight fasting using standardized methods, as detailed in our previous research [16]. All participating physicians received prior training before the study on how to interview the participants and assist them in completing the questionnaires.

Statistical analysis

The data were analyzed using SPSS software (version 17.0, Chicago, IL.) Independent t-tests were employed to examine the difference in anthropometrics, biochemical characteristics, obesity-related hormone peptides, and life-quality scores between EGCG group and placebo group. Paired t-tests were employed to examine the difference between before and after intervention for 16 weeks in both groups. All p values were two-tailed and α level of significance was set at 0.05. Our own experience suggested a standard deviation (SD) of 3.5% in a previous series of 60 patients with diabetes. It was calculated that to detect a reduction in

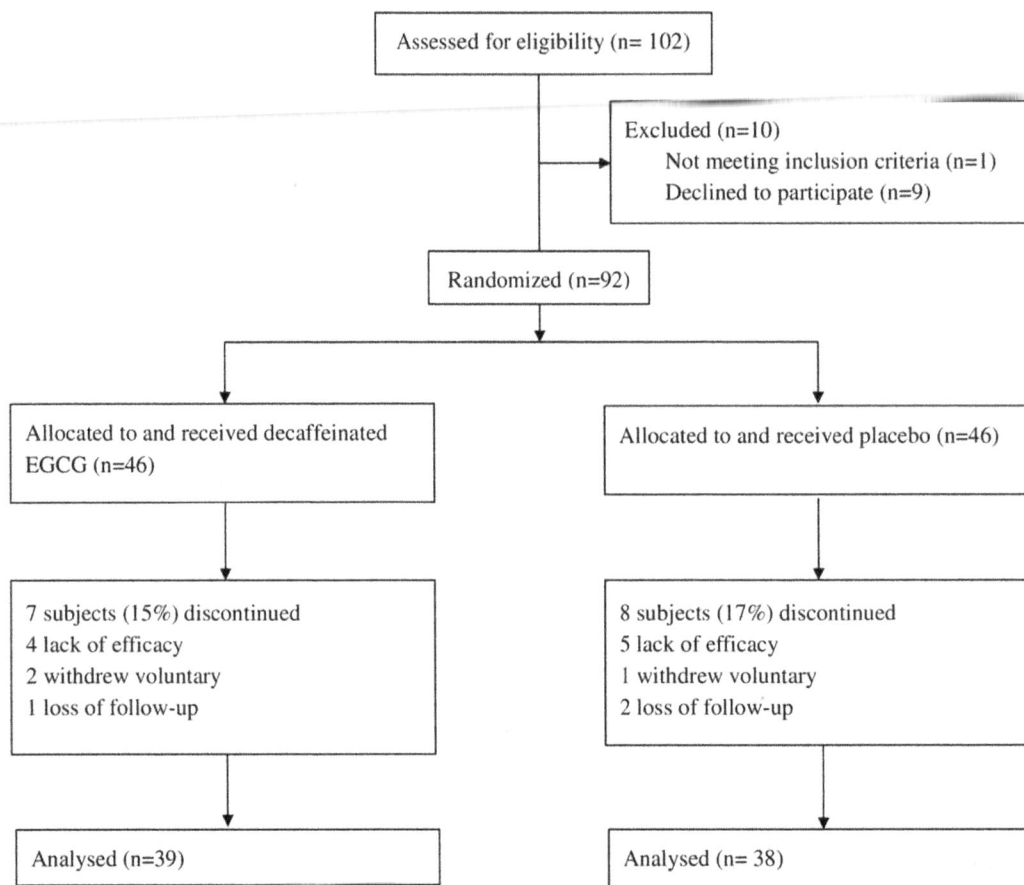

Figure 1. Study Flow Diagram.

triglyceride level of 2.4% with a significance level of 0.05 and a power of 0.8, that 64 patients would be required. Allowing for a 10% dropout, 70 patients would be needed in this study.

Results

Data were analyzed on a per-protocol basis, with subject exclusion occurring before release of the double-blind procedure. A total of 102 subjects were enrolled. Nine subjects did not receive their allocated intervention as they failed to attend study visit

because of work commitments or moving out of the area. One subject with poor blood sugar control (fasting plasma glucose values ≥ 500 mg/dL) at baseline was excluded as the primary investigator considered the risk of hyperglycemic hyperosmolar nonketotic coma. In the end, 92 subjects were randomly assigned. Further 7 subjects in the EGCG group and 8 subjects in the placebo group discontinued the intervention. Consequently, the data reported here came from 77 subjects (Fig. 1).

Baseline characteristics for both placebo and EGCG groups are shown in Table 2. No significant differences between any of the group means were detected in demographic, disease duration, glycemic, and lipid parameters (Table 2). To monitor compliance, subjects were required to return all packaging and unused capsules. Each subject received 336 capsules and on average 9.9 ± 13.0 capsules per subject (12.3 ± 15.0 capsules from the EGCG group and 7.5 ± 10.1 capsules from the placebo group) were returned, indicating that more than 95% of doses were taken.

To clarify the effect of concomitant medications on blood pressure, sugar and lipid levels, medications taken by the subjects were reviewed (Table 3). More than half of the participants, 21 subjects (53.8%) in the EGCG group and 23 subjects (60.5%) in the placebo group, took the oral antidiabetes medications. Although the percentage of antidiabetes medication usage was higher in the placebo group, the difference was not statistically significant ($p = 0.097$). Moreover, 6 subjects (15.4%) in the EGCG group and 4 subjects (10.5%) in the placebo group took

Table 1. The composition of green tea extracts.

Component	% in weight	Daily dose (in mg)
EGCG (Epigallocatechin gallate)	57.12	856.8
ECG (Epicatechin gallate)	15.74	236.1
EGC (Epigallocatechin)	7.70	115.5
EC (Epicatechin)	4.80	71.9
GCG (Gallocatechin gallate)	4.25	63.7
GC (Gallocatechin)	<0.07	<1.05
Caffeine	<0.07	<1.05
Cellulose	10.3	155.0

Table 2. Demographic data of participants.

	Decaffeinated EGCG (n = 39)	Placebo(cellulose) (n = 38)	P value
Gender (male/female)*	14/25	18/20	0.307
Age (years)	55.0±6.6	53.5±7.0	0.328
Body weight (kg)	66.4±13.2	68.8±13.6	0.442
Body mass index (kg/m²)	26.2±4.2	26.4±4.6	0.786
Time since diagnosis of diabetes (years)	5.2±5.9	4.1±4.3	0.339
Family history of diabetes, yes (n)*	27	27	0.861
Fasting blood sugar (mg/dL)	139.2±45.1	152.2±53.5	0.252
Glycemic hemoglobin, HbA1c (%)	7.5±1.6	7.7±1.8	0.591
Low density lipoprotein (mg/dL)	109.7±31.9	115.2±35.4	0.478
Triglyceride (mg/dL)	178.2±105.3	198.3±127.9	0.453
Remnants of capsules, No.	12.3±15.0	7.5±10.1	0.102
(Ratio, remnants/total, %)	(4±4.5)	(2±3)	

* Data analyzed by Chi-square test.

antihypertensive medications; while 6 subjects (15.4%) in the EGCG group and 2 subjects (5.3%) in the placebo group took the lipid modifying medications. There was no statistically significant difference in any concomitant medication between the two groups.

The 16-week treatment with decaffeinated GTE resulted in decreasing body weight and BMI (p <0.1), compared with baseline measurements, as shown in Table 4a. On the other hands, there is no significant changes in other anthropometric data, including waist circumference, hip circumference, and blood pressure after the 16-week course. Between-group comparison results are listed in Table 5a. There were no statistically significant differences detected for any of the variables assessed after 16 weeks of decaffeinated GTE versus placebo treatment.

Regarding serum lipid profiles, fasting TG decreased from 178.2±105.3 to 159.3±91.6 with statistical significance in the EGCG group (p = 0.03). However, fasting TG increased from 198.3±127.9 to 208.2±118.2 in the placebo group. In spite of the 2.1±38.5 percent of decrement in EGCG group and the 18.8±58.3 percent of increment in placebo group, decaffeinated EGCG led to a decreasing trend in serum TG (p<0.1). The total cholesterol level decreased slightly from 195.5±37.4 to 193.6±40.0 without statistically significant difference in EGCG group. HDL increased significantly from 49.5±13.6 to 52.2±15.7 in the EGCG group (p = 0.04), but the level after cellulose treatment was almost the same. In the between-group analysis, the percentages of increment in HDL were 6.1±16.0 in the EGCG

Table 3. Concomitant medications usage of participants.

Concomitant medication	Decaffeinated EGCG (n = 39)	Placebo(cellulose) (n = 38)	P value
Antidiabetic medications users, %	53.8	60.5	0.097
Sulfonylureas, %	35.9	34.2	0.877
Biguanides, %	43.6	44.7	0.919
Alpha glucosidase inhibitors, %	2.6	5.3	0.541
Thiazolidinediones, %	12.8	5.3	0.249
Dipeptidyl peptidase 4 (DPP-4) inhibitors, %	10.3	5.3	0.414
Meglitinide, %	2.6	0	0.320
Combination, %	35.9	26.3	
Antihypertensives users, %	15.4	10.5	0.787
Angiotensin-converting enzyme inhibitors, %	2.6	2.6	0.985
Angiotensin receptor blockers, %	10.3	7.9	0.719
Calcium channel blockers, %	7.7	2.6	0.317
Combination, %	5.1	2.6	
Lipid modifying agents users, %	15.4	5.3	0.146
HMG CoA reductase inhibitors,%	12.8	5.3	0.249
Fibrates, %	2.6	0	0.320
Combination, %	0	0	

Data analyzed by Chi-square test, except the mean of different medication analyzed by independent t-test.

Table 4.

Within-group analysis of anthropometrics and biochemical data at baseline and 16 weeks of study

Variable	Decaffeinated EGCG (n = 39)			Placebo (cellulose) (n = 38)		
	baseline	After 16 weeks	p-value	baseline	After 16 weeks	p-value
Anthropometric data						
Weight, kg	66.4±13.2	66.0±13.3	0.09*	68.8±13.6	68.6±13.7	0.69
Body mass index, kg/m²	26.2±4.2	26.0±4.0	0.06*	26.4±4.6	26.4±4.4	0.54
Waist circumference, cm	83.9±9.8	85.2±12.1	0.17	87.8±11.0	87.5±8.4	0.69
Hip circumference, cm	96.4±9.5	96.9±9.3	0.30	99.3±4.0	98.9±10.5	0.30
Waist hip ratio	0.9±0.1	0.9±0.1	0.60	0.9±0.6	0.9±0.5	0.63
Systolic blood pressure, mmHg	133.4±18.6	135.3±18.1	0.48	133.3±16.7	131.6±14.5	0.38
Diastolic blood pressure, mmHg	78.9±10.8	78.1±11.1	0.68	84.5±15.3	80.5±9.1	0.05*
Heart rate, bpm	76.9±13.0	77.6±13.7	0.59	75.9±10.9	76.6±13.1	0.56
Biochemical data						
Alanine transaminase (IU/L)	31.1±17.6	31.8±19.9	0.71	28.1±12.1	28.3±13.1	0.87
Creatinine, mg/dL	0.74±0.17	0.74±0.19	0.68	0.77±0.18	0.77±0.17	1.0
eGFR, %	75.8±13.5	75.2±14.2	0.57	75.6±13.0	75.7±13.3	0.91
Triglyceride, mg/dL	178.2±105.3	159.3±91.6	0.03 **	198.3±127.9	208.2±118.2	0.38
Total cholesterol, mg/dL	195.5±37.4	193.6±40.0	0.67	206.7±47.6	207.4±55.6	0.89
Low density lipoprotein, mg/dL	109.7±31.9	111.8±37.7	0.55	115.2±35.4	111.9±32.4	0.48
High density lipoprotein, mg/dL	49.5±13.6	52.2±15.7	0.04 **	46.7±11.6	46.8±11.4	0.94
Fasting blood sugar, mg/dL	139.2±45.1	148.2±48.1	0.07*	152.2±53.5	151.6±61.7	0.88
Glycemic hemoglobin, HbA1c, %	7.5±1.6	7.5±1.7	0.70	7.7±1.8	7.5±1.7	0.054
HSCRP, mg/L	0.26±0.27	0.36±0.36	0.013*	0.21±0.21	0.28±0.27	0.04*

Within-group analysis of hormone peptides and WHOQOL-BREF at baseline and 16 weeks of study

Variable	Decaffeinated EGCG (n = 39)			Placebo (cellulose) (n = 38)		
	baseline	After 16 weeks	p-value	baseline	After 16 weeks	p-value
Hormone peptides						
Insulin, IU/L	15.6±10.4	9.3±4.2	0.000**	17.0±14.8	12.3±7.5	0.039*
HOMA-IR index	5.4±3.9	3.5±2.0	0.004**	5.9±4.5	4.7±3.4	0.11
Leptin, ng/mL	7.7±5.4	8.3±5.8	0.46	7.6±7.6	8.1±6.5	0.51
Ghrelin, pg/mL	537.8±255.1	499.7±172.1	0.44	598.4±227.8	440.3±184.3	0.002**
Adiponectin, ug/mL	20.2±5.1	21.7±5.1	0.046**	18.6±2.9	20.3±3.8	0.000**
Apolipoprotein A1, mg/dL	137.9±34.5	191.7±74.5	0.000**	134.5±30.3	165.9±54.5	0.002**
Apolipoprotein B100, mg/dL	95.6±27.6	130.0±62.0	0.001**	99.4±25.9	116.7±40.5	0.006**
Glucagon-like peptide-1 (7–36), pmol/L	1.4±1.2	2.6±1.6	0.001**	1.9±2.3	2.2±1.8	0.60
WHOQOL-BREF						
Physical	62.1±14.1	68.1±12.3	0.001**	66.6±10.8	69.3±14.3	0.08
Psychological	70.9±15.5	72.3±12.1	0.42	74.1±14.5	74.2±12.8	0.95
Social	74.5±13.9	77.4±10.4	0.12	74.8±18.8	76.7±13.6	0.49
Environment	74.6±13.5	79.5±8.9	0.01	75.6±14.1	76.2±11.9	0.75

*p<0.1, **p<0.05

group and 1.9±17.9 in the placebo group, though without statistical significance. LDL increased from 109.7±31.9 to 111.8±37.7 in the EGCG group but declined from 115.2±35.4 to 111.9±32.4 in the placebo group; and neither difference was statistically significant.

As for blood sugar and insulin resistance, fasting glucose increased from 139.2±45.1 to 148.2±48.1 in the EGCG group, but decreased slightly from 152.2±53.5 to 151.6±61.7 in the placebo group. Neither group showed statistical significance in within-group analysis. With respect to glycohemoglobin, no statistically significant difference existed between the two groups. Interestingly, insulin decreased markedly from 15.6±10.4 to 9.3±4.2 (p = 0.000) in the EGCG group and from 17.0±14.8 to 12.3±7.5 (p = 0.039) in the placebo group. But the difference between groups didn't was not statistically significant. This study evaluates insulin resistance by HOMA-IR index. The HOMA-IR

Table 5.

Between-group analysis of anthropometrics and biochemical data at baseline and 16 weeks of study

	Reduction		
Variable	**Decaffeinated EGCG (n = 39)**	**Placebo (cellulose) (n = 38)**	**p-value**
Anthropometric data			
Weight, kg	−0.7±2.2	−0.2±3.5	0.45
Body mass index, kg/m²	−0.2±0.6	−0.1±0.9	0.61
Waist circumference, cm	0.7±4.2	−0.3±4.7	0.35
Hip circumference, cm	0.5±3.2	−0.5±2.6	0.14
Waist hip ratio	−0.0±0.0	0.0±0.0	0.71
Systolic blood pressure, mmHg	1.9±16.9	−1.7±11.7	0.28
Diastolic blood pressure, mmHg	−0.7±11.1	−4.1±12.6	0.23
Heart rate, bpm	0.8±9.1	0.7±7.3	0.96
Biochemical data			
Alanine transaminase (IU/L)	0.7±12.0	0.2±9.1	0.84
Creatinine, mg/dL	0.0±0.1	0.0±0.1	0.76
eGFR, %	−0.7±7.7	0.1±6.9	0.62
Uric acid, mg/dL	0.1±0.8	0.3±0.9	0.34
Triglyceride, mg/dL	−2.1±38.5	16.4±56.6	0.097*
Total cholesterol, mg/dL	−1.9±26.9	0.7±33.6	0.71
Low density lipoprotein, mg/dL	2.1±21.2	−3.3±29.0	0.36
High density of lipoprotein, mg/dL	2.7±7.8	0.1±6.3	0.11
Fasting blood sugar, mg/dL	9.0±30.3	−0.6±25.2	0.13
Glycemic hemoglobin, HbA1c, %	−0.0±5.5	−0.2±0.6	0.24
HSCRP	0.1±0.2	0.1±0.2	0.53

Between-group analysis of hormone peptides and WHOQOL-BREF at baseline and 16 weeks of study

	Reduction		
Variable	**Decaffeinated EGCG (n = 39)**	**Placebo (cellulose) (n = 38)**	**p-value**
Hormone peptides			
Insulin, IU/L	−6.3±10.0	−4.7±13.5	0.54
HOMA-IR index	−2.0±4.0	−1.3±4.8	0.50
Leptin, ng/mL	0.7±5.6	0.5±4.5	0.88
Ghrelin, pg/mL	−38.1±306.0	−158.1±292.0	0.08*
Adiponectin, ug/mL	1.5±4.4	1.6±2.2	0.24
Apolipoprotein A1, mg/dL	53.9±64.3	31.3±58.7	0.11
Apolipoprotein B100, mg/dL	34.4±57.7	17.3±37.0	0.13
Glucagon like peptide-1 (7-36), pmol/L	1.1±2.0	0.3±3.0	0.14
WHOQOL-BREF			
Physical	6.0±10.6	2.8±9.5	0.16
Psychological	1.4±10.7	0.1±12.3	0.63
Social	3.0±11.5	1.9±16.8	0.75
Environment	4.9±11.2	0.6±11.1	0.10

*P<0.1

in the EGCG group decreased from 5.4±3.9 to 3.5±2.0 with statistical significance (p = 0.004), while that in the placebo group decreased from 5.9±4.5 to 4.7±3.4 without statistical significance.

Among the obesity-related hormone peptides, ghrelin in the placebo group decreased from 598.4±227.8 to 440.3±184.3 with statistical significance (p = 0.002), as shown in table 4b. Ghrelin in the EGCG group also decreased after the 16-week course but did not achieve statistical significance. Adiponectin increased markedly in both groups but showed no statistically significant difference between groups. There was also no statistically significant difference in leptin level in the two groups. The hsCRP significantly increased in both groups with difference of 0.1±0.2.

Apo AI increased significantly in both groups and the differences were 53.9±64.3 in the EGCG group and 31.3±58.7 in the placebo group. Apo B-100 also increased significantly in both groups and the differences are 34.4±57.7 in the EGCG group and 17.3±57.0 in the placebo group. GLP-1 in EGCG group increased from 1.4±1.2 to 2.6±1.6 with statistical significance (p = 0.001), but the difference in GLP-1 in the placebo group didn't achieve statistical significance. However, none of the differences between the groups reached statistical significance (table 5b).

Adverse Effects

In the experimental group, one subject in the experimental group experienced symptoms of epigastric dullness and two developed mild constipation, while one subject in the placebo group had abdominal discomfort. All these symptoms were relieved in the first week after treatment. No major adverse effects of either experimental or placebo group were noted.

Discussion

The present initial results revealed no statistically significant difference between the EGCG and placebo groups in any of the anthropometric, glycemic, lipid or hormone peptide variables assessed. Despite of adequate sample size after calculation, the metabolic responses to EGCG in those patients with type 2 diabetes were various. Because the small sample size, the difference between the randomized groups was non-significant in our study. But our within-group analysis explored some new findings on GLP-1, insulin resistance, and lipid profile such as triglyceride and HDL, which were less affected by current antidiabetic medications.

The worldwide prevalence of diabetes has continued to increase dramatically instead of the improvement in outcomes for individual patients with diabetes. Lifestyle modification will undoubtedly play a key role in the ultimate solution to the problem of diabetes [17]. The anti-diabetic effect of green tea extracts may raise the potential of green tea to be the lifestyle modification for diabetic prevention. People who drink at least 4 cups of tea per day may have a 16% lower risk of developing type 2 diabetes than non-tea drinkers [18]. However, green tea catechins alone do not positively alter anthropometric measurements. A meta-analysis showed that GTE have a positive effect on weight loss and weight maintenance in obese people (BMI between 25 and 30) [19,20]. To understand the effect of green tea catechins in anthropometrics of diabetic subjects, and to avoid the potential confounding effect caused by caffeine in green tea, this study used decaffeinated GTE. Although a decreasing trend in body weight and BMI was observed, GTE did not significantly reduce body weight and BMI of diabetic subjects (BMI around 26) in our study. This result is similar to other studies for diabetic rats and diabetic population (BMI around 30) [21,22]. The difference may be due to the degree of obesity or disease nature, and it merits further investigation.

To our knowledge, this is the first study on the effect of GTE on GLP-1. Our results showed significant within-group changes in GLP-1 level and HOMA-IR index after 16 weeks of treatment only in the GTE group, despite there being no significant change in fasting glucose and HbA1c. Previous research reported a significant interaction between circulating GLP-1, serum HDL, and triglyceride concentrations but not waist circumference, fasting glucose, HbA1c, or presence of diabetes [23]. This result is consistent with the within-group findings in the present study. GLP-1 could lower blood sugar with insulin resistance through up-

regulating the pancreatic β-cell to enhance insulin secretion and suppressing glucagon secretion with gastric emptying. Therefore, the incretin therapy has been used in different stages of diabetes in recent years [24–26]. Several studies have shown that T2DM patients generally exhibit attenuated GLP-1 secretion [27–29]. In our patients, GLP-1 secretion was lower in both groups and enhanced only in GTE group, but whether the levels of GLP-1 secretion were sufficient could not be determined. Thondam et al. reported that metformin increased serum GLP-1 level in T2DM patients [30], and metformin could also enhance GLP-1 secretion in GLP-1 producing cell line [31]. This study has avoided the confounding effects of chronic antidiabetic treatment, because these treatments did not show any significant difference between GTE and placebo groups. Although several studies demonstrated the glucose-lowering effects of GTE, the fasting glucose and HbA1c did not decrease after GTE supplementation in our study. This discrepancy might be due to the more obvious patients with diabetes in our study, whose mean disease duration was around 5 years. The glucose-lowering effects of GTE supplementation are better in patients with diabetes history of less than 5 years than those with a history of more than 5 years. The increased GLP-1, lower insulin, and decreased HOMA-IR were only significant in the population with disease duration of less than 5 years (data was not shown). Future studies with larger numbers of patients will be required to investigate the clinical characteristics of patients with a better GLP-1 response to GTE.

Virtually every lipid and lipoprotein is affected by insulin resistance and diabetes mellitus, but control of hyperglycemia is unlikely to correct existing dyslipidemia. Although plasma glucose control is important in reducing microvascular complications due to diabetes, lipid management is also essential in these patients to decrease the incidence of cardiovascular events [32]. In this study, EGCG significantly reduced fasting triglyceride and increased HDL in within-group analysis and caused a decreasing trend of fasting triglycerides in between-group analysis. Adiponectin, apoA1 and apoB-100 increased significantly in both groups in within-group comparison. Whether adiponectin is positively associated with green tea consumption or not remains controversial [33–36]. Green tea extracts also could reduced fat deposit and ameliorated in high fat-fed rats via the adiponectin associated pathway [37]. Since adiponectin plays a role in regulating insulin function and is negatively associated with risk factors for cardiovascular disease, the clinical effects of GTE on adiponectin merits further clarification. ApoAI and apoB-100 are the major apolipoproteins of HDL and LDL, respectively[38]. In vitro study revealed that EGCG decreased apoB-100 secretion [39,40], which is inconsistent with our findings. Increased serum LDL, rather than decreased triglyceride, possibly leads to this discrepancy. However, the increase in apoAI after EGCG supplementation is compatible with that in HDL. Current guidelines recommend statin therapy and lifestyle modification as primary intervention for reducing cardiovascular risk in patients with T2DM. However, even with intensive lowering of LDL cholesterol, patients remain at high residual risk because of low HDL cholesterol and/or elevated triglycerides, justifying the need for additional therapy specifically aimed at the management of these abnormalities [3]. EGCG may be the logical dietary supplement for combination with a statin in this setting. Large prospective studies are needed to evaluate the clinical benefits and tolerability of these combinations.

Although the literature reported several suspected green tea-related hepatic reactions [41], the hepatotoxicity is probably due to metabolism or concomitant medications of a particular patient. Neither impaired liver/renal function nor major adverse effects were seen in our study. As for the limitation of this study, the relatively small sample size and relatively large variance of the metabolic measurements made the outcome non-significant. Besides, the compliance was monitored only by counting the returned packages and unused capsules. This study didn't measure the participants' serum level of EGCG to confirm the bioavailability and the effects on metabolism. Further research on the bioavailability and pharmacokinetics of EGCG in human studies is needed.

In conclusion, the present study showed no statistically significant difference between decaffeinated GTE and placebo in anthropometrics, glycemic and lipid profiles, as well as obesity-related hormone peptides after 16 weeks of treatment. Daily taking decaffeinated GTE with dose of 856 mg EGCG for 16 weeks is safe and free of severe adverse effects. The metabolic effects on

GLP-1 and insulin response of decaffeinated GTE in humans warrant continued investigation.

Acknowledgments

We thank Miao-Mei Chen and all colleagues at Branch of Linsen and Chinese Medicine, Taipei City Hospital, Taiwan, for their help with this study.

Author Contributions

Conceived and designed the experiments: CYL CHH. Performed the experiments: CYL CJH CHH. Analyzed the data: CYL CHH. Contributed reagents/materials/analysis tools: LHH IJC JPC. Wrote the paper: CYL.

References

1. Badulescu O, Badescu C, Ciocoiu M, Badescu M (2013) Interleukin-1-Beta and dyslipidemic syndrome as major risk factors for thrombotic complications in type 2 diabetes mellitus. Mediators Inflamm 2013: 169420.
2. Kreisberg RA (1998) Diabetic dyslipidemia. Am J Cardiol 82: 67U-73U; discussion 85U-86U.
3. Davidson M (2008) A review of the current status of the management of mixed dyslipidemia associated with diabetes mellitus and metabolic syndrome. Am J Cardiol 102: 19L-27L.
4. Khan N, Mukhtar H (2007) Tea polyphenols for health promotion. Life Sci 81: 519-533.
5. Jing Y, Han G, Hu Y, Bi Y, Li L, et al. (2009) Tea consumption and risk of type 2 diabetes: a meta-analysis of cohort studies. J Gen Intern Med 24: 557-562.
6. Ortsater H, Grankvist N, Wolfram S, Kuehn N, Sjoholm A (2012) Diet supplementation with green tea extract epigallocatechin gallate prevents progression to glucose intolerance in db/db mice. Nutr Metab (Lond) 9: 11.
7. Hursel R, Viechtbauer W, Dulloo AG, Tremblay A, Tappy L, et al. (2011) The effects of catechin rich teas and caffeine on energy expenditure and fat oxidation: a meta-analysis. Obes Rev 12: e573-581.
8. Hsu CH, Liao YL, Lin SC, Tsai TH, Huang CJ, et al. (2011) Does supplementation with green tea extract improve insulin resistance in obese type 2 diabetics? A randomized, double-blind, and placebo-controlled clinical trial. Altern Med Rev 16: 157-163.
9. Agin A, Jeandidier N, Gasser F, Grucker D, Sapin R (2006) Use of insulin immunoassays in clinical studies involving rapid-acting insulin analogues: Bi-insulin IRMA preliminary assessment. Clin Chem Lab Med 44: 1379-1382.
10. Starr JI, Mako ME, Juhn D, Rubenstein AH (1978) Measurement of serum proinsulin-like material: cross-reactivity of porcine and human proinsulin in the insulin radioimmunoassay. J Lab Clin Med 91: 683-692.
11. Matthews DR, Hosker JP, Rudenski AS, Naylor BA, Treacher DF, et al. (1985) Homeostasis model assessment: insulin resistance and beta-cell function from fasting plasma glucose and insulin concentrations in man. Diabetologia 28: 412-419.
12. Heijboer AC, Frans A, Lomecky M, Blankenstein MA (2011) Analysis of glucagon-like peptide 1; what to measure? Clin Chim Acta 412: 1191-1194.
13. Deacon CF, Holst JJ (2009) Immunoassays for the incretin hormones GIP and GLP-1. Best Pract Res Clin Endocrinol Metab 23: 425-432.
14. Yao G, Chung CW, Yu CF, Wang JD (2002) Development and verification of validity and reliability of the WHOQOL-BREF Taiwan version. J Formos Med Assoc 101: 342-351.
15. Pan HJ, Cole BM, Geliebter A (2011) The benefits of body weight loss on health-related quality of life. J Chin Med Assoc 74: 169-175.
16. Hsu CH, Tsai TH, Kao YH, Hwang KC, Tseng TY, et al. (2008) Effect of green tea extract on obese women: a randomized, double-blind, placebo-controlled clinical trial. Clin Nutr 27: 363-370.
17. Polonsky KS (2012) The past 200 years in diabetes. N Engl J Med 367: 1332-1340.
18. Consortium TI (2012) Tea consumption and incidence of type 2 diabetes in Europe: the EPIC-InterAct case-cohort study. PLoS One 7: e36910.
19. Phung OJ, Baker WL, Matthews LJ, Lanosa M, Thorne A, et al. (2010) Effect of green tea catechins with or without caffeine on anthropometric measures: a systematic review and meta-analysis. Am J Clin Nutr 91: 73-81.
20. Hursel R, Viechtbauer W, Westerterp-Plantenga MS (2009) The effects of green tea on weight loss and weight maintenance: a meta-analysis. International Journal of Obesity 33: 956-961.
21. Hsu CH, Liao YL, Lin SC, Tsai TH, Huang CJ, et al. (2011) Does supplementation with green tea extract improve insulin resistance in obese type 2 diabetics? A randomized, double-blind, and placebo-controlled clinical trial. Alternative Medicine Review 16: 157-163.
22. Ikeda I, Hamamoto R, Uzu K, Imaizumi K, Nagao K, et al. (2005) Dietary gallate esters of tea catechins reduce deposition of visceral fat, hepatic triacylglycerol, and activities of hepatic enzymes related to fatty acid synthesis in rats. Biosci Biotechnol Biochem 69: 1049-1053.
23. Yamaoka-Tojo M, Tojo T, Takahira N, Matsunaga A, Aoyama N, et al. (2010) Elevated circulating levels of an incretin hormone, glucagon-like peptide-1, are associated with metabolic components in high-risk patients with cardiovascular disease. Cardiovasc Diabetol 9: 17.
24. Baggio LL, Drucker DJ (2007) Biology of incretins: GLP-1 and GIP. Gastroenterology 132: 2131-2157.
25. Drucker DJ, Nauck MA (2006) The incretin system: glucagon-like peptide-1 receptor agonists and dipeptidyl peptidase-4 inhibitors in type 2 diabetes. Lancet 368: 1696-1705.
26. Cernea S (2011) The role of incretin therapy at different stages of diabetes. Rev Diabet Stud 8: 323-338.
27. Kishimoto M, Noda M (2011) A pilot study of the efficacy of miglitol and sitagliptin for type 2 diabetes with a continuous glucose monitoring system and incretin-related markers. Cardiovasc Diabetol 10: 115.
28. Vilsboll T, Krarup T, Deacon CF, Madsbad S, Holst JJ (2001) Reduced postprandial concentrations of intact biologically active glucagon-like peptide 1 in type 2 diabetic patients. Diabetes 50: 609-613.
29. Rask E, Olsson T, Soderberg S, Johnson O, Seckl J, et al. (2001) Impaired incretin response after a mixed meal is associated with insulin resistance in nondiabetic men. Diabetes Care 24: 1640-1645.
30. Thondam SK, Cross A, Cuthbertson DJ, Wilding JP, Daousi C (2012) Effects of chronic treatment with metformin on dipeptidyl peptidase-4 activity, glucagon-like peptide 1 and ghrelin in obese patients with Type 2 diabetes mellitus. Diabet Med 29: e205-210.
31. Kappe C, Patrone C, Holst JJ, Zhang Q, Sjoholm A (2012) Metformin protects against lipoapoptosis and enhances GLP-1 secretion from GLP-1-producing cells. J Gastroenterol.
32. Brown AS (2005) Lipid management in patients with diabetes mellitus. Am J Cardiol 96: 26E-32E.
33. Imatoh T, Tanihara S, Miyazaki M, Momose Y, Uryu Y, et al. (2011) Coffee consumption but not green tea consumption is associated with adiponectin levels in Japanese males. Eur J Nutr 50: 279-284.
34. Sone T, Kuriyama S, Nakaya N, Hozawa A, Shimazu T, et al. (2011) Randomized controlled trial for an effect of catechin-enriched green tea consumption on adiponectin and cardiovascular disease risk factors. Food Nutr Res 55.
35. Wu AH, Spicer D, Stanczyk FZ, Tseng CC, Yang CS, et al. (2012) Effect of 2-month controlled green tea intervention on lipoprotein cholesterol, glucose, and hormone levels in healthy postmenopausal women. Cancer Prev Res (Phila) 5: 393-402.
36. Wu AH, Yu MC, Stanczyk FZ, Tseng CC, Pike MC (2011) Anthropometric, dietary, and hormonal correlates of serum adiponectin in Asian American women. Nutr Cancer 63: 549-557.
37. Tian C, Ye X, Zhang R, Long J, Ren W, et al. (2013) Green Tea Polyphenols Reduced Fat Deposits in High Fat-Fed Rats via erk1/2-PPARgamma-Adiponectin Pathway. PLoS One 8: e53796.
38. Olofsson SO, Wiklund O, Boren J (2007) Apolipoproteins A-I and B: biosynthesis, role in the development of atherosclerosis and targets for intervention against cardiovascular disease. Vasc Health Risk Manag 3: 491-502.

Common Genetic Variants of Surfactant Protein D (SP-D) are Associated with Type 2 Diabetes

Neus Pueyo[1,9], Francisco J. Ortega[1,9], Josep M. Mercader[2], José M. Moreno-Navarrete[1], Monica Sabater[1], Sílvia Bonàs[2], Patricia Botas[4], Elías Delgado[4], Wifredo Ricart[1], María T. Martinez-Larrad[5], Manuel Serrano-Ríos[5], David Torrents[2,3], José M. Fernández-Real[1]*

1 Service of Diabetes, Endocrinology and Nutrition (UDEN), Institut d'Investigació Biomédica de Girona (IdIBGi), CIBER de la Fisiopatología de la Obesidad y la Nutrición (CIBERobn, CB06/03/0010) and Instituto de Salud Carlos III (ISCIII), Girona, Spain, 2 Joint IRB-BSC Program on Computational Biology, Barcelona Supercomputing Center, Barcelona, Spain, 3 Institució Catalana de Recerca i Estudis Avançats (ICREA), Barcelona, Spain, 4 Hospital Central de Asturias, Oviedo, Spain, 5 Department of Internal Medicine II, Hospital Clínico San Carlos, CIBER de Diabetes y Enfermedades Metabólicas Asociadas (CIBERDEM), Madrid, Spain

Abstract

Context: Surfactant protein-D (SP-D) is a primordial component of the innate immune system intrinsically linked to metabolic pathways. We aimed to study the association of single nucleotide polymorphisms (SNPs) affecting *SP-D* with insulin resistance and type 2 diabetes (T2D).

Research Design and Methods: We evaluated a common genetic variant located in the *SP-D* coding region (rs721917, Met^{31}Thr) in a sample of T2D patients and non-diabetic controls (n = 2,711). In a subset of subjects (n = 1,062), this SNP was analyzed in association with circulating SP-D concentrations, insulin resistance, and T2D. This SNP and others were also screened in the publicly available Genome Wide Association (GWA) database of the Meta-Analyses of Glucose and Insulin-related traits Consortium (MAGIC).

Results: We found the significant association of rs721917 with circulating SP-D, parameters of insulin resistance and T2D. Indeed, G carriers showed decreased circulating SP-D (p = 0.004), decreased fasting glucose (p = 0.0002), glycated hemoglobin (p = 0.0005), and 33% (p = 0.002) lower prevalence of T2D, estimated under a dominant model, especially among women. Interestingly, these differences remained significant after controlling for origin, age, gender, and circulating SP-D. Moreover, this SNP and others within the *SP-D* genomic region (i.e. rs10887344) were significantly associated with quantitative measures of glucose homeostasis, insulin sensitivity, and T2D, according to GWAS datasets from MAGIC.

Conclusions: SP-D gene polymorphisms are associated with insulin resistance and T2D. These associations are independent of circulating SP-D concentrations.

Editor: Massimo Federici, University of Tor Vergata, Italy

Funding: This work was supported by research grants from the Spanish Ministry of Science and Innovation (FIS 2011-0214), CIBER de la Fisiopatología de la Obesidad y la Nutrición (CIBERobn), and by research grants from the Spanish Ministry of Science and Education (SAF 2005-02073). Dr. Josep M. Mercader was supported by Sara Borrell fellowship from the Instituto de Salud Carlos III. The funders had no role in study design, data collection and analysis, decision to publish, or preparation of the manuscript.

Competing Interests: The authors have declared that no competing interests exist.

* E-mail: jmfreal@idibgi.org

9 These authors contributed equally to this work.

Introduction

Over nutrition and sedentary activities, in combination with repeated exposure to infectious agents and external injuries, could compromise the homeostasis of the innate immune system, leading to chronic subclinical inflammation, which is intrinsic to the metabolic syndrome [1]. Insulin resistance seems to be central to the pathophysiology of these alterations [2]. Approaches to this hypothesis have been made through the study of acute phase and innate immune proteins in association with insulin resistance and type 2 diabetes (T2D) [3]. Bactericidal/permeability-increasing protein, lipopolysaccharide binding protein, complement factors, α-defensins, and lactoferrin are examples of proteins from the

innate immune system closely associated with metabolic parameters [4,5,6,7].

Surfactant protein-D (SP-D) is a key-factor of the innate immunity system which develops its principal activity in lungs, protecting from inhaled microorganisms, organic antigens, and toxins [8]. SP-D modulates the leukocyte action contributing to the inflammatory response [9], and interacts with compounds such as bacterial lipopolysaccharides (LPS), oligosaccharides, and fatty acids [10]. The *SP-D* single nucleotide polymorphism (SNP) rs721917 (NC_000010.10: g.81706324A>G) is a *missense* substitution which leads the replacement in position 31 of an ancestral metionine by a threonine (Met^{31}Thr) [10]. This polymorphic variation in the N-terminal domain of the SP-D molecule influences oligomerization, function, and circulating concentrations [11], leading to decreased immunologic capacity against bacteria [10]. Indeed, subjects carrying AA-genotype (Met/Met) have increased concentrations of SP-D in plasma [12], and show multimers, dodecamers, and monomers of subunits, whereas GG-carriers (Thr/Thr) produce almost exclusively monomers [11].

Previous evidence disclosed associations of low vital capacity and low weight at birth with an increased risk of T2D [13]. The close relationship between pulmonary acute phase proteins, the inflammatory state, and the development of metabolic complications has been also demonstrated [14,15,16,17,18]. However, the mechanisms of these interactions depend on scarcely known factors. In a previous manuscript, we provided data according to which low circulating SP-D concentrations were associated with increased fat accumulation and decreased insulin sensitivity [19]. Given the relationships among SP-D, insulin resistance and T2D, we hypothesized that genetic alteration in the former could be also associated with the prevalence of insulin resistance and T2D.

Methods

Subject Recruitment

Data and samples from 2,711 Caucasian subjects were obtained from population based prospective studies performed in three regions of Spain between 1996 and 1999:680 subjects were recruited from the North-West (Asturias) [20], 1,341 from the

center (Madrid) [21], and 690 from the North-East (Girona) [7]. Eligible participants were selected at random from the census and, after a screening visit, they were invited to participate. The participation rate was higher than 70%. The mean age of the participants was 51+/−12 years; 1,344 were men and 1,367 were women. Baseline studies included a standardized questionnaire, physical examination, and laboratory tests. Height and weight were measured with the participant in light clothing and without shoes by trained personnel using calibrated scales and a wall-mounted stadiometer, respectively. BMI was calculated by dividing weight in kilograms by the square of the height in meters. Waist circumference was measured to the nearest 0.5 cm midway between the lowest rib and the iliac crest using an anthropometric tape. Blood pressure was measured in the supine position on the right arm after a 10-min rest; a standard sphygmomanometer of appropriate cuff size was used and the first and fifth phases were recorded. Values used in the analysis are the average of three readings taken at 5 min intervals. Fasting serum and plasma was withdrawn and stored at −80°C until analysis. According to the American Diabetes Association Criteria a 75 g oral glucose tolerance test was performed in all subjects. Type 2 diabetes (T2D) was diagnosed in subjects having fasting plasma glucose >7 mM and two-hour post-load plasma glucose >11.1 mM after the oral glucose tolerance test. T2D patients were also prospectively recruited from outpatient clinics on the basis of a stable metabolic control in the previous 6 months, as defined by

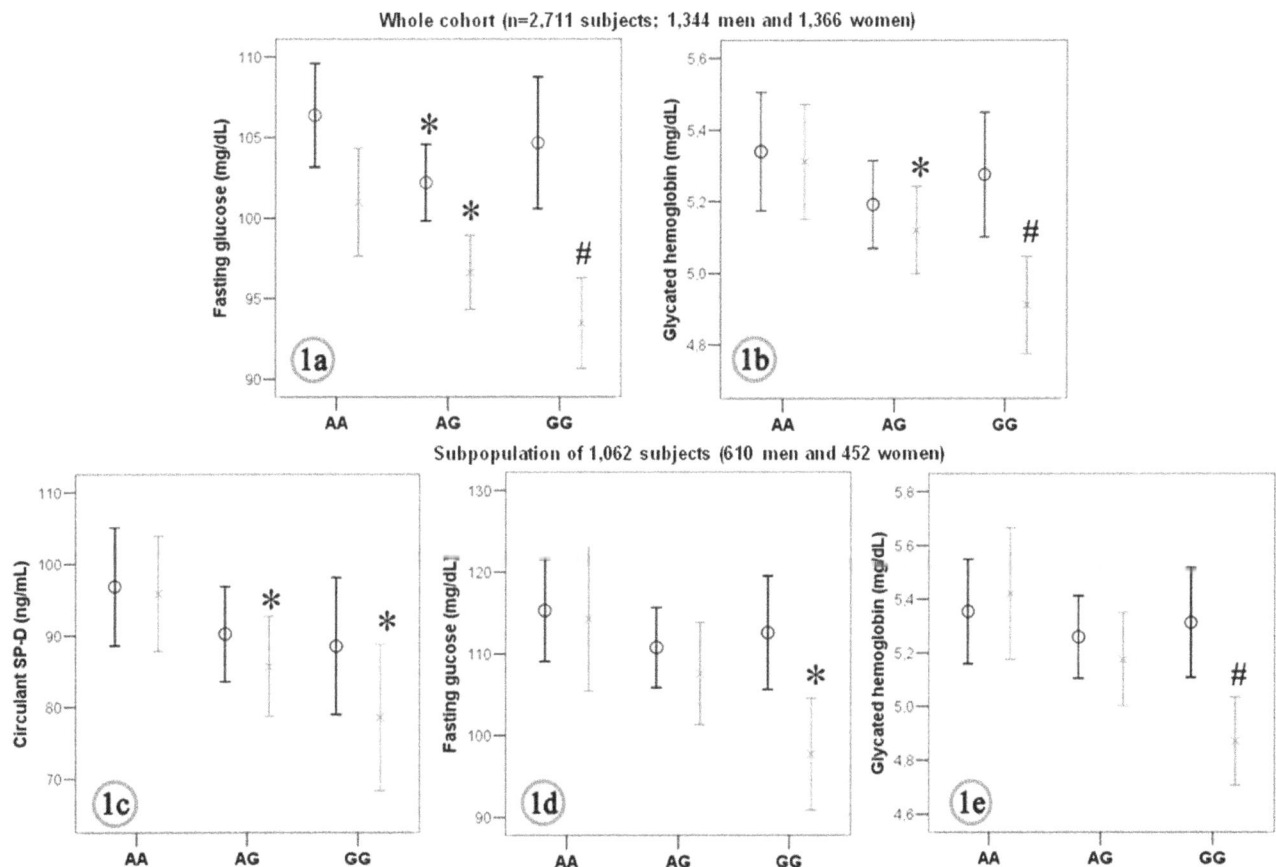

Figure 1. Genotypes for rs721917 and measures of impaired glucose tolerance and circulating SP-D. Mean and 95% confidence interval for fasting glucose (**Fig. 1a**) and glycated hemoglobin (**Fig. 1b**) for the whole cohort (n = 2,711), and for circulating SP-D concentration (**Fig. 1c**), fasting glucose (**Fig. 1d**) and glycated hemoglobin (**Fig. 1d**) in a subpopulation of subjects (n = 1,062) according to the genotypes for rs721917. Men: black bars, women: grey bars. *p<0.05 and #p<0.0001 for comparisons with AA-genotype.

Table 1. Subjects' characteristics according to the single nucleotide polymorphism rs721917 (NC_000010.10:g.81706324A>G, Met[31]Thr) for *SP-D* gene.

Genotype	AA	AG	GG	p[†]	p*	p**
Subjects (M)	468	664	212			
Smokers (%)	37	33	36			
T2D (%)	14	13	16			
Age (years)	51±12	52±12	53±12	0.431	0.275	0.215
BMI (kg/m^2)	27.9±4.3	27.8±4.3	28.3±4.5	0.27	0.974	0.238
WHR	0.95±0.07	0.96±0.08	0.95±0.06	0.111	0.158	0.868
Fasting Glucose (mg/dL)	106.5±35.5	102.1±31.1	104.3±29.8	0.083	**0.048**	0.438
Glucose 2 h post-overload (mg/dL)	108.5±39.4	110.8±46.7	121.6±49.4	**0.006**	0.076	**0.003**
Fasting Insulin (mU/L)	11.2±9	10.2±6.4	12.2±10.8	**0.011**	0.353	0.225
Insulin 2 h post-overload (mU/L)	50.2±55.5	43.3±49.5	66±70.3	**0.003**	0.894	**0.036**
HOMA$_{IR}$	2.74±2.26	2.49±1.69	3.04±3.03	**0.008**	0.383	0.186
HbA$_{1c}$ (%)	5.3±1.4	5.2±1.2	5.3±1.1	0.363	0.217	0.562
SP-D (ng/mL)[#]	98.9±68.3	92.5±67.8	91.5±62.4	0.498	0.24	0.336
Subjects (F)	501	641	225			
Smokers (%)	17	17	17			
T2D (%)	13	10	8			
Age (years)	52±12	51±12	52±12	0.478	0.415	0.942
BMI (kg/m^2)	29.5±7.3	28.8±6.4	29±6.2	0.189	0.073	0.339
WHR	0.84±0.07	0.84±0.07	0.85±0.08	0.627	0.542	0.344
Fasting Glucose (mg/dL)	100.9±37.8	96.6±29.6	93.5±21.4	**0.007**	**0.008**	**0.001**
Glucose 2 h post-overload (mg/dL)	108.6±38.9	102±31.7	103.7±32.5	**0.023**	**0.011**	0.152
Fasting Insulin (mU/L)	11.1±12	10.4±6.4	10.5±6.3	0.606	0.32	0.593
Insulin 2 h post-overload (mU/L)	37.2±35.2	35.4±35.7	32.2±42.5	0.67	0.523	0.384
HOMA$_{IR}$	2.58±2.71	2.38±1.59	2.39±1.56	0.311	0.187	0.374
HbA$_{1c}$ (%)	5.3±1.3	5.1±1.1	4.9±0.7	**0.006**	**0.01**	**<0.0001**
SP-D (ng/mL)[#]	95.9±52.8	85.7±51.2	78.6±44.4	**0.03**	**0.015**	**0.009**

T2D: Type 2 diabetes; **BMI:** Body mass index; **WHR:** Waist-to-hip ratio; **HbA$_{1c}$:** Glycated hemoglobin; **HOMA$_{IR}$:** Homeostasis model assessment of insulin resistance; **SP-D:** Surfactant protein-D.
[#]These determinations were performed in a subpopulation of 1,062 subjects.
[†]for the comparison by ANOVA among the different genotypes;
*for the comparison by test *t*-student between AA and non-AA individuals, and
between AA and GG carriers in the whole cohort. Significant differences are shown in **bold.

stable HbA1c values. Inclusion criteria were: 1) absence of systemic and metabolic disease other than obesity and T2D, and 2) absence of infection within the previous month. Liver disease and thyroid dysfunction were specifically excluded by biochemical work-up. Other exclusion criteria included the following: 1) clinically significant hepatic, neurological, endocrinologic, or other major systemic disease, including malignancy; 2) history or current clinical evidence of hemochromatosis; 3) history of drug or alcohol abuse, defined as >80 g/day in men and >40 g/day in women; 4) elevated serum creatinine concentration; 5) acute major cardio-vascular event in the previous 6 months; 6) acute illnesses and current evidence of acute or chronic inflammatory or infective diseases; and 7) mental illness rendering the subjects unable to understand the nature, scope, and possible consequences of the study. All participants were requested to withhold alcohol and

caffeine during at least 12 h prior to the different tests. All subjects gave written informed consent after the purpose of the study was explained to them. The experimental protocol was approved by the Ethics Committee of all participant institutions, including the *Hospital Central de Asturias* (Asturias, Spain), the *Hospital Clínico San Carlos* (Madrid, Spain), and the *Hospital Universitari de Girona Dr. Josep Trueta* (Girona, Spain), respectively, so we certify that all applicable institutional regulations concerning the ethical use of information and samples from human volunteers were followed during this research.

SP-D Gene Polymorphisms

The *SP-D* gene polymorphism rs721917 (NC_000010.10:g.81706324A>G) was analyzed using iPLEX^{TM} chemistry on a MALDI-TOF Mass Spectrometer (*Sequenom Inc.,*

Table 2. Codominant, dominant, and Log-additive models for *SP-D* gene polymorphism rs721917 (NC_000010.10:g.81706324A>G, Met^{31}Thr) in the whole cohort after correcting by origin of the sample, age, and sex-effects.

Model	No Type 2 Diabetes		Type 2 Diabetes		OR	OR CI (95%)	P (> |z|)
	N	%	N	%			
Codominant							
A/A	790	34.8	178	40.5	**1**		**0.009**
A/G	1102	48.5	203	46.1	**0.82**	**[0.65/1.04]**	
G/G	378	16.7	59	13.4	**0.6**	**[0.43/0.84]**	
Dominant							
A/A	790	34.8	178	40.5	**1**		**0.016**
A/G-G/G	1480	65.2	262	59.5	**0.76**	**[0.61/0.95]**	
Log-Additive							
(1, 2, 3)	2270	83.8	440	16.2	**0.79**	**[0.67/0.92]**	**0.002**

Model	Fasting Glucose (mg/dL)						
	N	Median	SE	Variation		CI (95%)	P (> |z|)
Codominant							
A/A	967	103.6	1.18				**0.001**
A/G	1305	99.5	0.84	**−3.57**		**[−6.1/−1.1]**	
G/G	437	98.9	1.27	**−5.8**		**[−9.2/−2.4]**	
Dominant							
A/A	967	103.6	1.18				**<0.001**
A/G-G/G	1742	99.3	0.71	**−4.13**		**[−6.4/−1.8]**	
Log-Additive							
(1, 2, 3)	−3.03	−4.66	−1.41				**<0.001**

Model	HbA1c (mg/dL)						
	N	Median	SE	Variation		CI (95%)	P (> |z|)
Codominant							
A/A	537	5.33	0.059				**0.003**
A/G	710	5.16	0.044	**−0.15**		**[−0.27/−0.03]**	
G/G	256	5.11	0.058	**−0.27**		**[−0.44/−0.11]**	
Dominant							
A/A	537	5.33	0.058				**0.002**
A/G-G/G	966	5.15	0.036	**−0.18**		**[−0.30/−0.07]**	
Log-Additive							
(1, 2, 3)	−0.14	−0.22	−0.06				**<0.001**

Model	SP-D (ng/mL)						
	N	Median	SE	Variation		CI (95%)	P (> |z|)
Codominant							
A/A	377	96.4	2.95				**0.014**
A/G	494	88.3	2.45	**−8.18**		**[−15.3/−1.1]**	
G/G	191	84.6	3.57	**−12.48**		**[−21.7/−3.2]**	
Dominant							
A/A	377	96.4	2.95				**0.005**
A/G-G/G	685	87.3	2.03	**−9.38**		**[−16.1/−2.7]**	
Log-Additive							
(1, 2, 3)	−6.65	−11.05	−2.06				**0.004**

OR are odd ratios and **OR CI (95%)** are their respective 95% confidence interval (CI). P (> \|z\|) is the P-value of the z-test that tests if the regression coefficients of the model can be assumed to be zero. Significant differences are shown in **bold**.

Table 3. Codominant, dominant, and Log-additive models for *SP-D* gene polymorphism rs721917 (NC_000010.10:g.81706324A>G, Met[31]Thr) after correcting by origin of the sample, age, sex, and concentrations of SP-D in plasma.

Model	No Type 2 Diabetes		Type 2 Diabetes		OR	OR CI (95%)	P (> |z|)
	N	%	N	%			
Codominant							
A/A	272	34.1	105	39.6	**1**		**0.039**
A/G	373	46.8	121	45.7	**0.81**	[0.58/1.13]	
G/G	152	19.1	39	14.7	**0.57**	[0.36/0.89]	
Dominant							
A/A	272	34.1	105	39.6	1		0.051
A/G-G/G	525	65.9	160	60.4	0.73	[0.54/1.00]	
Log-Additive							
(1, 2, 3)	797	75	265	25	**0.76**	[0.62/0.94]	**0.012**

Model	Fasting Glucose (mg/dL)						
	N	Median	SE	Variation		CI (95%)	P (> |z|)
Codominant							
A/A	377	114.9	2.6				**0.016**
A/G	494	109.4	1.97	**−5.61**		[−11.3/0.1]	
G/G	191	106.7	2.57	**−10.42**		[−17.8/−3.0]	
Dominant							
A/A	377	114.9	2.66				**0.011**
A/G-G/G	685	108.7	1.59	**−6.94**		[−12.3/−1.6]	
Log-Additive							
(1, 2, 3)	−5.28	−8.88	−1.68				**0.004**

Model	HbA1c (mg/dL)						
	N	Median	SE	Variation		CI (95%)	P (> |z|)
Codominant							
A/A	372	5.38	0.078				**0.014**
A/G	488	5.22	0.058	**−0.15**		[−0.31/0.01]	
G/G	189	5.14	0.072	**−0.302**		[−0.51/−0.09]	
Dominant							
A/A	372	5.38	0.078				**0.012**
A/G-G/G	677	5.2	0.047	**−0.192**		[−0.34/−0.04]	
Log-Additive							
(1, 2, 3)	−0.15	−0.25	−0.05				**0.003**

OR are odd ratios and **OR CI (95%)** are their respective 95% confidence interval (CI). P (> \|z\|) is the P-value of the z-test that tests if the regression coefficients of the model can be assumed to be zero. Significant differences are shown in **bold**.

San Diego, CA, USA), which is a multiple assay format. This SNP was mixed with other SNPs corresponding to different genes that are under study in our laboratories. The remaining procedure was similar to a previously described method for PCR reactions [22]. The products were spotted on a SpectroChip (Sequenom Inc.), processed and analysed in a Compact Mass Spectrometer by Mass-ARRAY Workstation (version 3.3) software (*Sequenom Inc.*). The high-throughput genotyping assays were performed at the genotyping facilities of *Centro Nacional de Genotipado* (CeGen), in the Node of Santiago.

The intergenic gene polymorphism rs10887344

(NC_000010.10:g.81768162G >A) was genotyped in the subpopulation of subjects recruited at the North-West of Spain (Asturias) by means of allelic discrimination assays using an ABI Prism 7000 sequence detector and TaqMan technology (Applied Biosystems, Foster City, CA, USA). The reaction was performed in a final volume of 25 µl. DNA was amplified after 50 cycles with an initial denaturation of 10 min at 95°C. The cycle program consisted of 15 sec denaturation at 92°C and 1 min annealing and extension at 60°C. Positive and negative controls, which were correctly identified, were included in all reactions.

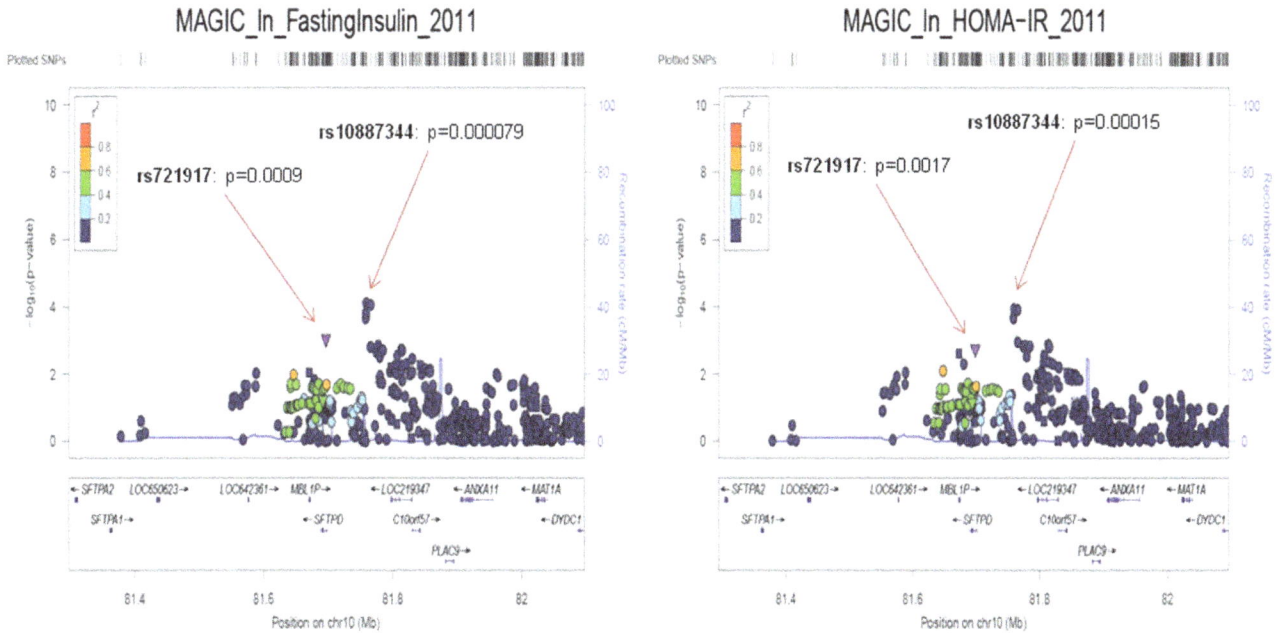

Figure 2. Regional association plot of chr.10. Regional association plot of the chromosome 10 region for fasting insulin and HOMA-IR in MAGIC GWA.

Analytical Determinations

Commercially available (BioVendor GmbH, Heidelberg, Germany) solid-phase enzyme-linked immunosorbent assays (ELISA) based on the sandwich principle were used for the in vitro quantitative determination of human surfactant protein-D (n = 1,065) concentrations in plasma. Intra- and inter- assay coefficients of variation for these determinations were between 5–10%. Other biochemical measurements were performed as previously described [6].

Statistical Analyses

The statistical association between the *SP-D* gene polymorphism rs721917 and type 2 diabetes (T2D) was assessed using custom-written software based on R environment [23]. Departures from Hardy-Weinberg equilibrium were tested in controls using a chi-square goodness of fit test with one degree of freedom. The risk of developing T2D under exposure to this *SP-D* SNP was evaluated using logistic regression to estimate Odd Ratios (OR), considering the AA genotype as the reference group. Hereby, codominant and dominant (fitting a dominant model for AA-genotype carriers) models that included the origin of the samples, age, and sex effects was fitted to estimate the ORs between the exposure to the GG, AG, and AA genotype. An additional model (Log-additive) was also fitted under these conditions. In a second assay of significance, circulating SP-D concentrations were also included as covariate. Other statistical analyses and graphics were performed using the program SPSS (IBM SPSS Statistics, Chicago, IL, USA). One-way ANOVA for multiple comparisons, using post-hoc by Bonferroni's test and the test t-Student when equal variances could be assumed, was used to compare groups with respect to continuous variables.

In order to replicate the associations found in our population, we evaluated the *SP-D* gene polymorphism rs721917 (NC_000010.10: g.81706324A>G) and screened for other associations within the *SP-D* genome region in data from publicly available datasets from the Meta-Analyses of Glucose

and Insulin-related traits Consortium (MAGIC). Seven glycemic traits were evaluated in genome wide association (GWA) databases of MAGIC, which includes data on continuous glycaemic traits in a sample of T2D patients and non-diabetic controls [24,25,26,27,28]. Standard Chi-Squared Tests and logistic regression tests were used to estimate ORs.

Results

Gene Association Results

The frequency of the G allele in the chromosome 10 at the position rs721917 NC_000010.10: g.81706324A>G (Contig position) of the *surfactant protein-D* (*SP-D*) gene was lower in subjects with impaired glucose tolerance and T2D (IGT, *Table 1*). Indeed, the increased prevalence of the A allele run in parallel to increased circulating SP-D concentrations (*Table 1*), fasting glucose, and glycated hemoglobin in women, but not in men (*Figure 1a and 1b*).

The study had a power >75% for estimating ORs >1.7 with a MAFs >0.70 and α = 0.05. The similar ORs for the AG and GG genotypes obtained for the codominant model suggest the possibility of fitting a dominant model for AA-genotype carriers (*Table 2*). In this case, the residual deviance of the genotype, once origin, age, and gender were added to the model, reached a p-value <0.001. An additional model (Log-additive) that included origin, age, and gender effects was also fitted. GG homozygotes had 40% (p = 0.0025) lower prevalence of T2D than A-allele carriers, estimated by the Log-additive model (*Table 2*). In agreement, significantly decreased fasting glucose (p = 0.0003) and glycated hemoglobin (p = 0.0006) was found in the whole cohort of G allele carriers (*Table 2*). No significant differences between genotypes were found for fasting insulin in this population. Similar results were found in additional models that included the effect of BMI or other anthropometrical parameters. Some T2D participants were under treatment (fibrates, statins, oral hypoglycemic drugs, and/or insulin). However, it should be noted that the main

Subpopulation of 633 subjects (284 men and 339 women)

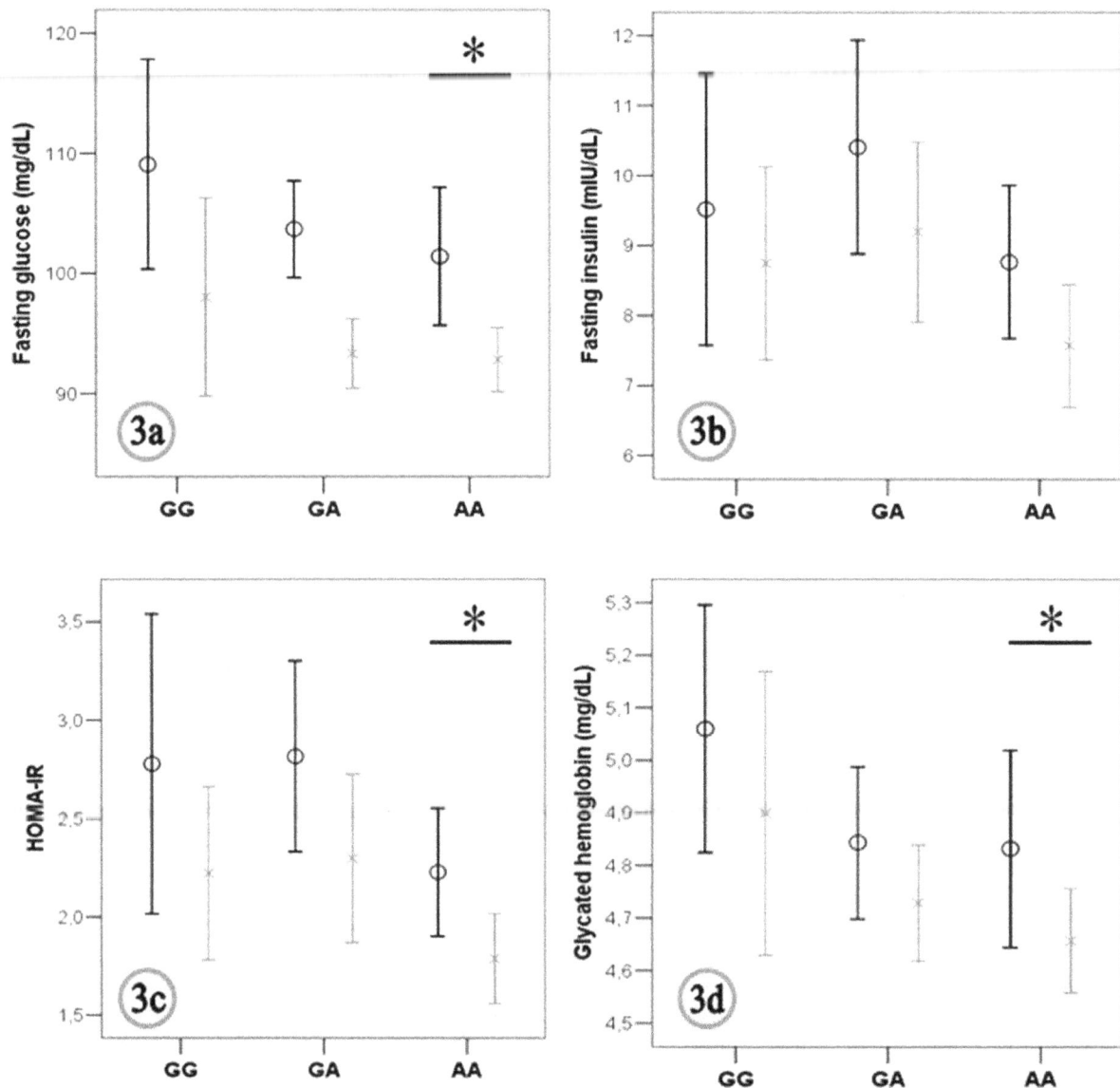

Figure 3. Genotypes for rs10887344 and measures of impaired glucose tolerance. Mean and 95% confidence interval for fasting glucose (**Fig. 3a**), fasting insulin (**Fig. 3b**), HOMA-IR (**Fig. 3c**), and glycated hemoglobin (**Fig. 3d**) according to the genotypes for rs10887344. Men: black bars, women: grey bars. *p<0.05 for comparisons with GG-genotype.

findings remained essentially unchanged after the exclusion of these subjects (data not shown).

Circulating SP-D Concentrations

To further study the possible biological significance of this association we hypothesized a link among the *SP-D* gene polymorphism rs721917, circulating SP-D concentrations, and risk factors for T2D. In this sample of subjects (n = 1,062), G-allele carriers had decreased circulating SP-D than AA-subjects (p-additive = 0.0042, *Table 1*). Currently, the increased frequency of the A allele run in parallel to increased sex-adjusted SP-D concentrations (*Fig. 1c*), fasting glucose (p additive = 0.004, *Fig. 1d*), and glycated hemoglobin (p-additive = 0.0035, *Fig. 1e*), especially among women. Of note, the significance of differences in fasting glucose between groups after controlling for origin, age, and

gender remained significant when correcting for SP-D concentrations in plasma (*Table 3*).

On the other hand, circulating SP-D concentrations were significantly decreased in T2D when compared to non-diabetic subjects in both non-obese and obese individuals, and inversely associated with BMI, fat mass, fasting glucose, and fasting triglycerides, as previously reported [19], and independently of genetic variations.

Validation of the Association through Screening of MAGIC GWA Databases

In order to validate the association between *SP-D* gene variants and T2D we explored the data generated in genome wide association (GWA) databases from the Meta-Analyses of Glucose and Insulin-related traits Consortium (MAGIC), who measures

Table 4. Subjects' characteristics according to the intergenic single nucleotide polymorphism rs10887344 (NC_000010.10:g.81768162G >A).

Genotype	GG	GA	AA	p*	p†
Subjects (M/F)	65/82	135/145	84/112		
Smokers (%)	20	29	24		
T2D (%)	**14**	**8**	**8**		
Age (years)	52±13	53±12	51±13	0.139	0.251
BMI (kg/m²)	28.2±4.7	28.2±4.8	27.6±4.5	0.295	0.227
WHR	0.88±0.07	0.89±0.09	0.87±0.09	0.054	0.382
Fasting Glucose (mg/dL)	**102.9±36.8**	**98.3±21.3**	**96.5±20.8**	0.065	**0.041**
Glucose 2 h-post overload (mg/dL)	117.1±56.7	116.8±50.3	108.4±43.2	0.166	0.128
Fasting insulin (mUI/dL)	**9.1±7**	**9.8±8.4**	**8.1±4.8**	0.039	0.118
HOMA_IR	**2.5±2.5**	**2.5±2.7**	**2.1±1.4**	0.026	0.022
HbA_1c (%)	**5.0±1.1**	**4.8±0.8**	**4.7±0.7**	0.026	0.015
SP-D (ng/mL)	97.2±53.6	103.8±63.8	98.3±55.5	0.524	0.864

T2D: Type 2 diabetes; **BMI:** Body mass index; **WHR:** Waist-to-hip ratio; **HbA_1c:** Glycated hemoglobin; **SP-D:** Surfactant protein-D; **MBL:** Mannose binding lectin.
*for the comparison by ANOVA among the different genotypes, and
†for the comparison by test t-student between AA and GG carriers in the whole cohort. Significant differences are shown in **bold**.

continuous glycaemic traits [24]. In this larger cohort, fasting Insulin (p = 0.0009) and HOMA_IR (p = 0.0017) were associated to rs721917 *SP-D* SNP following the additive model (***Figure 2***). Contrary to what might be expected, no significant changes regarding glucose concentrations were found.

In addition to the association of the *SP-D* gene polymorphism rs721917, a second SNP (rs10887344; chr10:81768162), located between *SP-D* gene and *LOC219347*, 59.3 Kb upstream of the *SP-D* gene (but not in LD with the first polymorphism analyzed, the rs721917, $r^2 = 0.082$), was also associated with fasting insulin (p = 0.000078; ***Figure 2***) and HOMA_IR in this GWA. Of note, associations of this intergenic SNP (rs10887344) with parameters of insulin resistance were replicated in our sample (***Table 4***). Indeed, in agreement with results from MAGIC GWA, increased fasting glucose (p = 0.04; ***Fig. 3a***), fasting insulin (***Fig. 3b***), HOMA_IR (p = 0.022; ***Fig. 3c***), and glycated hemoglobin (p = 0.015; ***Fig. 3d***) was found in GG carriers for rs10887344 when compared with AA genotype (***Table 4***), independently of sex, BMI, and circulating SP-D. Then, according to results for this second SNP associated with *SP-D* gene (rs10887344), GG homozygotes had higher prevalence of T2D than A-allele carriers.

Discussion

Polymorphisms of common receptors in the innate immune system like mannose-binding lectin [29], and toll-like receptors [30] are associated with altered susceptibility to infection, and the risk of a variety of inflammatory diseases. Indeed, many genetic

variants in the innate immune factors are associated with several metabolic risk factors for T2D, an observation that provides a rationale for further studying their role as biomarkers for the early risk prediction of this disease [31,32].

Genetic variations in the coding region of *surfactant protein-D* (*SP-D*) are associated with an increased risk of T2D (current report). Surfactant collectins such as SP-D are well known to be involved in lung innate immunity, being a key factor in the prevention of respiratory infections (see [33] for a review). In a scenario of repeated injuries and exposure to infectious agents, a chronic inflammatory response has been proposed as a leading factor for the development of metabolic disturbances and insulin resistance [34]. Lipopolysaccharides (LPS), for example, are at the onset of high-fat diet-induced metabolic diseases by triggering low grade chronic inflammation [35].

Surfactant immune function is primarily attributed to SP-A and -D. These proteins opsonize pathogens, regulate the inflammatory response, and interact with the adaptive immune response, being involved in the susceptibility to inflammation and infection [36]. In a previous manuscript, we found cross-sectional and longitudinal associations of circulating SP-D concentrations with insulin resistance and T2D [19]. In this study, we describe that the 31 Met→Thr *SP-D* gene single nucleotide polymorphism (SNP) rs721917 was associated with insulin resistance and the prevalence of T2D. Interestingly, differences in fasting glucose between groups after controlling for origin, age, and gender remained significant when controlling for SP-D concentrations in plasma. This suggests that the possible influence of the SNP rs721917 on metabolism may arise from changes in the molecular structure and/or functional properties of SP-D protein rather than through changes in its circulating concentrations. Indeed, this non-synonymous polymorphic variation of the N-terminal domain of the SP-D affects oligomerization and function, as well as circulating concentrations [10,11], changes that may explain the relationship with insulin resistance and T2D. In fact, subjects carrying the AA genotype (Met/Met) showed increased circulating SP-D concentrations in parallel to increased fasting glucose and T2D prevalence, especially among women and independently of circulating SP-D.

The putative functional consequences of rs721917 were explored using the FastSNP SNP characterization online application (http://fastsnp.ibms.sinica. *edu.tw/*). The SNP rs721917 involves a *missense* variation leading to conservative changes that appeared not only to affect the amino acid sequence of the protein but also to cause a disruption of three Exonic Splicing Enhancer (ESE) sequences, according to the systematic analysis of ESE sequences by Fairbrother *et al.* [37]. As three ESE are disrupted by this SNP (***Figure S1***), it is very likely that this SNP has an effect on alternative splicing, altering stability and circulating concentrations and even affecting biological functions. Accordingly, Leth-Larsen *et al.* [11] demonstrated that GG-carriers (Thr/Thr) produce almost exclusively monomers of SP-D, whereas subjects carrying AA genotype show multimers such as dodecamers and trimers of subunits. These high weight polimers of SP-D may bind to viruses and both Gram-positive and negative bacteria, while the monomeric species seem to bind LPS almost exclusively [11]. Thereby, the different genotypes may predispose individuals to different buffering capacity of metabolic endotoxemia. Indeed, the codons corresponding to this amino acid residue in the mature protein, here found to be linked to T2D, were associated with increase susceptibility to immune-related diseases [38,39]. Interestingly, in a subpopulation of 71 subjects (25 AA, 31 AG, and 15 GG-subjects), we observed an inverse association between free LPS concentrations in plasma and circulating SP-D in GG subjects ($r = -0.50$, $p = 0.05$), but not among A allele carriers (data not shown).

On the other hand, our results indicated that gender may influence the degree of susceptibility to T2D of subjects who share the AA genotype. It is becoming increasingly recognized that there are gender differences in pulmonary disease susceptibility and severity, being women apparently more sensitive to pulmonary injury than men [40,41]. Indeed, there are well-known gender-related differences in the composition of surfactant lipids and lipoproteins such as the surfactant protein B and C [42,43]. Our results indicate that the presence of the variant *SP-D* allele (Met/Met) increases the odds of developing insulin resistance and T2D preferentially among women.

The analyses of SP-D variants in GWAS datasets from MAGIC reinforce the association with T2D. In these datasets, the associations of insulin resistance with this SNP, but also with different SNPs other than those genotyped for this study, suggest that the influence of rs721917 variant might be capturing the association of other variants, such as rs10887344. Concurrently, the effects of this variant on circulating SP-D and insulin sensitivity were tested in a subpopulation of this study confirming the association with the prevalence of T2D in both men and women, although not changing plasma SP-D concentrations. Then, the rs10887344 turns to be a promising variant to test in further large scale association studies. Unfortunately, we were not able to test this SNP in other large published case-control data, as this SNP was not directly typed by any of these studies and genotype data at the individual level was not available in order to impute it from the datasets.

Overall, the findings reported here suggest the implication of SP-D variants in the modulation of metabolic parameters. The *SP-D* gene polymorphism rs721917, beyond modifying circulating concentrations, may modify SP-D structure, changing its specificity against infectious agents and other external agents [11]. Triggering factors such as weight gain, aging, and repeated usual-life infections, among others, results in low grade chronic inflammation which would be amplified in A-allele carriers. In the long term this process worsens insulin resistance, leading to T2D. However, the mechanisms responsible for the different associations should be investigated further.

Acknowledgments

We greatly appreciate the technical assistance of Gerard Pardo, Ester Guerra, Adriana Perich, and Oscar Rovira. Dr. Josep M Mercader was supported by Sara Borrell fellowship from the Instituto de Salud Carlos III. Data on glycaemic traits have been contributed by MAGIC investigators and have been downloaded from www.magicinvestigators.org. **Disclaimers:** The authors have nothing to disclose. All authors of this manuscript have directly participated in the execution, and analysis of the study. All authors are aware of and agree to the content of the manuscript, and all authors have approved the final version submitted and their being listed as an author on the manuscript. The contents of this manuscript have not been copyrighted or published previously. There are no directly related manuscripts or abstracts, published or unpublished, by one or more authors of this manuscript. The contents of this manuscript are not now under consideration for publication elsewhere. The submitted manuscript nor any similar manuscript, in whole or in part, will be neither copyrighted, submitted, or published elsewhere while the Journal is under consideration.

Author Contributions

Conceived and designed the experiments: NP FJO DT JMF-R. Performed the experiments: NP FJO JMM-N MS SB. Analyzed the data: NP FJO JMM. Contributed reagents/materials/analysis tools: JMM PB ED WR MM-L MS-R DT. Wrote the paper: NP FJO JMF-R.

References

1. Hotamisligil GS (2006) Inflammation and metabolic disorders. Nature 444: 860–867.
2. Fernandez-Real JM, Pickup JC (2008) Innate immunity, insulin resistance and type 2 diabetes. Trends Endocrinol Metab 19: 10–16.
3. Fernandez-Real JM, Pickup JC (2012) Innate immunity, insulin resistance and type 2 diabetes. Diabetologia 55: 273–278.
4. Gubern C, Lopez-Bermejo A, Biarnes J, Vendrell J, Ricart W, et al. (2006) Natural antibiotics and insulin sensitivity: the role of bactericidal/permeability-increasing protein. Diabetes 55: 216–224.
5. Lopez-Bermejo A, Chico-Julia B, Castro A, Recasens M, Esteve E, et al. (2007) Alpha defensins 1, 2, and 3: potential roles in dyslipidemia and vascular dysfunction in humans. Arterioscler Thromb Vasc Biol 27: 1166–1171.
6. Moreno-Navarrete JM, Martinez-Barricarte R, Catalan V, Sabater M, Gomez-Ambrosi J, et al. (2010) Complement factor H is expressed in adipose tissue in association with insulin resistance. Diabetes 59: 200–209.
7. Moreno-Navarrete JM, Ortega FJ, Bassols J, Castro A, Ricart W, et al. (2008) Association of circulating lactoferrin concentration and 2 nonsynonymous LTF gene polymorphisms with dyslipidemia in men depends on glucose-tolerance status. Clin Chem 54: 301–309.
8. Sano H, Kuroki Y (2005) The lung collectins, SP-A and SP-D, modulate pulmonary innate immunity. Mol Immunol 42: 279–287.
9. Crouch EC (2000) Surfactant protein-D and pulmonary host defense. Respir Res 1: 93–108.
10. Sorensen GL, Hjelmborg JB, Kyvik KO, Fenger M, Hoj A, et al. (2006) Genetic and environmental influences of surfactant protein D serum levels. Am J Physiol Lung Cell Mol Physiol 290: L1010–1017.
11. Leth-Larsen R, Garred P, Jensenius H, Meschi J, Hartshorn K, et al. (2005) A common polymorphism in the SFTPD gene influences assembly, function, and concentration of surfactant protein D. J Immunol 174: 1532–1538.
12. Foreman MG, Kong X, DeMeo DL, Pillai SG, Hersh CP, et al. (2011) Polymorphisms in surfactant protein-D are associated with chronic obstructive pulmonary disease. Am J Respir Cell Mol Biol 44: 316–322.
13. Barker DJ, Godfrey KM, Fall C, Osmond C, Winter PD, et al. (1991) Relation of birth weight and childhood respiratory infection to adult lung function and death from chronic obstructive airways disease. Bmj 303: 671–675.
14. Engstrom G, Janzon L (2002) Risk of developing diabetes is inversely related to lung function: a population-based cohort study. Diabet Med 19: 167–170.
15. Ford ES, Mannino DM (2004) Prospective association between lung function and the incidence of diabetes: findings from the National Health and Nutrition Examination Survey Epidemiologic Follow-up Study. Diabetes Care 27: 2966–2970.
16. Reading PC, Allison J, Crouch EC, Anders EM (1998) Increased susceptibility of diabetic mice to influenza virus infection: compromise of collectin-mediated host defense of the lung by glucose? J Virol 72: 6884–6887.
17. Yeh HC, Punjabi NM, Wang NY, Pankow JS, Duncan BB, et al. (2005) Vital capacity as a predictor of incident type 2 diabetes: the Atherosclerosis Risk in Communities study. Diabetes Care 28: 1472–1479.
18. Engstrom G, Hedblad B, Nilsson P, Wollmer P, Berglund G, et al. (2003) Lung function, insulin resistance and incidence of cardiovascular disease: a longitudinal cohort study. J Intern Med 253: 574–581.
19. Fernandez-Real JM, Valdes S, Manco M, Chico B, Botas P, et al. (2011) Surfactant protein d, a marker of lung innate immunity, is positively associated with insulin sensitivity. Diabetes Care 33: 847–853.
20. Valdes S, Botas P, Delgado E, Alvarez F, Cadorniga FD (2007) Population-based incidence of type 2 diabetes in northern Spain: the Asturias Study. Diabetes Care 30: 2258–2263.
21. Mansego ML, Martinez F, Martinez-Larrad MT, Zabena C, Rojo G, et al. (2012) Common variants of the liver fatty acid binding protein gene influence the risk of type 2 diabetes and insulin resistance in Spanish population. PLoS One 7: e31853.
22. Fernandez-Real JM, Mercader JM, Ortega FJ, Moreno-Navarrete JM, Lopez-Romero P, et al. (2011) Transferrin receptor-1 gene polymorphisms are associated with type 2 diabetes. Eur J Clin Invest 40: 600–607.
23. Zeggini E, Scott LJ, Saxena R, Voight BF, Marchini JL, et al. (2008) Meta-analysis of genome-wide association data and large-scale replication identifies additional susceptibility loci for type 2 diabetes. Nat Genet 40: 638–645.
24. Dupuis J, Langenberg C, Prokopenko I, Saxena R, Soranzo N, et al. (2010) New genetic loci implicated in fasting glucose homeostasis and their impact on type 2 diabetes risk. Nat Genet 42: 105–116.

25. Prokopenko I, Langenberg C, Florez JC, Saxena R, Soranzo N, et al. (2009) Variants in MTNR1B influence fasting glucose levels. Nat Genet 41: 77–81.

26. Saxena R, Hivert MF, Langenberg C, Tanaka T, Pankow JS, et al. (2010) Genetic variation in GIPR influences the glucose and insulin responses to an oral glucose challenge. Nat Genet 42: 142–148.

27. Soranzo N, Sanna S, Wheeler E, Gieger C, Radke D, et al. (2010) Common variants at 10 genomic loci influence hemoglobin A(C) levels via glycemic and nonglycemic pathways. Diabetes 59: 3229–3239.

28. Strawbridge RJ, Dupuis J, Prokopenko I, Barker A, Ahlqvist E, et al. (2011) Genome-wide association identifies nine common variants associated with fasting proinsulin levels and provides new insights into the pathophysiology of type 2 diabetes. Diabetes 60: 2624–2634.

29. Heitzeneder S, Seidel M, Forster-Waldl E, Heitger A (2012) Mannan-binding lectin deficiency - Good news, bad news, doesn't matter? Clin Immunol 143: 22–38.

30. Noreen M, Shah MA, Mall SM, Choudhary S, Hussain T, et al. (2012) TLR4 polymorphisms and disease susceptibility. Inflamm Res 61: 177–188.

31. Muller YL, Hanson RL, Bian L, Mack J, Shi X, et al. (2010) Functional variants in MBL2 are associated with type 2 diabetes and pre-diabetes traits in Pima Indians and the old order Amish. Diabetes 59: 2080–2085.

32. Arora P, Garcia-Bailo B, Dastani Z, Brenner D, Villegas A, et al. (2011) Genetic polymorphisms of innate immunity-related inflammatory pathways and their association with factors related to type 2 diabetes. BMC Med Genet 12: 95.

33. Haagsman HP, Hogenkamp A, van Eijk M, Veldhuizen EJ (2008) Surfactant collectins and innate immunity. Neonatology 93: 288–294.

34. Moreno-Navarrete JM, Fernandez-Real JM (2011) Antimicrobial-sensing proteins in obesity and type 2 diabetes: the buffering efficiency hypothesis. Diabetes Care 34 Suppl 2: S335–341.

35. Cani PD, Amar J, Iglesias MA, Poggi M, Knauf C, et al. (2007) Metabolic endotoxemia initiates obesity and insulin resistance. Diabetes 56: 1761–1772.

36. Wright JR (2004) Host defense functions of pulmonary surfactant. Biol Neonate 85: 326–332.

37. Fairbrother WG, Yeh RF, Sharp PA, Burge CB (2002) Predictive identification of exonic splicing enhancers in human genes. Science 297: 1007–1013.

38. Lahti M, Lofgren J, Marttila R, Renko M, Klaavuniemi T, et al. (2002) Surfactant protein D gene associated with severe respiratory syncytial virus infection. Pediatr Res 51: 696–699.

39. Floros J, Lin HM, Garcia A, Salazar MA, Guo X, et al. (2000) Surfactant protein genetic marker alleles identify a subgroup of tuberculosis in a Mexican population. J Infect Dis 182: 1473–1478.

40. Lund MB, Kongerud J, Boe J, Nome O, Abrahamsen AF, et al. (1996) Cardiopulmonary sequelae after treatment for Hodgkin's disease: increased risk in females? Ann Oncol 7: 257–264.

41. Prescott E, Bjerg AM, Andersen PK, Lange P, Vestbo J (1997) Gender difference in smoking effects on lung function and risk of hospitalization for COPD: results from a Danish longitudinal population study. Eur Respir J 10: 822–827.

42. Trotter A, Hilgendorff A, Kipp M, Beyer C, Kueppers E, et al. (2009) Gender-related effects of prenatal administration of estrogen and progesterone receptor antagonists on VEGF and surfactant-proteins and on alveolarisation in the developing piglet lung. Early Hum Dev 85: 353–359.

43. Provost PR, Boucher E, Tremblay Y (2009) Apolipoprotein A-I, A-II, C-II, and H expression in the developing lung and sex difference in surfactant lipids. J Endocrinol 200: 321–330.

GCKR Variants Increase Triglycerides while Protecting from Insulin Resistance in Chinese Children

Yue Shen[1,2], Lijun Wu[2], Bo Xi[3], Xin Liu[4], Xiaoyuan Zhao[2], Hong Cheng[2], Dongqing Hou[2], Xingyu Wang[4]*, Jie Mi[2]*

1 Graduate School of Peking Union Medicine College, Beijing, People's Republic of China, 2 Department of Epidemiology, Capital Institute of Pediatrics, Beijing, People's Republic of China, 3 Institute of Maternal and Child Health Care, School of Public Health, Shandong University, Shandong, People's Republic of China, 4 Laboratory of Human Genetics, Beijing Hypertension League Institute, Beijing, People's Republic of China

Abstract

Background: Variants in gene encoding glucokinase regulator protein (*GCKR*) were found to have converse effects on triglycerides and glucose metabolic traits. We aimed to investigate the influence of *GCKR* variants for triglycerides and glucose metabolic traits in Chinese children and adults.

Methods and Results: We genotyped two *GCKR* variants rs1260326 and rs1260333 in children and adults, and analyzed the association between two variants and triglycerides, glucose, insulin and HOMA-IR using linear regression model, and estimated the effect on insulin resistance using logistic regression model. Rs1260326 and rs1260333 associated with increased triglycerides in children and adults ($p<0.05$). In children, both variants significantly reduced insulin ($p<0.05$. for rs1260326, $\beta = -0.07$; for rs1260333, $\beta = -0.07$) and HOMA-IR ($p<0.05$. for rs1260326, $\beta = -0.03$; for rs1260333, $\beta = -0.03$). There were significant associations between two variants and insulin resistance for children. Under co-dominant model, for CT vs. CC, OR is 0.83 (95%CI 0.69–1.00) for rs1260326, and 0.83 (95%CI 0.68–1.00) for rs1260333; for TT vs. CC, OR is 0.72 (95%CI 0.58–0.88) for rs1260326, and 0.72 (95%CI 0.58–0.89) for rs1260333. Under allele model, for allele T vs. C, the ORs are 0.85 (95%CI 0.76–0.94) and 0.85 (95%CI 0.76–0.94) for rs1260326 and rs1260333, respectively.

Conclusions: Our study confirmed the associations between *GCKR* variants and triglycerides in Chinese children and adults. Triglycerides-increasing alleles of *GCKR* variants reduce insulin and HOMA-IR index, and protect from Insulin resistance in children. Our results suggested *GCKR* has an effect on development of insulin resistance in Chinese children.

Editor: Jianping Ye, Pennington Biomedical Research Center, United States of America

Funding: This work was supported by National Nature Science Foundation of China (81172746), Beijing Key Science and Technology Program (D111100000611002), Beijing Health System Leading Talent Grant (2009-1-08), and the Beijing Training Project for the Leading Talents in S & T (2011LJ07). The funders had no role in study design, data collection and analysis, decision to publish, or preparation of the manuscript.

Competing Interests: The authors have declared that no competing interests exist.

* E-mail: xingyuw@yahoo.com (XW); jiemi2010@foxmail.com (JM)

Introduction

Type 2 diabetes is a worldwide heath problem. For Chinese, the prevalence of type 2 diabetes is increasing, Yang W, *et al.* reported that the prevalence of total diabetes and prediabetes in China were 9.7% and 15.5%, respectively [1]. Insulin resistance contributes to the pathogenesis of type 2 diabetes, and genetics plays an important role for insulin resistance [2].

Glucokinase regulatory protein (GKRP; gene symbol: *GCKR*) is a rate-limiting factor of glucokinase (GCK), which functions as a key glycolytic enzyme for maintaining glucose homeostasis [3]. Polymorphisms at the *GCKR* gene region were firstly identified to be associated with triglycerides levels by genome wide association studies [4], and the alleles which increasing triglycerides levels were found to lower the glucose, insulin levels and insulin resistance by different association studies[5–7]. Rs1260326, non-synonymous variant in *GCKR*, was reported to have inverse effects on triglycerides and glucose levels in French individuals[8;9], and other European descent populations [10]. Another common variant rs1260333 which located in downstream of *GCKR* gene

region, was reported to be associated with triglycerides in European by Waterworth *et al.* [11]. In Chinese, the association of *GCKR* variants with glucose, insulin, insulin resistance and the risk of type 2 diabetes was inconsistent with Europeans[12–16]. Three studies validated the association between *GCKR* SNP and type 2 diabetes mellitus, but Wen J. *et al.* didn't[12;13;15;16]. Qi Q. *et al.* found *GCKR* SNPs (rs780094 and rs1260326) to be associated with glucose and HOMA-beta function index, but others didn't[12–16]. To better understand the metabolism of glucose-lipid, it is necessary to investigate the relationship of *GCKR* variants with triglycerides and glucose metabolic traits (glucose, insulin, HOMA-IR) for Chinese adults or children.

In the present study, we genotyped two *GCKR* variants rs1260326 and rs1260333 in larger population including two Chinese non-diabetic groups: 1) a children and adolescents population; 2) an adult population. We aimed to investigate the possible effects of rs1260326 and rs1260333 on triglycerides, fasting glucose, insulin and HOMA-IR index, and estimate their effects on the risk of insulin resistance in Chinese non-diabetic children and adults population.

Methods

Study Population and Measurements

All subjects are unrelated northern Chinese of the Han ethnicity living in the area of Beijing.

1. Children and adolescents. subjects were recruited from a cross-sectional population-based survey: the BCAMS study [17]. The study population and measurement of anthropometric parameters were collected, which introduced in our previous papers in details[18;19].Within this large group, pubertal development was assessed by Tanner stage of breast development (girls) and testicle volume (boys) [20]. The BCAMS study was approved by the Ethics Committee and Institutional Review Board at Capital Institute of Pediatrics (CIP). All participating children and their parents gave written informed consent under protocols provided by the CIP that clearly stated that the blood samples will be used for scientific research purposes including genetic studies. There were 3,518 children and adolescents were recruited and collected venipuncture blood for further tests. In this study, 33 individuals were excluded for FPG≥7.0 mmol/L and/or self-report diabetes during analysis.

2. Adults. subjects were consists of 1,773 non-diabetic participants by OGTT(oral glucose tolerance test, from a community-based health screening program and recruited by local community hospitals of Beijing, which are the cooperation loci of Beijing Hypertension League Institute(BHLI), during 2001–2003. General information was recorded, including age, sex, height, weight, disease history. All subjects gave written informed consent under protocols provided by BHLI that clearly stated that individual data and blood samples will be used for scientific research purposes including genetic studies. The informed consent forms and study purposes were approved by the Ethics Committee and Institutional Review Board of BHLI.

After fasted more than 8 hours or overnight, venous blood from each of these subjects was collected for further tests. All biochemical measurements were performed using commercially available kits. Triglycerides and fasting glucose were measured by enzymatic methods (Roche, Basel, Switzerland)by 7060 chemistry analyzer (Hitachi, Tokyo, Japan), and fasting insulin was measured by enzyme-linked immunosorbent assay. All experiments were carried out according to standard operating procedures. Body mass index (BMI) was calculated according to the formula: weight (kg) divided by squared height (m^2). Homeostasis model assessment of insulin resistance (HOMA-IR) index was calculated by the formula: (fasting glucose (mmol/l)* fasting insulin (μU/ml)/22.5) [21]. HOMA-IR index was divided into quartiles, and the top quartile was defined as insulin resistance (IR) [22], other three quartiles as controls. The cutoff of HOMA-IR index was 2.79 and 3.38 for insulin resistance diagnosis in our children and adults population, respectively.

Genome DNA Extraction and Genotyping

Genomic DNA was isolated from peripheral blood white cells using the salt fractionation method. All genotyping were performed by TaqMan probes Allelic Discrimination Assays (Assay number are C___2862880_1_ for rs1260326 and C___8724522_10 for rs1260333) with the GeneAmp 7900 Sequence Detection System (Applied Biosystems, Foster City, CA, USA). Genotyping call rates for all variants were greater than 99%. Duplicate samples were assayed with a concordance rate >99%.

Statistical Analysis

Quantitative variables were expressed as mean ± standard deviation (SD). The chi square test was used to compare the genotype distribution in the children and adults groups, and perform the Hardy-Weinberg equilibrium test for two variants. Differences between genotypes were tested with multiple linear regression analysis under an additive effect model, for children, adjusted for age, sex, BMI and puberty, and for adults, adjusted for age, sex and BMI. Triglycerides, fasting insulin and HOMR-IR index were square root transformed for approximate normality distribution. Odds ratios (ORs) were calculated using logistic regression analysis model to evaluate the possible associations of *GCKR* variants with insulin resistance. Statistical analyses were performed with SPSS, version 13.0 (SPSS, Inc., Chicago, Illinois), and $p<0.05$ was considered statistically significant.

Results

The major clinical and metabolic characteristics of children and adults are displayed in Table 1. Both of rs1260326 and rs1260333 were in Hardy-Weinberg equilibrium for each group ($p>0.05$) (Table 2). There is no difference of genotype distribution between children and adults for two variants ($p>0.05$) (Table 2).

The T alleles of rs1260326 and rs1260333 increased triglycerides for children (for rs1260326, $\beta=0.03$, $p=3.36\times10^{-9}$; for rs1260333, $\beta=0.03$, $p=1.00\times10^{-9}$) and adults (for rs1260326, $\beta=0.06$, $p=8.92\times10^{-7}$; for rs1260333, $\beta=0.06$, $p=4.81\times10^{-6}$) (Table 3). In children, T alleles of rs1260326 and rs1260333 strongly lowered fasting insulin (for rs1260326, $\beta=-0.07$, $p=0.003$; for rs1260333, $\beta=-0.07$, $p=0.003$) and HOMA-IR index (for rs1260326, $\beta=-0.03$, $p=0.002$; for rs1260333, $\beta=-0.03$, $p=0.002$) (Table 3). No associations were observed with fasting glucose in children (Table 3). For adults, it didn't reach statistically significance for relationships between the two *GCKR* variants and fasting glucose, insulin and HOMA-IR index (Table 3).

Table 4 showed the association between two *GCKR* variants and insulin resistance in children and adults groups. There were significant associations between two *GCKR* variants and insulin resistance for children (Table 4).

Table 1. Characteristic of children and adults.

	children	adults
n	3,485	1,773
male,%	51	49.3
Age (years)	12.4±3.1	45.1±9.1
BMI (kg/m^2)	21.9±4.9	25.1±3.7
triglycerides (mmol/L)	0.89(0.66–1.22)	1.29(0.88–1.94)
TC(mmol/L)	4.09±0.79	5.02±0.90
HDL-C(mmol/L)	1.40±0.32	1.43±0.34
LDL-C(mmol/L)	2.54±0.73	3.38±0.88
fasting blood glucose (mmol/L)	5.07±0.45	5.13±0.55
Fasting blood insulin (μU/ml)	8.35(5.12–12.99)	10.18(7.21–14.60)
HOMA-IR (mmol/L×μU/ml)	1.90(1.13–2.79)	2.28(1.59–3.38)

Data are mean±SD, or median (25%quatile-75%quatile).
HOMA-IR: (fasting blood glucose [mmol/L] * fasting blood insulin [μU/ml])/22.5.
TC: total cholesterol; HDL-C: high density lipoprotein cholesterol; LDL-C: low density lipoprotein cholesterol.

Table 2. Genotypes distribution in children and adults population.

SNP	population	genotype			MAF	H-W-P	chi square	p value
		CC	CT	TT				
rs1260326	children	726	1,711	1,048	0.45	0.57	0.11	0.95
	adults	371	860	538	0.45	0.43		
		CC	CT	TT				
rs1260333	children	744	1,682	1,059	0.45	0.11	1	0.61
	adults	397	845	522	0.46	0.12		

H-W-P: p value for Hardy-Weinberg equilibrium test.

For rs1260326, adjusted for age, sex, BMI and puberty, under co-dominant model, for CT vs. CC, OR (odds ratio) is 0.83(95%CI (confidence interval) 0.69–1.00, $p = 0.024$); for TT vs. CC, OR is 0.72(95%CI 0.58–0.88, $p = 0.002$). Under dominant model, OR is 0.78(95%CI 0.66–0.94, $p = 0.004$) for CT+TT vs. CC. And under allele model, compared with C allele, OR is 0.85(95%CI 0.76–0.94, $p = 0.002$) for T allele. Similar associations were observed for rs1260333 and insulin resistance in children, for CT vs. CC, OR is 0.83 (95%CI 0.68–1.00, $p = 0.012$); for TT vs. CC, OR is 0.72(95%CI 0.58–0.89, $p = 0.002$). For CT+TT vs. CC, OR is 0.78(95%CI 0.66–0.94, $p = 0.002$). For T allele vs. C allele, OR is OR = 0.85(95%CI 0.76–0.94, $p = 0.003$) (Table 4). No significant association between the two GCKR variants and insulin resistance was observed for adults (Table 4).

Discussion

To our knowledge, the present study firstly investigated the effects of GCKR variants rs1260326 and rs1260333 on glucose metabolism traits in Chinese population including children and adults. We replicated the association between rs1260326 and rs1260333 and triglycerides in Chinese children and adults, it suggested that the effects of GCKR variants rs1260326 and rs1260333 on triglycerides are similar in Chinese and Europeans. Our data firstly find that the triglycerides-increasing alleles of GCKR variants rs1260326 and rs1260333 lowered insulin and HOMA-IR, and reduced the risk of insulin resistance in Chinese descent children.

Both of GCKR variants rs1260326 and rs1260333, locate in a strong LD in our population ($r^2 = 0.88$, 0.89 for children and adults, respectively), and similar to the HapMap data (for CHB, $r^2 = 0.86$). For this, it is understandable that the variant rs1260333 has similar effects with rs1260326.

GKRP can activate GCK, which functions as a glucose sensor responsible for glucose phosphorylation in the first step of glycolysis [23]. As a coding variant (P446L), rs1260326 was well described as a potential causal polymorphism. Beer et al. reported an in vitro experiment that the T allele of rs1260326 had increased the activity of GCK [24]. Higher GCK activity could lead to increase triglycerides but lower glucose [23]. For adults, the association between rs1260326 and glucose, insulin and HOMA-IR were reported by European studies[8;9], among Indian Asians, the similar effect was observed by a genome wide association study [25]. In Japanese adults, rs1260326 associated with fasting glucose [26]. For children, effect of rs1260326 with glucose metabolism wasn't detected, although it associated with triglycerides levels [27]. In our study, the T alleles of GCKR increased the triglycerides levels in children and adults didn't lower glucose levels. This result

on glucose was consistent with studies conducted by other Chinese researchers for another GCKR variant rs780094[12;13], which is in the high LD block with rs1260326 (HapMap CHB $r^2 = 0.82$). For the inconsistent results on glucose within Chinese, Europeans and Japanese, we thought it should be due to the different genetic background and life styles with three populations.

We firstly observed that the GCKR variants of increasing triglycerides had lower the levels of insulin and HOMA-IR index, and reduce the risk of insulin resistance for Chinese children. There are some limitations in our study. For adults, it displayed similar trends, but didn't reach the significance. Given that limited sample size of adults, the power wasn't sufficient (under genetic additive model, to achieve power>80%, OR is 0.85, it needs >800 adult cases with insulin resistance in our study). It is one limitation of our study. Whether or not the GCKR variants associate with insulin resistance in Chinese adults, it needs larger-sample population to verify. Another limitation is that there was possible misclassification for diagnosing insulin resistance for children. We only excluded the subjects with FPG> = 7.0 mmol/L and/or self-report diabetes and treatment with anti-diabetic agents, and didn't considered 2 h postprandial glucose, that maybe introduced misclassification bias.

A transient insulin resistance develops in children during puberty [28]. For children, the insulin resistance emerging during pubertal maturation is accepted as a physiological condition rather than pathologic [29]. Pubertal insulin resistance was accompanied by greater fasting serum insulin concentrations while serum glucose concentrations were unchanged[30;31]. Insulin resistance in young adults is often accompanied by a dyslipidemic profile [32]. Prevailing theories for the pathogenesis of insulin resistance focus on lipid-mediated mechanisms [33]. Puberty is a high risk developmental period for type 2 diabetes [34], because the transient physiological status in insulin resistance induces an extra stress on the beta cells in the pancreas(29).Although insulin resistance declines in late puberty [31], the associations between GCKR variants and insulin resistance in Chinese children are still important to understand the mechanism of pubertal insulin resistance.

In conclusion, our study confirmed the association between GCKR variants and triglycerides levels in Chinese children and adults. The triglycerides-increasing alleles of GCKR variants can reduce blood insulin and HOMA-IR index, and the risk of insulin resistance in Chinese children. Our results suggested GCKR has an effect on development of insulin resistance in Chinese children. It's well-known that insulin resistance plays an important role in development of type 2 diabetes, prospective study is needed to

Table 3. Clinical and metabolic characteristics of Chinese children and adults stratified according to genotypes of rs1260333 and rs1260326.

SNP	parameters	children genotypes			p value[a] (β)	Adults genotypes			p value[b] (β)
		CC	CT	TT		CC	CT	TT	
rs1260326	n	726	1,711	1,048		371	860	538	
	BMI (kg/m²)	21.9±5.1	22.0±4.9	21.8±4.9	0.60(−0.06)[c]	25.2±3.8	25.1±3.7	25.1±3.6	0.74(−0.04)[d]
	Triglycerides(mmol/L)	0.82(0.63–1.16)	0.87(0.65–1.21)	0.94(0.71–1.30)	3.36×10^{-9}(0.03)	1.20(0.78–1.65)	1.28(0.88–1.96)	1.40(0.95–2.09)	8.92×10^{-7}(0.06)
	Fasting glucose(mmol/L)	5.08±0.48	5.07±0.44	5.05±0.45	0.10(−0.02)	5.14±0.56	5.14±0.55	5.09±0.54	0.10(−0.03)
	Fasting insulin(μU/ml)	8.56(5.02–13.69)	8.40(5.17–12.95)	8.13(5.09–10.28)	0.003(−0.07)	10.50(7.45–15.05)	10.18(7.17–14.13)	9.95(7.16–14.19)	0.34(−0.03)
	HOMA-IR (mmol/L×μU/ml)	1.96(1.11–3.20)	1.91(1.15–2.91)	1.83(1.10–2.75)	0.002(−0.03)	2.35(1.65–3.58)	2.30(1.60–3.37)	2.22(1.52–3.27)	0.27(−0.02)
		CC	CT	TT		CC	CT	TT	
rs1260333	n	744	1,682	1,059		397	845	522	
	BMI (kg/m²)	21.9±5.1	22.0±4.9	21.8±4.9	0.52 (−0.07)[c]	25.3±4.0	25.1±3.6	25.1±3.6	0.41 (−0.10)[d]
	Triglycerides(mmol/L)	0.82(0.62–1.15)	0.88(0.66–1.21)	0.94(0.70–1.30)	1.00×10^{-9}(0.03)	1.22(0.79–1.74)	1.28(0.88–14.28)	1.29(0.94–2.05)	4.81×10^{-6}(0.06)
	Fasting glucose(mmol/L)	5.08±0.48	5.07±0.44	5.05±0.45	0.11(−0.02)	5.14±0.56	5.14±0.55	5.09±0.54	0.10(−0.03)
	Fasting insulin(μU/ml)	8.65(5.02–13.66)	8.44(5.24–12.94)	8.10(2.04–12.30)	0.003(−0.07)	10.23(7.46–14.86)	10.23(7.21–14.28)	10.18(7.14–14.61)	0.85(−0.01)
	HOMA-IR (mmol/L×μU/ml)	1.97(1.11–3.17)	1.92(1.16–2.91)	1.81(1.09–2.75)	0.002(−0.03)	2.29(1.66–3.55)	2.31(1.60–3.36)	2.29(1.52–3.30)	0.67(−0.01)

Data are mean±SD, or median (25%quatile–75%quatile).
[a]adjusted for age, sex, BMI and puberty for children.
[b]adjusted for age, sex and BMI for adults.
[c]adjusted for age, sex and puberty for children.
[d]adjusted for age, sex for adults.
HOMA-IR = (fasting blood glucose [mmol/L] * fasting blood insulin [μU/ml])/22.5. During linear regression analyzing, triglycerides, fasting insulin and HOMR IR index were square root transformed for approximate normality distribution.
p values were calculated from linear regression assuming an additive model. P values<0.05 were shown in bold.

Table 4. Logistic regression analysis models of rs1260333 and rs1260326 for insulin resistance (IR).

SNP			children					adults				
			Control	IR	OR(95%CI)	p1	p2	Control	IR	OR(95%CI)	p1	p2
rs1260326	genotype	CC	497	228	1			266	105	1		
		CT	1,232	468	0.83(0.69–1.00)	0.051	**0.024**	649	211	0.82(0.63–1.08)	0.17	0.19
		TT	785	258	0.72(0.58–0.88)	**0.002**	**0.002**	411	127	0.78(0.58–1.06)	0.11	0.13
		CT+TT	2,017	726	0.78(0.66–0.94)	**0.008**	**0.004**	1,060	338	0.81(0.62–1.04)	0.10	0.12
	allele	C	2,226	924	1			1,181	421	1		
		T	2,802	984	0.85(0.76–0.94)	**0.002**	**0.002**	1,471	465	0.89(0.76–1.03)	0.13	0.15
rs1260333	genotype	CC	508	233	1			287	110	1		
		CT	1,214	460	0.83(0.68–1.00)	**0.047**	**0.012**	641	204	0.83(0.63–1.09)	0.18	0.35
		TT	792	261	0.72(0.58–0.89)	**0.002**	**0.002**	395	127	0.84(0.62–1.13)	0.25	0.42
		CT+TT	2,006	721	0.78(0.66–0.94)	**0.007**	**0.002**	1,036	331	0.83(0.65–1.07)	0.16	0.33
	allele	C	2,230	926	1			1,215	424	1		
		T	2,798	982	0.85(0.76–0.94)	**0.002**	**0.003**	1,431	458	0.92(0.79–1.07)	0.28	0.45

p1 unadjusted.
p2 adjusted for age, sex, BMI and puberty for children, adjusted for age, sex, and BMI for adults.
P values<0.05 were shown in bold.

estimate whether the variants associate with development of type 2 diabetes in Chinese descent population.

Acknowledgments

We gratefully acknowledge the contributions of the data collection team and the individuals who participated in this study, both children and adults. We thank Zhang Meixian (Department of Epidemiology, Capital Institute of Pediatrics, Beijing) and Zhang Yongzhi (Shantou University Medical College) for technical assistance.

Author Contributions

Researched data: YS LW XL XZ HC DH. Contributed to discussion: YS XL XW. Reviewed/edited manuscript: YS LW BX XL XZ HC DH. Interpreted data: LW BX JM. Contributed to design: XW. Made critical revisions of this manuscript: XW JM. Designed the study: JM. Collected data: JM. Analyzed the data: BX JM. Wrote the paper: YS.

References

1. Yang W, Lu J, Weng J, Jia W, Ji L, et al. (2010) Prevalence of diabetes among men and women in China. N Engl J Med 362: 1090–1101.
2. Staiger H, Machicao F, Fritsche A, Haring HU (2009) Pathomechanisms of type 2 diabetes genes. Endocr Rev 30: 557–585.
3. Van SE, Detheux M, Veiga da CM (1994) Short-term control of glucokinase activity: role of a regulatory protein. FASEB J 8: 414–419.
4. Saxena R, Voight BF, Lyssenko V, Burtt NP, de Bakker PI, et al. (2007) Genome-wide association analysis identifies loci for type 2 diabetes and triglyceride levels. Science 316: 1331–1336.
5. Teslovich TM, Musunuru K, Smith AV, Edmondson AC, Stylianou IM, et al. (2010) Biological, clinical and population relevance of 95 loci for blood lipids. Nature 466: 707–713.
6. Sparso T, Andersen G, Nielsen T, Burgdorf KS, Gjesing AP, et al. (2008) The GCKR rs780094 polymorphism is associated with elevated fasting serum triacylglycerol, reduced fasting and OGTT-related insulinaemia, and reduced risk of type 2 diabetes. Diabetologia 51: 70–75.
7. Willer CJ, Sanna S, Jackson AU, Scuteri A, Bonnycastle LL, et al. (2008) Newly identified loci that influence lipid concentrations and risk of coronary artery disease. Nat Genet 40: 161–169.
8. Vaxillaire M, Cavalcanti-Proenca C, Dechaume A, Tichet J, Marre M, et al. (2008) The common P446L polymorphism in GCKR inversely modulates fasting glucose and triglyceride levels and reduces type 2 diabetes risk in the DESIR prospective general French population. Diabetes 57: 2253–2257.
9. Orho-Melander M, Melander O, Guiducci C, Perez-Martinez P, Corella D, et al. (2008) Common missense variant in the glucokinase regulatory protein gene is associated with increased plasma triglyceride and C-reactive protein but lower fasting glucose concentrations. Diabetes 57: 3112–3121.
10. Perez-Martinez P, gado-Lista J, Garcia-Rios A, Mc MJ, Gulseth HL, et al. (2011) Glucokinase regulatory protein genetic variant interacts with omega-3 PUFA to influence insulin resistance and inflammation in metabolic syndrome. PLoS One 6: e20555.
11. Waterworth DM, Ricketts SL, Song K, Chen L, Zhao JH, et al. (2010) Genetic variants influencing circulating lipid levels and risk of coronary artery disease. Arterioscler Thromb Vasc Biol 30: 2264–2276.
12. Ling Y, Li X, Gu Q, Chen H, Lu D, et al. (2011) Associations of common polymorphisms in GCKR with type 2 diabetes and related traits in a Han Chinese population: a case-control study. BMC Med Genet 12: 66.
13. Tam CH, Ma RC, So WY, Wang Y, Lam VK, et al. (2009) Interaction effect of genetic polymorphisms in glucokinase (GCK) and glucokinase regulatory protein (GCKR) on metabolic traits in healthy Chinese adults and adolescents. Diabetes 58: 765–769.
14. Qi Q, Wu Y, Li H, Loos RJ, Hu FB, et al. (2009) Association of GCKR rs780094, alone or in combination with GCK rs1799884, with type 2 diabetes and related traits in a Han Chinese population. Diabetologia 52: 834–843.
15. Wen J, Ronn T, Olsson A, Yang Z, Lu B, et al. (2010) Investigation of type 2 diabetes risk alleles support CDKN2A/B, CDKAL1, and TCF7L2 as susceptibility genes in a Han Chinese cohort. PLoS One 5: e9153.
16. Hu C, Zhang R, Wang C, Yu W, Lu J, et al. (2010) Effects of GCK, GCKR, G6PC2 and MTNR1B variants on glucose metabolism and insulin secretion. PLoS One 5: e11761.
17. Mi J, Cheng H, Hou DQ, Duan JL, Teng HH, et al. (2006) [Prevalence of overweight and obesity among children and adolescents in Beijing in 2004]. Zhonghua Liu Xing Bing Xue Za Zhi 27: 469–474.
18. Xi B, Shen Y, Zhang M, Liu X, Zhao X, et al. (2010) The common rs9939609 variant of the fat mass and obesity-associated gene is associated with obesity risk in children and adolescents of Beijing, China. BMC Med Genet 11: 107.
19. Wu L, Xi B, Zhang M, Shen Y, Zhao X, et al. (2010) Associations of six single nucleotide polymorphisms in obesity-related genes with BMI and risk of obesity in Chinese children. Diabetes 59: 3085–3089.
20. Marshall WA, Tanner JM (1986) Puberty. In: Falkner F, Tanner JM, eds. Human Growth. II. Postnatal Growth. New York, NY: Plenum Press. 209 p.
21. Wallace TM, Levy JC, Matthews DR (2004) Use and abuse of HOMA modeling. Diabetes Care 27: 1487–1495.
22. Ford ES, Giles WH (2003) A comparison of the prevalence of the metabolic syndrome using two proposed definitions. Diabetes Care 26: 575–581.
23. Stoeckman AK, Ma L, Towle HC (2004) Mlx is the functional heteromeric partner of the carbohydrate response element-binding protein in glucose regulation of lipogenic enzyme genes. J Biol Chem 279: 15662–15669.

24. Beer NL, Tribble ND, McCulloch LJ, Roos C, Johnson PR, et al. (2009) The P446L variant in GCKR associated with fasting plasma glucose and triglyceride levels exerts its effect through increased glucokinase activity in liver. Hum Mol Genet 18: 4081–4088.

25. Chambers JC, Zhang W, Zabaneh D, Sehmi J, Jain P, et al. (2009) Common genetic variation near melatonin receptor MTNR1B contributes to raised plasma glucose and increased risk of type 2 diabetes among Indian Asians and European Caucasians. Diabetes 58: 2703–2708.

26. Hishida A, Morita E, Naito M, Okada R, Wakai K, et al. (2012) Associations of apolipoprotein A5 (APOA5), glucokinase (GCK) and glucokinase regulatory protein (GCKR) polymorphisms and lifestyle factors with the risk of dyslipidemia and dysglycemia in Japanese - a cross-sectional data from the J-MICC Study. Endocr J.

27. Windholz J, Kovacs P, Tonjes A, Dittrich K, Bluher S, et al. (2011) Effects of genetic variants in ADCY5, GIPR, GCKR and VPS13C on early impairment of glucose and insulin metabolism in children. PLoS One 6: e22101.

28. Amiel SA, Sherwin RS, Simonson DC, Lauritano AA, Tamborlane WV (1986) Impaired insulin action in puberty. A contributing factor to poor glycemic control in adolescents with diabetes. N Engl J Med 315: 215–219.

29. Goran MI, Ball GD, Cruz ML (2003) Obesity and risk of type 2 diabetes and cardiovascular disease in children and adolescents. J Clin Endocrinol Metab 88: 1417–1427.

30. Roemmich JN, Clark PA, Lusk M, Friel A, Weltman A, et al. (2002) Pubertal alterations in growth and body composition. VI. Pubertal insulin resistance: relation to adiposity, body fat distribution and hormone release. Int J Obes Relat Metab Disord 26: 701–709.

31. Moran A, Jacobs DR Jr, Steinberger J, Hong CP, Prineas R, et al. (1999) Insulin resistance during puberty: results from clamp studies in 357 children. Diabetes 48: 2039–2044.

32. Moran A, Jacobs DR Jr, Steinberger J, Steffen LM, Pankow JS, et al. (2008) Changes in insulin resistance and cardiovascular risk during adolescence: establishment of differential risk in males and females. Circulation 117: 2361–2368.

33. Savage DB, Petersen KF, Shulman GI (2007) Disordered lipid metabolism and the pathogenesis of insulin resistance. Physiol Rev 87: 507–520.

34. Dietz WH (1994) Critical periods in childhood for the development of obesity. Am J Clin Nutr 59: 955–959.

Increased Plasma DPP4 Activity is an Independent Predictor of the Onset of Metabolic Syndrome in Chinese over 4 Years: Result from the China National Diabetes and Metabolic Disorders Study

Fan Yang[1,2,9], Tianpeng Zheng[1,2,9], Yun Gao[1], Attit Baskota[1], Tao Chen[1], Xingwu Ran[1], Haoming Tian[1]*

1 Department of Endocrinology and Metabolism, West China Hospital of Sichuan University, Sichuan, P. R. China, 2 Department of Endocrinology and Metabolism, Affiliated Hospital of Guilin Medical University, Guangxi, P. R. China

Abstract

Aims: To determine whether fasting plasma Dipeptidyl Peptidase 4 (DPP4) activity and active Glucagon-Like Peptide-1 (GLP-1) were predictive of the onset of metabolic syndrome.

Methods: A prospective cohort study was conducted of 2042 adults (863 men and 1,179 women) aged 18-70 years without metabolic syndrome examined in 2007(baseline) and 2011(follow-up). Baseline plasma DPP4 activity was determined as the rate of cleavage of 7-amino-4- methylcoumarin (AMC) from the synthetic substrate H-glycyl-prolyl-AMC and active GLP-1 was determined by enzymoimmunoassay.

Results: During an average of 4 years of follow-up, 131 men (15.2%) and 174 women (14.8%) developed metabolic syndrome. In multiple linear regression analysis, baseline DPP4 activity was an independent predictor of an increase in insulin resistance over a 4-year period (P<0.01). In multivariable-adjusted models, the odds ratio (OR) for incident metabolic syndrome comparing the highest with the lowest quartiles of DPP4 activity and active GLP-1 were 2.82, 0.45 for men and 2.48, 0.36 for women respectively. Furthermore, plasma DPP4 activity significantly improved the area under the ROC curve for predicting new-onset metabolic syndrome based on information from metabolic syndrome components (Both P<0.01).

Conclusions: DPP4 activity is an important predictor of the onset of insulin resistance and metabolic syndrome in apparently healthy Chinese men and women. This finding may have important implications for understanding the aetiology of metabolic syndrome.

Editor: Giuseppe Biagini, University of Modena and Reggio Emilia, Italy

Funding: This study was supported by grants from the Chinese Medical Association Foundation and Chinese Diabetes Society (No. 07020470055). The funders had no role in study design, data collection and analysis, decision to publish, or preparation of the manuscript.

Competing Interests: The authors have declared that no competing interests exist.

* E-mail: w19831120@126.com

9 These authors contributed equally to this work.

Introduction

The metabolic syndrome is characterized by abnormal glucose tolerance, elevated blood pressure, hypertriglyceridemia, low HDL cholesterol, central obesity, microalbuminuria and insulin resistance, subjects with metabolic syndrome are at increased risk for type 2 diabetes and cardiovascular disease [1–2].Given the high prevalence of the metabolic syndrome and its severe consequences, it is essential to understand its biomarkers in population-based longitudinal studies. It is well established that central obesity is the hallmark of the metabolic syndrome [3]. A complex cross-talk scenario between adipose tissue and other organs has been found to underlie the progression of the metabolic syndrome [4]. This is mainly attributed to the huge number of adipokines which are proteins and peptides released by various adipose tissue cells.

Enlargement of adipose tissue leads to dysregulation of adipokine secretion, representing major link between obesity and metabolic syndrome. Since the metabolic syndrome is closely linked to obesity and adipose tissue dysfunction, adipokines are strong candidates to predict the development of metabolic syndrome.

Dipeptidyl peptidase-4 (DPP4) or T-cell activation antigen CD26 (EC 3.4.14.5.) is a serine exopeptidase belonging to the S9B protein family that cleaves X-proline dipeptides from the N-terminus of polypeptides, such as chemokines, neuropeptides, and peptide hormones [5]. Previous studies have documented that circulating DPP4 originate from cells of the immune system and differentiated adipocytes [6–7]. It is found to be a novel adipokine potentially linking obesity to the metabolic syndrome [6]. Recent data suggest that the protein level of DPP4 is significantly associated with insulin resistance factors and components of metabolic syndrome [6]. However, most of the observations come from cross-sectional studies and focus on the protein level of DPP4, until recently, little is known about the ability of circulating DPP4 activity as a predictor of insulin resistance and metabolic syndrome or about its ability to predict incident metabolic syndrome beyond the information provided by each of its components among healthy individuals.

We thus studied the prospective association of plasma DPP4 activity with the risk of incident metabolic syndrome and its components, as well as the predictive value of plasma DPP4 activity in identifying in individuals who will develop incident metabolic syndrome among healthy individuals. Since DPP4 is involved in the degradation of circulating active GLP-1 to biologically inactive fragments, plasma active GLP-1 level is also studied in our research. In our study, the homeostasis model assessment of insulin resistance (HOMA-IR) was used to estimate insulin resistance.

Methods

Subjects

The study population was men and women, aged 18–70 years, who participated in the China National Diabetes and Metabolic Disorders Study [8], a 4-year follow-up study that aims to clarify the prevalence and development of the type2 diabetes and metabolic disorders. Subjects are volunteers who came from 3 health examination centers in Sichuan province. The Medical Research Ethics Committee of the China–Japan Friendship Hospital (Location:2 Cherry Park Street, Chaoyang District, Beijing 100029, China) reviewed and approved the present study. The written informed consent was obtained from each participant before data collection. This study was registered on the Chinese clinical trial registry (#TR-CCH-Chi CTR -CCH-00000361).

The final sample size for the present analysis was 2042 participants (863 men and 1,179 women) without metabolic syndrome at baseline. Inclusion criteria: (1) Age between 18-70 years old. (2) Long-term residing (≥5 years) in China's Sichuan province. Exclusion criteria: (1) All subjects having past history of metabolic syndrome or have been diagnosed with metabolic syndrome at baseline during screening. (2) Using varieties of drugs to control blood glucose, blood pressure, blood lipid and other drugs used in preventing complications during natural process of metabolic syndrome. (3) Subjects deprived of personal safety and presence of any of the chronic diseases including stroke, myocardial infarction, other heart, liver, renal and respiratory dysfunction were excluded as progression of these in any stage may hinder our study. (4) Pregnant subjects and subjects with malignancy. (5) Does not need assistance from the medical staffs to complete the survey done twice at baseline and during follow-up. (6) Subjects with incomplete data. The diagnostic criteria of the metabolic syndrome were based on the criteria recommended by the WHO. We used the criteria by the WHO (1999), which require presence of one of diabetes mellitus(indicated by FPG ≥7.0 mmol/L or 2 h-PG≥11.1 mmol/L), impaired glucose tolerance(IGT,indicated by 2 h-PG between 7.8–11.09 mmol/L and FPG <6.1 mmol/L), or impaired fasting glucose(IFG,indicated by FPG between 6.10–6.99 mmol/L and 2 h-PG <7.8 mmol/L),and two of the following: blood pressure≥140/ 90 mmHg, dyslipidemia(triglycerides[TG] >1.7 mmol/L and HDL cholesterol <0.9 mmol/L [male] or <1.0 mmol/L[female]), central obesity(waist-to-hip ratio [WHR]>0.90 [male],>0.85 [female], or BMI >30 kg/m^2), or microalbuminuria.

Study design

A standard questionnaire was administered by trained staff to participants to record demographic characteristics and life style risk factors [9]. Blood pressure, body weight, height, waist and hip circumference, body mass index (BMI), and waist/hip ratio (WHR) were measured and calculated using standard methods, as previously described [8]. Participants were instructed to maintain their usual physical activity and diet for at least 3 days before undergoing an oral glucose tolerance test (OGTT). After an overnight fast≥10 h, venous blood samples were collected to measure FPG, fasting insulin, blood lipids (including TC, TG, LDL-C, and HDL-C), DPP4 activity and active GLP-1. Blood samples were also drawn at 30 and 120 min after a 75 g glucose load to measure glucose and insulin concentrations. Demographic characteristics, life style risk factors, anthropometric parameters and venous blood samples were both collected or determined at baseline and four years later.

Data collection

Plasma glucose levels were measured using a hexokinase enzymatic method. Insulin was measured by a radioimmunoassay with human insulin as a standard (Linco, St Charles, MO). TG, TC, LDL-C, and HDL-C levels were determined enzymatically. Plasma DPP4 activity was determined as the rate of cleavage of 7-amino-4- methylcoumarin (AMC) from the synthetic substrate H-glycyl-prolyl-AMC (H-Gly-Pro-AMC; Biovision, San Francisco, California, U.S.A.). It is expressed as the amount of cleaved AMC per minute per mL (nmol/min/mL). DPP4 activity was measured in the absence or the presence of sitagliptin, a specific DPP4 inhibitor, to test the specificity of the enzymatic assay. In our samples, sitagliptin inhibited the assayed activity by >95%. The intra-assay and inter-assay coefficients of variation were 2.13% and 8.56%, respectively. Samples for active GLP-1 were collected into iced Vacutainer tubes prepared with EDTA and DPP4 inhibitor for preventing degradation of active GLP into truncated, inactive GLP-1. Active GLP-1 which includes GLP-1(7-37) and GLP-1(7-36) was measured by enzyme-linked immunosorbent assay (Millipore, U.S.A.). The intra-assay and inter-assay coefficients of variation were 1.74% and 9.87%, respectively. Blood samples for measuring DPP4 activity and active GLP-1 levels were stored at −80 °C and subsequently DPP4 activity and active GLP-1 levels of all samples were measured within six months after the sample collection. The homeostasis model assessment of insulin resistance (HOMA-IR) was calculated from FPG and fasting insulin levels using the equation: FPG (mmol/L) × fasting insulin (μIU/ml)/22.5.

Statistical analysis

All of the statistical analyses were performed using the SPSS 16.0 software (SPSS Inc., Chicago, IL, USA). Data were expressed as means ± standard deviation, median (interquartile range), or percentage for normally distributed continuous various, abnormally distributed continuous variables, and categorical variables, respectively. Abnormally distributed variables including fasting insulin, 2-hour insulin, HOMA-IR and TG were logarithmically transformed before analysis. We divided the study population into quintiles of plasma DPP4 activity with cut points 5.57, 6.05, 6.50, 7.00 for men and 5.11, 5.95, 6.39, 7.02 for women, and plasma active GLP-1 with cut points 2.55, 2.80, 3.14, 3.71 for men and 2.45, 2.80, 3.13, 3.82 for women respectively. We evaluated the association of baseline DPP4 activity and active GLP-1 with the incidence of new cases of metabolic syndrome and with the incidence of new cases of each component of the metabolic syndrome at the follow-up visit. To evaluate the incidence of new

Table 1. Baseline characteristics of study population by incident metabolic syndrome.

	Men			Women		
	No metabolic syndrome	Metabolic syndrome	P	No metabolic syndrome	Metabolic syndrome	P
N(%)	732(84.8)	131(15.2)	-	1005(85.2)	174(14.8)	-
Age(years)	43.6±14.6	48.8±13.5	0.000	42.4±13.4	50.2±13.4	0.000
Current smoking, n (%)	168(23.0)	41 (31.3)	0.040	51(5.1)	18(10.3)	0.006
Alcohol consumption, n (%)	328(44.8)	64(48.9)	0.640	141(14.0)	30(17.2)	0.267
Leisure-time physical activity, n (%)	358(48.9)	87(66.4)	0.000	661(65.8)	118(67.8)	0.599
Family history of diabetes, n (%)	111(15.2)	23(17.6)	0.486	157(15.6)	24(13.8)	0.537
BMI(kg/m^2) [a]	22.61±3.36	26.03±4.99	0.000	22.68±3.86	24.76±4.64	0.000
WHR[a]	0.86±0.08	0.92±0.06	0.000	0.83±0.08	0.91±0.10	0.000
SBP(mmHg) [a]	114.1±14.9	128.0±21.4	0.000	112.4±16.7	126.9±25.0	0.000
DBP(mmHg) [a]	74.8±9.7	83.2±12.0	0.000	74.0±10.3	81.9±13.9	0.000
FPG (mmol/L) [a]	4.61±0.60	4.75±0.57	0.068	4.61±0.55	4.74±0.64	0.082
2 h-PG (mmol/L) [a]	5.30±1.21	5.80±1.19	0.000	5.46±1.10	5.92±1.06	0.000
Fasting insulin((μIU/ml) [a]	6.48(4.88,8.41)	8.00(5.45,10.08)	0.000	6.56(4.95,8.59)	7.30(5.46,9.52)	0.086
2 h-insulin(μIU/ml) [a]	18.37(10.70,30.47)	27.72(15.82,46.28)	0.027	21.20(13.11,37.25)	25.78(13.22,50.23)	0.021
TG (mmol/L) [a]	1.16(0.82,1.60)	2.07(1.57,2.87)	0.000	1.07(0.81,1.47)	1.77(1.27,2.32)	0.000
TC (mmol/L) [a]	4.47±1.00	5.00±0.90	0.000	4.57±1.48	4.96±1.32	0.019
LDL-C (mmol/L) [a]	2.65±0.78	2.96±0.76	0.001	2.65±0.76	2.85±0.98	0.203
HDL-C (mmol/L) [a]	1.24±0.33	1.09±0.25	0.000	1.33±0.34	1.21±0.39	0.000
HOMA-IR [a]	1.32(0.99, 1.69)	1.67(1.13,2.25)	0.000	1.32(0.99,1.80)	1.53(1.15,2.07)	0.032
Metabolic syndrome components, n (%)						
High blood pressure	85(11.6)	60(45.8)	0.000	110(10.9)	79(45.4)	0.000
High TG	157(21.4)	92(70.2)	0.000	164(16.3)	96(55.2)	0.000
Low HDL-C	79(10.8)	33(25.2)	0.000	139(13.8)	68(39.1)	0.000
Central obesity	180(24.6)	101(77.1)	0.000	360(35.8)	140(80.5)	0.000
Microalbuminuria	78(10.7)	42(32.1)	0.000	135(13.4)	69(39.7)	0.000

Data were expressed as means ± standard deviation, median (interquartile range), or percentage for normally distributed continuous various, abnormally distributed continuous variables, and categorical variables, respectively. Cigarette smoking was defined as having smoked at least 100 cigarettes in one's lifetime. Alcohol consumption was defined as consumption of ≥30 g of alcohol per week for 1 year or more. Regular leisure-time physical activity was defined as participation in ≥30 min of moderate or vigorous activity per day at least 3 days per week. [a] adjusted for age.

cases of each component, we excluded subjects with the presence of that specific component at baseline. Clinical and biochemical characteristics were compared by ANCOVA or χ2 tests. The DPP4 activity and active GLP-1'S predictive value for insulin resistance were quantified by multiple linear regressions. Logistic regression models were calculated to identify independent relations between DPP4 activity, active GLP-1 and incident metabolic syndrome. Five models were calculated: one crude model was adjusted for age, sex, BMI, and a fifth model was additionally adjusted for SBP, FPG, fasting insulin, TG, HDL-C, family history of diabetes, physical activity, smoking and alcohol consumption (fully adjusted model). Odds ratios (ORs) and 95% CIs are reported. To evaluate the added discrimination provided by DPP4 activity or active GLP-1 to predict incident cases of metabolic syndrome beyond the information provided by the components of the metabolic syndrome, we compared the areas under the receiver operating characteristic (ROC) curve in models that included BMI HDL cholesterol, TG, systolic blood pressure (SBP), fasting plasma glucose (FPG), and urine albumin-creatinine ratio(ACR) with and without DPP4 activity or active GLP-1.

Results

During 4 years follow-up, 131men (15.2%) and 174 women (14.8%) developed metabolic syndrome. Baseline BMI, WHR, SBP, diastolic blood pressure (DBP), 2 h-PG, 2 h-insulin, TG, total cholesterol (TC), HOMA-IR were significantly higher and HDL cholesterol was significantly lower in men and women who developed metabolic syndrome compared with those who did not (Table 1).

As per male and female, there was no significant statistical difference between the levels of DPP4 activity and active GLP-1 (as shown in Table S3 in File S1). Both in male and female, in comparison to the age group ≤30 years, age ≥61 years have increased level of DPP4 activity. Further, in comparison to the women between the age group 31–40 years, age group ≥51-years-old has significantly lower level of active GLP-1 (Figure S2 in File S1). DPP4 activity at baseline were significantly higher in subjects who developed metabolic syndrome compared with those who did not in both men and women whereas active GLP-1 levels was significantly lower (all P<0.001). A similar association was observed between DPP4 activity, active GLP-1 and each component of the metabolic syndrome except for high diastolic

Table 2. Baseline DPP4 activity and active GLP-1 according to presence or absence of components of new-onset metabolic syndrome.

	Men(n = 863)			Women(n = 1179)		
	Present	Absent	P	Present	Absent	P
DPP4 activity (nmol/min/ml)						
Metabolic syndrome	7.39±3.34	5.80±2.04	0.000	7.77±3.49	5.73±2.09	0.000
High SBP	6.91±2.96	5.95±2.26	0.001	7.20±3.41	5.90±2.29	0.000
High DBP	6.01±2.95	6.04±2.25	0.753	6.98±3.19	5.89±2.31	0.000
High TG	6.55±2.81	5.83±2.11	0.000	6.62±3.18	5.86±2.19	0.000
Low HDL-C	6.65±3.22	5.95±2.18	0.003	6.42±3.04	5.94±2.31	0.012
Central obesity	6.43±2.93	5.85±1.99	0.003	6.66±3.01	5.93±1.95	0.002
Microalbuminuria	6.01±2.66	6.04±2.30	0.785	7.99±1.55	6.11±1.33	0.000
No. of components						
0	5.82±1.92			5.70±1.87		
1	5.56±1.96			5.77±2.03		
2	6.45±2.24			5.98±2.47		
3	7.17±3.72			7.16±3.36		
>=4	7.71±4.32			8.40±4.69		
P for trend	0.000			0.000		
Active GLP-1 (pmol/L)						
Metabolic syndrome	2.82±0.87	3.17±1.00	0.000	2.77±0.95	3.19±1.07	0.000
High SBP	2.85±0.99	3.14±0.99	0.022	2.80±1.04	3.14±1.07	0.000
High DBP	2.85±0.92	3.15±0.99	0.004	3.01±1.06	3.15±1.06	0.273
High TG	2.96±0.86	3.18±1.03	0.006	2.96±1.04	3.18±1.06	0.015
Low HDL-C	2.89±0.89	3.13±1.00	0.017	2.99±0.91	3.16±1.09	0.030
Central obesity	2.99±0.95	3.17±1.00	0.021	2.71±1.09	3.17±1.04	0.000
Microalbuminuria	3.06±1.09	3.12±0.97	0.625	3.05±1.05	3.15±1.06	0.284
No. of components						
0	3.24±1.01			3.21±1.03		
1	3.11±0.98			3.15±1.06		
2	3.16±1.01			3.17±1.14		
3	2.61±0.72			2.93±0.99		
>=4	2.66±0.87			2.56±0.68		
P for trend	0.000			0.000		

Data were expressed as means ± standard deviation.

blood pressure and microalbuminuria (all P<0.05). Furthermore, plasma DPP4 activity progressively increased with the number of metabolic syndrome components developed by study participants over follow-up whereas active GLP-1 decreased progressively (P for trend <0.001 in both men and women) (Table 2).

Four-year longitudinal studies showed that baseline DPP4 activity was an independent predictor of an increase in fasting insulin and HOMA-IR in both men and women after adjustment for age, BMI, SBP, TG, HDL-C(all P<0.01) (Table 3). After a follow-up of over 4 years, the proportions of subjects who developed new-onset metabolic syndrome, high blood glucose, high blood pressure, high TG, low HDL cholesterol, high WHR, and high urine ACR were 14.9, 19.5, 15.0, 24.1, 18.0, 20.1 and 15.9%, respectively. In multivariable -adjusted models [model 5 (Table 4 and Table 5)], the OR for developing metabolic syndrome comparing subjects in the highest with those in the lowest quintile of baseline DPP4 activity and active GLP-1 were 2.82, 0.45 for men and 2.48, 0.36 for women respectively. The

corresponding ORs for high blood pressure, high TG, low HDL cholesterol, high WHR and high urine ACR according to baseline DPP4 activity were 3.66, 2.30, 2.84, 2.53 and 1.90, according to baseline active GLP-1 were 0.51, 0.19, 0.29, 0.38 and 1.10 respectively (Table S1-S2 in File S1).

We then evaluated how well baseline DPP4 activity and active GLP-1 levels predict incident metabolic syndrome beyond the information provided by baseline levels of metabolic syndrome components. The area under the ROC curve to predict incident metabolic syndrome using BMI HDL-C, TG, SBP, FPG and ACR was 0.783(95% CI 0.756–0.810). After DPP4 activity or active GLP-1 were added to the model, the corresponding areas under the ROC curve were 0.827(0.801–0.852) and 0.795(0.770–0.821) respectively. The P values for the comparison in areas under the ROC curve for the models with and without DPP4 activity or active GLP-1 levels were 0.021and 0.53(Figure S1 in File S1).

Table 3. Standardized coefficients (β) from the multiple linear regression analysis of glucose metabolism in the 4-year longitudinal study.

	Change in insulin(μU/ml)		Change in glucose(mmol/L)		Change in HOMA-IR	
	β	p	β	p	β	p
All[a]						
DPP4 activity	0.113	0.000	0.105	0.000	0.131	0.000
Active GLP-1	−0.048	0.031	0.001	0.949	−0.030	0.184
Men[b]						
DPP4 activity	0.116	0.001	0.095	0.006	0.108	0.002
Active GLP-1	−0.062	0.071	−0.015	0.672	−0.033	0.337
Women[b]						
DPP4 activity	0.105	0.000	0.112	0.000	0.157	0.000
Active GLP-1	−0.041	0.166	0.013	0.647	−0.030	0.313

[a]Sex,age,SBP, BMI,TG,HDL-C were included in the regeression model.
[b]Age,SBP, BMI,TG,HDL-C were included in the regression model.

Discussion

In this prospective study, we demonstrate, for the first time, that plasma DPP4 activity predict the onset of IR and metabolic syndrome. Plasma DPP4 activity is also a strong positive predictor of the total number of components of the metabolic syndrome developed and of each individual component of the metabolic syndrome

Lamers et al. [6]have proved that enlargement of visceral adipocytes and adipose tissue inflammation enhance the release of DPP4 from the fat cell to circulation, moreover, they found that circulating DPP4 concentrations correlated with various classic markers for the metabolic syndrome, namely, waist circumference, BMI, plasma triglycerides, HOMA-IR and fat cell volume. Kirino et al. [10] also reported that plasma DPP4 activity correlates with BMI in healthy young people. In our study, we found that plasma DPP4 activity was significantly higher in subjects who had higher WHR, blood pressure, blood lipid and HOMA-IR, furthermore, we also found that increased DPP4 activity is an independent predictor of metabolic syndrome and its components in our prospective study. Consequently, we speculated that in a relatively early stage, the various factors of insulin resistance or the

Table 4. ORs for new-onset metabolic syndrome in men according to baseline DPP4 activity and active GLP-1.

	Q 1	Q2	Q3	Q 4	Q5
DPP4 activity(nmol/ml/min)	≤5.57	5.58–6.05	6.06–6.50	6.51–7.00	>7.00
New-onset metabolic syndrome	13(7.6)	17(9.8)	29(16.1)	27(16.5)	45(26.0)
Metabolic syndrome					
Model 1	1	1.40(0.64–3.06)0.397	2.64(1.29–5.41)0.008	2.76(1.34–5.69)0.006	3.79(1.91–7.52)0.000
Model 2	1	1.27(0.58–2.78)0.558	2.58(1.26–5.29)0.009	2.76(1.33–5.70)0.006	3.40 (1.71–6.80)0.001
Model 3	1	1.31(0.59–2.89)0.508	2.62(1.28–5.36)0.009	2.73(1.32–5.64)0.007	3.04(1.51–6.13)0.002
Model 4	1	1.36(0.60–3.09)0.459	2.73(1.29–5.76)0.009	2.67(1.25–5.71)0.012	2.78(1.35–5.75)0.006
Model 5	1	1.36(0.60–3.10)0.463	2.80(1.32–5.93)0.007	2.73(1.27–5.84)0.010	2.82(1.36–5.85)0.005
Active GLP-1 (pmol/L)	≤2.55	2.56–2.80	2.81–3.14	3.15–3.71	≥3.72
New-onset metabolic syndrome	35(20.0)	27(14.9)	26(16.0)	29(16.5)	14(8.3)
Metabolic syndrome					
Model 1	1	0.84(0.47–1.50)0.551	0.94(0.52–1.70)0.849	1.00(0.56–1.78)0.999	0.37(0.18–0.73)0.004
Model 2	1	1.04(0.57–1.90)0.902	1.09(0.60–2.00)0.772	1.15(0.64–2.08)0.630	0.43(0.22–0.87)0.018
Model 3	1	1.12(0.61–2.05)0.723	1.16(0.63–2.13)0.637	1.21(0.67–2.16)0.534	0.42(0.21–0.86)0.017
Model 4	1	1.06(0.57–1.99)0.856	1.23(0.65–2.33)0.526	1.17(0.67–2.19)0.621	0.46(0.22–0.95)0.035
Model 5	1	1.03(0.55–1.94)0.924	1.30(0.68–2.48)0.427	1.23(0.66–2.29)0.517	0.45(0.22–0.94)0.034

Data are OR (95% CI) P or n (%).
Model 1 (adjusted for Age, BMI).
Model 2 (Model 1+ SBP).
Model 3 (Model 2 + FPG + Fasting insulin).
Model 4 (Model 3 + TG +HDL-C).
Model 5 (Model 4+ family history + physical activity + smoking + alcohol consumption).

Table 5. ORs for new-onset metabolic syndrome in women according to baseline DPP4 activity and active GLP-1.

	Q 1	Q2	Q3	Q 4	Q5
DPP4 activity(nmol/ml/min)	≤5.11	5.12–5.95	5.96–6.39	6.40–7.02	>7.02
New-onset metabolic syndrome	21(8.8)	24(10.2)	25(10.6)	45(19.1)	59(25.2)
Metabolic syndrome					
Model 1	1	1.26(0.67–2.34)0.476	1.26(0.68–2.34)0.466	2.54(1.45–4.45)0.001	3.21(1.86–5.52)0.000
Model 2	1	1.24(0.66–2.32)0.501	1.27(0.68–2.37)0.447	2.51(1.43–4.42)0.001	2.74(1.57–4.75)0.000
Model 3	1	1.25(0.67–2.34)0.487	1.28(0.69–2.38)0.435	2.55(1.45–4.48)0.001	2.71(1.56–4.71)0.000
Model 4	1	1.37(0.72–2.60)0.336	1.22(0.64–2.32)0.541	2.58(1.45–4.61)0.001	2.43(1.38–4.29)0.002
Model 5	1	1.40(0.74–2.66)0.306	1.27(0.66–2.42)0.474	2.67(1.49–4.78)0.001	2.48(1.40–4.39)0.002
Active GLP-1 (pmol/L)	≤2.45	2.46–2.80	2.81–3.13	3.14–3.82	≥3.83
New-onset metabolic syndrome	55(23.3)	36(14.8)	40(17.2)	23(9.9)	20(8.5)
Metabolic syndrome					
Model 1	1	0.56(0.35–0.91)0.018	0.69(0.43–1.09)0.114	0.37(0.22–0.63)0.000	0.34(0.19–0.59)0.000
Model 2	1	0.57(0.35–0.92)0.021	0.72(0.45–1.15)0.163	0.36(0.21–0.61)0.000	0.35(0.20–0.62)0.000
Model 3	1	0.56(0.35–0.91)0.019	0.70(0.44–1.12)0.138	0.35(0.20–0.60)0.000	0.35(0.20–0.62)0.000
Model 4	1	0.60(0.37–0.99)0.047	0.66(0.40–1.07)0.092	0.36(0.21–0.63)0.000	0.37(0.21–0.65)0.001
Model 5	1	0.62(0.37–1.01)0.057	0.66(0.40–1.08)0.100	0.36(0.20–0.63)0.000	0.36(0.20–0.64)0.001

Data are OR (95% CI) P or n (%).
Model 1 (adjusted for Age, BMI).
Model 2 (Model 1+ SBP).
Model 3 (Model 2 + FPG + Fasting insulin).
Model 4 (Model 3 + TG +HDL-C).
Model 5 (Model 4+ family history + physical activity + smoking + alcohol consumption).

components of the metabolic syndrome not only have a close relationship with DPP4 protein level, but they may also be closely related with DPP4 activity. Lamers et al. have documented that DPP4 induce insulin resistance in an autocrine and paracrine fashion at the level of Akt in three different primary cell types, namely, adipocytes, skeletal muscle, and smooth muscle cells, enzymatic activity of DPP4 seems to be involved in this process. In our study, we demonstrated for the first time that baseline plasma DPP4 activity was an independent predictor of an increase in insulin resistance in population-based prospective study. However, our study did not explore much about the mechanism by which increase in DPP4 activity lead to insulin resistance, that's why we are still not sure that DPP4 activity can lead to increase in insulin resistance.

We performed ROC curve analyses to evaluate the additional predictive ability of DPP4 activity beyond the information provided by the components of the metabolic syndrome at baseline. Within a model including BMI HDL-C, TG, SBP, FBG and ACR, DPP4 activity did significantly increase the area under the ROC curve, thereby demonstrating that in Chinese population, plasma DPP4 activity may increase the predictive ability for identification of subjects at risk for developing new-onset metabolic syndrome beyond that of the information provided by the components of the metabolic syndrome.

GLP-1, a member of the incretin hormone family, is found to be involved in insulin secretion and beta-cell proliferation in preclinical studies [11–12]. There are two forms of circulating active GLP-1 secreted after meal ingestion: GLP-1(7-37) and GLP-1(7-36), both peptides are equipotent and exhibit identical plasma half-lives and biological activities acting through the same receptor [13]. Since DPP4 is involved in the degradation of circulating active GLP-1 to biologically inactive fragments, plasma active GLP-1 level could also be associated with the development of

insulin resistance and metabolic syndrome. In our study, we found that fasting active GLP-1 can not predict the development of insulin resistance and incident metabolic syndrome beyond the information provided by its components, although our multiple logistic regression analyses indicated that fasting active GLP-1 predict the onset of metabolic syndrome and some of its components. The specific reason for this inconsistency is still unknown, we speculate that this mismatch may be related to pattern of active GLP-1 secretion. Since plasma active GLP-1 level increase significantly after meal ingestion and since it is responsible for a large proportion of postprandial insulin secretion, we can not ignore the possibility that fasting active GLP-1 is not an effective predictor of the onset of insulin resistance and metabolic syndrome in apparently healthy Chinese, postprandial plasma active GLP-1 may play a more important role than fasting plasma active GLP-1 in predicting incident metabolic syndrome. Prospective studies are still needed to evaluate the predictive value of postprandial plasma active GLP-1 to identify individuals at high risk of new-onset metabolic syndrome.

Some limitations of our study should also be considered. Firstly, the follow-up period of our cohort was only 4 years, and we could not evaluate whether the association between DPP4 activity, active GLP-1 and incident metabolic syndrome would persist in longer follow up. Secondly, we did not evaluate the predictive value of postprandial plasma active GLP-1 to identify individuals at high risk of new-onset metabolic syndrome. Lastly, this study is an epidemiological study and somehow it fails to address the precise role of DPP4 and GLP1 in the pathogenesis of metabolic syndrome and insulin resistance which is needed to be elucidated by further basic investigation.

In summary, we have shown prospectively that increased fasting plasma DPP4 activity independently predict incident metabolic syndrome and insulin resistance in apparently healthy Chinese, and it may be considered as a novel marker of metabolic syndrome and insulin resistance. These findings have implications for increasing our understanding of the aetiology of metabolic syndrome and merit further study in future studies that help to clarify causality and advance this area of research.

Supporting Information

File S1 Table S1. ORs for new-onset metabolic syndrome components according to baseline DPP4 activity (nmol/ml/min); Table S2. ORs for new-onset metabolic syndrome components according to baseline active GLP-1(pmol/L); Table S3. Comparison of DPP4 activity and active GLP-1 between men and women according to age; Figure S1. The area under the ROC curve to predict incident metabolic syndrome using Model1, Model2 and Model3; Figure S2. Sex-specific DPP4 activity and active GLP-1 levels according to age.

Acknowledgments

We gratefully acknowledge the residents and nurses of Department of Endocrinology of Yulin Community Hospital, the First People's Hospital of Longquan, and the First People's Hospital of Liangshan Yi Nationality Autonomy District for their diligent work on collecting demographic data and blood samples.

Author Contributions

Conceived and designed the experiments: HT XR. Performed the experiments: YG TC TZ. Analyzed the data: FY TZ. Contributed reagents/materials/analysis tools: AB. Wrote the paper: FY TZ.

References

1. von Bibra H, Sutton MSJ (2010) Diastolic dysfunction in diabetes and the metabolic syndrome: promising potential for diagnosis and prognosis. Diabetologia 53: 1033–1045.
2. Sattar N, McConnachie A, Shaper AG, Blauw GJ, Buckley BM, et al. (2008) Can metabolic syndrome usefully predict cardiovascular disease and diabetes? Outcome data from two prospective studies. The Lancet 371: 1927–1935.
3. Wellen KE, Hotamisligil GS (2005) Inflammation, stress, and diabetes. Journal of Clinical Investigation 115: 1111–1119.
4. Sell H, Dietze-Schroeder D, Eckel J (2006) The adipocyte–myocyte axis in insulin resistance. Trends in Endocrinology & Metabolism 17: 416–422.
5. Matteucci E, Giampietro O (2009) Dipeptidyl peptidase-4 (CD26): knowing the function before inhibiting the enzyme. Current medicinal chemistry 16: 2943–2951.
6. Lamers D, Famulla S, Wronkowitz N, Hartwig S, Lehr S, et al. (2011) Dipeptidyl peptidase 4 is a novel adipokine potentially linking obesity to the metabolic syndrome. Diabetes 60: 1917–1925.
7. Cordero OJ, Salgado FJ, Nogueira M (2009) On the origin of serum CD26 and its altered concentration in cancer patients. Cancer immunology, immunotherapy 58: 1723–1747.
8. Yang W, Lu J, Weng J, Jia W, Ji L, et al. (2010) Prevalence of diabetes among men and women in China. New England Journal of Medicine 362: 1090–1101.
9. Luepker R, Evans A, McKeigue P, Reddy K (2004) Cardiovascular Survey Methods World Health Organization. Geneva, Switzerland.
10. Kirino Y, Sei M, Kawazoe K, Minakuchi K, Sato Y (2011) Plasma dipeptidyl peptidase 4 activity correlates with body mass index and the plasma adiponectin concentration in healthy young people. Endocrine journal 59: 949–953.
11. Li L, El-Kholy W, Rhodes C, Brubaker P (2005) Glucagon-like peptide-1 protects beta cells from cytokine-induced apoptosis and necrosis: role of protein kinase B. Diabetologia 48: 1339–1349.
12. Zhang J, Tokui Y, Yamagata K, Kozawa J, Sayama K, et al. (2007) Continuous stimulation of human glucagon-like peptide-1 (7–36) amide in a mouse model (NOD) delays onset of autoimmune type 1 diabetes. Diabetologia 50: 1900–1909.
13. Ørskov C, Wettergren A, Holst JJ (1993) Biological effects and metabolic rates of glucagonlike peptide-1 7–36 amide and glucagonlike peptide-1 7–37 in healthy subjects are indistinguishable. Diabetes 42: 658–661.

Normal Weight Obesity is Associated with Metabolic Syndrome and Insulin Resistance in Young Adults from a Middle-Income Country

Francilene B. Madeira[1], Antônio A. Silva[2]*, Helma F. Veloso[2], Marcelo Z. Goldani[3], Gilberto Kac[4], Viviane C. Cardoso[5], Heloisa Bettiol[5], Marco A. Barbieri[5]

1 Physical Education Undergraduate Course, State University of Piauí, Teresina, Brazil, 2 Department of Public Health, Federal University of Maranhão, São Luís, Brazil, 3 Department of Pediatrics and Puericulture, Faculty of Medicine, Federal University of Rio Grande do Sul, Porto Alegre, Brazil, 4 Department of Social and Applied Nutrition, Josué de Castro Nutrition Institute, Federal University of Rio de Janeiro, Rio de Janeiro, Brazil, 5 Department of Puericulture and Pediatrics, Faculty of Medicine of Ribeirão Preto, University of São Paulo, Ribeirão Preto, Brazil

Abstract

Objective: This population-based birth cohort study examined whether normal weight obesity is associated with metabolic disorders in young adults in a middle-income country undergoing rapid nutrition transition.

Design and Methods: The sample involved 1,222 males and females from the 1978/79 Ribeirão Preto birth cohort, Brazil, aged 23–25 years. NWO was defined as body mass index (BMI) within the normal range (18.5–24.9 kg/m^2) and the sum of subscapular and triceps skinfolds above the sex-specific 90th percentiles of the study sample. It was also defined as normal BMI and % BF (body fat) >23% in men and >30% in women. Insulin resistance (IR), insulin sensitivity and secretion were based on the Homeostasis Model Assessment (HOMA) model.

Results: In logistic models, after adjusting for age, sex and skin colour, NWO was significantly associated with Metabolic Syndrome (MS) according to the Joint Interim Statement (JIS) definition (Odds Ratio OR = 6.83; 95% Confidence Interval CI 2.84–16.47). NWO was also associated with HOMA2-IR (OR = 3.81; 95%CI 1.57–9.28), low insulin sensitivity (OR = 3.89; 95%CI 2.39–6.33), and high insulin secretion (OR = 2.17; 95%CI 1.24–3.80). Significant associations between NWO and some components of the MS were also detected: high waist circumference (OR = 8.46; 95%CI 5.09–14.04), low High Density Lipoprotein cholesterol (OR = 1.65; 95%CI 1.11–2.47) and high triglyceride levels (OR = 1.93; 95%CI 1.02–3.64). Most estimates changed little after further adjustment for early and adult life variables.

Conclusions: NWO was associated with MS and IR, suggesting that clinical assessment of excess body fat in normal-BMI individuals should begin early in life even in middle-income countries.

Editor: Reury F.P Bacurau, University of São Paulo, Brazil

Funding: This study was supported by the Brazilian Research Council (CNPq, Brazilian acronym), the University of São Paulo and the São Paulo Research Foundation (FAPESP, Brazilian acronym) grant number 00/09508-7. The funders had no role in study design, data collection and analysis, decision to publish, or preparation of the manuscript.

Competing Interests: The authors have declared that no competing interest exists.

* E-mail: aasilva@ufma.br

Introduction

The prevalence of obesity (Body Mass Index - BMI ≥30 kg/m^2) has increased worldwide over the past decades [1,2], although more recent data suggest a slowing or levelling off of this trend [3]. In Brazil, from 1974–1975 to 2008–2009, the prevalence rates of obesity increased more than fourfold among men (2.8% to 12.4%) and more than twofold among women (from 8.0% to 16.9%) [4].

Obesity, defined as excess body fat (BF) [5,6], has been evaluated in both clinical and epidemiological studies, using predominantly BMI [7,8]. Studies have shown an association between extreme values of BMI and increased mortality [9,10]. However, because BMI does not differentiate lean from fat mass, this indicator has limited accuracy for diagnosing individuals with excess BF presenting BMI within the normal range [11–13].

In the early eighties, Ruderman et al. described a specific type of obesity defined as metabolically obese normal weight subjects (MONW). These individuals were characterized by normal body weight and BMI, but presented hyperinsulinemia, insulin-resistance, and increased type 2 diabetes, hypertriglyceridemia and cardiovascular diseases predisposition [14,15]. Few years later, De Lorenzo et al. [16] among other authors [17,18] used the term normal weight obesity (NWO) to identify individuals who have normal body weight and BMI but high % BF, accompanied by total lean mass deficiency. Therefore, MONW is a subset of NWO and from a conceptual and clinical perspective it is important to differentiate these two conditions.

Some other studies have reported associations between NWO and metabolic disorders [16,18–27]. In a study of the US population, individuals aged >20 years with NWO were four times more likely to develop metabolic syndrome (MS) than those with normal BMI and normal BF [18]. In another study carried out in Switzerland, which included only females of Caucasian origin aged 35–75 years, women with NWO had a higher cardiometabolic risk and higher prevalences of low high-density lipoprotein (HDL) cholesterol, high waist circumference (WC), high triglycerides and hyperglycaemia but a similar prevalence of hypertension compared to lean women [20].

However, to our knowledge, there are few studies reporting an association between NWO and metabolic disorders exclusively in young adults or coming from low and middle-income countries [28–30]. Studies in young populations are important because if NWO is associated with metabolic imbalances at an early age, clinical evaluation should change and preventive public policy actions should be redrawn and begin earlier in order to limit complications, as NWO individuals get older [6,15,31].

The objective of the present study was to evaluate the association between NWO and MS and insulin resistance (IR) in young adults from a population-based birth cohort performed in a middle-income country undergoing rapid nutrition transition, with adjustment for several early and adult life variables.

Methods

Ethics Statement

The project was approved by the Research Ethics Committee of the Clinics Hospital, Faculty of Medicine of Ribeirão Preto, University of São Paulo, Brazil. All participants signed an informed consent form.

Study design and participants

Data were abstracted from the first Ribeirão Preto birth cohort study, Brazil, which started in 1978/79. Data were obtained at birth and at young adult age (23–25 years) [32].

A total of 9067 liveborn infants, delivered at the eight maternity hospitals of Ribeirão Preto, from June 1st 1978 to May 31, 1979 (corresponding to 98% of all live births), participated in this study. Losses due to refusal or early discharge amounted to 3.5%. All infants whose families did not reside in the city (2094) and twins (146) were excluded, leaving a total of 6827 live births [33].

From the original cohort of 6827 singleton liveborns, 343 participants were found to be deceased and 819 could not be traced, leaving 5665 singletons. One in three subjects belonging to the same geographic area was invited for medical examination. The first of every three names was selected from a list sorted by birth date in each geographic region and, if unavailable, the next name down was selected. In this traced group, losses to follow-up (N = 705) occurred because of refusal to participate, imprisonment, death after 20 years of age, or failure to attend the interview. Losses were replaced using the same sampling frame, resulting in 2,063 young adults (1,068 females) [32]. For this study, only subjects with normal BMI (18.5 to 24.9 kg/m^2)[6] were included, comprising a total of 1,222 young adults. Details of the methodology have been published elsewhere [32,33].

Variables and data collection

At the time of their children's birth, the mothers answered a standardized questionnaire. Maternal schooling (≤4, 5 to 8, 9 to 11, ≥12 years), parity (1, 2 to 4, ≥5), type of delivery (vaginal, caesarean) and maternal smoking during pregnancy (yes, regardless of the number of cigarettes smoked, and no) were abstracted from this questionnaire. Birth weight was measured within 30 minutes of birth. Newborns were weighed naked on weekly calibrated mechanical scales with 10-g precision (Filizola, São

Paulo, Brazil). Gestational age at birth in complete weeks was derived from the last normal menstrual period reported by the mother.

Participants answered a questionnaire containing information on socioeconomic, demographic and behavioural variables, and underwent physical examination when they were 23–25 years of age. The variables collected in adulthood were: age, sex, self-reported skin colour (classified as white/non-white), family income measured in minimum wages and classified into three categories (<5, 5 to 9.9 and ≥10), schooling in years (≤8, 9 to 11 and ≥12), marital status (single, cohabiting), smoking (yes, regardless of the number of cigarettes smoked and no), alcohol consumption in grams per day (none, ≤31 and >31), percentage of fat in the diet (measured with a food-frequency questionnaire and derived from equations using the Dietsys software, version 4.0 (National Cancer Institute, Bethesda, MD, USA) [34] and physical activity (sedentary, sufficiently active and active), according to the International Physical Activity Questionnaire (IPAQ) guidelines [35,36]. A missing category was added to the family income variable because 91 participants did not report their income. Anthropometric measurements were taken by physicians or trained nurses with individuals wearing light clothing and no shoes, using a standard protocol [37]. Weight was measured to the nearest 100 g using mechanical scales (Filizola, São Paulo, Brazil). Height was measured to the nearest 0.1 cm using a freestanding wood stadiometer (University of São Paulo, Ribeirão Preto, Brazil). BMI was calculated as weight in kilograms divided by height in meters squared (kg/m^2). A D-loop non-stretch fiberglass tape was used for WC and hip circumference (HC) measures. WC was measured as the smallest circumference between the ribs and the iliac crest while the participant was standing with the abdomen relaxed, at the end of a normal expiration. Where there was no natural waistline, the measurement was taken at the level of the umbilicus. HC was measured at the maximum circumference between the iliac crest and the crotch while the participant was standing. The triceps and subscapular skinfolds were measured with the Lange adipometer (Beta Technology, Santa Cruz, CA, USA), following Lohman's protocol [37]. Acceptable inter- and intra-observer agreement was achieved. For blood pressure measurements we used an Omron digital sphygmomanometer model 740 (Omron Healthcare, Lake Forest, IL, US), with 15-minute intervals between measurements, with the participants seated. This procedure was performed three times and the average of the last two measurements was used.

A 40 ml blood sample was collected from the subject after a 12 hour fast by a trained technician. Fasting blood glucose was measured by the GOD/PAP human diagnostic enzymatic calorimetric method (Chronolab AG, Zug, Germany) with a coefficient of variation of 4.2%. Low density lipoprotein (LDL) cholesterol, HDL-cholesterol and triglycerides were determined by an enzymatic calorimetric method using the Dade Behring XPand apparatus (Dade Behring, Liederbach, Germany) and reagents of Dade Behring Dimension clinical chemistry. Fasting insulin was measured by radioimmunoassay (insulin kit, DPC, Los Angeles, CA, USA) with a coefficient of variation of 7.9% [38].

MS was defined according to the Joint Interim Statement (JIS) of the IDF Task Force on Epidemiology and Prevention, National Heart, Lung and Blood Institute, American Heart Association, World Heart Federation, International Atherosclerosis Society and International Association for the Study of Obesity. The JIS criterion requires the presence of any three of the following: 1) central obesity (WC ≥90 cm for men and ≥80 cm for women, cut-off points used for South American populations); 2) increased triglycerides ≥150 mg/dL, use of lipid medications or self-reported diagnosis of hypertriglyceridemia; 3) low HDL-cholesterol (<40 mg/dL for men and <50 mg/dL for women); 4) increased blood pressure (BP) (systolic pressure ≥130 mmHg and/or diastolic pressure ≥85 mmHg, current usage of antihypertensive drugs or previous diagnosis of hypertension); and 5) high fasting blood glucose (≥100 mg/dL), current use of anti-diabetic medication or previously diagnosed diabetes [39].

IR was evaluated by the Homeostasis Model Assessment index [40]. HOMA2 insulin resistance, HOMA2 insulin sensitivity (the opposite of insulin resistance) and insulin secretor activity (HOMA2 β cell function) were determined using the HOMA2 computer model, which uses correctly solved nonlinear solutions (available from http://www.dtu.ox.ac.uk/index.php?maindocZ/homa/) and takes into account variations in hepatic and peripheral glucose resistance, increases in the insulin secretion curve for plasma glucose concentrations above 10 mmol/L (180 mg/dL) and the contribution of circulating proinsulin [41]. The cut-off proposed by the Brazilian Metabolic Syndrome Study (BRAMS) were used for the diagnosis of HOMA2-IR (>1.8) [42]. Since there were no cut-offs described for the Brazilian population, HOMA2 insulin sensitivity was considered to be low when <10th percentile and HOMA2 β cell function was considered to be high if >90th percentile of the study sample distribution.

The subjects whose BMI was 18.5 to 24.9 kg/m^2 and whose sum of triceps and subscapular skinfolds was >90th percentile of the study sample for each sex were classified as NWO, corresponding to >23.1% BF in men and >33.3% BF in women. We also defined NWO as a normal BMI and % BF >23% in men and >30% in women, using Slaughter's equations (derived for adolescents 8–18 years) from the sum of triceps and subscapular skinfolds [43].

Statistical analysis

Statistical analysis was performed using the statistical package Stata version 12.0. Mean ± standard deviation or the 1st quartile, median and the 3rd quartile were presented when appropriate. Differences in mean values of demographic, dietetic, anthropometric and metabolic parameters according to the presence or absence of NWO were tested by the Student t-test when variables had a normal distribution or by the Mann-Whitney nonparametric test otherwise. Statistical differences in categorical variables according to NWO were evaluated using the chi-square test. Subsequently, we fitted logistic regression models, using NWO as the explanatory variable and separate models for each response variable - MS, its components (high WC, low HDL-cholesterol, high triglycerides, high blood pressure and high blood glucose), insulin resistance, insulin sensitivity, and β cell function. Three sequential models were presented: model 1 (adjusted for age, sex and skin colour), model 2 (adjusted for age, sex, skin colour and early life variables - birth weight, gestational age at birth, maternal schooling, parity, type of delivery and maternal smoking during pregnancy) and model 3 (adjusted for age, sex, skin colour, early and adult life variables (alcohol consumption, family income, schooling, marital status, smoking, percentage of fat in the diet and physical activity). Additional models were also further adjusted for WC to verify if associations between NWO and low HDL-cholesterol, high triglycerides, high blood pressure, high blood glucose, insulin resistance, low insulin sensitivity and high insulin secretion were independent from measures of central obesity. The models were not stratified by sex because no significant interactions between NWO and sex on MS or IR were detected. Odds ratios (OR) and their 95% confidence intervals (CI) were estimated.

Results

The prevalence of MS according to the JIS definition was 3.1% (95%CI 1.8%–4.9%) for males and 0.9% (95%CI 0.3%–1.9%) for females. The prevalence of HOMA2-IR was 2.0% (95%CI 1.0%–3.6%) for men and 2.6% (95%CI 1.5%–4.1%) for women. The prevalence of MS was higher for males than for females (3.1% vs. 0.9%, P = 0.004). Low HDL-cholesterol was significantly higher among women (38.0%) than men (31.2%), whereas high blood pressure was much higher among men (28.9%) than women (3.3%). High blood glucose was also higher among men (4.4%) than women (1.7%). IR, high WC and triglycerides did not differ by sex (Table 1).

Table 1. Prevalences of metabolic syndrome, its components and insulin resistance by sex among young adults with body mass index within the normal range, 1978/79 Ribeirão Preto birth cohort.

Variables	Males (n = 546)		Females (n = 676)		P ^{a}
	n	%	n	%	
Metabolic Syndrome – JIS^b					0.004
No	529	96.9	670	99.1	
Yes	17	3.1	6	0.9	
Waist circumference^c					0.852
Normal	509	93.2	632	93.5	
High	37	6.8	44	6.5	
HDL-cholesterol^d					0.014
Normal	373	68.8	413	62.0	
Low	169	31.2	253	38.0	
Triglycerides^e					0.439
Normal	509	93.9	618	92.8	
High	33	6.1	48	7.2	
Blood pressure^f					<0.001
Normal	388	71.1	654	96.8	
High	158	28.9	22	3.3	
Blood Glucose^g					0.004
Normal	520	95.6	656	98.4	
High	24	4.4	11	1.7	
HOMA2-IR^h					0.539
≤1.8	528	98.0	643	97.4	
>1.8	11	2.0	17	2.6	

Abbreviations: HDL, High Density Lipoprotein; HOMA, Homeostasis Model Assessment; IR, Insulin Resistance. ^{a}P value calculated by the chi-square test. ^{b}defined according to the Joint Interim Statement (JIS) of the IDF Task Force on Epidemiology and Prevention, National Heart, Lung and Blood Institute, American Heart Association, World Heart Federation, International Atherosclerosis Society and International Association for the Study of Obesity. ^{c}waist circumference (≥90 cm for men and ≥80 cm for women). ^{d}increased triglycerides (≥150 mg/dL, use of lipid medications or self-reported diagnosis of hypertriglyceridemia). ^{e}low HDL-cholesterol (<40 mg/dL for men and <50 mg/dL for women). ^{f}increased blood pressure (BP) (systolic pressure ≥130 mmHg and/or diastolic pressure ≥85 mmHg, current usage of antihypertensive drugs or previous diagnosis of hypertension). ^{g}high fasting blood glucose (≥100 mg/dL), current use of anti-diabetic medication or previously diagnosed diabetes. ^{h}Cut-off point based on the Brazilian Metabolic Syndrome Study - BRAMS criterion (2009). Numbers may not add up to total because of missing values.

Subjects with NWO did not differ from those without NWO according to early life variables (Table 2). Subjects with NWO did not differ by sex, age, family income, schooling, marital status, smoking or alcohol consumption compared to those without NWO. Individuals of white skin colour (10.5% vs. 6.2%, P = 0.013) and with a sedentary life style (10.8% vs. 5.3%, P = 0.010) presented a higher prevalence of NWO than their counterparts. Mean percentage of fat in the diet was higher among NWO subjects than among their peers without NWO (Table 3).

Subjects with NWO presented higher mean values of BMI, WC, hip circumference, waist to hip ratio, LDL-cholesterol, triglycerides, diastolic blood pressure, subscapular and triceps skinfolds, blood glucose, HOMA2-IR and insulin secretion, and lower values of insulin sensitivity than those without NWO. There were no differences in mean systolic blood pressure. HDL-cholesterol was lower among men with NWO compared to their counterparts but there were no differences among women (Table 4).

NWO was significantly associated with MS according to the JIS definition (OR = 6.83; 95%CI 2.84-16.47, P<0.001). NWO was also significantly associated with HOMA2-IR (OR = 3.81; 95%CI 1.57-9.28, P = 0.003), low insulin sensitivity (OR = 3.89; 95%CI 2.39-6.33, P<0.001), and high insulin secretion (OR = 2.17; 95%CI 1.24-3.80, P = 0.007). Significant associations between NWO and some components of MS were also detected: high WC (OR = 8.46; 95%CI 5.09-14.04, P<0.001), low HDL-cholesterol (OR = 1.65; 95% 1.11-2.47, P = 0.014) and high triglycerides (OR = 1.93; 95% 1.02-3.64, P = 0.042). Most estimates changed little after adjustment for early and adult life variables: the associations of NWO with low HDL-cholesterol and high triglycerides lost statistical significance and the association of NWO with high blood glucose became statistically significant. After further adjustment for WC, associations of NWO with high

blood glucose and high insulin secretion were no longer significant whereas associations of NWO with HOMA2-IR and insulin sensitivity nearly halved but continued to be significant (Table 5).

Table 6 presents models using % BF >23% for men and >30% for women to define NWO. NWO was consistently associated with MS, IR, insulin sensitivity and secretion in all adjusted models.

Discussion

In our study, NWO, defined by the combination of excess BF (sum of triceps and subscapular skinfolds >P90 of the study sample) and normal BMI was associated with MS according to the JIS definition (OR = 6.83), HOMA2-IR (OR = 3.81), low insulin sensitivity (OR = 3.89) and high insulin secretion (OR = 2.17) in young adults (23–25 years) from Brazil, a middle-income country. Adjustment for early and adult life variables did not change the estimates appreciably. When we defined NWO as normal BMI and % BF>23% for men and >30 for women results were consistent. Our data suggest that counting only on BMI to identify subjects who are at risk of metabolic disorders later in life may fail to identify an important fraction of the population who, despite having a normal BMI, present excess BF and are also at high risk of metabolic imbalances. It seems that, together with the epidemic of high-BMI obesity [3], there is a normal-BMI obesity epidemic that begins at a young age and is also evident in middle-income countries.

Our study showed that NWO is associated with a high risk of having MS at an early adult age. A 2004 US study also reported that NWO individuals were at increased risk of having MS [21]. A more recent study, carried out in the US using data from the Third National Health and Nutrition Examination Survey (NHANES III), including adults >20 years, showed that NWO was associated with a four-fold increase in the prevalence of MS

Table 2. Normal weight obesity according to early life variables, 1978/79 Ribeirão Preto birth cohort.

Variables	Normal weight obesity[a]		P
	No (n = 1111) n (%)	Yes (n = 111) n (%)	
Maternal schooling (years)			0.786[b]
≤4	484 (91.7)	44 (8.3)	
5 to 8	284 (90.5)	30 (9.5)	
9 to 11	189 (90.9)	19 (9.1)	
≥12	130 (89.0)	16 (11.0)	
Maternal parity			0.101[b]
1	405 (88.6)	52 (11.4)	
2 to 4	595 (92.3)	50 (7.8)	
≥5	87 (92.5)	7 (7.5)	
Type of delivery			0.521[b]
Vaginal	768 (90.6)	80 (9.4)	
Cesarean	343 (91.7)	31 (8.3)	
Maternal smoking during pregnancy			0.384[b]
No	819 (91.3)	78 (8.7)	
Yes	268 (89.6)	31 (10.4)	
Birth weight (grams)	3238±500[c]	3299±436[c]	0.220[d]
Gestational age at birth (weeks)	39.0±1.8[c]	39.3±1.3[c]	0.071[d]

[a]Normal weight obesity defined as a BMI from 18.5 to 24.9 kg/m² and the sum of triceps and subscapular skinfolds >90th percentile of the study sample for each sex. [b]P values calculated by the chi-square test. [c]Values are mean ± standard deviation. [d]P values calculated by the Student t-test. Numbers may not add up to total because of missing values.

Table 3. Normal weight obesity according to adult life variables, 1978/79 Ribeirão Preto birth cohort.

Variables	Normal weight obesity[a]		P
	No (n = 1,111) n (%)	Yes (n = 111) n (%)	
Age	23.9 ± 0.71[b]	24.0 ± 0.68[b]	0.485[c]
Sex			0.935[d]
Male	496 (90.8)	50 (9.2)	
Female	615 (91.0)	61 (9.0)	
Skin colour			0.013[d]
White	731 (89.5)	86 (10.5)	
Non-white	380 (93.8)	25 (6.2)	
Family income (minimum wages)			0.563[d]
<5	329 (90.1)	36 (9.9)	
5 to 9.9	345 (89.9)	39 (10.1)	
≥10	353 (92.4)	29 (7.6)	
Missing	84 (92.3)	7 (7.7)	
Schooling (years)			0.303[d]
≤8	152 (92.1)	13 (7.9)	
9 to 11	551 (91.8)	49 (8.2)	
≥12	408 (89.3)	49 (10.7)	
Marital Status			0.307[d]
Single	792 (91.5)	74 (8.5)	
Cohabiting	319 (89.6)	37 (10.4)	
Smoking			0.065[d]
No	927 (90.3)	100 (9.7)	
Yes	185 (94.4)	11 (5.6)	
Physical activity			0.010[d]
Sedentary	544 (89.2)	66 (10.8)	
Sufficiently active	220 (89.4)	26 (10.6)	
Active	342 (94.7)	19 (5.3)	
Alcohol consumption (g/day)			0.723[d]
None	296 (90.2)	32 (9.8)	
≤31	595 (90.7)	61 (9.3)	
>31	212 (92.2)	18 (7.8)	
Percentage of fat in the diet	35.8 ± 5.6[b]	37.5 ± 5.4[b]	0.002[c]

[a]Normal weight obesity defined as a BMI from 18.5 to 24.9 kg/m^2 and the sum of triceps and subscapular skinfolds >90th percentile of the study sample for each sex.
[b]Values are mean ± standard deviation. [c]P values calculated by the Student t-test. [d]P values calculated by the chi-square test.

(16.6% vs. 4.8%) [18]. Our study has some different characteristics compared to that investigation. It is important to note that we measured BF by means of the sum of triceps and subscapular skinfolds, whereas in the American study BF was measured by bioelectrical impedance. Also the criterion for categorization of excess BF differed: we considered those above the sex-specific 90th percentile of the sum of skinfolds as presenting excess BF while in the US study excess BF was defined by the highest sex-specific tertiles of BF percentage. The US study included subjects >20 years old whereas in our study only young adults, aged 23–25 years were included. For the diagnosis of MS the updated NCEP-ATPIII definition was used in the American study [18], whereas in our study we used the new JIS definition. These factors may explain the differences in risk estimates between NWO and MS in the two studies.

We used the JIS definition because it reflects the new emerged consensus to define MS. Furthermore, because our study sample

only included young adults more stringent criteria for identification of central obesity would be more appropriate to detect metabolic disorders earlier [44]. Furthermore, the use of lower cut-off points increases the power to detect statistically significant differences in case they exist, while sensitivity increases albeit specificity decreases.

Our study also showed that NWO was associated with an increased risk of presenting high WC (OR = 8.46), high triglycerides (OR = 1.93), and low HDL-cholesterol (OR = 1.65) in young adults. However, no association was observed between NWO and high blood pressure or high blood glucose, although the latter was associated with NWO in the fully adjusted model. The US population-based study, which included a sample of males and females for a total of 6,171 subjects, also showed a significant association between NWO and higher risk of dysregulation of the components of MS (central obesity, high triglycerides, low HDL-cholesterol, high blood pressure and high fasting plasma glucose)

Table 4. Normal weight obesity according to anthropometric and metabolic parameters, 1978/79 Ribeirão Preto birth cohort.

Variables	Normal weight obesity[a]		P
	No (n = 1,111)	Yes (n = 111)	
Body mass index (kg/m^2)	21.7±1.7[b]	23.6±1.1[b]	< 0.001[c]
Waist circumference (cm)			
Males	80.4±5.3[b]	87.6±4.9[b]	< 0.001[c]
Females	71.5±4.7[b]	77.2±4.5[b]	< 0.001[c]
Hip circumference (cm)	96.8±4.9[b]	101.1±4.5[b]	< 0.001[c]
Waist to hip ratio (cm)			
Males	0.83±0.04[b]	0.86±0.05[b]	< 0.001[c]
Females	0.74±0.05[b]	0.77±0.05[b]	< 0.001[c]
High density lipoprotein (mg/dL)			
Males	46.2±11.0[b]	42.8±9.8[b]	0.033[c]
Females	54.6±13.1[b]	51.6±12.1[b]	0.092[c]
Low density lipoprotein (mg/dL)	91 (76–110)[d]	104 (88–129)[d]	< 0.001[e]
Triglycerides (mg/dL)	69 (52–95)[d]	89 (64–117)[d]	< 0.001[e]
Systolic blood pressure (mmHg)	115±13[b]	115±13[b]	0.851[c]
Diastolic blood pressure (mmHg)	68±8[b]	70±7[b]	0.008[c]
Subscapular skinfold (mm)	12.7±3.3[b]	20.9±3.5[b]	< 0.001[c]
Triceps skinfold (mm)	11.7±4.6[b]	18.9±4.6[b]	< 0.001[c]
Sum of triceps and subscapular skinfolds (mm)	24.3±6.9[b]	39.8±6.4[b]	< 0.001[c]
Blood glucose (mg/dL)	81 (77–87)[d]	87 (80–91)[d]	< 0.001[e]
HOMA-2 insulin resistance	0.54 (0.36–0.87)[d]	0.77 (0.49–1.22)[d]	< 0.001[e]
HOMA-2 insulin sensitivity	185.7 (115.3–275.5)[d]	129.1 (81.8–203.1)[d]	< 0.001[e]
HOMA-2 β cell function	78.3 (58.0–106.6)[d]	90.9 (65.4–130.1)[d]	0.002[e]

Abbreviations: HOMA, Homeostasis Model Assessment. [a] Normal weight obesity defined as a BMI from 18.5 to 24.9 kg/m^2 and the sum of triceps and subscapular skinfolds >90th percentile of the study sample for each sex. [b]Values are mean ± standard deviation. [c]P values calculated by the Student t-test. [d]Values are median (1st quartile – 3rd quartile). [e]P values calculated by the Mann-Whitney non-parametric test.

[18]. Another study, carried out in Switzerland, which included women only, also showed that NWO was associated with abnormalities in the components of MS [20]. In contrast to the American [18] and the Swiss study [20], our study did not observe an association between NWO and high blood pressure. This could be due to the much younger age of our sample.

Young adults with NWO showed a higher prevalence of IR, as measured by the HOMA-2 model, than those without NWO (OR = 3.81). NWO was also associated with increased IR and low insulin sensitivity. The reduced sensitivity to insulin has been a feature found in subjects with NWO [15,18,45]. We also found, in agreement with the American study [18], that increased β cell function was detected among individuals with NWO. Possibly the high insulin secretion is a compensatory response to the reduced insulin sensitivity found in individuals with NWO [46]. Associations between NWO with HOMA2-IR and insulin sensitivity were not totally explained by central obesity because after further adjustment for WC, these associations nearly halved although continued to be significant.

Another recent study, which measured BF with air displacement plethysmography, although not using clinical cut-off points to assess metabolic dysregulation, also reported that non-obese subjects by the BMI criterion but obese by % BF had higher values of WC, blood pressure, triglycerides, glucose, insulin, HOMA and lower values of HDL-cholesterol compared to those with normal BMI and non-obese based on % BF [23].

Strengths and limitations

We consider the strength of this study to be the fact that it is a population-based cohort study, conducted in a sample of young adults. Adjustment was performed for several adult life variables. In addition, this study incorporates early life factors that have been implicated in the pathogenesis of obesity and IR. These facts allowed us to estimate the association between excess BF and metabolic disorders at an early adult age in subjects with BMI in the normal range in a middle-income country that is undergoing rapid nutrition transition [47]. The narrow age group (from 23 to 25 years of age) shall not be considered a limitation but a particular strength because it eliminates the confounding effect of age and many other age-dependent covariates that may have affected the analysis. Standardized methods were used to assess IR and measurements of body weight, skinfolds, lipids and others.

A potential limitation of our study is related to the method of categorization of excess BF. The sum of subscapular and triceps skinfolds above the sex-specific 90th percentiles of the study sample was used as a proxy for estimating excess BF. It is an arbitrary cut-off, and a definition of NWO different from those used in other studies [18–20,23]. However, results using % BF >23% in men and >30% in women produced consistent results regarding MS and IR. Furthermore, agreement between these two definitions of NWO (>90th of the sum of triceps and subscapular skinfolds and high percent body fat estimated by Slaughter's formula-based equation) was high (kappa = 0.879). Although using three or more

Table 5. Associations between normal weight obesity defined as the sum of the triceps and subscapular skinfolds >90th percentile with metabolic syndrome and its components and insulin resistance, insulin sensitivity and β cell function, 1978/79 Ribeirão Preto birth cohort.

Normal weight obesity	%	Model 1[a] OR (95% CI)	P [e]	Model 2[b] OR (95% CI)	P [e]	Model 3[c] OR (95% CI)	P [e]	Model 4[d] OR (95% CI)	P [e]
Metabolic Syndrome – JIS[f]									
No	1.3	1		1		1			
Yes	8.1	6.83 (2.84–16.47)	<0.001	7.22 (2.92–17.85)	<0.001	8.89 (3.32–4.47)	<0.001		
High waist circumference[g]									
No	4.4	1		1		1			
Yes	28.8	8.46 (5.09–14.04)	<0.001	8.37 (5.01–13.99)	<0.001	9.27 (5.32–16.15)	<0.001		
Low High Density Lipoprotein[h]									
No	33.9	1		1		1		1	
Yes	45.0	1.65 (1.11 2.17)	0.014	1.55 (1.02–2.33)	0.038	1.53 (1.00–2.34)	0.053	1.09 (0.69–1.72)	0.721
High triglycerides[i]									
No	6.2	1		1		1		1	
Yes	11.9	1.93 (1.02–3.64)	0.042	1.91 (1.01–3.63)	0.048	1.89 (0.97–3.70)	0.062	1.18 (0.57–2.45)	0.649
High blood pressure[j]									
No	14.6	1		1		1		1	
Yes	16.2	1.11 (0.62–1.97)	0.729	1.19 (0.66–2.13)	0.565	1.17 (0.65–2.13)	0.598	0.87 (0.46–1.67)	0.680
High blood glucose[k]									
No	2.6	1		1		1		1	
Yes	5.5	2.10 (0.84–5.23)	0.110	2.24 (0.89–5.69)	0.089	2.68 (1.01–7.12)	0.048	1.60 (0.54–4.76)	0.395
HOMA2- Insulin resistance[l]									
No	1.9	1		1		1		1	
Yes	6.5	3.81 (1.57–9.28)	0.003	4.01 (1.63–9.87)	0.003	4.91 (1.85–13.04)	0.001	2.94 (1.00–8.68)	0.005
Low HOMA2- Insulin sensitivity[m]									
No	8.4	1		1		1		1	
Yes	26.2	3.89 (2.39–6.33)	<0.001	4.01 (2.45–6.57)	<0.001	4.14 (2.45–6.99)	<0.001	2.22 (1.25–3.96)	0.007
High HOMA2- β cell function[n]									
No	9.4	1		1		1		1	
Yes	16.8	2.17 (1.24–3.80)	0.007	2.48 (1.27–3.97)	0.005	2.26 (1.25–4.08)	0.007	1.58 (0.83–3.00)	0.162

Abbreviations: OR, Odds ratio; CI, Confidence Interval; HOMA, Homeostasis Model Assessment. [a]adjusted for age, sex and skin color. [b]adjusted for age, sex, skin colour and early life variables (birth weight, gestational age at birth, maternal schooling, parity, type of delivery and maternal smoking during pregnancy). [c]adjusted for age, sex, skin colour, early and adult life variables (alcohol consumption, family income, schooling, marital status, smoking, percentage of fat in the diet and physical activity). [d]adjusted for age, sex, skin colour, early and adult life variables plus WC. [e]P value calculated by the log-likelihood ratio test. [f]defined according to the Joint Interim Statement (JIS) of the IDF Task Force on Epidemiology and Prevention, National Heart, Lung and Blood Institute, American Heart Association, World Heart Federation, International Atherosclerosis Society and International Association for the Study of Obesity. [g]high waist circumference (≥90 cm for men and ≥80 cm for women). [h]low HDL-cholesterol (<40 mg/dL for men and <50 mg/dL for women). [i]increased triglycerides (≥150 mg/dL, use of lipid medications or self-reported diagnosis of hypertriglyceridemia) [j]increased blood pressure (BP) (systolic pressure ≥130 mmHg and/or diastolic pressure ≥85 mmHg, current usage of antihypertensive drugs or previous diagnosis of hypertension). [k]high fasting blood glucose (≥100 mg/dL), current use of anti diabetic medication or previously diagnosed diabetes. [l]Based on the Brazilian Metabolic Syndrome Study - BRAMS criterion (2009) - HOMA2- Insulin resistance >2.8. [m]HOMA2- Insulin sensitivity was considered low if <90th percentile and normal otherwise. [n]HOMA2- β cell function was considered high if >90th percentile and normal otherwise.

measures of skinfold thickness is a validated method to estimate % BF [48,49], measures of other skinfolds were not available in our database to estimate % BF in adults. We thus estimated % BF using the Slaughter's equations based on the sum of two skinfolds (triceps and subscapular). It is important to note that our sample is composed of young adults aged 23/25 years and the Slaughter's equations were derived for adolescents. We used these equations assuming that % BF would have changed little from 18 to 23/25 years of age. We did not find any other suitable equation to estimate % BF from the sum of triceps and subscapular skinfolds for young adults.

However, the use of subscapular and triceps skinfolds provides a valid indication of excess fat in young people [31]. Selective losses have occurred comparing subjects followed up with those not followed up. Follow-up rates were slightly higher for women, those born preterm, those from better-off families and those whose mothers smoked or were married at the time of the participant's birth. Although statistically significant, these differences were small [32].

Consequences

These results suggest important questions about the isolated use of BMI to assess obesity. After all, having a normal BMI does not

Table 6. Associations between normal weight obesity defined as high percent body fat[a] with metabolic syndrome and insulin resistance, insulin sensitivity and β cell function, 1978/79 Ribeirão Preto birth cohort.

Normal weight obesity	%	Model 1[b] OR (95% CI)	P [e]	Model 2[c] OR (95% CI)	P [e]	Model 3[d] OR (95% CI)	P [e]
Metabolic Syndrome – JIS[f]							
No	1.4	1		1		1	
Yes	7.5	5.40 (2.21–13.22)	<0.001	5.66 (2.26–14.20)	<0.001	7.36 (2.65–20.45)	<0.001
HOMA2- Insulin resistance[g]							
No	2.0	1		1		1	
Yes	5.8	3.23 (1.26–8.22)	0.014	3.83 (1.32–8.68)	0.011	4.69 (1.65–13.32)	0.004
Low HOMA2- Insulin sensitivity[h]							
No	8.8	1		1		1	
Yes	23.3	3.15 (1.90–5.24)	<0.001	3.28 (1.96–5.47)	<0.001	3.38 (1.96–5.83)	<0.001
High HOMA2- β cell function[i]							
No	9.6	1		1		1	
Yes	14.6	1.79 (0.98–3.25)	0.057	1.89 (1.03–3.45)	0.039	1.85 (1.01–3.49)	0.049

Abbreviations: OR, Odds ratio; CI, Confidence Interval; HOMA, Homeostasis Model Assessment. [a]high percent body fat>23% for males and >30% for females. Percent body fat was estimated based on the Slaughter's equations using the sum of triceps and subscapular skinfolds. [b]adjusted for age, sex and skin color. [c]adjusted for age, sex, skin colour and early life variables (birth weight, gestational age at birth, maternal schooling, parity, type of delivery and maternal smoking during pregnancy). [d]adjusted for age, sex, skin colour, early and adult life variables (alcohol consumption, family income, schooling, marital status, smoking, percentage of fat in the diet and physical activity). [e]P value calculated by the log-likelihood ratio test. [f]defined according to the Joint Interim Statement (JIS) of the IDF Task Force on Epidemiology and Prevention, National Heart, Lung and Blood Institute, American Heart Association, World Heart Federation, International Atherosclerosis Society and International Association for the Study of Obesity. [g]Based on the Brazilian Metabolic Syndrome Study - BRAMS criterion (2009) - HOMA2- Insulin resistance >2.8. [h]HOMA2- Insulin sensitivity was considered to be low if <90th percentile and normal otherwise. [i]HOMA2- β cell function was considered high if >90th percentile and normal otherwise.

mean no risk for metabolic disorders and consequently for cardiovascular diseases [45]. A BMI cut-off of ≥ 30 kg/m^2 has good specificity but misses more than half the people with excess fat [11,12]. This situation reveals the need for changes in routine clinical evaluation, requiring the incorporation of other simple low-cost measures, like skinfolds or WC, or bioelectrical impedance to evaluate excess BF percentage in individuals with BMI within the normal range. The strong associations found in this study reinforce the need to adopt screening for increased BF as early as possible[13], given that metabolic changes associated with NWO were observed in young adults with normal BMI early in the life course, even in a middle-income country where the burden of obesity-related diseases is not as high as in some developed countries. Although the prevalence rate of MS is low in this young population [50], changes in health care and educational programs, especially encouraging the adoption of a healthy lifestyle, including physical activity and the development of healthy eating habits, are highly advisable in an attempt to halt the spread of future epidemics of obesity in normal-BMI individuals [3,31].

Conclusion

In conclusion, our study found associations between NWO and MS and IR early in life in young adults with BMI within the

normal range. This implies that using only BMI for the assessment of risk factors for cardiovascular diseases may lead to false-negatives and suggests the need to include the assessment of BF in the routine clinical evaluation of individuals at an early age, even in middle-income countries. Even though prevalence rates of metabolic disorders are low in this population of young adults, as nutrition transition is rapid and as they get older, the burden of obesity-related diseases would tend to be high in the future. Thus, early detection and prevention of this epidemic of normal weight obesity is highly desirable.

Acknowledgments

The authors are indebted to the Laboratories of Endocrinology, Nutrition and Paediatrics of the University Hospital, Faculty of Medicine of Ribeirão Preto, which performed the biochemical tests in the blood samples.

Author Contributions

Review the manuscript for intellectual content: FBM AAS HFV MZG GK VCC HB MAB. Conceived and designed the experiments: AAS MAB HB. Analyzed the data: FBM AAS HFV. Contributed reagents/materials/analysis tools: AAS MZG GK HB MAB. Wrote the paper: FBM AAS HFV MZG GK VCC HB MAB.

References

1. Withrow D, Alter DA (2011) The economic burden of obesity worldwide: a systematic review of the direct costs of obesity. Obes Rev 12: 131–141.
2. Popkin BM, Doak CM (1998) The obesity epidemic is a worldwide phenomenon. Nutr Rev 56: 106–114.
3. Flegal KM, Carroll MD, Kit BK, Ogden CL (2012) Prevalence of obesity and trends in the distribution of body mass index among US adults, 1999-2010. JAMA 307: 491–497.
4. Instituto Brasileiro de Geografia e Estatística (IBGE) (2010) Pesquisa de Orçamentos Familiares 2008–2009: Antropometria e estado nutricional de crianças, adolescentes e adultos no Brasil. Rio de Janeiro: Instituto Brasileiro de Geografia e Estatística.
5. Yang Q, Cogswell ME, Flanders WD, Hong Y, Zhang Z, et al, (2012) Trends in cardiovascular health metrics and associations with all cause and CVD mortality among US adults. JAMA 307: 1273–1283.
6. World Health Organization (WHO) (2000) Obesity: preventing and managing the global epidemic. Report of a WHO consultation. World Health Organ Tech Rep Ser 894: 1–253.

7. Snijder MB, van Dam RM, Visser M, Seidell JC (2006) What aspects of body fat are particularly hazardous and how do we measure them? Int J Epidemiol 35: 83–92.

8. World Health Organization (WHO) (1995) Physical status: the use and interpretation of anthropometry. Geneva: World Health Organization.

9. Calle EE, Rodriguez C, Walker-Thurmond K, Thun MJ (2003) Overweight, obesity, and mortality from cancer in a prospectively studied cohort of U.S. adults. N Engl J Med 348: 1625–1638.

10. Flegal KM, Graubard BI, Williamson DF, Gail MH (2007) Cause-specific excess deaths associated with underweight, overweight, and obesity. JAMA 298: 2028–2037.

11. Romero-Corral A, Somers VK, Sierra-Johnson J, Thomas RJ, Collazo-Clavell ML, et al. (2008) Accuracy of body mass index in diagnosing obesity in the adult general population. Int J Obes 32: 959–966.

12. Okorodudu DO, Jumean MF, Montori VM, Romero-Corral A, Somers VK, et al. (2010) Diagnostic performance of body mass index to identify obesity as defined by body adiposity: a systematic review and meta-analysis. Int J Obes 34: 791–799.

13. De Lorenzo A, Bianchi A, Maroni P, Iannarelli A, Di Daniele N, et al. (2011) Adiposity rather than BMI determines metabolic risk. Int J Cardiol [Epub ahead of print].

14. Ruderman NB, Schneider SH, Berchtold P (1981) The "metabolically-obese," normal-weight individual. Am J Clin Nutr 34: 1617–1621.

15. Ruderman N, Chisholm D, Pi-Sunyer X, Schneider S (1998) The metabolically obese, normal-weight individual revisited. Diabetes 47: 699–713.

16. De Lorenzo A, Martinoli R, Vaia F, Di Renzo L (2006) Normal weight obese (NWO) women: an evaluation of a candidate new syndrome. Nutr Metab Cardiovasc Dis 16: 513–523.

17. Marques-Vidal P, Pecoud A, Hayoz D, Paccaud F, Mooser V, et al. (2008) Prevalence of normal weight obesity in Switzerland: effect of various definitions. Eur J Nutr 47: 251–257.

18. Romero-Corral A, Somers VK, Sierra-Johnson J, Korenfeld Y, Boarin S, et al. (2010) Normal weight obesity: a risk factor for cardiometabolic dysregulation and cardiovascular mortality. Eur Heart J 31: 737–746.

19. De Lorenzo A, Del Gobbo V, Premrov MG, Bigioni M, Galvano F, et al. (2007) Normal-weight obese syndrome: early inflammation? Am J Clin Nutr 85: 40–45.

20. Marques-Vidal P, Pecoud A, Hayoz D, Paccaud F, Mooser V, et al. (2010) Normal weight obesity: relationship with lipids, glycaemic status, liver enzymes and inflammation. Nutr Metab Cardiovasc Dis 20: 669–675.

21. St-Onge MP, Janssen I, Heymsfield SB (2004) Metabolic syndrome in normal-weight Americans: new definition of the metabolically obese, normal-weight individual. Diabetes Care 27: 2222–2228.

22. Di Renzo L, Galvano F, Orlandi C, Bianchi A, Di Giacomo C, et al. (2010) Oxidative stress in normal-weight obese syndrome. Obesity (Silver Spring) 18: 2125–2130.

23. Gomez-Ambrosi J, Silva C, Galofre JC, Escalada J, Santos S, et al. (2012) Body mass index classification misses subjects with increased cardiometabolic risk factors related to elevated adiposity. Int J Obes 36: 286–294.

24. Kim LJ, Nalls MA, Eiriksdottir G, Sigurdsson S, Launer LJ, et al. (2011) Associations of visceral and liver fat with the metabolic syndrome across the spectrum of obesity: the AGES-Reykjavik study. Obesity 19: 1265–1271.

25. Wildman RP, Muntner P, Reynolds K, McGinn AP, Rajpathak S, et al. (2008) The obese without cardiometabolic risk factor clustering and the normal weight with cardiometabolic risk factor clustering: prevalence and correlates of 2 phenotypes among the US population (NHANES 1999–2004). Arch Intern Med 168: 1617–1624.

26. Dvorak RV, DeNino WF, Ades PA, Poehlman ET (1999) Phenotypic characteristics associated with insulin resistance in metabolically obese but normal-weight young women. Diabetes 48: 2210–2214.

27. Kosmala W, Jedrzejuk D, Derzhko R, Przewlocka-Kosmala M, Mysiak A, et al. (2012) Left ventricular function impairment in patients with normal-weight obesity: contribution of abdominal fat deposition, profibrotic state, reduced insulin sensitivity, and proinflammatory activation. Circ Cardiovasc Imaging 5: 349–356.

28. Tsai CH (2009) Metabolic syndrome in non-obese Taiwanese: new definition of metabolically obese, normal-weight individual. Chin Med J (Engl) 122: 2534–2539.

29. Hosseinpanah F, Barzin M, Amiri P, Azizi F (2011) The trends of metabolic syndrome in normal-weight Tehranian adults. Ann Nutr Metab 58: 126–132.

30. Deurenberg-Yap M, Chew SK, Deurenberg P (2002) Elevated body fat percentage and cardiovascular risks at low body mass index levels among Singaporean Chinese, Malays and Indians. Obes Rev 3: 209–215.

31. Olds TS (2009) One million skinfolds: secular trends in the fatness of young people 1951–2004. Eur J Clin Nutr 63: 934–946.

32. Barbieri MA, Bettiol H, Silva AA, Cardoso VC, Simoes VM, et al. (2006) Health in early adulthood: the contribution of the 1978/79 Ribeirao Preto birth cohort. Braz J Med Biol Res 39: 1041–1055.

33. Cardoso VC, Simoes VM, Barbieri MA, Silva AA, Bettiol H, et al. (2007) Profile of three Brazilian birth cohort studies in Ribeirao Preto, SP and Sao Luis, MA. Braz J Med Biol Res 40: 1165–1176.

34. Molina MC, Bettiol H, Barbieri MA, Silva AA, Conceicao SI, et al. (2007) Food consumption by young adults living in Ribeirao Preto, SP, 2002/2004. Braz J Med Biol Res 40: 1257–1266.

35. International Physical Activity Questionnaire (IPAQ) (2004) Guidelines for Data Processing and Analysis of the International Physical Activity Questionnaire (IPAQ) - Short and Long Forms. Available: http://www.ipaq.ki.se/scoring.pdf. Accessed 23 Nov 2012.

36. Craig CL, Marshall AL, Sjostrom M, Bauman AE, Booth ML, et al. (2003) International physical activity questionnaire: 12-country reliability and validity. Med Sci Sports Exerc 35: 1381–1395.

37. Lohman T, Roche A, Martorell R (1991) Anthropometric standardization reference manual. Champaign, IL: Human Kinetics Books.

38. Silva AA, Santos CJ, Amigo H, Barbieri MA, Bustos P, et al. (2012) Birth weight, current body mass index, and insulin sensitivity and secretion in young adults in two Latin American populations. Nutr Metab Cardiovasc Dis 22: 533–539.

39. Alberti KG, Eckel RH, Grundy SM, Zimmet PZ, Cleeman JI, et al. (2009) Harmonizing the metabolic syndrome: a joint interim statement of the International Diabetes Federation Task Force on Epidemiology and Prevention; National Heart, Lung, and Blood Institute; American Heart Association; World Heart Federation; International Atherosclerosis Society; and international association for the Study of Obesity. Circulation 120: 1640–1645.

40. Matthews DR, Hosker JP, Rudenski AS, Naylor BA, Treacher DF, et al. (1985) Homeostasis model assessment: insulin resistance and beta-cell function from fasting plasma glucose and insulin concentrations in man. Diabetologia 28: 412–419.

41. Wallace TM, Levy JC, Matthews DR (2004) Use and abuse of HOMA modeling. Diabetes Care 27: 1487–1495.

42. Geloneze B, Vasques AC, Stabe CF, Pareja JC, Rosado LE, et al. (2009) HOMA1-IR and HOMA2-IR indexes in identifying insulin resistance and metabolic syndrome: Brazilian Metabolic Syndrome Study (BRAMS). Arq Bras Endocrinol Metabol 53: 281–287.

43. Slaughter MH, Lohman TG, Boileau RA, Horswill CA, Stillman RJ, et al. (1988) Skinfold equations for estimation of body fatness in children and youth. Human biology 60: 709–723.

44. Alberti KG, Zimmet P, Shaw J (2005) The metabolic syndrome--a new worldwide definition. Lancet 366: 1059–1062.

45. Karelis AD, St-Pierre DH, Conus F, Rabasa-Lhoret R, Poehlman ET (2004) Metabolic and body composition factors in subgroups of obesity: what do we know? J Clin Endocrinol Metab 89: 2569–2575.

46. Silva AA, Santos CJ, Amigo H, Barbieri MA, Bustos P, et al. (2011) Birth weight, current body mass index, and insulin sensitivity and secretion in young adults in two Latin American populations. Nutr Metab Cardiovasc Dis.

47. Monteiro CA, Conde WL, Popkin BM (2004) The burden of disease from undernutrition and overnutrition in countries undergoing rapid nutrition transition: a view from Brazil. Am J Public Health 94: 433–434.

48. Jackson AS, Pollock ML (1978) Generalized equations for predicting body density of men. Br J Nutr 40: 497–504.

49. Jackson AS, Pollock ML, Ward A (1980) Generalized equations for predicting body density of women. Med Sci Sports Exerc 12: 175–181.

50. Bustos P, da Silva AA, Amigo H, Bettiol H, Barbieri MA (2007) Metabolic syndrome in young adults from two socioeconomic Latin American settings. Nutr Metab Cardiovasc Dis 17: 581–589.

Does DNA Methylation of *PPARGC1A* Influence Insulin Action in First Degree Relatives of Patients with Type 2 Diabetes?

Linn Gillberg[1,2]*, Stine Jacobsen[1,2], Rasmus Ribel-Madsen[3], Anette Prior Gjesing[3], Trine W. Boesgaard[2,4], Charlotte Ling[5], Oluf Pedersen[3,4,6], Torben Hansen[3,7], Allan Vaag[1,2,8]

1 Department of Endocrinology, Rigshospitalet, Copenhagen, Denmark, 2 Steno Diabetes Center, Gentofte, Denmark, 3 Section of Metabolic Genetics, The Novo Nordisk Foundation Center for Basic Metabolic Research, Faculty of Health Sciences, University of Copenhagen, Copenhagen, Denmark, 4 Hagedorn Research Institute, Gentofte, Denmark, 5 Department of Clinical Sciences, Lund University, Malmoe, Sweden, 6 Faculty of Health Sciences, University of Aarhus, Aarhus, Denmark, 7 Faculty of Health Sciences, University of Southern Denmark, Odense, Denmark, 8 Faculty of Health Sciences, University of Copenhagen, Copenhagen, Denmark

Abstract

Epigenetics may play a role in the pathophysiology of type 2 diabetes (T2D), and increased DNA methylation of the metabolic master regulator peroxisome proliferator-activated receptor gamma coactivator 1 alpha (*PPARGC1A*) has been reported in muscle and pancreatic islets from T2D patients and in muscle from individuals at risk of T2D. This study aimed to investigate DNA promoter methylation and gene expression of *PPARGC1A* in skeletal muscle from first degree relatives (FDR) of T2D patients, and to determine the association with insulin action as well as the influence of family relation. We included 124 Danish FDR of T2D patients from 46 different families. Skeletal muscle biopsies were excised from *vastus lateralis* and insulin action was assessed by oral glucose tolerance tests. DNA methylation and mRNA expression levels were measured using bisulfite sequencing and quantitative real-time PCR, respectively. The average *PPARGC1A* methylation at four CpG sites situated 867-624 bp from the transcription start was associated with whole-body insulin sensitivity in a paradoxical positive manner ($\beta = 0.12$, $P = 0.03$), supported by a borderline significant inverse correlation with fasting insulin levels ($\beta = -0.88$, $P = 0.06$). Excluding individuals with prediabetes and overt diabetes did not affect the overall result. DNA promoter methylation was not associated with *PPARGC1A* gene expression. The familiality estimate of *PPARGC1A* gene expression was high ($h^2 = 79 \pm 27\%$ ($h^2 \pm SE$), $P = 0.002$), suggesting genetic regulation to play a role. No significant effect of familiality on DNA methylation was found. Taken together, increased DNA methylation of the *PPARGC1A* promoter is unlikely to play a major causal role for the development of insulin resistance in FDR of patients with T2D.

Editor: Anita Magdalena Hennige, University of Tübingen, Germany

Funding: This work was supported by The Danish Strategic Research Council, The Danish Council for Independent Research, EASD, Exgenesis, Rigshospitalets forskningsudvalg and Steno Diabetes Center. The funders had no role in study design, data collection and analysis, decision to publish, or preparation of the manuscript.

Competing Interests: The authors have declared that no competing interests exist.

* E-mail: linn.gillberg@rh.regionh.dk

Introduction

Type 2 diabetes (T2D) is a multifactorial and slowly progressing multiple organ disease where metabolic abnormalities eventually leading to hyperglycemia are established long before the overt T2D diagnosis has become manifest [1]. Both genetic and non-genetic factors influence the development of T2D, and it has been estimated that the susceptibility to develop T2D in individuals with a T2D parent is 3–4 times higher compared to the background population [2]. Indeed, significant defects of peripheral (muscle) and hepatic insulin action, as well as of pancreatic beta cell function, have been reported to be present decades before first degree relatives (FDR) of patients with T2D are supposed to develop the disease [3,4]. Genetic variants currently associated with susceptibility to T2D only explain up to 10% of the putative "primary" contribution to T2D risk [5] and it has therefore been debated whether the increased diabetes risk among FDR could be linked to epigenetic traits and not to classic genetic traits defined as

alterations of the DNA sequence. However, little is known about the influence of heritability on epigenetic variation.

DNA methylation represents the most studied epigenetic trait and it is generally believed that increased methylation in the promoter region of tissue specific genes may confer transcriptional repression [6,7]. This putative association has however been difficult to establish in several human studies [8–10]. Both DNA methylation and gene expression of the master metabolic regulator peroxisome proliferator-activated receptor gamma coactivator 1 alpha (*PPARGC1A*) has been extensively studied in relation to T2D. *PPARGC1A* upregulates transcription of genes involved in mitochondrial oxidative metabolism and biogenesis as well as skeletal muscle glucose transport [11,12], and because mitochondrial defects have been associated with peripheral insulin resistance in healthy subjects [13,14] it has been suggested that reduced *PPARGC1A* expression in skeletal muscle may be a primary feature of insulin resistance [11,15]. Furthermore, *PPARGC1A* may be involved in biological functions with implications for in vivo insulin action including protection against oxidative stress, formation of muscle fiber types as well as regulation of microvascular flow [16,17].

Reduced gene expression of *PPARGC1A* has been detected in skeletal muscle from both T2D patients [15,18–20] and non-diabetic, insulin resistant FDR [21]. However, other studies did not consistently find decreased *PPARGC1A* expression in either T2D patients [22] or in healthy [22,23] or insulin resistant [24] individuals with a family history of T2D.

In a study by Ling *et al.*, DNA methylation in a region of the *PPARGC1A* promoter located 867-624 base pairs (bp) upstream from the transcription start was higher in T2D patients, and furthermore showed a trend towards an inverse correlation with gene expression in pancreatic islets [25]. *PPARGC1A* gene expression as well as insulin secretion was reduced in T2D patients in this study, suggesting that DNA methylation in this distinct region of the promoter may influence the metabolic phenotype. Increased *PPARGC1A* promoter methylation has also been reported in skeletal muscle from individuals with impaired glucose tolerance (IGT) and T2D in a more proximal region of the *PPARGC1A* promoter located 337-37 bp upstream from the transcription start [18]. Collectively, increased methylation in the promoter region of *PPARGC1A* in individuals with T2D – or at increased risk of developing T2D – represent the hitherto most studied, and with some exceptions consistent, molecular epigenetic change potentially involved in the pathogenesis of insulin resistance and T2D.

To further investigate the role of DNA methylation in the development of T2D and insulin resistance, we examined *PPARGC1A* DNA promoter methylation in the two distinct regions previously examined and *PPARGC1A* gene expression in skeletal muscle from a unique population of 124 FDR of T2D patients from 46 different families. Furthermore, we determined the association between DNA methylation and clinical phenotypes including measures of insulin action. Finally, we evaluated whether DNA methylation and gene expression of *PPARGC1A* in muscle tissue demonstrate familial clustering and thus may be under genetic control.

Materials and Methods

Subjects

One-hundred-twenty-four Danish men and women from 46 different families were recruited in 2005–2007 as part of the EUGENE2 Consortium study population [26]. All individuals were FDR of patients with T2D and had either one parent with known T2D and the other parent with no family history of T2D and/or normal response to an oral glucose tolerance test (OGTT) (112 individuals), or a sibling (8 individuals) or child (4 individuals) with T2D at the time of recruitment. The common denominator of the study population was the known family history of T2D, and subjects were invited to participate irrespective of their glucose tolerance. The 46 families included 13 of size 1 (1 individual per family), 12 of size 2, 9 of size 3, 6 of size 4, 4 of size 5, 1 of size 6 and 1 of size 10. The study was approved by the Ethical Committee of Copenhagen and was in accordance with the principles of the Declaration of Helsinki II. All subjects signed an informed consent form prior to participation. Nine T2D patients received insulin treatment and were asked to discontinue the insulin treatment 12 hours prior to the clinical examination.

Clinical Examinations

Participants were examined by anthropometric measurements, and a standard OGTT was performed. Blood samples for measurements of plasma glucose and serum insulin were drawn every 30 min during the OGTT until 180 min after ingestion of the 75 g glucose solution. On another occasion after an overnight fast, skeletal muscle tissue was excised from the *vastus lateralis* muscle using a Bergström needle and snap frozen in liquid nitrogen at $-80°C$. Plasma glucose and serum insulin levels were measured as previously described [26]. Insulin sensitivity was estimated from plasma glucose and serum insulin levels obtained in the fasted state and during the OGTT, calculating the homeostatic model assessment of insulin resistance (HOMA-IR) [27] as well as the whole-body Matsuda insulin sensitivity index (ISI) [28]. Estimates of insulin secretion was reported as HOMA of β-cell function (HOMA-β) [27] and the corrected insulin response (CIR) calculated as (serum insulin$_{30 min}$ [pmol l^{-1}] ×0.144×100)/ (plasma glucose$_{30 min}$ [mmol l^{-1}] ×(plasma glucose$_{30 min}$ [mmol l^{-1}] −3.89)) [29].

DNA Methylation

Genomic DNA was isolated from muscle biopsies using the DNeasy Blood and Tissue Kit (Qiagen, Hilden, Germany). Bisulfite conversion of 500 ng DNA was performed using the EZ DNA Methylation-Gold Kit (Zymo Research, Orange, CA, USA). Site-specific DNA methylation at four CpG sites in a subpart of the *PPARGC1A* promoter located 867-624 bp upstream from the transcription start (Figure 1) was determined by bisulfite sequencing [30]. These CpG sites are identical to the CpG sites investigated by Ling *et al.* where the numbering of the CpG sites (-961, -936, -903, -772) was carried out based on the translational start site situated 120 bp from the transcriptional start site. The bisulfite treated DNA was amplified with forward primer 5'-TATTTTAAGGTAGTTAGGGAGGAAA-3' and reverse primer 5'-CCCATAACAATAAAAAATACCAACTC-3' designed by MethPrimer [31]. PCR amplicons were verified by electrophoresis through a 3% ethidium bromide stained agarose gel and treated with ExoSAP-IT (USB Corp, Cleveland, OH, USA) to remove small contaminating fragments. Sequencing PCR was performed using the BigDye Terminator v3.1 Cycle Sequencing Kit (Applied Biosystems, Foster City, CA, USA). DNA samples were precipitated with the BigDye XTerminator Purification Kit (Applied Biosystems), and the samples were sequenced in an ABI 3130xl Genetic Analyzer (Applied Biosystems). The sequence trace files were subjected to quality control and methylation quantification using the epigenetic sequencing methylation (ESME) analysis software version 3.2.1 (Epigenomics, Berlin, Germany). For each sample, the sequence regularity was checked manually by visualization of the ESME output picture files and exclusion of data among repeated measurements was set to a cut off of 10% for the largest methylation difference among the triplicate measurements. DNA methylation at four CpG sites in the proximal *PPARGC1A* promoter (-260, -136, -99, -94) was analyzed with pyrosequencing. Two primer assays covering the CpG of interest were designed using the PyroMark Assay Design 2.0 software (Qiagen). The PyroMark PCR kit (Qiagen) was used for amplifying bisulfite converted DNA according to manufacturer's protocol. The PyroMark Q96 Vacuum Workstation was used for preparing the samples and pyrosequencing was performed with the PyroMark Q96 ID instrument (Qiagen). Data were analyzed with the Pyrogram software v.2.5.8. Pyrograms for all samples were checked manually to validate the quality of the sequencing analysis and samples with unreliable methylation results based on warning messages given by the software (uncertainties due to baseline shift, low signal to-noise ratio, low peak height and high peak-height deviation at positions close to the CpG site analyzed) were re-run. DNA methylation results that

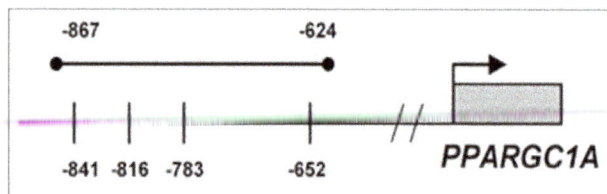

Figure 1. CpG sites analyzed in the *PPARGC1A* promoter. The CpG sites investigated are marked with a perpendicular line.

were subjected to these warning messages after the re-analysis were excluded.

Gene Expression

Total RNA was extracted from muscle tissue using TRI Reagent (Sigma-Aldrich, St. Louis, MO, USA) and converted to cDNA by use of the QuantiTect Reverse Transcription Kit (Qiagen). Gene expression was determined by quantitative real-time PCR with the ABI PRISM 7900HT Sequence Detection System (Applied Biosystems) using gene-specific primers and TaqMan probes for *PPARGC1A* (Hs00173304_m1) (Applied Biosystems). Each sample was measured in duplicate, and the standard curve approach was used for quantification. *PPARGC1A* mRNA samples with Ct values above 31 cycles or a Ct difference above 0.35 on repeated measurements were re-run. Samples that exceeded these cut-offs on the re-analysis were excluded. The *PPARGC1A* mRNA quantity was normalized to the relative amount of cDNA content in each sample as measured in triplicates with the Quant-iT OliGreen ssDNA Assay Kit (Invitrogen, Carlsbad, USA) in combination with the ABI PRISM 7900HT Sequence Detection System [32,33]. This method of normalization is based on the Oligreen dye, which binds with a preferential affinity to ssDNA and upon binding emits fluorescence that can be measured in a single step during adapted thermal conditions. The cDNA content of each sample was calculated after being plotted as a function of the cDNA concentration (i.e. to the linearity of a cDNA standard curve). Samples with a standard deviation divided by average of above 10% on triplicate measurements were re-run, and samples exceeding the cut-off of 10% on repeated measurements after the re-analysis were excluded. Also, *PPARGC1A* mRNA was normalized to cyclophilin (*PPIA*) gene expression of each sample (n = 105), but due to significant associations between *PPIA* mRNA expression and both age ($P = 0.04$) and gender ($P = 0.002$), the *PPARGC1A* mRNA normalized to the cDNA content was considered to be a more robust method for normalization.

Statistical Analysis

Quantitative data were analyzed with linear mixed models in RGui version 2.13.1 (http://www.r-project.org). Residuals from the mixed model analyses were checked for normality by qq-plots. Given that all participants included are of very high risk of developing T2D, and the fact that definition of prediabetic and overt diabetic status is based on arbitrary criteria, we analyzed the results of the study considering the total population of participants' altogether. In order to test the robustness of our findings, and due to the heterogeneous study population, we subsequently analyzed all results for the non-diabetic and the T2D subjects separately. All analyzes were adjusted for age, gender, body mass index (BMI) and glucose tolerance status (fixed effects). Pedigree (coded as a family number) was included as a random factor. Results from the mixed models are presented as effect estimates (β) with 95%

confidence intervals and *P*-values. Unpaired, non-parametric tests and Spearman's correlation tests (ρ) were performed in SAS 9.1 (SAS Institute Inc., Cary, NC). *P*-values ≤ 0.05 were considered significant in two-tailed testing. *PPARGC1A* DNA methylation and gene expression was analyzed in skeletal muscle biopsies from all 124 participants and reliable experimental data was obtained for 117 individuals (DNA methylation, region -867 to -624), 109 individuals (DNA methylation, CpG -260) and 102 individuals (gene expression) respectively. *PPARGC1A* DNA methylation of CpG -136, -99 and -94 was analyzed and obtained from 15 individuals. Because only one subject had a methylation percentage above 0% on one of the CpG sites (NGT subject, 3.87% on CpG -99), and the remaining 14 subjects had no (0%) methylation on all 3 CpG sites, we decided not to analyze methylation of these CpG sites in the remaining samples.

The influence of the familial relation on methylation and gene expression of *PPARGC1A* was estimated from a polygenic model as the proportion of the additive genetic variation on the total variation (variance component approach). The term familiality is used instead of (narrow sense) heritability to emphasize that the resulting estimate not only provides information about genetic similarity, but also shared environmental effects in the FDR group. The familiality of DNA methylation and gene expression was adjusted for age, gender, BMI and glucose tolerance status using the SOLAR software (http://solar.txbiomedgenetics.org).

Results

Subjects Characteristics

The study population consisted of 45 men and 79 women being 32–83 years old (Table 1). The group had varying degrees of BMI (18–47 kg/m^2) and 45 individuals were obese (BMI above 30 kg/m^2). According to the 1999 WHO diagnostic criteria, 80 individuals had normal glucose tolerance (NGT), 5 impaired fasting glucose (IFG), 12 IGT, 2 had both IFG and IGT and 25 individuals had T2D. In this study, the 19 individuals with IFG and/or IGT were grouped together. Individuals in the IFG/IGT subgroup had significantly higher age, fasting triglycerides, plasma glucose and serum insulin levels compared to the NGT subgroup, and were significantly more insulin resistant based on Matsuda ISI (Table 1). Individuals with T2D were characterized by higher age, BMI, HbA1C, fasting serum insulin and plasma triglyceride levels, and lower insulin sensitivity (Matsuda ISI) and insulin secretion (HOMA-β and CIR) compared to NGT subjects. Furthermore, they showed significantly higher HbA1C and lower 2 h OGTT related serum insulin and insulin secretion compared to IFG/IGT subjects. All subgroups differed in fasting and 2 h OGTT-related plasma glucose levels and in estimates of in vivo insulin resistance by HOMA-IR (Table 1). Insulin sensitivity based on Matsuda ISI was significantly lower in men than in women (6.3 vs. 8.7).

PPARGC1A mRNA Expression

Skeletal muscle gene expression of *PPARGC1A* was not significantly different between the NGT, IFG/IGT and T2D subgroups (Figure 2). *PPARGC1A* gene expression did not show any significant associations with age, gender, BMI, fasting glucose, insulin or triglyceride levels, or with insulin sensitivity based on HOMA-IR or Matsuda ISI indices in the whole FDR group (data not shown). When the FDR group was divided into non-diabetic and T2D subgroups, *PPARGC1A* gene expression in the T2D subgroup (n = 25) was significantly positively correlated with whole-body insulin sensitivity (Matsuda ISI) (β = 0.16 (0.03;0.29) $P = 0.02$). Similar results of *PPARGC1A* gene expression was obtained when *PPARGC1A* mRNA was normalized to *PPIA*

Table 1. Clinical characteristics of the FDR group (n = 124) stratified according to glucose tolerance status.

	NGT	IFG/IGT	T2D
n (total)	*80*	*19*	*25*
n (men/women)	*23/57*	*11/8*	*11/14*
Age (years)	51.5±10.0	54.8±10.7*	60.4±10.3++
BMI (kg/m²)	27.2±5.2	29.8±5.4	31.3±4.7++
HbA1C (%)	5.3±0.3	5.4±0.4	7.3±1.6++,§§
Fasting			
Plasma glucose (mmol l⁻¹)	5.4±0.4	5.8±0.5**	9.9±4.0++,§§
Serum insulin (pmol l⁻¹)	41.7±33.7	60.2±40.1*	64.9±50.6++
Plasma triglyceride (mmol l⁻¹)	1.2±0.6	1.7±0.7**	2.0±1.4+
2h OGTT related			
Plasma glucose (mmol l⁻¹)	5.8±1.1	8.1±1.7**	16.4±5.0++,§§
Serum insulin (pmol l⁻¹)	215±196	497±465*	257±318§
Insulin sensitivity			
HOMA-IR	1.5±1.3	2.2±1.5*	4.2±4.2++,§
Matsuda ISI	9.5±5.1	5.4±3.3**	4.3±2.1++
Insulin secretion			
HOMA-β	63.9±44.5	77.5±53.4	38.4±30.2++,§
CIR	8.6±5.4	6.1±4.0	1.6±1.9++,§§

Data are mean ± SD. Significant differences between NGT and IFG/IGT at *P<0.05, **P<0.001. Significant differences between NGT and T2D at +P<0.05, ++P<0.001. Significant differences between IFG/IGT and T2D at §P<0.05, §§P<0.001. All parameters except age and BMI were analyzed with unpaired non-parametric tests due to lack of normal distribution. Indices of insulin sensitivity and insulin secretion were calculated as described in subjects and methods. BMI, body mass index; CIR, corrected insulin response; HOMA-β, homeostatic model assessment of β-cell function; HOMA-IR, homeostatic model assessment of insulin resistance; IFG, impaired fasting glycemia; IGT, impaired glucose tolerance; NGT, normal glucose tolerance; OGTT, oral glucose tolerance test; T2D, type 2 diabetes.

mRNA expression as compared to cDNA content (data not shown).

PPARGC1A DNA Methylation

PPARGC1A DNA methylation in the region 867-624 bp upstream from the transcription start was not affected by gender, age, BMI, fasting plasma glucose or triglyceride levels, or with insulin resistance based on the HOMA-IR index. PPARGC1A methylation did not differ significantly between the NGT, IFG/IGT and T2D subgroups (Figure 3). Interestingly, the average degree of PPARGC1A DNA methylation for the whole FDR group was positively associated with whole-body insulin sensitivity (Matsuda ISI) ($\beta = 0.12$ (0.01;0.24) $P = 0.03$) (Figure 4). The positive correlation with insulin action was significant on one (site −783: $\beta = 0.12$ (0.002;0.23) $P = 0.05$), and borderline significant on two (site −841: $\beta = 0.08$ (−0.004;0.16) $P = 0.06$; site −816: $\beta = 0.09$ (−0.02;0.20) $P = 0.09$) out of the four CpG sites. This finding was also supported by a borderline significant inverse correlation between average DNA methylation and fasting serum insulin levels ($\beta = -0.88$ (−1.80;0.04) $P = 0.06$). When subjects were divided according to glucose tolerance status, the relation between average PPARGC1A methylation and whole-body insulin sensitivity remained significant in the NGT ($\beta = 0.14$ (0.006;0.28) $P = 0.04$) and the NGT/IFG/IGT (non-diabetic) group ($\beta = 0.14$

(0.02;0.27) $P = 0.02$), but not in the IFG/IGT or T2D group. Separate analyses of non-diabetic subjects (n = 99) also revealed significant inverse correlations between average PPARGC1A DNA methylation and fasting insulin ($\beta = -0.83$ (−1.64;−0.02) $P = 0.05$), fasting glucose ($\beta = -3.86$ (−7.80;0.07) $P = 0.05$) and insulin resistance based on HOMA-IR ($\beta = -1.65$ (−3.02;−0.27) $P = 0.02$). Finally, PPARGC1A promoter methylation in the region 867–624 bp upstream from the transcription start did not show a significant inverse correlation with PPARGC1A gene expression (Figure 5).

Familiality of PPARGC1A DNA Methylation and Gene Expression

The familiality for PPARGC1A gene expression ($h^2 = 79 \pm 27\%$, $P = 0.002$) ($h^2 \pm SE$) was higher than for PPARGC1A promoter methylation ($h^2 = 16 \pm 17\%$, $P = 0.16$), and only the gene expression showed a statistically significant influence by familiality.

Discussion

Several studies have suggested that skeletal muscle DNA methylation and gene expression of PPARGC1A may be involved in the pathogenesis of T2D [8,18,20,21,25]. Our current study including 124 Danish FDR of T2D patients did however not show any association between glucose tolerance status and PPARGC1A promoter methylation or gene expression in skeletal muscle. Unexpectedly, and opposite to our a priori hypothesis, the degree of PPARGC1A methylation correlated positively with whole-body insulin sensitivity, and inversely with fasting insulin levels. Our data furthermore indicate that genetics and/or shared environmental effects play a role in the regulation of PPARGC1A gene expression, whereas PPARGC1A DNA methylation seems less influenced by familiality factors. Overall, our data do not support the view that skeletal muscle PPARGC1A promoter methylation plays any major causal role in the pathogenesis of T2D, at least not among individuals with a family history of T2D.

Skeletal muscle gene expression of PPARGC1A and genes involved in oxidative phosphorylation has been extensively studied in relation to prediabetes and T2D, and increased skeletal muscle expression of PPARGC1A is believed to contribute to improved insulin sensitivity [15,34,35]. We were unable to establish an association between PPARGC1A gene expression and in vivo insulin resistance in the total population of FDR in our study. However, when analyzed according to glucose tolerance status, PPARGC1A gene expression in the T2D subgroup showed a significant positive correlation with whole-body insulin sensitivity, which was in accordance with our hypothesis.

The FDR subjects studied have increased risk of T2D due to having a parent, sibling or child diagnosed with the disease. Also the participants are subdivided into 46 different families, which makes our group more genetically homogenous compared to the general Danish population [26]. It could be argued that we lack a control group of individuals without a family history of T2D, making our results more difficult to contrast with some of the previous studies. However, in three previous studies the muscle PPARGC1A gene expression in healthy or insulin resistant individuals with a family history of T2D was similar to healthy matched controls without a family history of T2D [22–24].

The association between insulin sensitivity and PPARGC1A gene expression in skeletal muscle has been investigated in previous studies with conflicting results [21,24,36]. Patti et al. found reduced expression of PPARGC1A in insulin resistant compared to insulin sensitive offspring of parents with T2D [21], whereas Morino et al. found no alteration in gene expression or protein content of

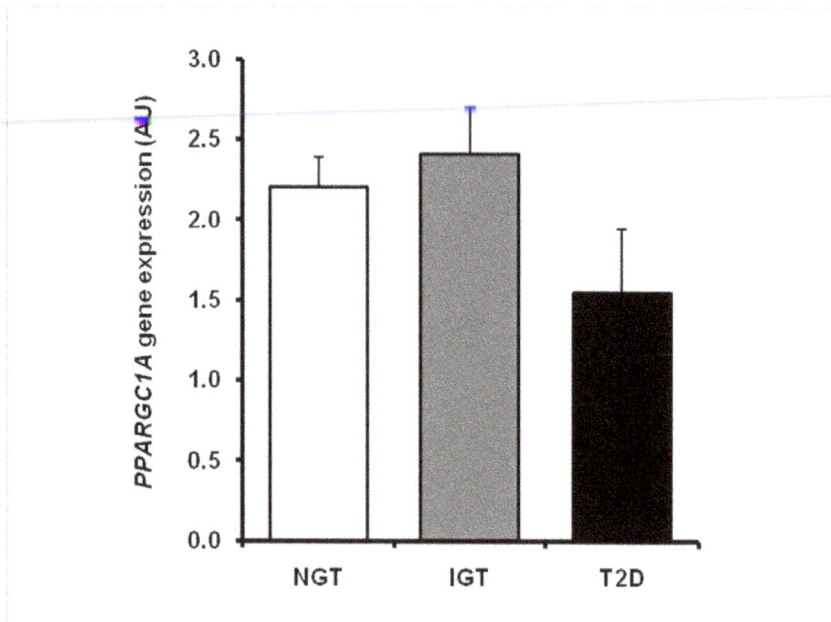

Figure 2. Skeletal muscle gene expression of *PPARGC1A.* Participants are stratified according to glucose tolerance status (NGT, IFG/IGT, T2D). Data are mean±SE.

PPARGC1A in young, insulin resistant offspring of T2D parents compared to controls [24]. Also, T2D has been associated with a reduced muscle *PPARGC1A* gene expression in some [18–21], but not all [22] studies. In accordance with our results, Palsgaard *et al.* found similar *PPARGC1A* gene expression in T2D compared to normoglycemic subjects [22]. Collectively, the present study together with previous studies suggests that the expected inverse relationship between skeletal muscle *PPARGC1A* gene expression and insulin resistance or T2D is not a consistent and reproducible finding. Interestingly, intervention studies have shown that skeletal muscle gene expression of *PPARGC1A* was downregulated in young healthy men after 9 days of bed rest [37], and after a 5 day high-fat high-calorie diet in low birth weight men with an

increased risk of T2D [8]. Moreover, the increase in *PPARGC1A* mRNA and protein content following exercise is reduced and delayed in muscle from insulin resistant subjects [38]. Therefore, a metabolic challenge could be necessary to unmask the association between *PPARGC1A* expression and prediabetes in the FDR subjects included in this study.

DNA promoter methylation could be one among several mechanisms regulating *PPARGC1A* gene transcription in not only skeletal muscle, but also in other primary diabetogenic tissues such as the pancreatic beta cell, liver or adipose tissue. Only muscle was addressed in this study, and indeed *PPARGC1A* DNA methylation

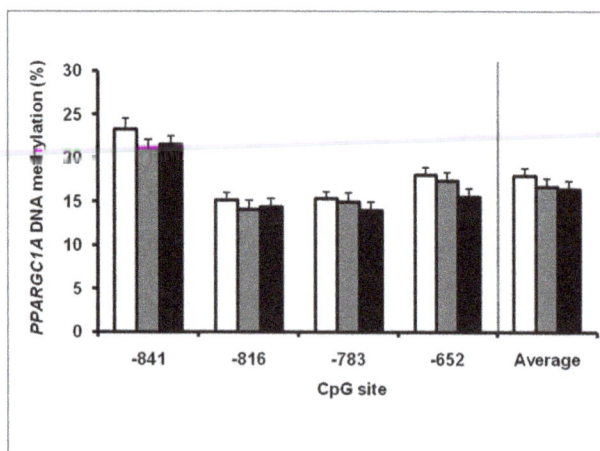

Figure 3. DNA methylation at different CpG sites in the promoter region of *PPARGC1A* **in skeletal muscle.** The FDR participants are stratified according to glucose tolerance status: NGT (*white bars*), IFG/IGT (*grey bars*), T2D (*black bars*). Data are mean ± SE.

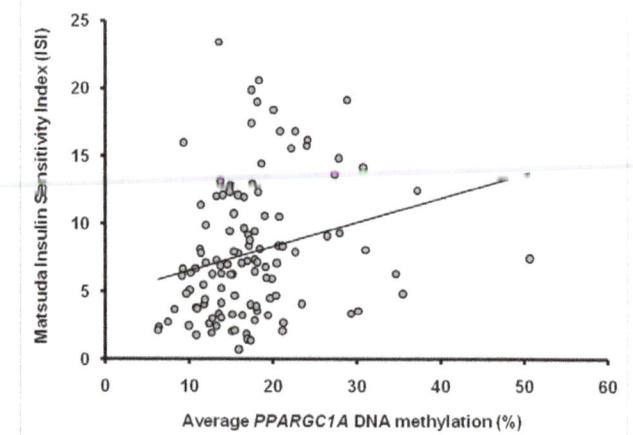

Figure 4. Correlation between average skeletal muscle DNA methylation of the *PPARGC1A* **promoter and whole-body insulin sensitivity.** Methylation is shown in percentage and Matsuda ISI was used as a marker of whole-body insulin sensitivity in the FDR group. β = 0.12 (0.01;0.24) *P* = 0.03, adjusted for age, gender, BMI, glucose tolerance and family pedigree. Unadjusted correlation (Spearman's correlation): ρ 0.31, *P* = 0.0007.

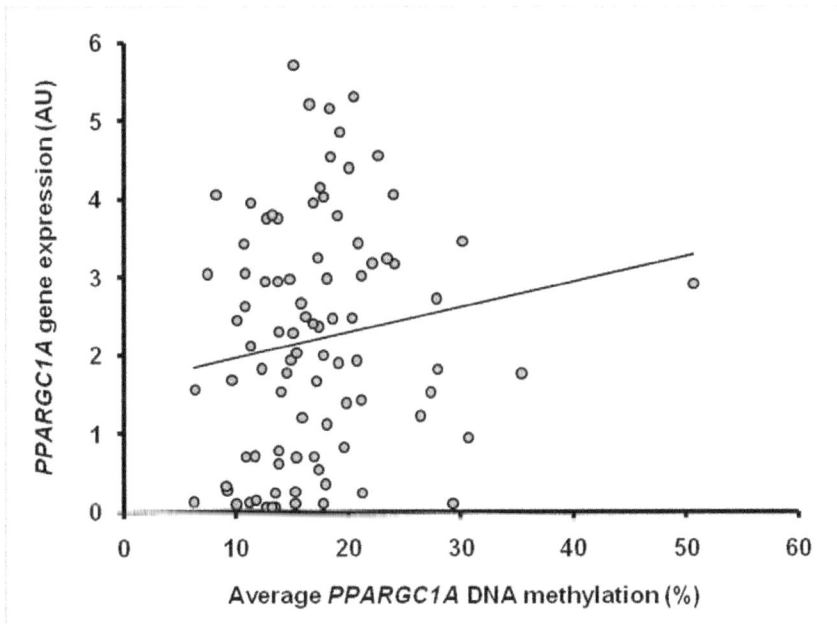

Figure 5. Correlation between average skeletal muscle DNA methylation and gene expression of *PPARGC1A*. Methylation is show in percentage and gene expression in arbitrary units (AU). $\beta = 0.013$ ($-0.034;0.059$), $P = 0.59$, adjusted for age, gender, BMI, glucose tolerance and family pedigree. Unadjusted (Spearman's correlation): ρ 0.22, $P = 0.04$.methylation at CpG site -260 in the *PPARGC1A* promoter was 0% in 98 individuals and 4–10% in 11 individuals (4 with T2D and 7 with NGT). The DNA methylation at CpG site -260 was not different among T2D (1.1 ± 1.7) compared to NGT subjects (0.74 ± 2.3), and there were no significant associations between DNA methylation and whole body insulin sensitivity, gene expression or any other clinical parameter (data not shown).

and/or gene expression could be more tightly linked and functionally important with respect to T2D pathogenesis in tissues other than muscle. Our recent study of skeletal muscle and subcutaneous adipose tissue from monozygotic twins showed that between these different tissues involved in peripheral glucose metabolism, numerous DNA methylation differences were found. However, between twin differences of DNA methylation in each specific tissue were modest [39]. These findings emphasize the robustness of the tissue specific DNA methylation patterns.

Importantly, the CpG sites analyzed in the *PPARGC1A* promoter were carefully selected based on previous studies where DNA methylation of these sites in skeletal muscle and pancreatic islets show signs of metabolic relevance [8,18,25,37]. We were however unable to establish this relationship in skeletal muscle from the FDR group despite the large number of participants. In spite of a fairly convincing belief among many that promoter DNA methylation causes transcriptional repression, poor correlations between these factors have been reported for most genes in large-scale studies such as the Human Epigenome Project, where one third of the differentially methylated promoter regions were found to correlate inversely with gene transcription [9]. Possible explanations of the lack of an inverse correlation between DNA promoter methylation and gene expression of *PPARGC1A* in our study may be that the amount of *PPARGC1A* mRNA analyzed by quantitative real-time PCR may not reflect *PPARGC1A* transcription in cases where the mRNA turnover rate is high. To this end, associations between *PPARGC1A* mRNA and promoter methylation might only be unmasked when the regulation is activated in response to metabolically challenged states, as for example during exposure to a diet rich in calories and/or after high-intense physical exercise. Cyclical, rapid changes in methylation status at promoter CpG dinucleotides of transcriptionally active genes may constitute another explanation of the lack of correlation with gene

expression, as previously shown in the promoter of estrogen receptor alpha [40]. Finally, we cannot exclude the possibility that other CpG sites in the *PPARGC1A* promoter may play a more important role in the regulation of gene expression and subsequent metabolic actions.

In a study by Barres *et al.* DNA methylation of non-CpG sites in a region -337 to -37 bp upstream from the transcription start was increased in skeletal muscle from both IGT and T2D compared to NGT subjects [18]. The promoter methylation was inversely correlated with gene expression and consequently suggested to be associated with impaired insulin sensitivity. Therefore, it was unexpected for us to observe that increased DNA methylation of CpG sites in the region -867 to -624 bp upstream from the transcription start was associated with in-creased (and not decreased) whole-body insulin sensitivity, supported by a borderline significant inverse association with insulin levels in the fasting state. Excluding individuals with glucose intolerance and/or overt diabetes did not affect the significance of these associations.

In this study, we focused primarily on the four methylation sites that we previously found to exhibit increased methylation in prediabetic and T2D subjects [8,25]. In order to address to potential impact of DNA methylation at the sites closer to transcription start, we measured these too in the present cohort. However, we found these sites to be without any detectable DNA methylation in the majority of the study subjects. Accordingly, we were unable to find any differences between groups and we furthermore could not determine any relationship with gene expression or insulin action.

Whole-body insulin sensitivity as estimated by the Matsuda ISI reflects insulin sensitivity in both liver and peripheral tissues, and has been shown to correlate with peripheral insulin sensitivity as measured by the gold standard hyperinsulinemic euglycemic clamp technique [28]. A possible explanation for the paradoxical association between increased *PPARGC1A* DNA methylation and improved insulin sensitivity, as well as reduced insulin levels, in the FDR group could be a counter-regulatory cellular mechanism. One could imagine that *de novo* methylation processes may become activated in FDR with an improved insulin sensitivity state of the body, such that the *PPARGC1A* promoter region is methylated to shut off pathways activated by *PPARGC1A*, all together balancing the regulation of the system by a feedback mechanism. Also, other studies by our group have shown that *PPARGC1A* promoter methylation at the identical CpG sites in muscle tissue from young, healthy men is sensitive to physiological and metabolic challenges such as 5-days high-fat high-calorie diet [8] and 9 days of bed rest [37]. Whatever the mechanism may be, the hypothesis that increased methylation of the *PPARGC1A* promoter is associated with insulin resistance seems questionable and needs further investigation.

The inclusion of families in the FDR group allowed us to estimate the influence of familiality (i.e. genetic effects and shared environmental effects) on DNA methylation and gene expression of *PPARGC1A*. Our data clearly demonstrate that *PPARGC1A* gene expression was highly influenced by familiality ($h^2 = 79\pm27\%$, $P = 0.002$), whereas the influence of familiality on *PPARGC1A* promoter methylation was low and insignificant ($h^2 = 16\pm17\%$, $P = 0.16$). We believe that polymorphisms either within, adjacent to or distant from the regulatory region and the gene body may be able to modulate *PPARGC1A* transcription and/or *PPARGC1A* mRNA degradation. Also, heritable effects of DNA methylation on other CpG sites than the ones investigated in this study could also possibly be involved in the regulation of *PPARGC1A* transcription. The influence of heritability on skeletal muscle *PPARGC1A* gene expression was previously investigated in young and elderly monozygotic and dizygotic twins and although the heritable effect was not statistically significant in either young or elderly twins, a polymorphism in *PPARGC1A*, the Gly482Ser variant, was associated with *PPARGC1A* gene expression [41]. Conversely, a genome-wide analysis of gene expression in lymphoblastoid cell lines from monozygotic twin pairs suggested a significant heritable component of gene expression levels with an average broad-sense heritability estimated to 31% [42]. Heritable effects of DNA methylation was recently investigated at 1760 CpG

sites in 186 regions in the human major histocompatibility complex in CD4+ lymphocytes from 49 monozygotic and 40 dizygotic Norwegian twin pairs [43]. In accordance with our data, they reported low heritability estimates for DNA methylation, ranging from 2% to 16% across four types of gene regions in the major histocompatibility complex. The limited genetic contribution to *PPARGC1A* DNA methylation variation in skeletal muscle from our group, together with our previous studies of *PPARGC1A* methylation in relation to physiological and dietary challenges [8,37], all together suggests that the CpG sites that we have investigated in the *PPARGC1A* promoter have a highly dynamic and relatively fast regulation of methylation that mainly is controlled by environmental effects such as the physiological/metabolic state of the body.

In conclusion, a paradoxical positive relationship between *PPARGC1A* DNA methylation and insulin action in skeletal muscle was demonstrated. These data challenge the notion of an adverse effect of *PPARGC1A* DNA methylation on insulin action, at least among individuals with a family history of T2D. Furthermore, data from the FDR group revealed a significant effect of familiality on *PPARGC1A* gene expression contrasting the absence of any significant familiality on degree of DNA methylation. Further studies are needed to increase our understanding of the impact of DNA methylation and gene expression of *PPARGC1A* as well as other candidate genes on the pathogenesis of T2D.

Acknowledgments

Marianne Modest and Lars Sander Koch from Steno Diabetes Center provided technical support for the experiments. We are especially appreciative of the cooperation of all individuals who participated in this study.

Author Contributions

Designed and/or supervised the human studies: TWB OP TH AV. Designed the DNA methylation assay: CL. Conceived and designed the experiments: AV SJ LG. Performed the experiments: LG SJ RR-M. Analyzed the data: LG APG. Contributed reagents/materials/analysis tools: AV OP TH. Wrote the paper: LG AV.

References

1. Perseghin G, Ghosh S, Gerow K, Shulman GI (1997) Metabolic defects in lean nondiabetic offspring of NIDDM parents: a cross-sectional study. Diabetes 46: 1001–1009.

2. Meigs JB, Cupples LA, Wilson PW (2000) Parental transmission of type 2 diabetes: the Framingham Offspring Study. Diabetes 49: 2201–2207.

3. Allbegovic AC, Hojbjerre L, Sonne MP, van HG, Stallknecht B, et al. (2009) Impact of 9 days of bed rest on hepatic and peripheral insulin action, insulin secretion, and whole-body lipolysis in healthy young male offspring of patients with type 2 diabetes. Diabetes 58: 2749–2756. db09–0369 [pii];10.2337/db09–0369 [doi].

4. Vaag A, Henriksen JE, Beck-Nielsen H (1992) Decreased insulin activation of glycogen synthase in skeletal muscles in young nonobese Caucasian first-degree relatives of patients with non-insulin-dependent diabetes mellitus. J Clin Invest 89: 782–788.

5. Voight BF, Scott LJ, Steinthorsdottir V, Morris AP, Dina C, et al. (2010) Twelve type 2 diabetes susceptibility loci identified through large-scale association analysis. Nat Genet 42: 579–589. ng.609 [pii];10.1038/ng.609 [doi].

6. Bird A (2007) Perceptions of epigenetics. Nature 447: 396–398.

7. Razin A, Riggs AD (1980) DNA methylation and gene function. Science 210: 604–610.

8. Brons C, Jacobsen S, Nilsson E, Ronn T, Jensen CB, et al. (2010) Deoxyribonucleic acid methylation and gene expression of PPARGC1A in human muscle is influenced by high-fat overfeeding in a birth-weight-dependent manner. J Clin Endocrinol Metab 95: 3048–3056.

9. Eckhardt F, Lewin J, Cortese R, Rakyan VK, Attwood J, et al. (2006) DNA methylation profiling of human chromosomes 6, 20 and 22. Nat Genet 38: 1378–1385.

10. Lomba A, Milagro FI, Garcia-Diaz DF, Marti A, Campion J, et al. (2010) Obesity induced by a pair-fed high fat sucrose diet: methylation and expression pattern of genes related to energy homeostasis. Lipids Health Dis 9: 60.

11. Michael LF, Wu Z, Cheatham RB, Puigserver P, Adelmant G, et al. (2001) Restoration of insulin-sensitive glucose transporter (GLUT4) gene expression in muscle cells by the transcriptional coactivator PGC-1. Proc Natl Acad Sci U S A 98: 3820–3825.

12. Wu Z, Puigserver P, Andersson U, Zhang C, Adelmant G, et al. (1999) Mechanisms controlling mitochondrial biogenesis and respiration through the thermogenic coactivator PGC-1. Cell 98: 115–124.

13. Petersen KF, Befroy D, Dufour S, Dziura J, Ariyan C, et al. (2003) Mitochondrial dysfunction in the elderly: possible role in insulin resistance. Science 300: 1140–1142.

14. Petersen KF, Dufour S, Befroy D, Garcia R, Shulman GI (2004) Impaired mitochondrial activity in the insulin-resistant offspring of patients with type 2 diabetes. N Engl J Med 350: 664–671.

15. Patti ME (2004) Gene expression in humans with diabetes and prediabetes: what have we learned about diabetes pathophysiology? Curr Opin Clin Nutr Metab Care 7: 383–390.

16. Arany Z, Foo SY, Ma Y, Ruas JL, Bommi-Reddy A, et al. (2008) HIF-independent regulation of VEGF and angiogenesis by the transcriptional coactivator PGC-1alpha. Nature 451: 1008–1012. nature06613 [pii];10.1038/nature06613 [doi].

17. Handschin C, Spiegelman BM (2008) The role of exercise and PGC1alpha in inflammation and chronic disease. Nature 454: 463–469. nature07206 [pii];10.1038/nature07206 [doi].

18. Barres R, Osler ME, Yan J, Rune A, Fritz T, et al. (2009) Non-CpG methylation of the PGC-1alpha promoter through DNMT3B controls mitochondrial density. Cell Metab 10: 189–198.

19. Carey AL, Petersen EW, Bruce CR, Southgate RJ, Pilegaard H, et al. (2006) Discordant gene expression in skeletal muscle and adipose tissue of patients with type 2 diabetes: effect of interleukin-6 infusion. Diabetologia 49: 1000–1007.

20. Mootha VK, Lindgren CM, Eriksson KF, Subramanian A, Sihag S, et al. (2003) PGC-1alpha-responsive genes involved in oxidative phosphorylation are coordinately downregulated in human diabetes. Nat Genet 34: 267–273.

21. Patti ME, Butte AJ, Crunkhorn S, Cusi K, Berria R, et al. (2003) Coordinated reduction of genes of oxidative metabolism in humans with insulin resistance and diabetes: Potential role of PGC1 and NRF1. Proc Natl Acad Sci U S A 100: 8466–8471.

22. Palsgaard J, Brons C, Friedrichsen M, Dominguez H, Jensen M, et al. (2009) Gene expression in skeletal muscle biopsies from people with type 2 diabetes and relatives: differential regulation of insulin signaling pathways. PLoS One 4: e6575.

23. Karlsson HK, Ahlsen M, Zierath JR, Wallberg-Henriksson H, Koistinen HA (2006) Insulin signaling and glucose transport in skeletal muscle from first-degree relatives of type 2 diabetic patients. Diabetes 55: 1283–1288.

24. Morino K, Petersen KF, Dufour S, Befroy D, Frattini J, et al. (2005) Reduced mitochondrial density and increased IRS-1 serine phosphorylation in muscle of insulin-resistant offspring of type 2 diabetic parents. J Clin Invest 115: 3587–3593.

25. Ling C, Del GS, Lupi R, Ronn T, Granhall C, et al. (2008) Epigenetic regulation of PPARGC1A in human type 2 diabetic islets and effect on insulin secretion. Diabetologia 51: 615–622.

26. Boesgaard TW, Gjesing AP, Grarup N, Rutanen J, Jansson PA, et al. (2009) Variant near ADAMTS9 known to associate with type 2 diabetes is related to insulin resistance in offspring of type 2 diabetes patients–EUGENE2 study. PLoS One 4: e7236.

27. Matthews DR, Hosker JP, Rudenski AS, Naylor BA, Treacher DF, et al. (1985) Homeostasis model assessment: insulin resistance and beta-cell function from fasting plasma glucose and insulin concentrations in man. Diabetologia 28: 412–419.

28. Matsuda M, DeFronzo RA (1999) Insulin sensitivity indices obtained from oral glucose tolerance testing: comparison with the euglycemic insulin clamp. Diabetes Care 22: 1462–1470.

29. Sluiter WJ, Erkelens DW, Reitsma WD, Doorenbos H (1976) Glucose tolerance and insulin release, a mathematical approach I. Assay of the beta-cell response after oral glucose loading. Diabetes 25: 241–244.

30. Frommer M, McDonald LE, Millar DS, Collis CM, Watt F, et al. (1992) A genomic sequencing protocol that yields a positive display of 5-methylcytosine residues in individual DNA strands. Proc Natl Acad Sci U S A 89: 1827–1831.

31. Li LC, Dahiya R (2002) MethPrimer: designing primers for methylation PCRs. Bioinformatics 18: 1427–1431.

32. Rhinn H, Marchand-Leroux C, Croci N, Plotkine M, Scherman D, et al. (2008) Housekeeping while brain's storming Validation of normalizing factors for gene expression studies in a murine model of traumatic brain injury. BMC Mol Biol 9: 62.

33. Rhinn H, Scherman D, Escriou V (2008) One-step quantification of single-stranded DNA in the presence of RNA using Oligreen in a real-time polymerase chain reaction thermocycler. Anal Biochem 372: 116–118.

34. Finck BN, Kelly DP (2006) PGC-1 coactivators: inducible regulators of energy metabolism in health and disease. J Clin Invest 116: 615–622.

35. Lin J, Handschin C, Spiegelman BM (2005) Metabolic control through the PGC-1 family of transcription coactivators. Cell Metab 1: 361–370.

36. Hammarstedt A, Jansson PA, Wesslau C, Yang X, Smith U (2003) Reduced expression of PGC-1 and insulin-signaling molecules in adipose tissue is associated with insulin resistance. Biochem Biophys Res Commun 301: 578–582.

37. Alibegovic AC, Sonne MP, Hojbjerre L, Bork-Jensen J, Jacobsen S, et al. (2010) Insulin resistance induced by physical inactivity is associated with multiple transcriptional changes in skeletal muscle in young men. Am J Physiol Endocrinol Metab 299: E752–E763.

38. De FE, Alvarez G, Berria R, Cusi K, Everman S, et al. (2008) Insulin-resistant muscle is exercise resistant: evidence for reduced response of nuclear-encoded mitochondrial genes to exercise. Am J Physiol Endocrinol Metab 294: E607–E614.

39. Ribel-Madsen R, Fraga MF, Jacobsen S, Bork-Jensen J, Lara E, et al. (2012) Genome-wide analysis of DNA methylation differences in muscle and fat from monozygotic twins discordant for type 2 diabetes. PLOS ONE 7: e51302. 10.1371/journal.pone.0051302 [doi];PONE-D-12–16067 [pii].

40. Metivier R, Gallais R, Tiffoche C, Le PC, Jurkowska RZ, et al. (2008) Cyclical DNA methylation of a transcriptionally active promoter. Nature 452: 45–50.

41. Ling C, Poulsen P, Carlsson E, Ridderstrale M, Almgren P, et al. (2004) Multiple environmental and genetic factors influence skeletal muscle PGC-1alpha and PGC-1beta gene expression in twins. J Clin Invest 114: 1518–1526.

42. McRae AF, Matigian NA, Vadlamudi L, Mulley JC, Mowry B, et al. (2007) Replicated effects of sex and genotype on gene expression in human lymphoblastoid cell lines. Hum Mol Genet 16: 364–373.

43. Gervin K, Hammero M, Akselsen HE, Moe R, Nygard H, et al. (2011) Extensive variation and low heritability of DNA methylation identified in a twin study. Genome Res 21: 1813–1821.

Associations between Serum Apelin-12 Levels and Obesity-Related Markers in Chinese Children

Hong-Jun Ba, Hong-Shan Chen*, Zhe Su, Min-Lian Du, Qiu-Li Chen, Yan-Hong Li, Hua-Mei Ma

Pediatric Department, The First Affiliated Hospital, Sun Yat-sen University, Guangzhou, Guangdong Province, China

Abstract

Objective: To investigate possible correlations between apelin-12 levels and obesity in children in China and associations between apelin-12 and obesity-related markers, including lipids, insulin sensitivity and insulin resistance index (HOMA-IR).

Methods: Forty-eight obese and forty non-obese age- and gender-matched Chinese children were enrolled between June 2008 and June 2009. Mean age was 10.42 ± 2.03 and 10.86 ± 2.23 years in obesity and control groups, respectively. Main outcome measures were apelin-12, BMI, lipids, glucose and insulin. HOMA-IR was calculated for all subjects.

Results: All obesity group subjects had significantly higher total cholesterol (TC), triglycerides (TG), low-density lipoprotein cholesterol (LDL-C), insulin levels and HOMA-IR (all $P<0.05$). In separate analyses, obese girls had significantly higher LDL-C, insulin and HOMA-IR than controls, and obese boys had significantly higher TC, TG, insulin and HOMA-IR than controls (all $P<0.05$). Apelin-12 levels were significantly higher in obese girls compared to controls ($P=0.024$), and correlated positively with TG in all obese subjects. Among obese girls, apelin-12 levels correlated positively with TG, insulin and HOMA-IR after adjusting for age and BMI. In all boys (obese and controls) apelin-12 was positively associated with fasting plasma glucose (FPG). No significant correlations were found in either group between apelin-12 levels and other characteristics after adjusting for age, sex, and BMI.

Conclusions: Apelin-12 levels are significantly higher in obese vs. non-obese girls in China and correlate significantly with obesity-related markers insulin, HOMA-IR, and TG. Increased apelin-12 levels may be involved in the pathological mechanism of childhood obesity.

Editor: Ayyalasomayajula Vajreswari, National Institute of Nutrition, India

Funding: This study was supported by Grant 2007B031500006 from the Technology Program of Guangdong Province in China. The funders had no role in study design, data collection and analysis, decision to publish, or preparation of the manuscript.

Competing Interests: The authors have declared that no competing interests exist.

* E-mail: hongshand@163.com

Introduction

The rapidly increasing prevalence of childhood obesity has alarmed public health agencies, healthcare clinicians and researchers, and the general public globally [1]. In China, the prevalence of obesity and overweight among children was 2% and 5%, respectively, in the 1980s; in 2002, 155 million children worldwide were overweight or obese, including 12 million in China [2]. Obesity is a multifactorial disease and its development is attributed to genetic predisposition, misregulation of energy balance, and environmental and social factors [3]. Obesity in childhood is associated with a variety of metabolic disorders, including insulin resistance [4], dyslipidemia [5], hyperglycemia [6], type 2 diabetes mellitus [7], and risk of cardiovascular complications [8]. Furthermore, obese children tend to become obese adults [9]. Clearly, understanding childhood obesity is critical in order to reduce its incidence and the development of related metabolic disorders.

Adipose tissue stores triglycerides and also secretes polypeptides, adipocyte-produced hormones called adipokines (or adipocytokines), including leptin, visfatin, vaspin, apelin, adiponectin and resistin, which all play important roles in metabolism and energy

homeostasis [10–12]. Apelin, identified by Tatemoto et al. [12], is a novel bioactive peptide expressed in adipocytes of humans; it is encoded by the APLN gene and is the endogenous ligand of the orphan G protein-coupled receptor, APJ, now known as apelin receptor, APLNR. The gene encodes a 77 amino acid polypeptide [12], and all isoforms are derived from a common 77-amino acid precursor, preproapelin [13]. To date, 46 fragments of active apelin peptides have been identified from apelin-55 to apelin-12, all generated by the proproteins of 55 amino acids [14]. Active forms of apelin are expressed in many peripheral tissues (heart, lung, kidney, liver, adipose tissue, gastrointestinal tract, and endothelium) and brain regions (hypothalamus) [15]. Apelin-12 is a 12-amino peptide fragment that has been implicated in reducing blood pressure via a nitric oxide mechanism [16], and is involved in feeding mechanisms via stimulation of cholecystokinin secretion [17]. The synthesis of apelin in adipocytes is triggered by insulin and its plasma levels are reported to increase in association with insulin resistance and hyperinsulinemia [18]. Apelin-12 is considered to be one of the more potent forms of apelin [14].

Apelin expression participates in regulation of blood pressure [16], cardiac contractility [19], fluid balance [20] and stimulation of ACTH release by the pituitary [21]. Expression of apelin in adipocytes is shown to be increased in mouse models of obesity associated with hyperinsulinemia, and apelin levels paralleled plasma insulin levels during fasting and refeeding of mice [17]. Tumor necrosis factor-alpha (TNF-α) [22], growth hormone [23], insulin and glucocorticoids [24] all up-regulate the expression of apelin in adipocytes. Tasci et al. [25] have also found that plasma apelin-12 was lower in patients with elevated LDL-C. While Erdem et al. [26] found significantly reduced plasma apelin levels in obese subjects with untreated type 2 diabetes compared to non-diabetic subjects, Li et al. [27] have found elevated plasma apelin levels in people with impaired glucose tolerance and type 2 diabetes mellitus.

All studies cited above indicate that controversy exists around the levels and the associations of apelin in metabolic disorders. Although associations have been shown between apelin-12 and atopic dermatitis [28] and insulin resistance in adolescents with polycystic ovary syndrome [29], studies are lacking about associations of this adipocyte-secreted factor in obese children, and there is no agreement to date on whether apelin levels correlate with childhood obesity. Therefore, the purpose of the present study was to investigate possible correlations between apelin-12 levels and obesity in children in China and identify associations between apelin-12 and obesity-related markers, including lipids, insulin sensitivity and insulin resistance index.

Patients and Methods

Study Population and Anthropometric Measurements

Between June 2008 and June 2009, 88 (48 obese and 40 non-obese) Chinese children, matched for age and sex, were enrolled in this cross-sectional study. All participants were from Guangzhou, China, and recruited from patients receiving regular health check-ups or evaluation of obesity. Their demographic and clinical data were analyzed retrospectively. Using criteria developed in China, obesity was defined as BMI for age- and sex-specific categories at the 95th percentile or higher [30]. Exclusion criteria were the presence of endocrine diseases, infections, chronic illnesses, and use of prescription medication for any reason. BMI was calculated for all subjects (weight in kilograms divided by the square of height in meters). Waist circumference (WC) was measured with a tape measure at the level of the umbilicus to the nearest 0.1 cm as previously described [31]. Detailed personal and family medical history was obtained for each participant. All subjects underwent a complete physical examination. The stage of puberty was determined according to the Tanner criteria [32]. The nature and purpose of the study were carefully explained to both parents and subjects before obtaining written informed consent from parents and voluntary assent from the children. This study was approved by the Institutional Ethics Board of the First Affiliated Hospital of Sun Yat-sen University.

Clinical Laboratory Determinations

Venous blood samples were drawn from all subjects in the morning between 8:00 AM and 9:00 AM after a 12-hour overnight fast. Blood samples were collected according to recommendations of the individual assay kits' manufacturers. Serum and plasma samples were frozen and stored at −70°C until the tests were performed.

Laboratory determinations of plasma glucose (FPG, mg/dl), total cholesterol (TC, mmol/l) high-density lipoprotein cholesterol (HDL, mmol/l) and triglycerides (TG, mmol/l) were assessed by standard laboratory methods using commercially available test kits (Roche Diagnostics GmbH, Mannheim, Germany). Low-density

lipoprotein cholesterol (LDL-C, mmol/l) value was obtained using the Friedwald formula. Other assays were performed as follows:

Insulin assay protocol. Insulin (µU/ml) was measured by an enzyme-linked immunoassay kit (DRG Instruments GmbH, Marburg, Germany), with a lower limit of sensitivity of 1.76 µU/ml and intra- and inter-assay CVs of 2.2% and 4.4%, respectively. Protocol was as follows: Add 25 µl/well of standard, sample, and positive control followed by 25 µl/well conjugate reagent and mix well for 10 sec. Incubate at room temperature (20–23°C) for 0.5 hours. Wash immunoplate 3 times with 400 µl/well of 1×assay buffer. Add 50 µl/well of enzyme complex and incubate at room temperature for 0.5 hours. Wash immunoplate 3 times with 400 µl/well of 1×assay buffer. Add 50 µl/well of TMB substrate solution and incubate at room temperature for 15 minutes. Terminate reaction with 50 µl/well of H_2SO_4. Read absorbance OD at 450 nm and calculate results.

Apelin-12 assay protocol. Serum apelin-12 levels were determined by enzyme-linked immunosorbent assay (ELISA) (Human Apelin-12 ELISA Kit. Phoenix Pharmaceuticals, Belmont, CA) Intra- and inter-assay CVs were 5%, and 14%, respectively. Protocol was as follows: Add 50 µl/well of standard, sample, or positive control, 25 µl primary antibody and 25 µl biotinylated peptide. Incubate at room temperature (20–23°C) for 2 hours. Wash immunoplate 4 times with 350 µl/well of 1×assay buffer. Add 100 µl/well of SA-HRP solution and incubate at room temperature for 1 hour. Wash immunoplate 4 times with 350 µl/well of 1×assay buffer. Add 100 µl/well of TMB substrate solution and incubate at room temperature for 1 hour. Terminate reaction with 100 µl/well of 2N HCl. Read absorbance OD at 450 nm and calculate results.

Estradiol & testosterone assays. Serum hormone levels (estradiol and testosterone) were measured by chemiluminescence microparticle immunoassay kits (CMIA) (ARCHITECT Integrated System, Abbott Laboratories, Lake Forest, IL, USA), with lower limits of sensitivity of 10 pg/ml for estradiol and 0.14 ng/mL for testosterone. Intra- and inter-assay CVs were 4.5% and 6.1% for estradiol, and 2.6% and 4.9% for testosterone, respectively. Protocols for both assays were performed as follows: Load reagents (estradiol/testosteron) onto the ARCHITECT i System. Mix calibrators and controls by gentle inversion prior to use. Hold bottles vertically and dispense 15 drops (400 µl) of each calibrator or 10 drops (250 µl) of each control into each respective sample cup. Load samples and press RUN. The ARCHITECT i System performs all mixing and reaction functions, incubation, washing, measurements and calculations.

Insulin resistance index (HOMA-IR). The index of insulin resistance, HOMA-IR, was calculated according to the following homeostasis model assessment (HOMA), as previously described [33]: HOMA-IR = FINS×FPG/22.5, where FINS is fasting insulin (µU/mL), and FPG is fasting plasma glucose level (mmol/l).

Statistical Analysis

Subjects' demographics and clinical characteristics were summarized as mean with standard deviation (mean±SD) for continuous data and n(%) for categorical data by group; differences between groups were compared using two-sample t-test for continuous data, Pearson Chi-square test for sex and Mann-Whitney U test for non-normally distributed data (Tanner criteria for stage of puberty). Correlations of apelin-12 levels with demographics and clinical characteristics were presented as coefficients of correlation (r) with respective P-values through partial correlation analysis after adjusting for age, sex, and BMI overall, and by adjusting for age and BMI in boys and girls separately. General linear regression analysis was performed to identify associations of apelin-12 levels with obesity-related markers by adjusting for age, sex, and BMI in groups overall, and by adjusting for age and BMI in boys and girls separately. Results were presented as estimated β with standard error (SE) and P-value. All statistical assessments were two-tailed and P<0.05 was set as statistical significance. All statistical analyses were performed using SPSS 17.0 statistics software (SPSS Inc, Chicago, IL, USA).

Results

A total of 88 subjects were enrolled in this study, including 48 subjects (20 girls/28 boys) in an obesity group and 40 subjects (16 girls/24 boys) in a non-obese control group. Average ages were 10.42 (SD = 2.03) years and 10.86 (SD = 2.23) years in the obesity group and control group, respectively. Table 1 summarizes subjects' demographics and clinical characteristics by groups overall and in males and females separately. Among all subjects, those in the obesity group had significantly higher TC, TG, LDL-C, insulin, and HOMA-IR (all P<0.05) than the control group. When males and females were analyzed separately, obese girls had significantly higher LDL-C, insulin, HOMA-IR, and apelin-12 than controls; obese boys had significantly higher TC, TG, insulin, and HOMA-IR than controls. No significant differences were found in apelin-12 levels between obese and non-obese groups. (Table 1).

Apelin-12 levels correlated positively with insulin (A), TG (B) and HOMA-IR (C) in girls, however apelin-12 levels were not correlated significantly with insulin, TG and HOMA-IR in boys (D–F) (Fig. 1). Table 2 represents partial correlation analysis of apelin-12 levels with other characteristics after adjusting for age, sex, and BMI in all subjects, and girls and boys in the obese and control groups separately, adjusting for age and BMI. In the obesity group overall, apelin-12 correlated positively with TG but no other significant correlations were found in either of the groups between apelin-12 levels and other characteristics after adjusting for age, sex, and BMI. Among females in the obese group, apelin-12 levels correlated positively with TG, insulin, and HOMA-IR after adjusting for age and BMI.

Table 3 shows results of general linear regression analysis of the association of apelin 12 levels with group effect, presenting subjects' characteristics after adjusting for age, sex and BMI. Apelin-12 levels increased as TG increased in all subjects and in girls alone [β(SE) = 0.336 (0.142) in all subjects, P = 0.021; β(SE) = 0.074(0.263) in boys, P = 0.780; β(SE) = 0.499 (0.129), P = 0.001 in girls]. When the data were segregated by gender, apelin-12 in obese girls was positively associated with TG, insulin, and HOMA-IR. [TG: β(SE) = 0.579 (0.143), P = 0.002; insulin: β(SE) = 0.056 (0.019), P = 0.008; β(SE) = 0.243 (0.088), P = 0.015]. In all male subjects (control and obesity groups), apelin-12 was

Table 1. Demographics and clinical characteristics of all subjects by obese and control groups and boys and girls separately.

Variables	Overall			Girls			Boys		
	Control (n = 40)	Obesity (n = 48)	P-value	Control (n = 16)	Obesity (n = 20)	P-value	Control (n = 24)	Obesity (n = 28)	P-value
Age, years	10.86±2.23	10.42±2.03	0.334	10.85±2.23	9.73±2.08	0.129	10.87±2.28	10.91±1.88	0.941
Sex			0.874						
Girls	16 (40%)	20 (41.7%)							
Boys	24 (60%)	28 (58.3%)							
BMI, Kg/m2	16.80±1.83	25.65±4.18	<.001*	16.76±2.21	24.02±3.90	<.001*	16.83±1.58	26.86±4.04	<.001*
Tanner stage			0.085			0.223			0.351
1	23 (57.5%)	18 (37.5%)		9 (56.3%)	6 (60%)		14 (58.3%)	12 (42.9%)	
2	7 (17.5%)	11 (22.9%)		1 (6.3%)	0 (0%)		6 (25%)	11 (39.3%)	
3	4 (10%)	11 (22.9%)		1 (6.3%)	8 (40%)		3 (12.5%)	3 (10.7%)	
4	4 (10%)	3 (6.3%)		3 (18.8%)	1 (5%)		1 (4.2%)	2 (7.1%)	
5	2 (5%)	5 (10.4%)		2 (12.5%)	5 (25%)		0 (0%)	0 (0%)	
TC, mmol/L	4.08±0.76	4.69±0.64	0.003*	4.37±0.36	4.77±0.74	0.097	3.92±0.88	4.63±0.55	0.007*
TG mmol/L	0.89±0.30	1.27±0.62	0.003*	1.14±0.32	1.30±0.75	0.613	0.75±0.20	1.25±0.51	<.001*
LDL-C, mmol/L	2.38±0.75	2.90±0.73	0.037*	2.34±0.55	3.11±0.71	0.041*	2.40±0.91	2.75±0.72	0.308
HDL-C mmol/L	1.56±0.23	1.46±0.57	0.579	1.58±0.25	1.39±0.24	0.149	1.54±0.23	1.52±0.73	0.930
Insulin, μU/ML	7.62±4.93	23.63±17.57	<.001*	7.48±4.03	16.09±7.63	<.001*	7.71±5.53	29.01±20.59	<.001*
FPG, mmol/L	4.86±0.52	4.80±0.54	0.593	4.65±0.36	4.58±0.62	0.683	5.01±0.57	4.96±0.42	0.745
HOMA-IR	1.72±1.10	4.73±3.17	<.001*	1.42±0.51	3.21±1.78	<.001*	1.91±1.33	5.80±3.50	<.001*
Apelin-12 level, ng/Ml	1.13±0.55	1.20±0.59	0.576	0.84±0.28	1.19±0.57	0.024*	1.31±0.60	1.20±0.61	0.537
Serum estradiol level	32.04±41.06	24.80±24.26	0.437	50.00±54.40	32.33±32.07	0.328	15.46±6.24	17.27±8.04	0.509
Serum testosterone level	1.08±1.62	0.65±0.69	0.181	0.47±0.77	0.53±0.46	0.762	1.51±1.92	0.72±0.80	0.123

BMI, body mass index; FPG, fasting plasma glucose; HOMA-IR, homeostasis model assessment of insulin resistance; HDL-C, high density lipoprotein cholesterol; LDL-C, low density lipoprotein cholesterol; TC, total cholesterol; TG, triglycerides.
Continuous data are summarized as mean±SD and categorical data as n (%); differences between the groups were compared using two-sample t-test for continuous data, Pearson Chi-square test for sex, and Mann-Whitney U test for Tanner stage.
*indicates significant difference between groups. (P<0.05).

1A

1B

1C

1D

1E

1F

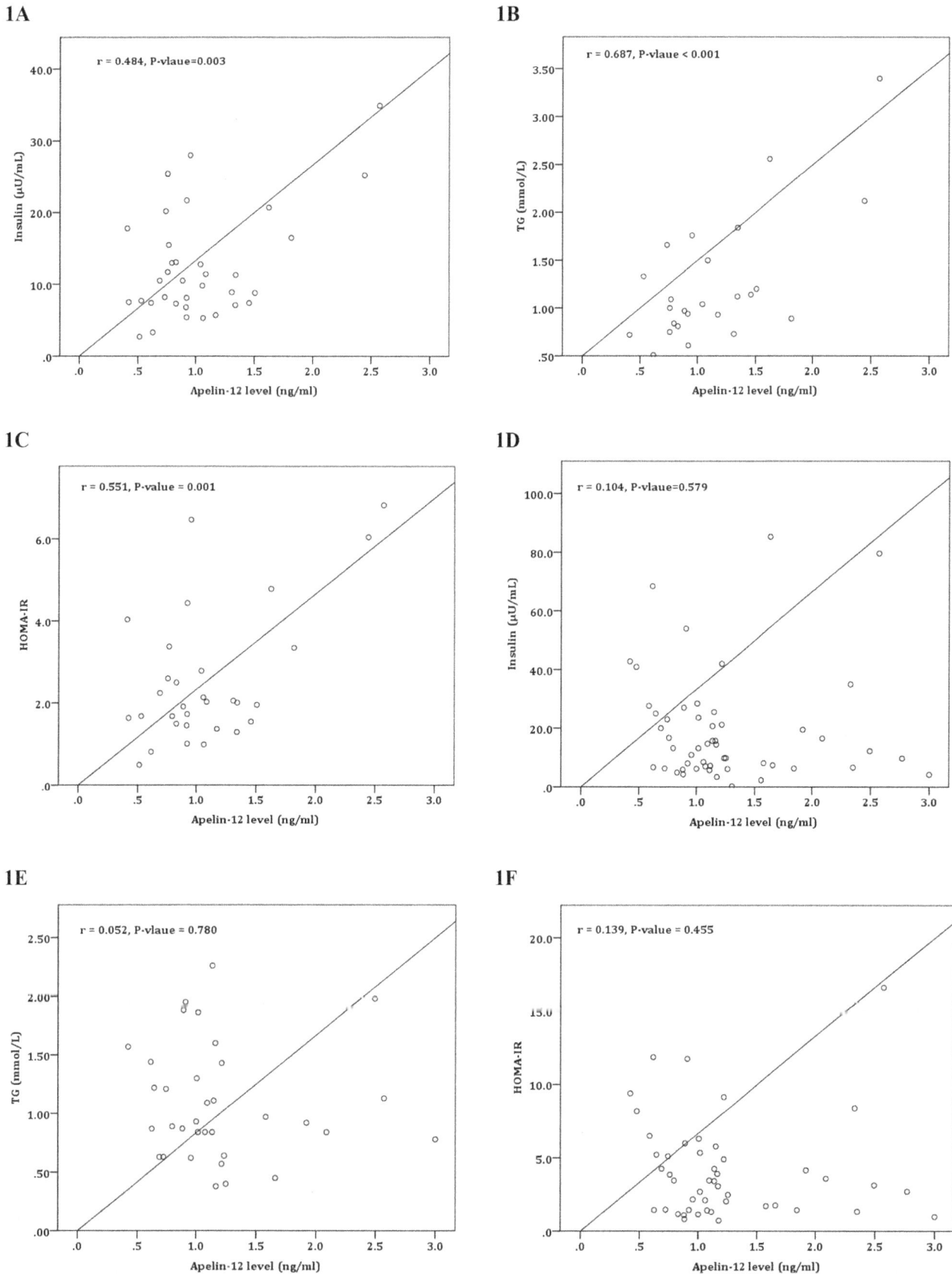

Figure 1. Associations between apelin levels, fasting insulin, triglycerides and HOMA-IR. Figure 1 depicts the association between apelin levels and (A) fasting insulin, (B) TG, and (C) HOMA-IR in female subjects and the association between apelin levels and (D) fasting insulin, (E) TG, and

(F) HOMA-IR in male subjects. Correlation coefficients with respective P-values are presented through partial correlation analysis after adjusting for age and BMI. The apelin levels were positively correlated with fasting insulin, TG, and HOMA-IR in females; No significant results were observed in males. TG, triglycerides; HOMA_IR, homeostasis model assessment of insulin resistance; BMI, body mass index.

positively associated with FPG. [β(SE) = 0.448(0.191), P = 0.024] (Table 3).

Correlation Analysis of Apelin in Obese and Nonobese Subjects

Correlation analysis of apelin-12 levels with anthropometric and biochemical indices, demonstrated significant correlations between apelin-12 and BMI-SDS, TG, FINS, and HOMA-IR in all girl subjects (obese and non-obese groups). No correlations were found between apelin-12 levels and estradiol and testosterone; no significant differences were found in estradiol and testosterone levels between girls and boys in both groups. In boys, FPG levels correlated positively with apelin-12 levels (Table 2). Stepwise linear regression analysis with apelin-12 as a dependent variable

Table 2. Correlation of apelin-12 levels with demographics and clinical characteristics by obesity and control groups, and boys and girls separately.

	Overall		Girls		Boys	
	r	P-value	r	P-value	r	P-value
Obesity group						
TC, mmol/L	0.162	0.337	0.121	0.642	0.194	0.427
TG mmol/L	0.436	0.006*	0.723	0.001*	0.003	0.728
LDL-C, mmol/L	0.165	0.351	−0.063	0.830	0.299	0.214
HDL-C mmol/L	−0.190	0.289	−0.387	0.172	−0.130	0.607
Insulin, μU/ML	0.186	0.226	0.600	0.008*	0.152	0.467
FPG, mmol/L	0.207	0.183	0.017	0.947	0.207	0.333
HOMA-IR	0.217	0.168	0.580	0.015*	0.130	0.546
Serum estradiol level	0.289	0.121	0.384	0.158	0.384	0.175
Serum testosterone level	−0.030	0.852	−0.386	0.140	−0.047	0.827
Control group						
TC, mmol/L	0.48	0.082	0.882	0.118	0.592	0.093
TG mmol/L	−0.058	0.843	0.833	0.167	−0.045	0.908
LDL-C, mmol/L	0.525	0.147	0.913	0.268	0.709	0.180
HDL-C mmol/L	0.104	0.633	−0.703	0.445	0.239	0.699
Insulin, μU/ML	−0.112	0.514	0.129	0.675	−0.130	0.565
FPG, mmol/L	0.385	0.037*	0.246	0.467	0.448	0.062
HOMA-IR	−0.066	0.733	0.094	0.796	0.13	0.546
Serum estradiol level	−0.152	0.500	−0.331	0.350	0.275	0.412
Serum testosterone level	0.075	0.718	0.393	0.261	0.034	0.904

BMI, body mass index; FPG, fasting plasma glucose; HOMA-IR, homeostasis model assessment of insulin resistance; HDL-C, high density lipoprotein cholesterol; LDL-C, low density lipoprotein cholesterol; TC, total cholesterol; TG, triglycerides.
Results are presented as coefficients of correlation (r) with respective P-value through partial correlation analysis after adjusting for age, sex, and BMI overall, and after adjusting for age and BMI in boys and girls separately.
*indicates significant correlation. (P<0.05).

and BMI-SDS, TG, FINS, and HOMA-IR as independent variables revealed that only TG was an important determinant of apelin-12 levels in female subjects. (Table 3).

Discussion

The present study analyzed the data of obese and non-obese children in Guangzhou, China, aiming to determine whether correlations could be found between apelin-12 levels of the groups and obesity in this population and to identify associations, if any, between apelin-12 and obesity-related markers, especially lipids, insulin sensitivity and insulin resistance index. In obese subjects, TC, TG, LDL-C, insulin, and HOMA-IR were significantly higher than in non-obese controls. When boys and girls were analyzed separately, altogether different results were shown: obese girls had significantly higher LDL-C, insulin, and HOMA-IR than controls; on the other hand, obese boys had significantly higher TC, TG, insulin, and HOMA-IR than controls. Notably, apelin-12 levels were significantly higher in obese girls compared to controls (p = 0.024). Age-, sex- and BMI-adjusted correlation analysis of apelin-12 levels with all other obesity-related factors revealed a positive correlation only between apelin-12 and TG, but no other significant correlations were found in either group between apelin-12 levels and the other characteristics. Most importantly, apelin-12 levels correlated positively with TG, insulin, and HOMA-IR in obese girls, indicating clinical significance although the mechanism remains to be explained. Also, linear regression analysis showed that apelin-12 levels increased as TG increased in all subjects and in girls alone, showing again that apelin-12 was positively associated with TG, insulin, and HOMA-IR. Among all boys in the control and obese groups, apelin-12 was positively associated with FPG only.

To the best of our knowledge, this is the first study on apelin-12 and obesity-related markers in children in China. Our results showed significantly higher TC, TG, LDL-C, insulin, and HOMA-IR in all obese subjects versus non-obese controls, but results vary among other international studies of apelin and obesity-related markers. Boucher et al. [17] reported increased plasma apelin levels in obese adult males and suggested further that, since adipose tissue is an important source of apelin production, and the expression of apelin and APJ both increase in adipose tissue in obese individuals, elevated serum apelin of obese subjects might be attributable to augmented adipose tissue. Minor changes in plasma apelin were associated with changes in BMI in obese subjects during 8-weeks of a very-low-calorie diet [34]. Those authors have suggested that apelin may not correlate as strongly with fat mass as with more abundant adipokines such as leptin and adiponectin. Li et al. [27] have found a correlation between apelin and BMI, and Heinonen et al. [35] have also found that apelin plasma concentration was significantly higher in morbidly obese patients compared to normal-weight controls. In contrast, Reinehr and colleagues (2011) evaluated apelin concentration, weight status, body fat, insulin resistance, leptin and obesity-related cardiovascular risk factors before and after one-year lifestyle intervention, demonstrating that weight loss in obese children was not associated with changes in apelin concentration as the authors have hypothesized, and no significant relationships were found between apelin, insulin resistance, cardiovascular risk factors and obesity in children [36]. Results of these studies

Table 3. Linear regression analysis of associations of apelin-12 levels with obesity-related markers.

Variables	Overall (Adjusted for age, sex, BMI)		Control group (Adjusted for age, sex, BMI)		Obesity group (Adjusted for age, sex, BMI)	
	β(SE)	P-value	β(SE)	P-value	β(SE)	P-value
Total (N = 88)						
Group						
Obesity	0.208 (0.224)	0.356	–		–	
Control	1					
Tanner stage	0.070 (0.073)	0.343	0.057 (0.115)	0.614	0.012 (0.112)	0.918
TC, mmol/L	0.178 (0.112)	0.118	0.399 (0.210)	0.082	0.146 (0.150)	0.973
TG mmol/L	0.336 (0.142)	0.021*	−0.161 (0.793)	0.843	0.415 (0.143)	0.006*
LDL-C, mmol/L	0.191 (0.112)	0.096	0.429 (0.263)	0.147	0.129 (0.136)	0.351
HDL-C mmol/L	−0.173 (0.169)	0.313	0.480 (0.967)	0.497	−0.186 (0.172)	0.289
Insulin, µU/ML	0.005 (0.005)	0.373	−0.012 (0.018)	0.514	0.007 (0.006)	0.226
FPG, mmol/L	0.303 (0.131)	0.024*	0.442 (0.193)	0.037*	0.215 (0.101)	0.183
HOMA-IR	0.035 (0.031)	0.267	−0.034 (0.100)	0.733	0.049 (0.035)	0.168
Serum estradiol level	0.002 (0.003)	0.382	−0.002 (0.002)	0.500	0.009 (0.005)	0.121
Serum testosterone level	0.041 (0.068)	0.547	0.030 (0.083)	0.718	−0.031 (0.163)	0.852
Boys (N = 52)						
Group						
Obesity	0.044 (0.336)	0.895				
Control	1					
Tanner stage	0.166 (0.140)	0.242	0.190 (0.224)	0.407	0.161 (0.200)	0.430
Total cholesterol, mmol/L	0.250 (0.154)	0.115	0.490 (0.252)	0.093	0.216 (0.265)	0.427
TG, mmol/L	0.074 (0.263)	0.780	−0.163 (1.354)	0.908	0.096 (0.273)	0.728
LDL-C, mmol/L	0.258 (0.148)	0.093	0.588 (0.337)	0.180	0.242 (0.187)	0.214
HDL-C mmol/L	−0.062 (0.196)	0.754	0.774 (1.821)	0.699	0.103 (0.196)	0.607
Insulin, µU/ML	0.003 (0.006)	0.587	−0.016 (0.027)	0.565	0.005 (0.006)	0.467
FPG, mmol/L	0.448 (0.191)	0.024*	0.533 (0.266)	0.062	0.301 (0.304)	0.333
HOMA-IR	0.017 (0.036)	0.644	−0.039 (0.130)	0.767	0.024 (0.039)	0.546
Serum estradiol level	0.038 (0.019)	0.056	0.027 (0.032)	0.412	0.041 (0.028)	0.175
Serum testosterone level	0.001 (0.087)	0.991	0.016 (0.131)	0.904	−0.043 (0.193)	0.827
Girls (N = 36)						
Group						
Obesity	0.182 (0.301)	0.549				
Control						
Tanner stage	−0.010 (0.088)	0.909	−0.049 (0.101)	0.638	−0.022 (0.131)	0.871
TC, mmol/L	0.099 (0.163)	0.548	0.354 (0.134)	0.118	0.091 (0.192)	0.642
TG, mmol/L	0.499 (0.129)	0.001*	0.465 (0.218)	0.167	0.579 (0.143)	0.002*
LDL-C, mmol/L	−0.022 (0.171)	0.898	0.312 (0.140)	0.268	−0.047 (0.214)	0.830
HDL-C mmol/L	−0.635 (0.522)	0.240	−0.659 (0.554)	0.445	−1.089 (0.750)	0.172
Insulin, µU/ML	0.035 (0.015)	0.027*	0.009 (0.022)	0.675	0.056 (0.019)	0.008*
FPG, mmol/L	0.076 (0.167)	0.654	0.208 (0.274)	0.467	0.018 (0.257)	0.947
HOMA-IR	0.210 (0.074)	0.009*	0.056 (0.210)	0.796	0.243 (0.088)	0.015*
Serum estradiol level	0.002 (0.003)	0.352	−0.002 (0.002)	0.350	0.007 (0.005)	0.158
Serum testosterone level	−0.056 (0.167)	0.743	0.140 (0.116)	0.261	−0.579 (0.370)	0.140

BMI, body mass index; FPG, fasting plasma glucose; HOMA-IR, homeostasis model assessment of insulin resistance; HDL-C, high density lipoprotein cholesterol; LDL-C, low density lipoprotein cholesterol; TC, total cholesterol; TG, triglycerides.
Results are presented as estimated β with standard error (SE) and P-value through general linear regression analysis after adjusting for age, sex, and BMI overall, and after adjusting for age and BMI in boys and girls separately.
*indicates significant association. ($P<0.05$).

indicate that agreement is still lacking on the relationship between apelin levels and obesity, especially in children.

Gender differences in relation to apelin-12 levels have not been fully explored or explained. Significantly lower apelin levels reported in pubertal obese children compared to normal-weight pubertal children suggests a link between sex hormones and apelin levels [37]. A study focused on gender differences of pubertal adiponectin levels in association with serum androgen levels found significantly reduced serum adiponectin concentration in boys, which was in parallel to physical and pubertal development compared to those adiponectin concentrations of age-matched female counterparts [38]. The decline was inversely related to testosterone and dehydroepiandrosterone sulfate levels, and the authors reported a strong association between adiponectin levels and obesity, pubertal development and metabolic parameters. The present study found significantly different results between boys and girls of the obese group: in this group, girls had significantly higher LDL-C, insulin, and HOMA-IR vs. controls while obese boys had significantly higher TC, TG, insulin and HOMA-IR vs. controls. Most importantly, apelin-12 levels were significantly higher in all obese female children vs. non-obese controls, which was not true for boys. Gender differences in our study require further investigations, however evidence pertaining to adioponectin and pubertal development sheds light on the differences between male and female apelin-12 levels and and its association with other biochemical parameters.

Correlations between apelin and insulin resistance, a major characteristic of obesity and type 2 diabetes, have been demonstrated by several authors. Erdem et al. [26] demonstrated a negative correlation with HOMA-IR in newly diagnosed type 2 diabetes mellitus. Tasci et al. [25] have reported a mild to moderate negative correlation between apelin and HOMA-IR in patients with elevated LDL-C. In contrast, Li et al. [27] described a positive correlation with HOMA-IR in patients with impaired glucose tolerance and type 2 diabetic subjects, and Hosoya et al. [18] have shown that plasma apelin levels increased markedly in insulin resistance and hyperinsulinemia. In the present study, HOMA-IR was significantly higher in all obese subjects compared to that in non-obese controls. Taken together, our results and those reported previously indicate that different associations between apelin and insulin resistance may depend on the extent of insulin resistance. Insulin resistance is common to both obesity and type 2 diabetes, and apelin is linked with obesity-associated variations of insulin sensitivity status [17]. In view of these associations, Castan-Laurell et al. [15] suggest that apelin may act as an insulin sensitizing agent and may be a potential target for diabetes treatment, that is, given its potent activity in energy metabolism and ability to improve insulin sensitivity.

In the present study, positive correlations were found between apelin-12 levels and TG, insulin, and HOMA-IR in obese girls. TG, as one of the components of metabolic syndrome, plays an important role in predicting impaired glucose tolerance in adolescents at risk for type 2 diabetes mellitus [39], and it has been suggested as a surrogate to identify insulin resistance in apparently healthy subjects [40]. In the present study, although we found a strong correlation between TG and serum apelin concentration in obese girls after adjusting for BMI and age, the relationship was insignificant in non-obese subjects, suggesting that the association may be more pronounced above a certain threshold determined by the extent of obesity, or that TG may affect apelin levels by inducing insulin resistance. Than et al. [41] proposed that apelin inhibits both adipogenesis and lipolysis through specific molecular pathways, acting through apelin APJ receptors expressed in adipocytes and resulting in decreased levels of free fatty acids in plasma and the release of free fatty acids from adipocytes. Yue et al. showed that mice deficient in apelin signaling also have increased circulating levels of free fatty acids and glycerol along with increased adiposity, and these effects can be reversed by exogenous apelin [42]. Since high levels of free fatty acid can lead to insulin resistance, this may help to explain the beneficial role of apelin in regulating metabolic homeostasis, although further study is needed to describe the underlying mechanism.

This study has some limitations, including that the data were cross-sectional and analyzed retrospectively from a relatively small cohort. Also, we did not investigate the mechanisms underlying apelin-12 levels in association with weight status and obesity-related markers. Further prospective studies with large samples are needed to clarify the role and mechanisms of apelin in association with obesity-related markers in a sub-population of obese children.

In conclusion, apelin-12 levels are significantly higher in obese female children in China compared to non-obese and correlate significantly with the obesity-related markers insulin, HOMA-IR and TG in this population. Increased apelin-12 levels may be involved in the pathological mechanism of obesity. Our results suggest beneficial effects of apelin in maintaining metabolic homeostasis and its potential clinical utility as a biomarker or therapeutic target.

Author Contributions

Conceived and designed the experiments: H-SC. Performed the experiments: H-JB. Analyzed the data: H-SC H-JB ZS M-LD. Wrote the paper: H-JB H-SC. Critical revision of the article: H-SC H-JB ZS M-LD Q-LC Y-HL H-MM.

References

1. Barlow SE, Expert Committee (2007) Expert Committee Recommendations Regarding the Prevention, Assessment, and Treatment of Child and Adolescent Overweight and Obesity: Summary Report. (suppl 4): 164–192.

2. Liu WJ, Lin R, Liu AL, Du L, Chen Q (2010) Prevalence and association between obesity and metabolic syndrome among Chinese elementary school children: a school-based survey. BMC Public Health 10: 780.

3. Rashid MN, Fuentes F, Touchon RC, Wehner PS (2003) Obesity and the risk for cardiovascular disease. Preventive Cardiology 6: 42–47.

4. Caprio S (2001) Insulin resistance in childhood obesity. Pediatric Endocrinology and Metabolism (suppl 1): 487–492.

5. Kwiterovich PO Jr (2008) Recognition and management of dyslipidemia in children and adolescents. Journal of Clinical Endocrinology and Metabolism 93: 4200–4209.

6. Weiss R, Kaufman FR (2008) Metabolic complications of childhood obesity: identifying and mitigating the risk. Diabetes Care 31 (Suppl 2): 310–316.

7. Arslanian S (2002) Type 2 diabetes in children: clinical aspects and risk factors. Hormone Research (Suppl 1): 19–28.

8. Mattsson N, Rönnemaa T, Juonala M, Viikari JS, Raitakari OT (2008) Childhood predictors of the metabolic syndrome in adulthood. The Cardiovascular Risk in Young Finns Study. Annals of Medicine 40(7): 254–252.

9. Pietrobelli A, Espinoza MC, De Cristofaro P (2008) Childhood obesity: looking into the future. Angiology (Suppl 2): 30–33.

10. Berg AH, Combs TP, Scherer PE (2002) ACRP30/adiponectin: an adipokine regulating glucose and lipid metabolism. Trends in Endocrinology and Metabolism 13: 84–89.

11. Steppan CM, Bailey ST, Bhat S, Brown EJ, Banerjee RR, et al. (2001) The hormone resistin links obesity to diabetes. Nature 409: 307–312.

12. Tatemoto K, Hosoya M, Habata Y, Fujii R, Kakegawa T, et al. (1998) Isolation and characterization of a novel endogenous peptide ligand for the human APJ receptor. Biochemical and Biophysical Research Communication 251: 471–476.

13. Lee DK, Cheng R, Nguyen T, Fan T, Kariyawasam AP, et al. (2000) Characterization of apelin, the ligand for the APJ receptor. Journal of Neurochemistry 74: 34–41.

14. Mesmin C, Fenaille F, Becher F, Tabet JC, Ezan E (2011) Identification and characterization of apelin peptides in bovine colostrum and milk by liquid

chromatography-mass spectrometry. Journal of Proteome Research 10: 5222–5231.

15. Castan-Laurell I, Dray C, Knauf C, Kunduzova O, Valet P (2012) Apelin, a promising target for type 2 diabetes treatment? Trends in Endocrinology and Metabolism 23: 234–241.

16. Tatemoto K, Takayama K, Zou MX, Kumaki I, Zhang W, et al. (2001) The novel peptide apelin lowers blood pressure via a nitric oxide-dependent mechanism. Regulatory Peptides 99: 87–92.

17. Boucher J, Masri B, Daviaud D, Gesta S, Guigné C, et al. (2005) Apelin, a newly identified adipokine up-regulated by insulin and obesity. Endocrinology 146: 1764–1771.

18. Hosoya M, Kawamata Y, Fukusumi S, Fujii R, Habata Y, et al. (2000) Molecular and functional characteristics of APJ. Tissue distribution of mRNA and interaction with the endogenous ligand apelin. Journal of Biological Chemistry 275: 21061–21067.

19. Szokodi I, Tavi P, Földes G, Voutilainen-Myllylä S, Iives M, et al. (2002) Apelin, the novel endogenous ligand of the orphan receptor APJ, regulates cardiac contractility. Circulation Research 91: 434–440.

20. Taheri S, Murphy K, Cohen M, Sujkovic E, Kennedy A, et al. (2002) The effects of centrally administered apelin-13 on food intake, water intake and pituitary hormone release in rats. Biochemical and Biophysical Research Communications 291: 1208–1212.

21. Reaux-Le Goazigo A, Alvear-Perez R, Zizzari P, Epelbaum J, BLuet-Pajot MT, et al. (2007) Cellular localization of apelin and its receptor in the anterior pituitary: evidence for a direct stimulatory action of apelin on ACTH release. American Journal of Physiology, Endocrinology, and Metabolism 292: E7–15.

22. Daviaud D, Boucher J, Gesta S, Dray C, Guigne C, et al. (2006) TNFalpha up-regulates apelin expression in human and mouse adipose tissue. The Okodi FASEB Journal 20: 1528–1530.

23. Kralisch S, Lossner U, Bluher M, Paschke R, Stumvoll M, et al. (2007) Growth hormone induces apelin mRNA expression and secretion in mouse 3T3-L1 adipocytes. Regulatory Peptides 139: 84–89.

24. Wei L, Hou X, Tatemoto K (2005) Regulation of apelin mRNA expression by insulin and glucocorticoids in mouse 3T3-L1 adipocytes. Regulatory Peptides 132: 27–32.

25. Tasci I, Dogru T, Naharci I, Erdem G, Yilmaz MI, et al. (2007) Plasma apelin is lower in patients with elevated LDL-cholesterol. Experimental and Clinical Endocrinology & Diabetes 115: 428–432.

26. Erdem G, Dogru T, Tasci I, Sonmez A, Tapan S (2008) Low plasma apelin levels in newly diagnosed type 2 diabetes mellitus. Experimental and Clinical Endocrinology & Diabetes 116: 289–292.

27. Li L, Yang G, Li Q, Tang Y, Yang M, et al. (2006) Changes and relations of circulating visfatin, apelin, and resistin levels in normal, impaired glucose tolerance, and type 2 diabetic subjects. Experimental and Clinical Endocrinology & Diabetes 114: 544–548.

28. Machura E, Szczepanska M, Ziora K, Ziora D, Swietochowska E, et al. Evaluation of adipokines: apelin, visfatin, and resistin in children with atopic dermatitis. Mediators of Inflammation 2013; doi10.1155/2013/760691.

29. Cekmez F, Cekmez Y, Pirgon O, Canpolat FE, Aydoniz S, et al. (2011) Evaluation of new adipocytokines and insulin resistance in adolescents with polycystic ovary syndrome. European Cytokine Network 22: 32–37.

30. Ji CY, Ma J, He ZH, Chen TJ, Song Y, et al. (2010) [Reference norms of waist circumference for Chinese school age children and adolescents]. Chinese Journal of School Health 2010; 31: 257–259. Article in Chinese.

31. Zannolli R, Morgese G (1996) Waist percentiles: a simple test for atherogenic disease? Acta Paediatrics 85: 1368–1369.

32. Tanner JM (1981)Growth and maturation during adolescence. Nutrition Review 39: 43–55.

33. Ten S, Maclaren N (2004) Insulin resistance syndrome in children. Journal of ClinicalEndocrinology & Metabolism 2004; 89: 2526–2539.

34. Heinonen MV, Lääksönen DE, Karhu T, Karhunen L, Laitinen T, et al. (2009) Effect of diet-induced weight loss on plasma apelin and cytokine levels in individuals with the metabolic syndrome. Nutrition Metabolism and Cardio-vascular Disease 2009; Mar 9. [Epub ahead of print].

35. Heinonen MV, Purhonen AK, Miettinen P, Pääkkönen M, Pirinen E, et al. (2005) Apelin, orexin-A and leptin plasma levels in morbid obesity and effect of gastric banding. Regulatory Peptides 130: 7–13.

36. Reinehr T, Woelfle J, Roth CL (2011) Lack of association between apelin, insulin resistance, cardiovascular risk factors, and obesity in children: a longitudinal analysis. Metabolism Clinical and Experimental 60: 1349–1354.

37. Tapan S, Tacilar E, Abaci A, Sonmez A, Kilic S, et al. (2010) Decreased plasma apelin levels in pubertal obese children. Journal of Pediatric Endocrinology & Metabolism 23: 1039–1046.

38. Böttner A, Katzsch J. Müller G, Kapellen TM, Blüher S, et al. (2004) Gender differences of adiponectin levels develop during the progression of puberty and are related to serum androgen levels. Journal of Clinical Endocrinology & Metabolism 89: 4053–4061.

39. Love-Osborne K, Butler N, Gao D, Zeitler P (2006) Elevated fasting triglycerides predict impaired glucose tolerance in adolescents at risk for type 2 diabetes. Pediatric Diabetes 7: 205–210.

40. Simental-Mendía LE, Rodríguez-Morán M, Guerrero-Romero F (2008) The product of fasting glucose and triglycerides as surrogate for identifying insulin resistance in apparently healthy subjects. Metabolic Syndrome and Related Disorders 6: 299–304.

41. Than A, Chen Y, Foh LC, Leow MKS, Lim SC, et al. (2012) Apelin inhibits adipogenesis and lipolysis through distinct molecular pathways. Molecular and Cellular Endocrinology 362: 227–241.

42. Yue P, Jin H, Xu S, Allaud M, Deng AC, et al. (2011) Apelin decreases lipolysis via G_q G_1 and AMPK-dependent mechanisms. Energy Balance–Obesity 152: 59–68.

Waist Circumference Independently Associates with the Risk of Insulin Resistance and Type 2 Diabetes in Mexican American Families

Manju Mamtani*, Hemant Kulkarni, Thomas D. Dyer, Laura Almasy, Michael C. Mahaney, Ravindranath Duggirala, Anthony G. Comuzzie, John Blangero, Joanne E. Curran

Department of Genetics, Texas Biomedical Research Institute, San Antonio, Texas, United States of America

Abstract

Objective: In spite of the growing recognition of the specific association of waist circumference (WC) with type 2 diabetes (T2D) and insulin resistance (IR), current guidelines still use body mass index (BMI) as a tool of choice. Our objective was to determine whether WC is a better T2D predictor than BMI in family-based settings.

Research Design and Methods: Using prospectively collected data on 808 individuals from 42 extended Mexican American families representing 7617.92 person-years follow-up, we examined the performance of WC and BMI as predictors of cumulative and incident risk of T2D. We used robust statistical methods that accounted for the kinships and included polygenic models, discrete trait modeling, Akaike information criterion, odds ratio (OR), relative risk (RR) and Kullback-Leibler R^2. SOLAR software was used to conduct all the data analyses.

Results: We found that in multivariate polygenic models, WC was an independent predictor of cumulative (OR = 2.76, p = 0.0002) and future risk of T2D (RR = 2.15, p = 3.56×10^{-9}) and outperformed BMI when compared in a head-to-head fashion. High WC ($\geq$94.65 cm after adjusting for age and sex) was also associated with high fasting glucose, insulin and triglyceride levels and low high-density lipoprotein levels indicating a potential association with IR. Moreover, WC was specifically and significantly associated with insulin resistant T2D (OR = 4.83, p = 1.01×10^{-13}).

Conclusions: Our results demonstrate the value of using WC as a screening tool of choice for future risk of T2D in Mexican American families. Also, WC is specifically associated with insulin resistant T2D.

Editor: Raffaella Buzzetti, Sapienza, University, Italy

Funding: This work was supported in part by National Institutes of Health (NIH) grants R01 DK082610 and R01 DK079169. Data collection for the San Antonio Family Heart Study was supported by NIH grant R01 HL045522. The development of the analytical methods and software used in this study was supported by NIH grant R37 MH059450. The AT&T Genomics Computing Center supercomputing facilities used for this work were supported in part by a gift from the AT&T Foundation and with support from the National Center for Research Resources Grant Number S10 RR029392. This investigation was conducted in facilities constructed with support from Research Facilities Improvement Program grants C06 RR013556 and C06 RR017515 from the National Center for Research Resources of the National Institutes of Health. The funders had no role in study design, data collection and analysis, decision to publish, or preparation of the manuscript.

Competing Interests: The authors have declared that no competing interests exist.

* E-mail: mmamtani@txbiomedgenetics.org

Introduction

The prevalence of Type 2 diabetes (T2D) is rapidly increasing worldwide.1–3] This upsurge is concomitant with the sudden global increase in the prevalence of obesity, an established risk factor in the pathogenesis of T2D.4–7] This concomitance indicates that the operationally easy-to-measure and accurate anthropometric indexes that characterize obesity may also closely associate with the risk of T2D and may therefore be used for the screening of T2D. Such a public health intervention can be expected to augment the programmatic yield of T2D detection strategies and provide more opportunities for effective prevention and control of T2D. Indeed, current guidelines by various agencies like the WHO, ADA and German Diabetes Society (Deutsche Diabetes Gesellschaft, DDG) recommend body mass index (BMI) as the primary screening anthropometric index for T2D.8]

There is now a growing recognition that central rather than general obesity is more contributory to and therefore better correlates with the risk of T2D.9–13] Interestingly, BMI is an indicator of generalized obesity while waist circumference (WC) shows an excellent correlation with central obesity.13,14] Thus, WC should be theoretically more useful than BMI to predict the risk of T2D. In this context, we 15] and others have demonstrated the superiority of WC over BMI for screening of T2D in epidemiological settings.16–19] Such a paradigmatic shift from the use of BMI to WC for screening of T2D entails that the screening efficacy of WC should also be demonstrated in other settings such as family studies. This is important since WC has been shown to be a highly heritable trait 20–22]. In this regard, Gao et al. 23] have recently shown that using WC as a monitoring tool for T2D may be beneficial in family settings. Additional studies are required that robustly demonstrate the screening performance of WC in family studies across the world. Further, the relative importance of BMI and WC in screening for T2D risk in the families is unknown.

We conducted this study with the following research questions: 1) Is WC associated with an increased risk of current or future T2D and its related traits in pedigreed Mexican American individuals; and 2) Is WC better than BMI for predicting T2D risk? To answer these two questions, we used the rich resource of Mexican American subjects enrolled in the San Antonio Family Heart Study (SAFHS) and examined the absolute and relative performance of WC for the prediction of T2D in family settings.

Materials and Methods

Ethics Statement

Informed written consent was obtained from all participants before collection of samples. The Institutional Review Board of the University of Texas Health Sciences Center at San Antonio approved the study.

Study subjects

The SAFHS is an ongoing endeavor that focuses on 1,431 members of 42 large and extended Mexican American families in San Antonio. Details of this study have been described elsewhere.[24,25] Briefly, this collaborative research effort involving the Texas Biomedical Research Institute and the University of Texas Health Science Center at San Antonio began in 1991 and currently includes data on ~2000 individuals. The SAFHS aims to quantify the relative contributions of genetic and environmental factors to the risk of developing cardiovascular diseases and metabolic syndrome. Extensive phenotypic assessment for a number of traits related to metabolic syndrome has been performed in these individuals. As a part of this study, the participants were also followed up prospectively. Currently data for the baseline and two follow-up visits is available. We used this prospectively collected data for the longitudinal component of this study.

Outcomes and predictors

We studied three primary outcomes: cumulative risk of T2D, risk of incident T2D and risk of future insulin resistance (IR). Cumulative risk of T2D was defined as concurrent existence or future development of T2D. T2D was diagnosed according to American Diabetes Association criteria.[26] Participants who reported to be under treatment with either oral anti-diabetic agents or insulin, or who gave a history of diabetes were also considered to have T2D. Incident T2D was defined as detection of new cases of T2D during follow-up. IR was measured by the Homeostasis Model of Assessment–Insulin Resistance (HOMA-IR). The HOMA-IR was estimated as follows – fasting glucose (mmol/L) x fasting insulin (µU/ml)/22.5.[27] For defining IR we used HOMA-IR cut-points of 2.6 (the commonly used clinical cut-point for IR) and 3.8 (as specifically recommended for Mexican-American populations).[28] We also examined associations with several T2D-related traits as secondary outcomes. These included fasting glucose, fasting glucose adjusted for anti-diabetic drug use, serum insulin, triglycerides, total serum cholesterol, high density lipoprotein cholesterol (HDL-C), directly measured low density lipoprotein cholesterol (LDL-C), LDL-C fraction 1 and LDL-C fraction 2. Blood samples were obtained after a 12-hour fast for measurement of various phenotypes including glucose, total cholesterol, triglycerides, LDL and HDL cholesterol, and they were collected again 2 h after a standardized oral glucose load to measure plasma glucose. All the secondary outcomes and insulin resistance were assessed prospectively at the second follow-up visit.

We examined the association of the following 15 anthropometric indexes with one or more of the aforementioned outcomes. The anthropometric indexes included skin-fold thicknesses (biceps, triceps, forearm, subscapular, abdominal, suprailiac, medial calf and lateral calf), waist and hip circumferences, weight, height and three composite indexes: BMI, waist/hip ratio (WHR) and subscapular/triceps ratio (STR). Methods for measurements of these indexes have been described previously.[22,25]

Statistical analysis

We used univariate and multivariate polygenic models to study the association of various anthropometric indexes with cumulative risk of T2D. All the polygenic models used in this study were of the form:

$$O_i = m + \sum b_k a_{ik} + g_i + e_i$$

where, O is the outcome of interest; m is the trait mean; a is the covariate vector of dimension k with b as the corresponding regression coefficients; g is the polygenic effect and e is the residual error for an individual indexed by i. In all of these models we included age, age^2, age*sex, age^2*sex and sex as covariates. For univariate analyses the polygenic models included the above-mentioned covariates and each anthropometric index separately. Model fits were compared using log-likelihoods (for all outcomes) and the Kullback-Leibler R^2 (K-L R^2, for dichotomous outcomes only). For multivariate analyses, all the anthropometric indexes were simultaneously included in a single model along with the abovementioned covariates. However, since WHR is highly correlated with WC by definition, we could not use a single multivariate model including all the composite indexes (BMI, WHR and STR) as covariates. Instead, we ran univariate polygenic models for each of these indexes and then compared the model fits using K-L R^2. For comparing regression coefficients of different indexes, we estimated the standardized regression coefficient for each index as the regression coefficient divided by its standard error.

Statistical significance of the regression coefficient estimated from a polygenic model was determined by constraining the regression coefficient to zero, estimating the difference in log-likelihoods between the constrained and unconstrained models and applying a chi-square test. For dichotomous outcomes, the discrete trait modeling procedure was used. The odds ratio (OR) of a dichotomous outcome was determined as $e^{-\sqrt{\pi}\beta}$ since the SOLAR software [29] returns a negative regression coefficient from a probit model for a positively associated covariate.

For ease of clinical usage, we estimated the optimal cut-point for WC as a predictor of the cumulative risk of T2D. We dichotomized WC by sliding cut-points over the observed range. At each cut-point we used age and sex adjusted polygenic models with the dichotomized WC as a covariate. From each model we determined the Akaike Information Criterion (AIC) [estimated as -2×Loglikelihood – 2*(number of fitted parameters)] and the OR. The optimal cut-point was estimated as that at which the AIC was minimum and OR was maximum. SOLAR software was employed in all the statistical analyses and statistical significance was assessed at a type I error rate of 0.05.

Results

Study subjects

We studied 808 participants from 42 extended Mexican American families on whom data for various metabolic, anthropometric and demographic variables was available. One hundred and seventy eight (22.02%) subjects developed T2D by visit 3 of whom 100 subjects were detected as new diabetes cases during follow-up. The total length of follow-up was 7617.92 person-years, translating to an incidence rate of 13.13 T2D cases/1000 population/year. The mean age of the study sample was 37.0 (SD = 14.39) years and there were 292 (36.1%) males. Prevalence of insulin resistance was 74.6% based on a HOMA-IR cut-off of 2.6 and 56.1% using a cut-off of 3.8.

Anthropometric indexes and cumulative risk of T2D

We first studied the associations of various anthropometric indexes like skin-fold thicknesses (biceps, triceps, forearm, subscapular, abdominal, suprailiac, medial calf and lateral calf), waist and hip circumferences, and weight and height with the cumulative risk of T2D (Table 1). We used univariate and multivariate polygenic regression models adjusting for age, sex and their interaction to evaluate these associations. In univariate polygenic analyses, all the anthropometric indexes except lateral calf thickness and height were independently and significantly associated with the cumulative risk of T2D (Table 1). Interestingly, WC showed the strongest association with the cumulative risk of T2D ($\beta = -0.4761$, $p = 4.30 \times 10^{-14}$). In the multivariate polygenic model (i.e. including all the anthropometric indexes in the single model), we observed that only biceps skinfold thickness, lateral calf skinfold thickness and WC were significantly associated with the cumulative risk of T2D (Table 1). Notably, the strength of association of WC with cumulative risk of T2D increased in the multivariate context as compared to that in the univariate context ($\beta = -0.5746$ and -0.4761; OR = 2.76 and 2.32 for multivariate and univariate models, respectively).

WC as a predictor of future T2D

As WC was strongly associated with the cumulative risk of T2D, we next assessed whether WC can also predict the future risk of T2D. For this we studied the association of WC with the incident cases of T2D (new cases during follow-up) using the polygenic model. Indeed, WC was also significantly associated with an increased risk of incident T2D [$\beta = -0.43$, RR (95% CI) = 2.15 (1.64–2.82) $p = 3.56 \times 10^{-9}$]. Thus WC was not only associated with the cumulative risk of T2D but also predicted the future risk of T2D.

Comparison of WC with composite anthropometric indexes

Subsequently, we compared the performance of WC with other composite anthropometric indexes like BMI, WHR and STR for predicting the cumulative risk of T2D using univariate polygenic models. We observed that the K-L R^2 values for WC, BMI, WHR and STR were 0.20, 0.18, 0.19 and 0.13, respectively. The standardized regression coefficients (p) for these indexes were -7.1034 (4.20×10^{-14}), -6.3093 (2.44×10^{-11}), -6.5005 (9.17×10^{-13}) and -2.2081 (0.0456), respectively. Importantly, WC was strongly correlated with the cumulative T2D risk. However, the heritability of WC was marginally lower than that of BMI (0.54 versus 0.56).

To address our second research question, we further compared the associative performance of WC and BMI in a head-to-head fashion. In a multivariate polygenic model we included both WC and BMI as correlates of cumulative T2D risk. To ensure that these analyses were not influenced by potential collinearity between WC and BMI, we first estimated the total phenotypic correlation between these two traits. For this reason, we used

bivariate trait analyses in which the kinship structure, age, sex and their interactions were accounted for. We found that 23.29% of the model variance was unique and not accounted for by the phenotypic correlation between WC and BMI, thus mitigating the possible influence of collinearity on our results. We estimated from the polygenic model that WC (standardized $\beta = -3.67$, $p = 0.0002$) was a more powerful predictor of cumulative T2D risk than BMI (standardized $\beta = -0.09$, $p = 0.9269$). Moreover, when we compared the performance of WC and BMI for predicting the future risk of T2D in a multivariate polygenic model, we observed that WC [standardized $\beta = -7.29$, RR (95% CI) = 2.12 (1.65–2.71) $p = 0.0066$] was a better and stronger predictor of incident T2D than BMI [standardized $\beta = -0.41$, RR (95% CI) = 1.05 (0.84–1.32) $p = 0.8480$].

Determination of the optimal cut-point for WC

We aimed to find an age- and sex-adjusted cut-point that can simply yet informatively dichotomize WC as a correlate of the cumulative T2D risk. The best cut-point (as indicated by the minimum AIC of 669.05) in this population was 94.65 cm (Figure 1). At this cut-point the OR (95% CI) for cumulative T2D risk was 4.53 (2.98–6.87). Interestingly, another peak in OR was observed at a WC cut-point of 118.5 cm. While this peak could be construed as representing a cut-point for males, we found that the AIC at this cut-off was quite high (698.55) as compared to that for the gender-nonspecific cut-point of 94.65 cm.

Arguably, use of a gender-agnostic cut-point may lose diagnostic information as compared to the strategy of using a gender-specific cut-point. To directly contrast these two strategies, we compared the predictive performance of the gender-agnostic cut-point with that of the recommended gender-specific WC cut-points for the US population (≥ 102 cm for males and ≥ 88 cm for females).[30] We found that the strategy of using a single cut-point demonstrated predictive performance comparable to the strategy of using the gender-specific cut-points (AIC of 669.05 versus 658.25, that is an information loss of 1.6% due to gender-agnostic cut-point). Moreover, the OR for T2D risk associated with the single cut-point strategy (4.53) was better than that associated with the strategy of gender-specific cut-points (3.98).

Association of dichotomized WC with T2D-related traits

We observed that dichotomized WC was significantly associated with high fasting glucose ($\beta = 0.5251$, $p = 3.81 \times 10^{-14}$), fasting glucose adjusted for anti-diabetic drug use ($\beta = 0.3659$, $p = 2.64 \times 10^{-8}$), high serum insulin ($\beta = 0.6025$, $p = 5.44 \times 10^{-11}$), high triglycerides ($\beta = 0.3422$, $p = 2.38 \times 10^{-5}$) and low HDL-C ($\beta = -0.3142$, $p = 0.0001$) (Figure 2). Only 1.8% of study subjects were receiving lipid-lowering drugs, and adjustment for the use of these drugs did not alter the results significantly (Table S1).

Association of dichotomized WC with IR and insulin resistant T2D

The abovementioned associations are interesting because high fasting glucose, high serum insulin, high triglycerides and low HDL-C are all indicators of insulin resistance.[31,32] Therefore, we next assessed whether dichotomized WC is associated with IR in general and insulin resistant T2D (defined as presence of IR as well as T2D) in particular. We observed that dichotomized WC was highly predictive of both IR and insulin resistant T2D (Figure 3). Interestingly, dichotomized WC strongly predicted T2D with HOMA-IR >3.8 [$\beta = -0.8902$, OR (95% CI) = 4.83 (3.12–7.49), $p = 1.01 \times 10^{-13}$, Figure 3].

Table 1. Univariate and multivariate association of anthropometric indexes with cumulative risk of T2D.

Anthropometric Index	Univariate Analysis			Multivariate Analysis		
	B	OR (95% CI)	P	β	OR (95% CI)	P
Skinfold Thickness						
Biceps	−0.3795	1.96 (1.52–2.52)	5.83×10^{-9}	−0.3842	1.97 (1.19–3.28)	0.0083
Forearm	−0.1795	1.37 (1.10–1.71)	0.0041	0.1711	0.74 (0.48–1.13)	0.1588
Triceps	−0.2345	1.51 (1.18–1.94)	0.0007	0.0999	0.84 (0.53–1.33)	0.4469
Subscapular	−0.3420	1.83 (1.47–2.29)	2.75×10^{-8}	−0.0925	1.18 (0.79–1.76)	0.4210
Abdominal	−0.3072	1.72 (1.36–2.17)	6.79×10^{-7}	0.1790	0.73 (0.47–1.14)	0.1560
Suprailiac	−0.3949	2.01 (1.59–2.54)	4.38×10^{-10}	−0.1341	1.27 (0.76–2.12)	0.3549
Medail Calf	−0.1672	1.34 (1.08–1.67)	0.0073	−0.0456	1.08 (0.69–1.69)	0.7196
Lateral Calf	0.0117	0.98 (0.94–1.02)	0.851	0.3676	0.52 (0.35–0.77)	0.0008
Circumferences						
Waist	−0.4761	2.32 (1.84–2.93)	4.30×10^{-14}	−0.5746	2.76 (1.59–4.81)	0.0002
Hip	−0.3410	1.83 (1.46–2.30)	2.89×10^{-8}	0.2734	0.62 (0.33–1.16)	0.1232
Others						
Weight	−0.3828	1.97 (1.58–2.46)	4.52×10^{-10}	−0.2439	1.54 (0.78–3.06)	0.2144
Height	0.0208	0.96 (0.72–1.29)	0.8061	0.1595	0.75 (0.51–1.11)	0.1501

β, regression coefficient; OR, odds ratio; CI, confidence interval; p, significance value

The definition of HOMA-IR used in our study did not consider the concurrent use of anti-diabetic agents. To safeguard against the potential confounding due to this, we repeated the above-mentioned analyses by adjusting for the use of anti-diabetic drugs. Our results still concurred with earlier interpretations (compare the purple and red bars in Figure 3).

Discussion

Our results clearly demonstrate that WC is the strongest anthropometric index that associates with insulin resistance and T2D in Mexican American families whether examined longitudi-

nally or cumulatively. Irrespective of age and gender, WC exceeding 94.65 cm was most informative with regard to a cumulative risk of T2D. Of note, in univariate or multivariate contexts, WC was more strongly related to cumulative or incident risk of T2D as compared to BMI. The implications of our results need to be considered in the light of three important aspects of research related to metabolic syndrome and T2D.

First, there is an ongoing debate on the use of WC or BMI in screening programs for early detection of T2D.8,33] Various clinical guidelines primarily favor the use of BMI in screening programs, while a recent meta-analysis 33] indicates that BMI and

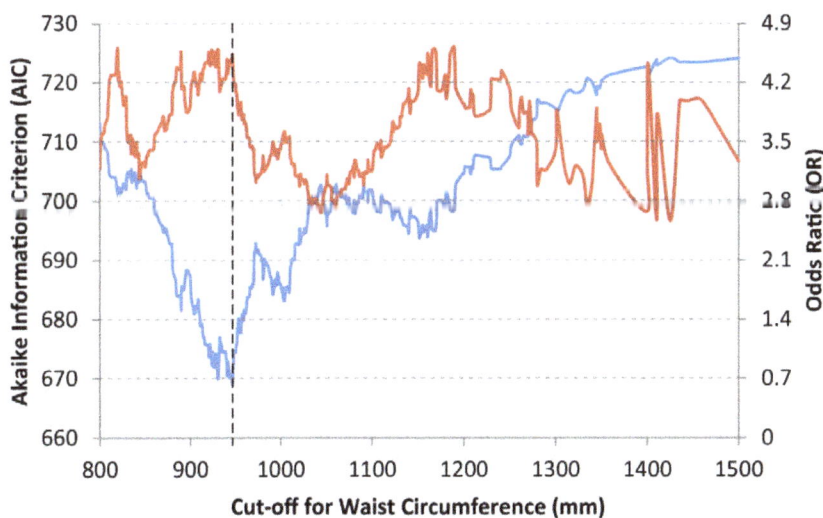

Figure 1. Determination of the optimal cut-point for waist circumference as a predictor of cumulative T2D risk. Figure shows Akaike information criterion (left y-axis) and odds ratio (right y-axis) for a cut-point of waist circumference indicated on the x-axis. Dashed vertical line indicates the optimal cut-point.

T2D-related traits	Polygenic regression coefficient	Statistical Significance
Fasting glucose		3.81×10^{-14}
Fasting glucose adjusted for antidiabetic drug use		2.64×10^{-8}
Serum Insulin		5.44×10^{-11}
Triglycerides		2.38×10^{-5}
Total serum cholesterol		0.4252
High density lipoprotein cholesterol (HDL-C)		0.0001
Low density lipoprotein cholesterol directly measured (LDL-C)		0.3423
Low density lipoprotein cholesterol fraction 1 (LDL-C f1)		0.3386
Low density lipoprotein cholesterol fraction 2 (LDL-C f2)		0.4117

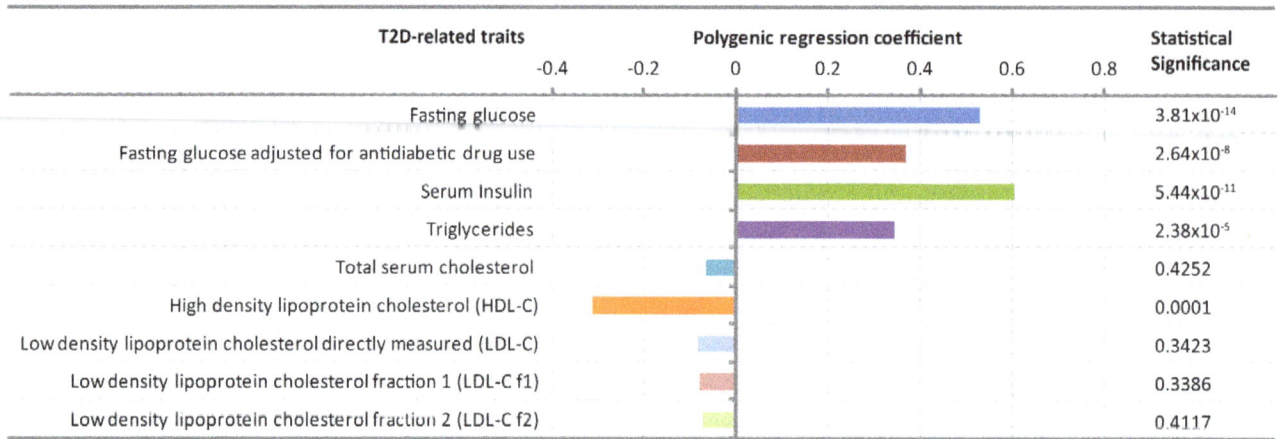

Figure 2. Association of dichotomized WC with T2D-related traits. The bars represent regression coefficients estimated using polygenic regression models.

WC can be used interchangeably since they have similar predicting abilities for future risk of T2D. On the other hand, there is now a growing recognition that WC may be more suited than BMI as a predictor of T2D risk.34] Studies in various populations 15,18,35] have demonstrated the superiority of WC over BMI in this regard. Our findings support the view that WC should be used in screening programs instead of BMI because 1)

WC is strongly associated with the risk of both prevalent and incident T2D; 2) WC is also an indicator of insulin resistance (irrespective of the presence of T2D) and insulin resistant T2D (i.e. insulin resistance with the presence of T2D); 3) In a single multivariate model WC outperformed BMI as a predictor of cumulative as well as incident risk of T2D; and 4) In spite of its high heritability WC still independently predicted the risk of T2D

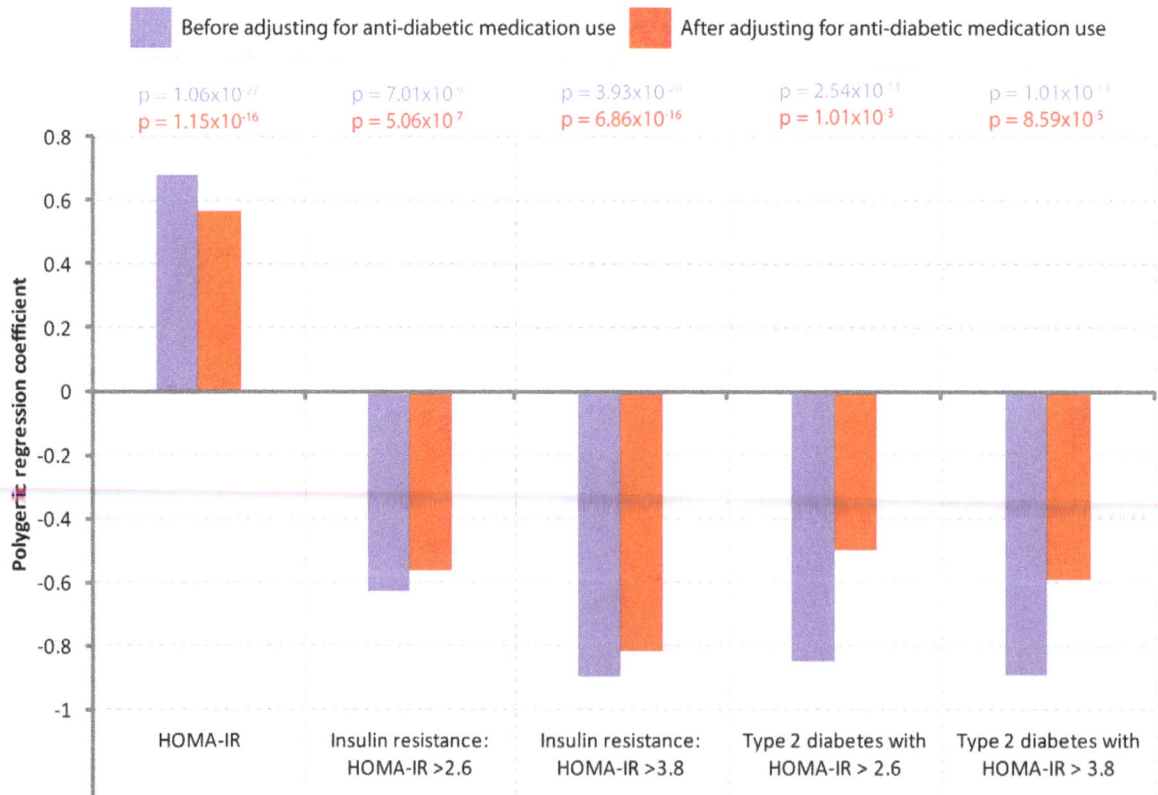

Figure 3. Association of dichotomized WC with IR and insulin resistant T2D. The bars represent regression coefficients estimated using polygenic regression models. Results are shown before (purple bars) and after (red bars) adjusting for the use of antidiabetic medication which includes the oral antidiabetic drugs as well as insulin. Statistical significance of a regression coefficient is shown in color-coded fashion at the top of the graph.

in pedigreed Mexican American families. Moreover, WC is as simple, convenient, inexpensive and easy to use in clinical practice as BMI and it can be easily monitored by patients themselves. For these reasons we believe that reevaluation of existing guidelines for screening of T2D is needed.

Second, the role of WC for prediction of T2D risk in families has been understudied. To our knowledge, a prospective evaluation of the importance of WC in diabetes pathogenesis in extended pedigrees has not been studied. Our results therefore proffer novel evidence in that regard. Since use of families as units can improve outcomes of diabetes screening programs,36] our findings point towards the possibility of further refining such strategies by inclusion of WC as the primary screen. WC is one of the requirements for the diagnosis of metabolic syndrome and the International Diabetes Federation (IDF) recommends that WC cut-points specific for different populations are needed.30] Our results demonstrate that an age-, sex-adjusted cut-point of 94.65 cm was highly informative in this ethnic population. While the generalizability of this cut-point remains limited, it is noteworthy that the optimal WC cut-point observed in this study for the prediction of T2D risk is practically close to the average of the recommended gender specific cut-points (102 cm for males and 88 cm for females) for the diagnosis of metabolic syndrome.30] This would therefore indicate that the recommended WC cut-point for the diagnosis of metabolic syndrome might also be useful for predicting the future risk of T2D. Further, our results suggest that use of a single population-specific WC cut-point may be at least as informative as gender-specific cut-points.

Third, we found that WC was specifically associated with future risk of insulin resistance as well as insulin resistant T2D. WC is associated with IR since it closely associates with visceral obesity, which is a critical determinant of IR. Indeed, WC in itself is considered to be a strong predictor of visceral fat.12] Mechanistically, increased secretion of free fatty acids and inflammatory cytokines combined with decreased secretion of adiponectin orchestrate in the multivariate culmination in visceral obesity and insulin resistance.37] At the level of the adipocyte, hyperinsulinaemia characteristic of IR activates 11-hydroxysteroid dehydrogenase in the omental adipose tissue and is followed by release of active cortisol. These changes induce a cushingoid fat distribution and increase in WC.38] Our observations afford a strong support to these biological underpinnings. Recent past has seen an accretion of epidemiological evidence that bolsters the

associative/causal link between WC and IR. However, prospective family-based studies that show such a link have generally been lacking.

The clear strengths of our approach are a family-based prospective study design, an ethnically homogenous sample, a large sample size, extensive follow-up data and robust statistical methods. However, our study suffers from limitations inherent in any observational study of this type. First, the attrition rate in the present study was 33.1%, which is slightly higher than that seen in typical prospective studies. Since information on metabolic syndrome related traits was not available for the individuals who did not complete the follow up, it was not possible to predict the direction of effect of this potential attrition bias on the strength of tested associations. However, assuming that the attrition pattern was missing-at-random, we believe that the attrition would only under-power our interpretations and not bias them either-way. Second, due to the nature of the periodically scheduled visits, the exact time of event (i.e. the date of T2D occurrence) in the study participants is unknown. Instead, we used the cumulative risk of T2D as our primary outcome. This outcome variable captures the existing and prospective risk of T2D development. Lastly, our study sample represents a high risk population for metabolic syndrome and therefore these results cannot be directly applied to the general population.

Notwithstanding these limitations, our results provide compelling support to the burgeoning notion that WC is a simple and accurate predictor of ensuing and impending T2D especially if IR is concomitantly present. These results further highlight a need for reexamination, reappraisal and revision of existing guidelines with an aim to improve assessment of T2D risk.

Acknowledgments

We are grateful to the participants of the San Antonio Family Heart Study for their continued involvement. We also thank Ms. Cindy Tumiel for editorial assistance.

Author Contributions

Conceived and designed the experiments: MM JEC JB. Performed the experiments: HK TDD LA MCM RD AGC JB JEC. Analyzed the data: MM HK. Contributed reagents/materials/analysis tools: JB JEC. Wrote the paper: MM.

References

1. Ginter E, Simko V (2010) Diabetes type 2 pandemic in 21st century. Bratisl Lek Listy 111: 134–137.
2. Lam DW, LeRoith D (2012) The worldwide diabetes epidemic. Curr Opin Endocrinol Diabetes Obes 19: 93–96.
3. Osei K (2003) Global epidemic of type 2 diabetes: implications for developing countries. Ethn Dis 13: S102–106.
4. Garber AJ (2012) Obesity and type 2 diabetes: which patients are at risk? Diabetes Obes Metab 14: 399–408.
5. Keller U (2006) From obesity to diabetes. Int J Vitam Nutr Res 76: 172–177.
6. Naser KA, Gruber A, Thomson GA (2006) The emerging pandemic of obesity and diabetes: are we doing enough to prevent a disaster? Int J Clin Pract 60: 1093–1097.
7. Seidell JC (2000) Obesity, insulin resistance and diabetes--a worldwide epidemic. Br J Nutr 83 Suppl 1: S5–8.
8. Feller S, Boeing H, Pischon T (2010) Body mass index, waist circumference, and the risk of type 2 diabetes mellitus: implications for routine clinical practice. Dtsch Arztebl Int 107: 470–476.
9. Appel SJ, Jones ED, Kennedy-Malone L (2004) Central obesity and the metabolic syndrome: implications for primary care providers. J Am Acad Nurse Pract 16: 335–342.

10. Despres JP, Lemieux I, Bergeron J, Pibarot P, Mathieu P, et al. (2008) Abdominal obesity and the metabolic syndrome: contribution to global cardiometabolic risk. Arterioscler Thromb Vasc Biol 28: 1039–1049.
11. Kim MK, Jang EH, Son JW, Kwon HS, Baek KH, et al. (2011) Visceral obesity is a better predictor than generalized obesity for basal insulin requirement at the initiation of insulin therapy in patients with type 2 diabetes. Diabetes Res Clin Pract 93: 174–178.
12. Korsic M, Fister K, Ivankovic D, Jelcic J (2011) [Visceral obesity]. Lijec Vjesn 133: 284–287.
13. Wang Y, Rimm EB, Stampfer MJ, Willett WC, Hu FB (2005) Comparison of abdominal adiposity and overall obesity in predicting risk of type 2 diabetes among men. Am J Clin Nutr 81: 555–563.
14. He Y, Zhai F, Ma G, Feskens EJ, Zhang J, et al. (2009) Abdominal obesity and the prevalence of diabetes and intermediate hyperglycaemia in Chinese adults. Public Health Nutr 12: 1078–1084.
15. Mamtani MR, Kulkarni HR (2005) Predictive performance of anthropometric indexes of central obesity for the risk of type 2 diabetes. Arch Med Res 36: 581–589.

16. Schulze MB, Thorand B, Fritsche A, Haring HU, Schick F, et al. (2012) Body adiposity index, body fat content and incidence of type 2 diabetes. Diabetologia 55: 1660–1667.

17. Stevens J, Couper D, Pankow J, Folsom AR, Duncan BB, et al. (2001) Sensitivity and specificity of anthropometrics for the prediction of diabetes in a biracial cohort. Obes Res 9: 696–705.

18. Warren TY, Wilcox S, Dowda M, Baruth M (2012) Independent association of waist circumference with hypertension and diabetes in African American women, South Carolina, 2007–2009. Prev Chronic Dis 9: E105.

19. Wei M, Gaskill SP, Haffner SM, Stern MP (1997) Waist circumference as the best predictor of noninsulin dependent diabetes mellitus (NIDDM) compared to body mass index, waist/hip ratio and other anthropometric measurements in Mexican Americans--a 7-year prospective study. Obes Res 5: 16–23.

20. Bastarrachea RA, Kent J, Comuzzie AG (2007) [Study of the genetic component of cardiovascular risk phenotypes in a Mexican population]. Med Clin (Barc) 129: 11–13.

21. Bayoumi RA, Al-Yahyaee SA, Albarwani SA, Rizvi SG, Al-Hadabi S, et al. (2007) Heritability of determinants of the metabolic syndrome among healthy Arabs of the Oman family study. Obesity (Silver Spring) 15: 551–556.

22. Voruganti VS, Lopez-Alvarenga JC, Nath SD, Rainwater DL, Bauer R, et al. (2008) Genetics of variation in HOMA-IR and cardiovascular risk factors in Mexican-Americans. J Mol Med (Berl) 86: 303–311.

23. Gao JB, Cheng JL, Ding HP, Shen MY (2011) [The disease characteristics and risk factors of type 2 diabetes mellitus in pedigrees]. Zhonghua Nei Ke Za Zhi 50: 474–477.

24. MacCluer JW, Stern MP, Almasy L, Atwood LA, Blangero J, et al. (1999) Genetics of atherosclerosis risk factors in Mexican Americans. Nutr Rev 57: S59–65.

25. Mitchell BD, Kammerer CM, Blangero J, Mahaney MC, Rainwater DL, et al. (1996) Genetic and environmental contributions to cardiovascular risk factors in Mexican Americans. The San Antonio Family Heart Study. Circulation 94: 2159–2170.

26. (2003) Report of the expert committee on the diagnosis and classification of diabetes mellitus. Diabetes Care 26 Suppl 1: S5–20.

27. Hanley AJ, Williams K, Stern MP, Haffner SM (2002) Homeostasis model assessment of insulin resistance in relation to the incidence of cardiovascular disease: the San Antonio Heart Study. Diabetes Care 25: 1177–1184.

28. Qu HQ, Li Q, Rentfro AR, Fisher-Hoch SP, McCormick JB (2011) The definition of insulin resistance using HOMA-IR for Americans of Mexican descent using machine learning. PLoS One 6: e21041.

29. Almasy L, Blangero J (1998) Multipoint quantitative-trait linkage analysis in general pedigrees. Am J Hum Genet 62: 1198–1211.

30. Alberti KG, Eckel RH, Grundy SM, Zimmet PZ, Cleeman JI, et al. (2009) Harmonizing the metabolic syndrome: a joint interim statement of the International Diabetes Federation Task Force on Epidemiology and Prevention; National Heart, Lung, and Blood Institute; American Heart Association; World Heart Federation; International Atherosclerosis Society; and International Association for the Study of Obesity. Circulation 120: 1640–1645.

31. Bardini G, Dicembrini I, Pala L, Cresci B, Rotella CM (2011) Hypertriglyceridaemic waist phenotype and beta-cell function in subjects with normal and impaired glucose tolerance. Diabet Med 28: 1229–1233.

32. Gonzalez-Chavez A, Simental-Mendia LE, Elizondo-Argueta S (2011) Elevated triglycerides/HDL-cholesterol ratio associated with insulin resistance. Cir Cir 79: 126–131.

33. Qiao Q, Nyamdorj R (2010) Is the association of type II diabetes with waist circumference or waist-to-hip ratio stronger than that with body mass index? Eur J Clin Nutr 64: 30–34.

34. Freemantle N, Holmes J, Hockey A, Kumar S (2008) How strong is the association between abdominal obesity and the incidence of type 2 diabetes? Int J Clin Pract 62: 1391–1396.

35. Feng RN, Zhao C, Wang C, Niu YC, Li K, et al. (2012) BMI is Strongly Associated With Hypertension, and Waist Circumference is Strongly Associated With Type 2 Diabetes and Dyslipidemia, in Northern Chinese Adults. J Epidemiol 22: 317–323.

36. Pancoska P, Buch S, Cecchetti A, Parmanto B, Vecchio M, et al. (2009) Family networks of obesity and type 2 diabetes in rural Appalachia. Clin Transl Sci 2: 413–421.

37. Tabata S, Yoshimitsu S, Hamachi T, Abe H, Ohnaka K, et al. (2009) Waist circumference and insulin resistance: a cross-sectional study of Japanese men. BMC Endocr Disord 9: 1.

38. Wahrenberg H, Hertel K, Leijonhufvud BM, Persson LG, Toft E, et al. (2005) Use of waist circumference to predict insulin resistance: retrospective study. BMJ 330: 1363–1364.

Identification of Direct and Indirect Social Network Effects in the Pathophysiology of Insulin Resistance in Obese Human Subjects

Christian H. C. A. Henning[1]*, **Nana Zarnekow**[1], **Johannes Hedtrich**[1], **Sascha Stark**[1], **Kathrin Türk**[2], **Matthias Laudes**[2]

1 Institute of Agricultural Economics, University of Kiel, Kiel, Germany, **2** Department of Internal Medicine 1, University of Kiel, Kiel, Germany

Abstract

Objective: The aim of the present study was to examine to what extent different social network mechanisms are involved in the pathogenesis of obesity and insulin-resistance.

Design: We used nonparametric and parametric regression models to analyse whether individual BMI and HOMA-IR are determined by social network characteristics.

Subjects and Methods: A total of 677 probands (EGO) and 3033 social network partners (ALTER) were included in the study. Data gathered from the probands include anthropometric measures, HOMA-IR index, health attitudes, behavioural and socio-economic variables and social network data.

Results: We found significant treatment effects for ALTERs frequent dieting (p<0.001) and ALTERs health oriented nutritional attitudes (p<0.001) on EGO's BMI, establishing a significant indirect network effect also on EGO's insulin resistance. Most importantly, we also found significant direct social network effects on EGO's insulin resistance, evidenced by an effect of ALTERs frequent dieting (p = 0.033) and ALTERs sport activities (p = 0.041) to decrease EGO's HOMA-IR index independently of EGO's BMI.

Conclusions: Social network phenomena appear not only to be relevant for the spread of obesity, but also for the spread of insulin resistance as the basis for type 2 diabetes. Attitudes and behaviour of peer groups influence EGO's health status not only via social mechanisms, but also via socio-biological mechanisms, i.e. higher brain areas might be influenced not only by biological signals from the own organism, but also by behaviour and knowledge from different human individuals. Our approach allows the identification of peer group influence controlling for potential homophily even when using cross-sectional observational data.

Editor: Kathrin Maedler, University of Bremen, Germany

Funding: The study is funded by the federal ministry of education and research (BMBF), Number: 0315540A, DRKS00005285. The funders had no role in study design, data collection and analysis, decision to publish, or preparation of the manuscript.

Competing Interests: The authors have declared that no competing interests exist.

* E-mail: chenning@ae.uni-kiel.de

Introduction

Obesity is becoming a major health problem in many countries throughout the world with the increasing prevalence reaching almost epidemic proportions [1]. Of particular concern, obesity associated co-morbidities such as type 2 diabetes and cardiovascular disease are driving a progressive increase in biomedical and also socio-economic problems.

In the past, epidemiological studies revealed a significant correlation of the risk of childhood obesity with parental BMI, suggesting a genetic impact in the development of this important metabolic disease [2]. Subsequently, several studies identified risk alleles for obesity, with most of them being involved in central appetite regulation in distinct brain areas in the hypothalamus. These risk alleles included SNPs in Proopiomelanocortin [3], Neuropeptide-Y [4], Leptin [5], Agouti-related Peptide (AgRP) [6]

and, of particular importance, in the Melanocortin-4-receptor (MC4R) [7]. The identification of a central role of specific neurons within the hypothalamus in the pathophysiology of obesity lead to further experimental studies in affected human subjects in order to investigate if also distinct areas in the cerebral cortex are somehow involved in the abnormal regulation of eating behaviour. These studies identified regions in the medial frontal and middle frontal gyrus, which are important in dysregulation of reward activity in the brains of obese human subjects [8]. In contrast to the basal brain functions organised in the hypothalamus, these higher brain areas might be influenced not only by biological signals from the own organism, but also, for example, by behaviour and knowledge from different human individuals [8,9].

Beyond these intrinsic neurobiological mechanisms, a broad set of social and environmental explanations have been provided for surging rates of obesity [10]. In particular, recent studies support the role of social networks as a determinant of the prevalence of obesity [11,12,13,14,15] or health outcomes in general [16,17]. One of the seminal studies showing that social networks are important in the spread of obesity was reported by Christakis and Fowler in 2007 [11]. In this analysis, based on the Framingham Heart Study, it was reported that the risk for becoming obese for a human subject is increased by 57% if he or she had a friend who became obese in a given interval. This finding was particularly interesting, since in the same analysis, the risk of developing obesity was only 40% increased if a sibling became obese. Interpreting their results Christakis and Fowler argue that obesity is "contagious", transmission being mediated by changing weight–related behaviour (diet, exercise, lifestyle, etc.) [11]. However, the specific mechanisms by which networks influence behaviour are not fully understood, yet, although social norms [11,16,18], imitation [11,19], belief formation as well as social capital have been implicated [20]. Moreover, at the methodological level the social network 'contagion' hypothesis has also been critically discussed [12,21,22,23]. Existing empirical studies try to identify network effects using observational data, hence these studies are plagued by serious identification problems, which can be best summarized by Manski's reflection problem [24]. In this regard Shoham et al. [10] applied the Stochastic Actor-Based Model (SABM) as an innovative statistical approach developed by Snijders [25] to distinguish homophily from social contagion (see table 1: glossary). Although we consider the SABM as an appropriate statistical model to solve the identification problem between contagion and homophily, a drawback of this approach, however, can be seen in the fact that it demands longitudinal data, while many clinical studies provide only cross-sectional data.

In this context, the aim of the present study was to develop an innovative approach using cross-sectional observational data (1) to test empirically the effect of social networks on the development of obesity in an independent European cohort and, most important-ly, (2) to examine the effect of social networks on insulin resistance in obese human subjects.

Material and Methods

Data collection and measurement

We conducted a clinical and social survey [Food Chain Plus Study, funded by the federal ministry of education and research (BMBF), Number: 0315540A, DRKS00005285]. The survey started in September 2011 and has enrolled to date a subsample of 327 obese people with a BMI >30, and a randomized control group of 350 probands. The study was approved by the local ethics committee (Number: 156/03, Ethics committee of the University of Kiel, Germany) and written informed consent was obtained for every subject before inclusion into the study. For each proband we collected anthropometric (weight, height, blood pressure, waist circumference, sensory testing, testing for muscular strength), and biochemical data [fasting insulin serum levels, fasting glucose serum levels, serum C-reactive protein levels, serum triglyceride levels] as well as behavioural data. The biochemical analysis was performed by routine measurements within the department of laboratory medicine at the University Medical Centre in Kiel. The Homeostasis Model Assessment Index for Insulin Resistance (HOMA-IR) was calculated as follows: fasting insulin (μU/ml)*fasting glucose (mg/dl)/405. Probands visited the University Medical Centre in Kiel where relevant anthropometic and biochemical data has been collected. Moreover, diabetes type 2 was diagnosed. In total 28 of the 677 probands had diabetes type 2. Since medication for diabetes type 2 might reduce the HOMA-IR index we explicitly checked the HOMA-IR index of the 28 EGOs with diabetes type 2 (for the term EGO see table 1: glossary). None of the 28 probands had a normal HOMOR-IR index below or equal to 2. A contrario, for most EGOs with diabetes type 2 an extremely high HOMA-IR index is reported resulting in an average HOMA-IR index of 19.1 for this specific subgroup. Accordingly, we concluded that including the 28 EGOs with diabetes type 2 in our sample will not bias our results (We thank an anonymous reviewer for pointing out the potential impact of medication for diabetes type 2 in the HOMA-IR index.).

Further, data on nutrition and activity behaviour as well as relevant socio-economic characteristics of probands were collected. For further details please see table 2. Socio-economic data included age, sex, education, household size, and household

Table 1. Glossary.

Term	Definition
EGO	The actor whose network and behavior choices are being modeled.
ALTER	A person connected to the ego who may influence the behavior of the ego. An actor who is named as a friend by the ego.
Actor	A respondent.
Homophily	The tendency for people to choose relationships with people who have similar attributes.
Peer influence	The effect of alters' behavior on ego's behavior.
Social Influences	Synonym for peer influence.
Tie	A connection between two individuals (nodes) that can be either one-way (directed) or two-way (bilateral)
Node	An object that may or may not be connected to other objects in a network.
EGO-centric network	Subset of social relations among all persons (ALTERS) to whom a specific individual person (EGO) has a social tie. The EGO-centric network is also called the neighborhood or peer group of EGO.
Network multiplier	The value of similar behaviors or attitudes, averaged across all of the EGO's ALTERs; network multiplier is used as a measure of peer influence.
PSM	Propensity Score Matching is a non-parametric econometric estimation method of treatment effects controlling for potential selection bias.
SABM	Stochastic Actor-Based Model.

income. Behavioural and lifestyle data that were collected for ALTER including frequency of undertaking diets (DIET), attitude towards food (AT), nutritional knowledge (KNOW), frequency of physical activities (SPORT). The data were collected for EGO as well as for all of EGO's social network contacts (ALTER). The collected data is reported in table 2. Moreover, in a special social network survey we collected EGO-centric network data from each proband. Moreover, EGO-centric network data had been collected when probands visited the study center using a specific computer based social network questionnaire. The collected ego-centric network data were applied to the name generator concept, the state-of-the-art methodology to collect social network data [26]. To implement this, the following three name generator questions were asked:

G1: With whom do you regularly discuss personal problems?

G2: To whom can you turn for help if you have a problem?

G3: With whom do you regularly discuss health-related (especially weight-related) problems?

For all ALTER mentioned by EGO in response, we also asked for their *gender, age, education,* and *profession.* Further, we asked EGO to estimate for each ALTER the following characteristics: (1) ALTER-*BMI* measured in five categories (1–5) ranging from very slim to very fat, for details see table 2; (2) *Nutrition knowledge (ALTER-KNOW)*: 1 = very low, 2 = low, 3 = average, 4 = good, 5 = excellent; (3) *Nutritional attitude (ALTER-AT)*: 1 = food is mainly convenience; diet has to balance health and convenience aspects, 3 = diet has to be mainly healthy; (4) *Frequency of sport activities* (ALTER-SPORT) longer than 30 minutes: 1 = never; 2 = 1–2 per month, 3 = 1 per week, 4 = several times per week; 5 = every day; (5) *Diet behaviour (ALTER-DIET)*, we ask how often ALTER has made a specific diet to lose weight: 1 = never, 2 = 1 time, 3 = 2–3 times; 4 = 4–5 times, 5 = >5 times. At the end of the questionnaire, we also asked questions about the *strength, length,* and *importance* of the relation with the named individuals. Following the concept of Krackhardt (for further explanations see [26]), we asked interviewees to describe the pairwise relations of the ten most important individuals mentioned on a 3 point scale with 0 = do not know each other, 1 = know each other, 2 = know each other very well.

Data management and statistical analysis

We calculated different network multiplier (NET-Z) measuring the field strength of different health-relevant behaviours and attitudes (Z = KNOW, DIET, BMI, AT, SPORT) prevalent in EGO's social network and operating on EGO [27]:

$$NET - Z_i = \overline{fr_i} \sum_{j \in N^i} t_{ij} X_j,$$

where t_{ij} is the relative strength of a network tie between EGO j and ALTER i and $\overline{fr_i}$ is the average absolute strength of a network tie. We measure the relative strength of EGO-ALTER relations (t_{ij}) using the relation frequency of ALTER's network contact with EGO. Our network multiplier also corresponds to the *network force,* a measure suggested by [28] as well as to the position generator, a EGO-centric network measure suggested by [28,29].

First, we apply Propensity Score Matching (PSM) to identify the average treatment effect on treated (ATT) [30] of the different lifestyle attributes of EGO's social peer group (NET-Z).

To this end we define for each attribute NET-Z a binary treatment variable D_{NET-Z} as follows:

$$D_{NET-Z} = \begin{cases} 1 & \text{if } NET - Z > \text{Mean}(NET - Z) \\ 0 & \text{if } NET - Z \leq \text{Mean}(NET - Z) \end{cases}$$

Further, we estimated separate probit functions using each D_{NET-Z} as endogenous variable and relevant socio-economic characteristics (X^{EGO}) and lifestyle indicators of EGO (Z^{EGO}) as well as all relevant lifestyle multiplicators calculated for EGO's social network except the one corresponding to the endogenous variable D_{NET-Z}. In particular, socio-economic variables include EGO's age, sex, household size (HS), education (EDUC), while EGO's lifestyle indicators include EGO-attitude towards food (EGO-AT), EGO's nutrition knowledge (EGO-KNOW), EGO's diet behaviour (EGO-DIET). Based on each estimated probit function we calculated corresponding PSM-scores for all EGO's and used calculated PSM-scores to match the treatment group (l_1) with a corresponding control group (l_0) applying a Kernel Matching operator [31,32]. Finally, we calculated for each treatment variable NET-Z the average treatment effect on treated as follows:

$$ATT = \frac{1}{N_1} \sum_{i \in I_1} \left[Y_i^1 - \sum_{j \in I_0} W_{N_0}(i,j) Y_j^0 \right]$$

Using the Kernel matching operator implies that all members of the control group are used to estimate the ATT, but with different weights, where the following weight for each observation in the control group is used:

$$W_{N_0}^{KM}(i,j) = \frac{G_{ij}}{\sum_{k \in I_0} G_{ik}}; \quad with: \quad G_{ik} = \frac{G(b_i - b_j)}{a_{N_0}}$$

G denotes the Kernel function [31] with a_{N_0} and b_j being specific parameters of the Kernel function. The kernel weights decrease with the distance of the propensity score of a member of the control group to the propensity score of the member of the treatment group. Thus, treated EGOs are compared with non-treated EGOs who have the same socio-economic characteristics as well as the same health related attitudes and behavior as treated EGO and who also have the same peer group characteristics despite from the treatment variable. PSM-matching is a statistical procedure that allows the construction of a control group including other EGOs that are statistical siblings of the treated EGOs, but differ exactly regarding the considered treatment variable. Since, EGO's own characteristics are explicitly included in the statistical construction of the control group PSM matching controls for a potential selection bias due to dynamic peer group selection such as homophily, but also other potential selection biases assuming all relevant determinants of selection into treatment are taken into account ('selection on observables' see [31]).

Second, to analyze to what extend social networks have an influence on insulin resistance and thus on EGO's probability to develop type 2 diabetes and cardiovascular diseases, we regress EGO's HOMA-IR-index on EGO's obesity-status, socio-economic variables (X) and health related lifestyle attributes (EGO-Z) as well as on the corresponding social network multipliers (NET-Z) measuring the field strength of relevant lifestyle attributes of

Table 2. Summarized descriptive statistics of the FOCUS-sample.

	EGO (Std.deviation)	ALTERS
	mean values	*mean values*
Age	51.05	48.89
	(14.46)	(12.85)
Sex (1: male, 0: women)	1: 232, 0: 452	1: 1241 , 0:1759
Household-Size (HS)	2.35	
	(1.62)	
Income[1]	8.92 (4.01)	
Education[2] (EDUC)	5.32 (2.32)	[3]3.92 (1.84)
BMI	32.88 (10.98)	42.8° (0.71)
HOMA-IR	4.93 (7.15)	
N	684	3033
Behavior		
Knowledge[5] (KNOW)	4.93 (1.85)	3.64 (0.74)[6]
Attitude[7] (AT)	4.14 (1.58)	1.75 (0.54)[8]
Diet[9]	4.93 (1.85)	2.30 (1.08)[10]
Sport		2.55 (1.01)[11]
Network		
Size	5.54 (2.93)	
Duration (years)	25.56 (11.33)	
Type (0: family, 1: friends)	0: 1186; 1: 1847	
Frequency[12]	3.11 (0.61)	
Intensity[13]	2.55 (0.41)	
Multiplier		
Knowldge (KNOW)	6.83 (2.39)	
Attitude (AT)	3.34 (1.39)	
Diet	4.04 (2.53)	
Sport	4.66 (2.33)	
BMI	5.07 (2.09)	

[1]Income level: 1: <499 Euro to 16: >4000 Euro.
[2]Education: 1 = means no educational achievement; 10 = PhD.
[3]Education: 1 = means no educational achievement; 8 = PhD.
[4]Nutritional status: 1 = very slim; 5 = very fat.
[5]Reading of food information is important: 1 (not agree)-7 (agree completely).
[6]Knowledge: 1 = no; 5 = excellent.
[7]Low fat food is important: 1 (not agree)-7 (agree completely).
[8]Attitude: 1 = food has to be tasty, 2 = food has to balance enjoyment of eating and health, 3 = food has to be mainly healthy.
[9]I always eat healthy and well balanced: 1 (not agree)-7 (agree completely)
[10]Diet: 1 = never; 5 = more than 5 times.
[11]Sport: 1 = never; 5 = daily.
[12]Contact frequency: 1 = never to 5 = daily.
[13]Intensity: 1 = no talk about private issues; 3 = often.

EGO's social network operating on EGO. EGO's obesity status is measured by a dummy variable, where OBS-EGO = 1 indicates a BMI>30 and OBS-EGO = 0 indicates a BMI<30. Regression models are estimated applying a two-stage IV-estimator to take potential endogeneity of EGO's BMI into account. We used EGO's lifestyle attributes (EGO-Z), the relevant network multipliers of EGO's social network (NET-Z) and EGO's socio-economic variables (X-EGO) as instruments for EGO's obesity status (OBS-EGO). Moreover, we use the second stage estimation to analyze the indirect impact of social networks on EGO's HOMA-IR-index via influencing EGO's obesity status (OBS-EGO), while the main regression at the first stage includes direct

effects of social peer groups on EGO's insulin resistance, i.e. direct peer group effects correspond to effects operating via the direct influence of higher brain areas by the behaviour of other human individuals [8] that do not operate via a change in EGO's behaviour or obesity status.

However, since an average of 39% of EGO's network contacts are family ties, estimations might be plagued by an endogeneity problem in the following sense. Insulin resistance is at least partly genetically determined [33]. Hence, assuming that health related behaviour and attitudes are also at least partly genetically determined might imply a spurious relationship between direct peer group effects induced by family ties and EGO's HOMA-

Table 3. Estimated treatment effects (ATT) of social network characteristics on obesity (BMI).

Treatment Variable	Selection	Treated Group	Control Group	ATT	t-values*	p
$D_{NET-DIET}$	unmatched	35.900	31.050	4.849	5.7	0.000
	matched	35.900	31.613	4.287	4.3	0.000
$D_{NET-BMI}$	unmatched	33.357	32.543	0.814	0.96	0.567
	matched	33.357	33.203	0.154	0.14	0.779
$D_{NET-Sport}$	unmatched	31.830	33.652	−1.822	−2.13	0.005
	matched	31.830	32.582	−0.752	−0.71	0.200
$D_{NET-Know}$	unmatched	32.939	32.871	0.068	0.08	0.900
	matched	32.939	34.342	−1.403	−0.8	0.200
D_{NET-AT}	unmatched	32.210	33.520	−1.310	−1.54	0.050
	matched	32.210	35.753	−3.543	−2.95	0.000

*t-values derived via bootstrapping.

index. Of course, we already control for this spurious relationship as well as for a potential spurious correlation due to homophily as a dynamic peer group selection since we explicitly include EGO's own health related behaviour and attitudes in our main regression equation. Nevertheless as an additional robustness check we undertake a three stage IV estimation where we instrumented EGO's family peer group behaviour and attitudes at a third stage using corresponding behaviour and attitude of EGO's non-family ties as instruments. Moreover, we re-estimate our two-stage IV regression model excluding family ties completely.

Results

Characteristics of the study cohort

N = 677 subjects designated as EGOs were included. Basic descriptive statistics of our sample are reported in table 2. Any person to whom EGOs are linked serve as a social contact, and is designated "ALTER" in the following. A total of n = 3033 ALTERS, observed family and social ties, were connected. This yields an average of 5.5 ties per EGO within the network. A total of 39.1% of the 3033 ALTERs were family contacts. The remaining 60.9% were connected through friendship to EGO. The average duration of relationship was 25.5 years with a standard deviation of 11.3. The minimum duration was 0.666 years and the maximum 61.5 years. The mean age of investigated EGOs was 51 years with a range from 19 to 84 years. The mean age of ALTERs was 48 years, ranging from 11 to 91. 34% of the EGOs were men, while 41% of ALTERs were male. The educational level was measured on a scale ranging from 1 to 10 (1 to 8 in case of ALTERs) with 1 indicating no formal education and a 10 (8) denoting a PhD-level. The average educational level of EGO's was 5.3 on a 10 point scale, while the mean education level of ALTERs was 4.1 on a 8 point scale. The frequency of EGO's network contacts ranged from 28% who meet daily, over 39% who meet weekly to 29% who meet only on a monthly basis. Only 4% of ALTERs did meet less than one time per month by EGO.

Treatment effects of social network characteristics on obesity

In table 3 the treatment effects (ATT) of social networks on EGO's BMI are reported, generated from PSM-Matching analysis for the five different network characteristics. As can be seen from table 3 the PSM-matching results imply that the average BMI of EGO's social peer group has no significant influence on EGO's own BMI, while we found significant network effects for the weight related behaviour and attitude of social peer groups. In particular, we found significant treatment effects for diet behaviour and nutritional attitude, while nutritional knowledge and sport activities of peer groups had no significant impact on EGO's BMI. In quantitative terms the impact was the highest for diet behaviour resulting in an average treatment effect of 4.3, i.e. having a social network that frequently engaged in diets implies an increase in BMI by 4.3 kg/m^2. Given an average BMI of 31 in our sample this corresponds to a remarkable effect of more than 13%, which is highly significant with a t-value of 4.3 (p<0.001). Analogously, we found a remarkably high effect on EGO's BMI of 3.5 kg/m^2 for health oriented attitude of EGO's social network corresponding to a reduction of over 10% of the average BMI. Furthermore, a high frequency of sport activities in EGO's social network reduces EGO's BMI by 0.75 kg/m^2, but this effect was statistically not significant.

Multiple regression analysis on social network effect on insulin resistance

Results of the second stage of the IV-estimations are reported in table 4 (Model A), while results of the probit estimation of the first stage of our IV-estimation are reported in table 5 (Model A). As can be seen from table 4 the main determinant of EGO's insulin resistance corresponds to EGO's obesity status with a normalized partial impact of *0.258*. In absolute terms an increase of 1% in the probability of becoming obese implies an increase of *0.07* units of the HOMA-IR index. However, beyond obesity status also sex has a significant effect on insulin resistance with a normalized coefficient of 0.101 (see table 4, model A). In particular, males generally have a higher HOMA-IR-index when compared to females, with an absolute difference of 1.44 between men and women.

The most remarkable finding of our analyses, however, was a significant and robust direct influence of social networks on EGO's insulin resistance, even correcting for EGO's BMI. In particular, a higher frequency of diet behaviour (p = 0.052) as well as sport activities (p = 0.038) in EGO's social network reduces significantly her/his HOMA-IR-index given normalized regression coefficient of −0.101 and −0.078, respectively. In quantitative terms a maximal difference in the diet behaviour of EGO's network changing from no diet to an average of more than 5 diets undertaken per network contact implies an absolute decrease of *1.16* units of the HOMA-IR-index. Taking the normal HOMA-

Table 4. Results of the IV-estimation: Dependent variable EGO's HOMA-IR.

	Model A-0			Model A			Model B		
	Coef.	P>|t|*	Beta	Coef.	P>|t|*	Beta	Coef.	P>|t|*	Beta
Male	1.388	0.009	0.098	1.439	0.007	0.101	1.459	0.005	0.103
EGO-DIET	0.140	0.436	0.038	0.140	0.433	0.038	0.184	0.045	0.051
EGO-AT	0.165	0.413	0.039	0.154	0.383	0.036	0.109	0.119	0.026
EGO-KNOW	-0.067	0.630	-0.020						
NET-AT	-0.051	0.840	-0.011						
NET-DIET	-0.291	0.040	-0.110	-0.267	0.053	-0.101	-0.082	0.671	-0.031
NET-BMI	0.284	0.060	0.088	0.332	0.014	0.103	0.245	0.022	0.076
NET-KNOW	0.126	0.465	0.045						
NET-SPORT	-0.264	0.040	-0.092	-0.225	0.038	-0.078	-0.202	0.015	-0.070
EGO-BMI	7.375	0.000	0.263	7.231	0.000	0.258	6.358	0.000	0.227
Prob >F =	0			0			0		
R-squared	0.386			0.385			0.374		
Adj R-squared	0.377			0.379			0.367		

*t-values derived via bootstrapping.

Table 5. Results of Logit-Model: Dependent variable EGO's BMI-status (OBS-EGO) (IV-first stage).

OBS-EGO	Model A			Model B		
	coef	P>|z|	Marginal effect	coef	P>|z|	Marginal effect
NET-KNOW	0.031	0.613	0.008	−0.044	0.725	−0.011
NET-AT	−0.134	0.145	−0.033	−0.186	0.340	−0.046
NET-BMI	−0.034	0.536	−0.009	−0.232	0.048	−0.057
NET-DIET	0.238	0.000	0.059	0.504	0.000	0.124
NET-SPORT	−0.001	0.988	0.000	0.026	0.783	0.006
Age	−0.011	0.110	−0.003	−0.014	0.039	−0.004
Male	−0.053	0.789	−0.013	0.009	0.965	0.002
Income	−0.053	0.041	−0.013	−0.066	0.012	−0.016
Education	−0.268	0.000	−0.067	−0.265	0.000	−0.065
HS	0.093	0.252	0.023	0.069	0.333	0.017
LGO DIET	0.294	0.000	0.073	0.280	0.000	0.069
EGO-AT	−0.384	0.000	−0.096	−0.378	0.000	−0.093
EGO-KNOW	0.144	0.002	0.036	0.149	0.002	0.037
Constant	1.170	0.030		1.883	0.014	

IR-value of <2.0 as a reference this corresponds to a remarkable change of 58%, and even if we compare this with the average HOMA-IR-index in our sample of 4.8 it still corresponds to a remarkable change of 24%. Analogously, a maximal change of the frequency of sport activities in EGO's network from no activities to an average sport activity of at least once per day decreases EGO's HOMA-IR-index *by 1.06* units, which still corresponds to remarkable 53% and 22% compared to the critical HOMA-IR-value of <2.0 and the average HOMA-IR-value of *4.8* in our sample, respectively.

Interestingly, in contrast to the lifestyle of EGO's social peer group EGO's own lifestyle indicators have no significant direct impact on EGO's HOMA-IR-index. However, EGO's lifestyle significantly influences EGO's BMI-status (see table 5, model A), where especially EGO's health oriented nutritional attitude (EGO-AT) reduces significantly EGO's probability to become obese (p = 0.000) with a marginal effect of −0.096 (see table 5, model A). Moreover, a high education (p = 0.000) and income level (p = 0.041) reduce EGO's probability to become obese. Peer group effects on EGO's BMI, however, are less pronounced in the multiple regression analysis. Only for diet behaviour of EGO's peer network a highly significant positive effect on EGO's BMI-status was observed (p = 0.000, see table 5). For all other network multipliers only an insignificant effect resulted from our multiple regression analysis.

Combining the strong and significant impact of the EGO's BMI on her/his HOMA-IR-index estimated at the second stage with the estimation results of the logit regression at the first stage implies a strong indirect social network effect on insulin resistance. We calculated the indirect network effect as the marginal effect of a network multiplier on EGO's probability of becoming obese multiplied by the marginal effect of EGO's obesity status on her HOMA-IR-index. Significant indirect and direct peer group effects were identified for diet behaviour, while sport behaviour and BMI-status of EGO's peer network impact only directly on EGO's insulin resistance (Model A, table 4, 5). In contrast, EGO's own health related lifestyle and nutritional knowledge impact only indirectly on his/her insulin resistance (Model A, table 4, 5). Please note that we essentially derived the same results, i.e. we observe

significant direct and indirect peer group effects on EGO's HOMA-IR-index, undertaking a three-stage IV estimation instrumenting behaviour and attitude of EGO's family ties (Model B, table 4, 5). Furthermore, results of our preferred model A do not change if we include insignificant lifestyle variables of EGO and his/her peer network (see model A-0 in table 4). Moreover, these results remain also robust if we re-estimate the two-stage IV regression model excluding family ties (estimation results are not presented here, but are available from the authors upon request). Therefore, we are confident that our main estimation results correspond to robust findings.

Discussion

In recent years biomedical research has been enormously extended in regard to the pathophysiology of obesity and its associated co-morbidities. In terms of body weight regulation, it was established early that genetic factors explain 30–50% of the obesity epidemic and that environmental factors are tremendously important [34]. While initial studies focused mainly on nutrition, eating behaviour and physical activity as important environmental factors, in 2007 Christakis and Fowler demonstrated that social network effects might even be more important than genetic polymorphisms in the development of obesity [11]. However, in contrast to what was found for obesity, until now no data exist on the impact of social network effects on insulin resistance, a key obesity-associated morbidity that is the mediator of obesity-associated type 2 diabetes, lipid disorders and atherosclerosis [35]. Therefore the aim of the present study was to (1) investigate the impact of social network effects on obesity development in an independent European cohort and (2) to examine potential direct and indirect social network effects on the development of insulin resistance.

The results reported here imply that specific lifestyles attributes of social peer groups, especially frequent diet and nutritional attitude in favour of healthy food, influence significantly EGO's BMI. These findings confirm the previously identified network effects on body weight gain in the US population [11]. Together, these findings provide evidence for the hypothesis that appetite regulation organised in the hypothalamus might be influenced not only by biological signals from the periphery (e. g. ghrelin and leptin [36]), but also via function of the cerebral cortex via knowledge and/or behaviour from different human individuals of the patients relatives and peer group [8,11].

In addition to what was examined in earlier reports, in the present social network study we also calculated the HOMA-IR index for the first time for each of the 677 individual subjects in order to obtain a measure for their insulin action. Applying our mathematical model, we identified for the first time that social networks can influence EGO's insulin resistance. This is in part explained by indirect effects of the peer group on EGO's BMI and the BMI determining EGO's insulin resistance. This finding is not unexpected since many clinical and experimental studies have shown insulin resistance of liver and skeletal muscle to be associated with obesity [37]. Ectopic lipid accumulation in liver and skeletal muscle in response to an excess of energy intake is postulated to explain this association, leading in turn to serine phosphorylation of insulin receptor substrate (IRS)-1 and thereby inhibition of intracellular insulin receptor signalling [35,38]. Therefore, as shown in this report, if the peer group influences EGO's BMI then one would expect that EGO's insulin resistance should also be affected. Hence, from a mathematical point of view, the fact that peer group effects on EGO's BMI are in line with peer group effects on EGO's insulin resistance indicates, that the associations found in our cohort are true sociobiological effects rather than statistical artefacts.

The most remarkable finding of our study corresponds to the fact that we also have been able to identify direct peer group effects on EGO's insulin resistance. That means that our regression analyses yield these significant network effects even when we control for EGO's BMI and for EGO's own weight-related attitudes and behaviour, respectively. This is particular interesting, since it has been shown that for example physical activity is able to improve insulin sensitivity in overweight subjects independently of significant changes in BMI [39]. Therefore, the fact that the degree of physical activity of the peer group beneficially affects directly EGO's insulin resistance suggests the existence of a potent sociobiological mechanism in the pathogenesis of insulin resistance.

At a methodological level PSM-matching as well as two-stage multiple regression analysis are adequate methods avoiding the problem of latent homophily even if only cross-sectional data can be used (no panel data). However these statistical analyses are based on certain assumptions that we could not test explicitly. In particular, PSM matching is based on the assumption of "selection on observables" [31], i.e. we have to assume that our analysis includes all relevant selection variables. Thus, to the extent that "selection on unobservables" occurs PSM would deliver biased results [31]. In contrast, our two-stage estimation is not plagued by

the problem of latent homophily as it appears rather unrealistic to assume that peer group selection occurs on the basis of insulin resistance. However, since an average of 39% of EGO's network contacts are family ties estimations might be plagued by an endogeneity problem resulting from spurious relationship between direct peer group effects and EGO's HOMA-index induced by genetic relations among family ties and EGO. Given our estimation design this spurious relationship could only occur if weight related behaviour and attitudes are determined by the same genes as the HOMA-index which we consider as rather unrealistic. Nevertheless we undertook an additional robustness check, i.e. we conducted a three stage IV estimation where we instrumented EGO's family peer group behaviour and attitudes at a third stage using corresponding behaviour and attitude of EGO's non-family ties as instruments. Moreover, we re-estimated our two-stage IV regression excluding family ties. Both alternative estimation strategies delivered in essence the same results. Hence, beyond theoretical considerations also on pure statistical grounds we are confident that we can exclude spurious relationships and that our main results correspond to robust findings.

In summary our study indicates for the first time that social network phenomena appear not only to be relevant for the spread of obesity, but also for the spread of insulin resistance. Direct and indirect social network mechanisms have been identified as significant factors determining the risk for impaired insulin signalling. Weight-related attitudes and behaviour of peer groups exert particularly significant impact not only on EGO's obesity status, but also directly on EGO's insulin resistance. These results might have important clinical implications for the design of future obesity therapy programs. Given the fact that many individual-level intervention strategies to prevent obesity, including nutritional education, behavioural therapy and physical activity [40,41], achieve very few sustained effects [41] our results might be used to design novel weight loss programs. These programs should include not only patients (EGOs) treatment but also education of the patients peer group to achieve more sustained results of multimodal obesity therapy programs in the future. Moreover, beyond designing innovative obesity therapy programs including peer group effects based on external peer group compositions, understanding the dynamics of peer group formation might also enable the design of peer group structures that amplify identified positive peer group effects on EGO's obesity and related co-morbidities.

Author Contributions

Conceived and designed the experiments: CH NZ ML. Performed the experiments: ML CH KT SS JH. Analyzed the data: CH NZ SS JH ML. Contributed reagents/materials/analysis tools: CH ML NZ JH SS. Wrote the paper: CH ML NZ.

References

1. Hedley AA, Ogden CL, Johnson CL, Carroll MD, Curtin LR, et al. (2004) Prevalence of overweight and obesity among US children, adolescents, and adults 1999–2002. JAMA 291: 2847–2850.
2. Turconi G, Guarcello M, Maccarini L, Bazzano R, Zaccardo A, et al. (2006) BMI values and other anthropometric and functional measurements as predictors of obesity in a selected group of adolescents. Eur J Nutr 45: 136–143.
3. Krude H, Biebermann H, Luck W, Horn R, Brabant G, et al. (1998) Severe early-onset obesity, adrenal insufficiency and red hair pigmentation caused by POMC mutations in humans. Nat Genet 19: 155–157.
4. Hung CC, Pirie F, Luan J, Lank E, Motala A, et al. (2004) Studies of the Peptide YY and Neuropeptide Y2 Receptor Genes in Relation to Human Obesity and Obesity-Related Traits. Diabetes 53: 2461–2466.
5. Montague CT, Farooqi S, Whitehead JP, Soos MA, Rau H, et al. (1997) Congenital Leptin Deficiency is associated with severe early-onset obesity in humans. Nature 387: 903–908.
6. Marks DL, Boucher N, Lanouette CM, Pérusse L, Brookhart G, et al. (2004) Ala67Thr polymorphism in the Agouti-related peptide gene is associated with inherited leanness in humans. Am J Med Genet A 126A: 267–271.
7. Yeo GS, Farooqi IS, Aminian S, Halsall DJ, Stanhope RG, et al. (1998) A frameshift mutation in MC4R associated with dominantly inherited human obesity. Nat Genet 20: 111–112.
8. Frankort A, Roefs A, Siep N, Roebroeck A, Havermans R, et al. (2012) Reward activity in satiated overweight women is decreased during unbiased viewing but increased when imagining taste: an event-related fMRI study. Int J Obesity 36: 627–637.
9. Fogassi L, Ferrari PF, Gesierich B, Rozzi S, Chersi F, et al. (2005) Parietal lobe: from action organization to intention understanding. Science 308: 662–667.
10. Shoham DA, Tong L, Lamberson PJ, Auchincloss AH, Zhang J, et al. (2012) An Actor-Based Model of Social Network Influence on Adolescent Body Size, Screen Time, and Playing Sports. PLoS ONE 7:e39795.

11. Christakis NA, Fowler JH (2007) The spread of obesity in a large social network over 32 years. N Eng J Med 357: 370–379.
12. Cohen-Cole E, Fletcher JM (2008) Is Obesity Contagious? Social Networks vs. Environmental Factors in the Obesity Epidemic. J Health Econ 27: 1382–1387.
13. Bahr DB, Browning RC, Wyatt HR, Hill JO (2009) Exploiting social networks to mitigate the obesity epidemic. Obesity 17: 723–728.
14. de la Haye K, Robins G, Mohrd P, Wilson C (2010) Obesity-related behaviors in adolescent friendship networks. Soc Networks 32: 161–167.
15. Fletcher A, Bonell C, Sorhaindo A (2011) You are what your friends eat: systematic review of social network analyses of young people's eating behaviours and bodyweight. J Epidemiol Commun H 65: 548–555.
16. Smith K, Christakis N (2008) Social networks and health. Annu Rev Sociol 34: 405–429.
17. Valente TW (2008) Social networks and health: models, methods, and applications. Oxford: University Press.
18. Berkman LA, Glass T (2000) Social integration, social networks, social support, and health. In: Berkman L, Kawachi I editors. Social epidemiology. Oxford: University Press. pp. 137–173.
19. Bandura A (1986) Social foundations of thought and action: a social cognitive theory. Upper Saddle River: Prentice-Hall.
20. Moore S, Daniel M, Paquet C, Dube L, Gauvin L (2009) Association of individual network social capital with abdominal adiposity, overweight and obesity. J Public Health 31: 175–183.
21. Shalizi CR, Thomas AC (2011) Homophily and Contagion Are Generally Confounded in Observational Social Network Studies. Socio Meth Res 40: 211–239.
22. Johns D (2010) Everything is contagious. Slate.com website. Available: http://www.slate.com/articles/health_and_science/science/features/2010/everything_is_contagious/has_a_plague_of_social_illness_struck_mankind.html http://www.slate.com/id/2250102/entry/2250103/. Accessed 2013 Dec 17.
23. Cohen-Cole E, Fletcher JM (2008) Detecting implausible social network effects in acne, height, and headaches: longitudinal analysis. BMJ 337:a2533.
24. Manski CF (1993) Identification of endogenous social effects: the reflection problem. Rev Econ Stud 60: 531–542.
25. Snijders T, van de Bunt G, Steglich G (2010) Introduction to stochastic actor-based models for network dynamics. Social Networks 32: 44–60.
26. Wasserman S, Faust K (1994) Social Network Analysis: Methods and Applications. Cambridge: University Press.

27. Battiston S, Bonabeau E, Weisbuch G (2004) Impact of Corporate Boards Interlock on the Decision Making Dynamics. In: Gallegati M, Kirman AP, Marsili M editors. The Complex Dynamics of Economic Interaction. Springer-Verlag. pp. 355–378.
28. Van der Gaag M, Snijders TAB (2005) The resource generator: Measurement of individual social capital. Soc Networks 27: 21–29.
29. Snijders TAB, Bosker RJ (1999) Multilevel Analysis: An Introduction to Basic and Advanced Multilevel Modeling. Thousand Oaks: Sage Publications Ltd.
30. Rosenbaum PR, Rubin DB (1983) The central role of the propensity score in observational studies for causal effects. Biometrika 70: 41–55.
31. Caliendo M, Kopeinig S (2008) Some practical guidance for the implementation of propensity score matching. J Econ Surv 22: 31–72.
32. Gu X, Rosenbaum PR (1993) Comparison of multivariate matching methods: Structures, distances, and algorithms. J Comp Graph Stat 2: 405–420.
33. George S, Rochford JJ, Wolfrum C, Gray SL, Schinner S, et al. (2004) A family with severe insulin resistance and diabetes due to a mutation in AKT2. Science 304: 1325–1328.
34. Stunkard AJ, Harris JR, Pedersen NL, McClearn GE (1990) The body-mass index of twins who have been reared apart. N Eng J Med 322: 1483–1487.
35. Samuel VT, Shulman GI (2012) Mechanisms for insulin resistance: common threads and missing links. Cell 148: 852–871.
36. Coll AP, Farooqi IS, O'Rahilly S (2007) The hormonal control of food intake. Cell 129: 251–262.
37. Kahn BB, Flier JS (2000) Obesity and insulin resistance. J Clin Invest 106: 473–481.
38. Morino K, Petersen KF, Shulman GI (2006) Molecular mechanisms of insulin resistance in humans and their potential links with mitochondrial dysfunction. Diabetes 55: 9–15.
39. Duncan GE, Perri MG, Theriaque DW, Hutson AD, Eckel RH, et al. (2003) Exercise training, without weight loss, increases insulin sensitivity and postheparin plasma lipase activity in previously sedentary adults. Diabetes Care 26: 557–562.
40. Golley RK, Maher CA, Matricciani L, Olds TS (2013) Sleep duration or bedtime? Exploring the association between sleep timing behavior, diet and BMI in children and adolescents. Int J Obes 37: 546–551.
41. Waters E, de Silva-Sanigorski A, Burford BJ, Brown T, Campbell KJ, et al. (2011) Interventions for preventing obesity in children. Cochrane Database Syst Rev 12:CD001871.

The Associations between Serum Zinc Levels and Metabolic Syndrome in the Korean Population: Findings from the 2010 Korean National Health and Nutrition Examination Survey

Jin-A Seo[1], Sang-Wook Song[1], Kyungdo Han[2], Kyung-Jin Lee[1], Ha-Na Kim[1]*

1 Department of Family medicine, St. Vincent's Hospital, College of Medicine, The Catholic University of Korea, Seoul, Korea, 2 Department of Biostatistics, College of Medicine, The Catholic University of Korea, Seoul, Korea; Department of Preventive Medicine, College of Medicine, The Catholic University of Korea, Seoul, Korea

Abstract

The prevalence of metabolic syndrome has been increasing rapidly worldwide. The functions of zinc may have a potential association with metabolic syndrome, but such associations have not been investigated extensively. Therefore, we examined the relationship between serum zinc levels and metabolic syndrome or metabolic risk factors among South Korean adults ≥20 years of age. The analysis used data from the Korean National Health and Nutrition Examination Survey, a cross-sectional survey of Korean civilians, conducted from January to December 2010. A total of 1,926 participants were analyzed in this study. Serum zinc levels in men were negatively associated with elevated fasting glucose (adjusted odds ratio [aOR], 0.58; 95% confidence interval [CI], 0.36–0.93) and positively associated with elevated triglycerides (aOR, 1.47; 95% CI, 1.01–2.13). A difference in serum zinc levels was detected in women, depending on the number of metabolic syndrome components (p = 0.002). Furthermore, serum zinc levels showed a decreasing trend with increasing numbers of metabolic syndrome components in women with metabolic syndrome. These findings suggest that serum zinc levels might be associated with metabolic syndrome or metabolic risk factors. Further gender-specific studies are needed to evaluate the effect of dietary or supplemental zinc intake on metabolic syndrome.

Editor: Stefan Kiechl, Innsbruck Medical University, Austria

Funding: The authors have no support or funding to report.

Competing Interests: The authors have declared that no competing interests exist.

* Email: onef01@catholic.ac.kr

Introduction

Zinc is the second most common trace metal in the body and, as an essential micronutrient, is important in growth and development. Zinc also has crucial roles in the synthesis, storage and secretion of insulin and in the actions of insulin on carbohydrate metabolism [1,2]; thus, zinc possesses an insulinomimetic effect [3,4]. Furthermore, zinc plays vital roles as a cofactor for metalloenzymes in antioxidant defense systems such as those involving superoxide dismutase, catalase, and glutathione peroxidase [5], and as reducing inflammatory cytokine production via regulation of a zinc-finger protein [6,7].

Metabolic syndrome (MetS), a cluster of metabolic risk factors including hyperglycemia, atherogenic dyslipidemia, elevated blood pressure and abdominal obesity, is associated with an increased risk of cardiovascular disease and all-cause mortality [8–10]. The prevalence of MetS has been increasing rapidly worldwide [11] such that MetS has become a major medical issue. The prevalence of MetS in U.S. adults was 27.9% according to the National Health and Nutrition Examination Survey (NHANES) of 1988–1994 and 34.1% according to the NHANES of 1999–2006 [12]. In Korea, the prevalence of MetS increased from 24.9% in 1998

to 31.3% in 2007, according to the Korean National Health and Nutrition Examination Survey (KNHANES) [13].

MetS represents a complex interaction of maladaptive characteristics related to impaired insulin action at target organs, suggesting that insulin resistance plays a key role in the pathogenesis of MetS [14]. The potential role of oxidative stress and chronic inflammation in MetS has also been reported, and increased oxidative stress or the presence of chronic inflammation may affect the development of MetS [15–17]. Despite the critical roles of insulin resistance and/or oxidative stress and chronic inflammation in MetS pathogenesis [14–17] and the functions of zinc related to insulin resistance [3,4], oxidative stress [5], or chronic inflammation [6,7], studies on the association between MetS and body zinc status are scarce and the results are controversial. In a cross-sectional study of Iranian participants, serum zinc levels were significantly higher in men with MetS as compared to those without MetS, but had a trend of a negative association in women with MetS [18]. In a study conducted in a Chinese population, Chinese men with MetS had a higher level of serum zinc [19]; however, serum zinc levels were not associated with MetS in European [20] or Persian populations [21]. Furthermore, no studies have been conducted on the association between MetS and serum zinc levels in a Korean population. Therefore, we evaluated whether serum zinc levels are associated with MetS and whether serum zinc levels differ according to MetS components in Korean adults using the data from KNHANES V-1.

Materials and Methods

Study population

We used data collected from the KNHANES V-1 conducted from January to December 2010. The KNHANES is implemented by the Korea Centre for Disease Control and Prevention (KCDC) during 3-year intervals to assess the status of public health and to provide baseline data for the development, establishment, and evaluation of public health policies in the Korean population. In KNHANES, participants comprise non-institutionalized individuals ≥1 year of age, selected using a stratified, multi-stage cluster probability sampling design to ensure an independent and homogeneous sampling each year in addition to a nationally representative sampling. Data are collected by a variety of means, including household interviews, anthropometric and biochemical measurements, and nutritional status assessments [22]. All the protocols were approved by the Institutional Review Board of the KCDC and the participants provided written informed consent at baseline.

In the KNHANES V-1, 10,938 participants were recruited, and 8,958 of them completed the survey (participation rate: 81.9%). In this cross-sectional study, we originally examined 1,988 adults ≥20 years of age by assessing serum zinc levels from data on 8,958 participants collected from KNHANES V-1. We excluded those participants with missing information or values for the major variables (n = 60) and with decreased kidney function (estimated glomerular filtration rate <30 mL/min/1.73 m²) (n = 2). The population for the current study thus consisted of 1,926 participants. The current study was approved by the Institutional Review Board of the Catholic University of Korea (IRB approval number: VC14EISI0070).

Definitions of variables

We used the revised criteria of the National Cholesterol Education Program Adult Treatment Panel III (NCEP-ATP III) to define MetS [23]. The NCEP-ATP III criteria define MetS as the presence of any three or more of the following five MetS components: waist circumference ≥90 cm (≥85 cm for women) according to the Korean Society for the Study of Obesity cut-off point for abdominal obesity [24]; triglyceride levels ≥150 mg/dL or taking medication for elevated triglycerides; high-density lipoprotein (HDL) cholesterol levels <40 mg/dL (<50 mg/dL for women) or taking medication to reduce HDL-cholesterol; systolic blood pressure ≥130 mmHg or diastolic blood pressure ≥ 85 mmHg or taking antihypertensive medication; fasting glucose levels ≥100 mg/dL or taking medication for elevated glucose levels. The MetS phenotypes represented any three or more combinations of the five MetS components. Serum zinc levels were categorized by quartiles with quartile 1 (Q1) representing the lowest zinc levels, Q2: low-medium zinc levels, Q3: high-medium zinc levels and Q4: the highest zinc levels.

Laboratory measurements

Blood samples were collected from the antecubital vein of each participant after at least 12 h of fasting, processed, refrigerated immediately and transported in cold storage to the Central Testing Institute in Seoul, Korea. All blood samples were analyzed within 24 h after arrival at the testing facility. Fasting plasma glucose, triglyceride, HDL-cholesterol, and creatinine levels were measured using an auto-analyzer (Hitachi Automatic Analyzer 7600, Hitachi, Japan). Analysis of serum insulin was performed using an immunoradiometric assay (1470 WIZARD Gamma Counter, PerkinElmer, Finland). Insulin resistance was assessed using the homeostasis model assessment of insulin resistance (HOMA-IR) index, which was calculated as follows: [fasting glucose (mg/dL) × fasting insulin (μIU/mL)]/405 [25]. The glomerular filtration rate (GFR) was estimated by the re-expressed "Modification of Diet in Renal Disease" study equation using calibrated serum creatinine values [26]; the formula used for estimated GFR (eGFR) was as follows:

$$175 \times (\text{serum creatinine concentration})^{-1.154} \times (\text{age})^{-0.203}.$$

For measuring serum zinc concentrations, a trace element tube was used and serum zinc concentration was determined by inductively coupled plasma mass spectrometry using PerkinElmer ICP-MS (PerkinElmer, MA, USA). Serum samples were diluted with 2% nitric acid, and serum zinc concentration was obtained from a linear relationship (r = 0.999) between concentrations of zinc stock standard (1000 μg/mL, SPEX CertiPrep, NJ, USA) and absorbance. The accuracy of the analytical methods was tested with standard reference material (ClinChek Serum Controls, lyophilised for trace elements, RECIPE, Munich, Germany). The standard deviation index was 0.50, and coefficients of variation for inter- and intra-assay were 2%, and 4%, respectively.

Clinical and anthropometric measurements

Anthropometric measurements of the participants were performed by specially trained examiners. Height and weight were measured after an overnight fast while the participants wore a lightweight gown, and waist circumference was measured using a measuring tape in the horizontal plane around the umbilical region after exhaling. Blood pressure measurements were taken in the sitting position after a rest period of at least 5 min. Body mass index (BMI) was calculated as each participant's weight (in kilograms) divided by the square of height (in meters).

Self-reported information regarding age, gender, smoking, alcohol consumption, and the amount of physical activity were obtained. Cigarette smoking was divided into three categories based on current use estimates: non-smoker, ex-smoker and current smoker. Alcohol consumption was classified into three categories: abstinence (no alcoholic drinks consumed within the last year), moderate drinking (less than 14 standard drinks consumed for men or 7 for women per week) and heavy drinking (more than 14 standard drinks consumed for men or 7 for women per week). Physical activity was classified as low or not. Low physical activity was defined as 150 min or less of moderate intensity or 75 min or less of vigorous intensity exercise per week [27].

Statistical analysis

To analyze the data using a complex sampling design, we used the SAS PROC SURVEY module, considering strata, clusters, and weights. All analyses were performed using the sample weights from KNHANES. Gender-specific characteristics of the study population were analyzed using independent t-tests for continuous variables and the chi-squared test for dichotomous variables. The data are expressed as means ± standard errors or percentages and as geometric means and 95% confidence intervals (CI) for skewed distributions. Variables with skewed distributions were analyzed after logarithmic transformation. The correlations between serum zinc levels, MetS components and insulin resistance were analyzed using Pearson's correlation analysis. The differences in the mean values of MetS components according to serum zinc level quartile were evaluated using analysis of covariance (ANCOVA) with age, smoking, alcohol consumption, physical activity, BMI, and eGFR levels as covariates. We also examined the relationship between serum zinc levels as the dependent variable and MetS components as the independent variable, using multiple logistic regression analysis. Model 1 was adjusted for age, and model 2 was adjusted for age, smoking, alcohol consumption, physical activity, BMI, and eGFR levels. Serum zinc levels and the percentage of participants in Q4 were analyzed according to the number of MetS components using ANCOVA after adjusting for the above-mentioned covariates and using the chi-squared test, respectively. The percentages of participants according to MetS phenotypes and serum zinc levels were analyzed using the chi-square test. All statistical analyses were performed using the SAS software (ver. 9.2; SAS Institute, Cary, NC, USA). P-values<0.05 were considered to indicate statistical significance.

Results

1. Characteristics of the participants according to serum zinc levels and the correlations between serum zinc levels and metabolic syndrome components

The present study was conducted using a total of 1,926 participants. In this population, the prevalence of MetS was 26.4% (n = 248) in men and 26.4% (n = 260) in women. Mean serum zinc levels in men with and without MetS were 142.0±2.4 µg/dL and 141.1±1.9 µg/dL (p = 0.717), respectively, and in women with and without MetS were 127.5±2.5 µg/dL and 129.6±1.9 µg/dL (p = 0.419), respectively. Table 1 shows the characteristics of the study participants according to serum zinc level quartiles, in particular, Q1-3 versus Q4. In men, significant differences in age and fasting glucose and insulin levels were observed according to serum zinc levels, while age, systolic blood pressure, and insulin levels were higher in women in serum zinc level Q1-3 than in Q4.

In both men and women, significant negative correlations were observed between serum zinc levels and fasting glucose (for men: r = −0.127, p = 0.003; for women: r = −0.078, p = 0.045) and the HOMA-IR index (r = −0.120, p = 0.003 for men, r = −0.113, p = 0.006 for women), and, in women, between serum zinc levels and systolic blood pressure (r = −0.082, p = 0.015) and insulin levels (r = −0.097, p = 0.023) (Table 2).

2. Mean metabolic syndrome component values according to serum zinc level quartile

The mean values of MetS components adjusted for age, smoking, alcohol consumption, physical activity, BMI, and eGFR levels according to serum zinc level quartile are shown in Table 3. In men, as serum zinc levels increased, fasting glucose levels decreased (p for trend = 0.013). HDL-cholesterol levels were not significantly different according to quartiles of serum zinc levels in both men and women (p = 0.398 and 0.308, respectively), but as serum zinc levels increased, HDL-cholesterol levels showed a decreasing trend (p for trend = 0.088 and 0.083, respectively).

3. Associations between serum zinc levels and metabolic syndrome and its components

Unadjusted odds ratios (ORs), age-adjusted ORs (model 1), and multivariate-adjusted ORs (model 2) of serum zinc levels according to the presence of MetS and its components are shown in Table 4. Men with elevated fasting glucose levels were more likely to have low serum zinc levels than were those with normal fasting glucose levels (unadjusted OR 0.50, 95% confidence interval [CI] 0.33–0.77, p = 0.001), and this negative association remained significant after adjusting for covariates (adjusted OR 0.58, 95% CI 0.36–0.93, p = 0.023). The multivariate-adjusted OR of serum zinc levels for elevated triglyceride levels in men was 1.47 (95% CI 1.01–2.13, p = 0.044). However, no significant association between MetS components and serum zinc levels was found in women. No association was detected between the presence of MetS and serum zinc levels in either men or women.

4. Serum zinc levels and the percentage of the highest zinc level group (Q4) according to the number of metabolic syndrome components

Figure 1 shows mean serum zinc levels, and the percentage of the highest zinc level group (Q4) according to the number of MetS components. After adjusting for age, smoking, alcohol drinking, physical activity, BMI, and eGFR levels, in women, a difference in serum zinc levels was observed based on the number of MetS components (p = 0.002). Furthermore, in women with MetS (the number of MetS components: 3, 4 and 5), serum zinc levels showed a decreasing trend as the number of MetS components increased. In terms of the percentage of Q4, the difference showed according to number of MetS components, and the percentage of Q4 in women with MetS showed a decreasing trend as the number of MetS components increased (p = 0.050). No differences in mean serum zinc levels and the percentages of Q4 according to number of MetS components were observed in men (p = 0.727 and p = 0.741, respectively).

5. Percentages of participants according to the MetS component combinations (MetS phenotypes) and serum zinc levels

The participant distribution according to the MetS component combinations and serum zinc levels (Q1-3, and Q4) is shown in Figure 2. In men with the MetS phenotype manifesting as increases in waist circumference, blood pressure and fasting glucose, the percentage of participants in Q4 was lower than in Q1-3 (p = 0.021); on the other hand, in men with the MetS phenotype manifesting as increased waist circumference, elevated triglyceride, and reduced HDL-cholesterol, the percentage in Q4 was higher than in Q1-3 (p = 0.012). There were no significant differences in the percentage of men with other MetS phenotypes. Among women of almost every MetS phenotype, the percentage of participants in Q4 was significantly lower than those in Q1-3, with the exception of the MetS phenotypes manifesting as increased waist circumference, elevated fasting glucose and reduced HDL-cholesterol, and as increased waist circumference, elevated triglycerides and reduced HDL-cholesterol.

Discussion

We investigated the associations of serum zinc levels with MetS or its metabolic risk factors in Korean adults. The results of this study showed associations between serum zinc levels and certain MetS components. Serum zinc levels in men were negatively associated with elevated fasting glucose and positively associated with elevated triglycerides. In both men and women, as serum zinc levels increased, HDL-cholesterol levels showed a decreasing trend. Although there was no significant association found between serum zinc levels and the prevalence of MetS in either men or women, there were differences in serum zinc levels

Table 1. Characteristics of the study participants according to serum zinc level quartile.

	Men			Women		
	Q1,2,3 (n = 704)	Q4 (n = 235)	p value	Q1,2,3 (n = 740)	Q4 (n = 247)	p value
Age (years)	44.8±0.9	41.2±1.0	0.009	46.4±0.8	42.7±1.3	0.012
Current smoking (%)	43.5	42.2	0.786	5.3	5.4	0.951
Heavy drinking (%)	9.1	9.7	0.811	6.3	6.5	0.932
Low physical activity (%)	72.0	68.7	0.425	81.2	78.7	0.526
Body mass index (kg/m^2)	24.1±0.1	24.0±0.3	0.837	23.5±0.2	23.2±0.3	0.457
Zinc (µg/dL)	128.8±1.3	180.0±2.0	<0.001	118.2±1.2	166.9±2.0	<0.001
Metabolic syndrome (%)	27.1	24.5	0.509	27.1	24.1	0.479
Waist circumference (cm)	84.0±0.5	84.3±0.8	0.715	78.3±0.5	77.2±0.9	0.252
SBP (mmHg)	123.4±0.7	121.3±1.0	0.105	118.7±0.8	114.2±1.0	0.002
DBP (mmHg)	80.7±0.6	80.9±0.8	0.850	75.1±0.5	73.4±0.7	0.071
Fasting glucose (mg/dL)	100.5+1.5	95.1±1.3	0.004	95.1±1.0	92.4±1.1	0.081
Triglycerides (mg/dL)	127.0±1.0	127.5±1.1	0.654	95.7±1.0	93.6±1.1	0.333
HDL-cholesterol (mg/dL)	50.0±0.6	49.0±0.9	0.378	56.1±0.6	55.5±1.0	0.618
Insulin (µIU/mL)*	9.7 (9.4–10.1)	9.4 (8.8–10.0)	0.037	10.0 (9.7–10.4)	9.6 (9.0–10.2)	0.018
HOMA-IR index*	2.4 (2.3–2.4)	2.2 (2.0–2.4)	0.078	2.3 (2.2–2.4)	2.2 (2.0–2.3)	0.077
eGFR (mL/min/1.73 m^2)	94.9±0.9	97.0±1.0	0.170	100.4±1.06	100.5±1.8	0.944

Values are expressed as means ± standard errors or percentages and as geometric means and 95% confidence intervals for skewed distributions*. Quartile 1 (Q1): the lowest zinc levels, Q2: low-medium zinc levels, Q3: high-medium zinc levels, and Q4: the highest zinc levels. SBP = systolic blood pressure; DBP = diastolic blood pressure; HDL = high-density lipoprotein; HOMA-IR = homeostasis model assessment of insulin resistance; eGFR = estimated glomerular filtration rate.

according to the number of MetS components in women; in particular, in women with MetS, serum zinc levels decreased as the number of MetS components increased, and low serum zinc levels (Q1-3) showed a greater prevalence than the highest serum zinc levels (Q4) among almost every MetS phenotype.

We used serum zinc concentration to assess body zinc status. Zinc status has been measured in a number of tissues such as serum or plasma, different blood cell types, hair, and nails [28]. However serum zinc concentration is viewed as the most appropriate indicator for evaluating individual's zinc status, as compared to other assessment [29], although the sensitivity and specificity of the serum zinc level might be limited by responsive-

ness to confounding factors such as acute stress, infection, or altered steroidal hormone levels [30]. Furthermore serum zinc concentration is the only biomarker to show a dose-response relationship to dietary zinc manipulations [29–31], so mean serum zinc level in a population may reflect the status of dietary zinc intakes or zinc supplementation, and could be used as an indicator of zinc deficiency at the population level [30].

Several studies have reported a relationship between serum zinc levels and MetS. However, the relationship between serum zinc levels and the prevalence of MetS is inconclusive. In this study, no differences in serum zinc levels were seen between participants with and without MetS. In line with our findings, serum zinc levels

Table 2. Correlations between serum zinc levels and metabolic syndrome components.

	Correlation coefficient (r) with zinc level	
	Men	Women
Waist circumference	0.052	−0.070
Systolic blood pressure	−0.047	−0.082*
Diastolic blood pressure	0.013	−0.066
Fasting glucose	−0.127**	−0.078*
Triglycerides	0.020	−0.016
HDL-cholesterol	−0.033	−0.041
Insulin[†]	−0.066	−0.097*
HOMA-IR index[†]	−0.120**	−0.113**

*p<0.05,
**p<0.01.
[†]Variables with skewed distributions performed log-transformation.
HDL = high-density lipoprotein; HOMA-IR = homeostasis model assessment of insulin resistance.

Table 3. Adjusted mean values of metabolic syndrome components according to serum zinc level quartile.

	Serum zinc levels				p value	p for trend
	Q1	Q2	Q3	Q4		
Men						
N	234	235	235	235		
Zinc (µg/dL)	107.6±11.0	130.5±4.5	147.7±5.5	180.3±23.8		
Range of zinc level (µg/dL)	69.7–122.5	122.6–133.3	138.4–157.6	157.8–333.2		
Waist circumference (cm)	83.3±0.7	84.4±0.8	84.5±0.8	84.9±0.8	0.487	0.168
SBP (mmHg)	124.0±1.3	122.3±1.2	124.4±1.3	122.6±1.1	0.586	0.705
DBP (mmHg)	80.9±1.1	80.6±0.9	80.7±0.9	80.9±0.8	0.993	0.997
Fasting glucose (mg/dL)	104.7±2.9	99.2±1.3	98.0±2.8	96.8±1.3	0.063	0.013
Triglycerides (mg/dL)	119.7±1.0	138.1±1.3	126.0±1.0	130.9±1.1	0.142	0.423
HDL-cholesterol (mg/dL)	50.5±0.9	50.1±1.1	49.2±1.0	48.4±0.9	0.398	0.088
Women						
N	246	248	246	247		
Zinc (µg/dL)	99.6±9.3	119.7±4.3	137.3±5.4	167.9±24.0		
Range of zinc level (µg/dL)	58.1–111.6	111.7–127.1	128.0–146.9	147.0–347.7		
Waist circumference (cm)	77.8±0.8	78.2±0.6	77.1±0.8	77.6±0.8	0.764	0.644
SBP (mmHg)	116.4±1.0	119.2±1.2	116.8±1.2	115.9±1.1	0.201	0.481
DBP (mmHg)	74.4±0.7	75.0±0.7	74.8±0.9	73.9±0.8	0.793	0.672
Fasting glucose (mg/dL)	94.2±1.0	97.2±2.5	91.5±1.0	93.2±1.2	0.074	0.080
Triglycerides (mg/dL)	89.2±1.0	93.3±1.0	94.8±1.0	96.9±1.0	0.565	0.162
HDL-cholesterol (mg/dL)	57.6±1.1	55.6±0.8	55.8±0.8	55.0±0.8	0.308	0.083

Values are means ± standard errors. Adjustment for age, smoking, alcohol consumption, physical activity, BMI, and eGFR levels. Quartile 1 (Q1): the lowest zinc levels, Q2: low-medium zinc levels, Q3: high-medium zinc levels, and Q4: the highest zinc levels. SBP = systolic blood pressure; DBP = diastolic blood pressure; HDL = high-density lipoprotein.

Table 4. Odds ratios and 95% confidence intervals of serum zinc level according to metabolic syndrome and its components.

	Men			Women		
	OR	95% CI	p value	OR	95% CI	p value
Elevated waist circumference						
Unadjusted	1.17	0.76–1.81	0.472	0.92	0.63–1.34	0.660
Model 1	1.27	0.81–1.97	0.294	1.13	0.74–1.73	0.572
Model 2	1.28	0.82–1.98	0.279	1.15	0.76–1.74	0.875
Elevated blood pressure						
Unadjusted	0.98	0.70–1.37	0.890	0.62	0.42–0.92	0.018
Model 1	1.17	0.79–1.74	0.442	0.78	0.41–1.49	0.446
Model 2	1.12	0.74–1.68	0.591	0.78	0.42–1.44	0.420
Elevated fasting glucose						
Unadjusted	0.50	0.33–0.77	0.001	0.60	0.36–1.02	0.059
Model 1	0.58	0.36–0.92	0.020	0.70	0.40–1.24	0.222
Model 2	0.58	0.36–0.93	0.023	0.75	0.43–1.32	0.318
Elevated triglycerides						
Unadjusted	1.34	0.94–1.91	0.110	0.74	0.45–1.21	0.224
Model 1	1.48	1.02–2.14	0.040	0.87	0.54–1.40	0.574
Model 2	1.47	1.01–2.13	0.044	0.91	0.58–1.42	0.667
Reduced HDL-cholesterol						
Unadjusted	1.29	0.87–1.91	0.201	0.92	0.61–1.40	0.702
Model 1	1.40	0.93–2.09	0.106	1.09	0.72–1.63	0.693
Model 2	1.42	0.94–2.14	0.097	1.13	0.74–1.71	0.577
Metabolic syndrome						
Unadjusted	0.87	0.58–1.31	0.509	0.85	0.54–1.34	0.483
Model 1	1.02	0.66–1.59	0.921	1.13	0.67–1.91	0.643
Model 2	1.01	0.65–1.58	0.956	1.21	0.72–2.05	0.478

Model 1: adjustment for age, Model 2: adjustment for age, smoking, alcohol consumption, physical activity, BMI and eGFR levels. HDL = high-density lipoprotein; OR = odds ratio; CI = confidence interval.

did not differ significantly between subjects with and without MetS in a cohort study of 2,233 Iranian subjects aged 15–65 years [21], and in a cross-sectional study conducted in 1,902 European participants, serum zinc levels did not show an association with MetS [20]. However, Yu et al. [19] reported significantly higher serum zinc levels in subjects with MetS compared with those without MetS in a study of 379 Chinese men aged 24–57 years. Furthermore, in a population-based study consisting of 2,401 Iranian adults, mean serum zinc levels were positively associated with men with MetS compared with those without MetS; however, in women, medium serum zinc levels were associated with a lower prevalence of MetS, compared with the lowest zinc levels [18].

Because of the diversity of MetS phenotypes, the treatment strategies used for this condition may be different [32]. In men, serum zinc levels were negatively associated with elevated fasting glucose, but positively correlated with elevated triglycerides. Thus, the different directions of associations with serum zinc levels and certain components of MetS might account for the variations in serum zinc status according to the MetS phenotype (Figure 2A). In women, on the other hand, no significant association between MetS components and serum zinc levels was found, but with almost every MetS phenotype, the percentage of participants with the highest zinc level (Q4) was significantly lower than the percentage of those with the lowest or medium zinc level (Q1-3) (Figure 2B). Furthermore, in women with MetS, serum zinc levels

showed a decreasing trend as the number of MetS components increased. Therefore, with regard to serum zinc levels in women, the presence or severity of MetS might be more useful than the MetS phenotype. Further investigations are warranted to clarify the gender difference in the association between serum zinc levels and MetS.

In this study, low serum zinc levels were associated with elevated fasting glucose levels in men, and significant negative correlations were found between serum zinc levels and fasting glucose as well as insulin resistance in both men and women. Similar to our findings, Islam et al. [33] reported that participants with pre-diabetes had lower zinc levels than did normal participants in a cross-sectional study of 280 Bangladesh adults aged ≥30 years, and Vashum et al. [34] showed that a higher serum zinc concentration was associated with increased insulin sensitivity in a cross-sectional study of 452 Australian adults aged 55–85 years. Insulin resistance is known to play a key role in the development of MetS, although the pathogenesis that unites the components of MetS is unclear. An overabundance of circulating fatty acids released by visceral fat might be a main contributor to the development of insulin resistance [35]. In an experimental study in rats, defects in insulin-stimulated tyrosine phosphorylation of insulin receptor substrates-1 and −2 by high levels of circulating fatty acids contributed to insulin resistance [36]. Zinc, however, is known to increase insulin receptor phosphorylation and downstream protein phosphorylation in insulin signaling pathways [1,2], such that a decrease in body zinc status might cause insulin resistance [33,34].

The issue of whether serum zinc levels are associated with plasma lipids is controversial. In agreement with our results, Ghasemi et al. [18] found a positive correlation between serum zinc levels and triglycerides in Iranian men whereas no association was observed between serum zinc concentrations and lipid profiles in a Kuwaiti population [37] or in Lebanese adults [38]. Although several studies have shown no association between serum zinc levels and HDL-cholesterol concentrations [18,37,38], we found a trend for a negative association between serum zinc and HDL-cholesterol levels in both men and women. Additionally, in a meta-analysis of 33 randomized controlled trials, no significant effects of zinc supplementation on serum lipids were observed, but zinc supplementation was associated with a significant decrease in HDL-cholesterol levels in a sub-group analysis of healthy participants, and HDL-cholesterol levels increased as a result of zinc supplementation in a sub-group analysis of subjects with type 2 diabetes mellitus [39]. However, the negative association between serum zinc and lipoprotein metabolism in our study should be considered cautiously, including the influence of zinc-rich foods such as red meat on plasma lipids [40] and various

health conditions known to influence zinc homeostasis [41–44], and further investigations considering these factors are warranted to confirm the association between serum zinc levels and lipid profiles.

Other factors not included in the clinical definition of MetS, such as chronic inflammation [16] or oxidative stress [15], may lead to the development of MetS. Inflammatory cytokines released by visceral fat [45], including tumor necrosis factor-α (TNF-α), interleukin-6 (IL-6) and plasminogen activator inhibitor-1 (PAI-1), stimulate C-reactive protein (CRP) production in the liver, and these processes are associated with MetS [17]. On the other hand, oxidative stress, which occurs when reactive oxygen species (ROS) exceed the antioxidant capacity, may play an important role in MetS [15]. Zinc reduces inflammatory cytokine production via up-regulation of a zinc-finger protein, which inhibits nuclear factor-κB (NF-κB) activation [6,7]. Furthermore, zinc, a cofactor for antioxidant enzymes, such as superoxide dismutase and glutathione peroxidase, decreases ROS generation and induces metallothionein, which decreases the ·OH burden [2], suggesting that a decrease in body zinc status may contribute to the development or aggravation of MetS. In addition, chronic inflammation or oxidative stress may contribute to the decreased serum zinc levels.

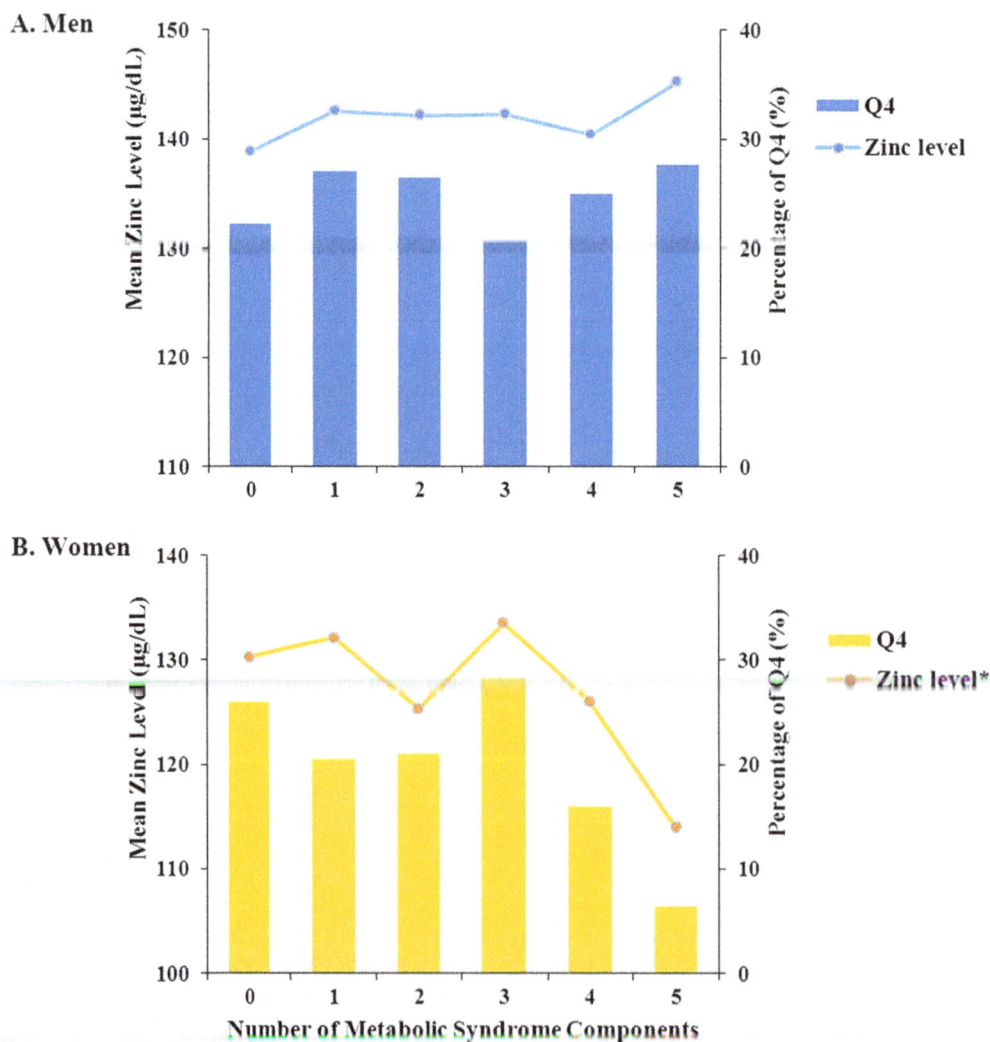

Figure 1. Serum zinc levels and the percentage of participants in the highest zinc level quartile according to the number of metabolic syndrome components. *p value<0.05.

A. Men

B. Women

Phenotypes of Metabolic Syndrome

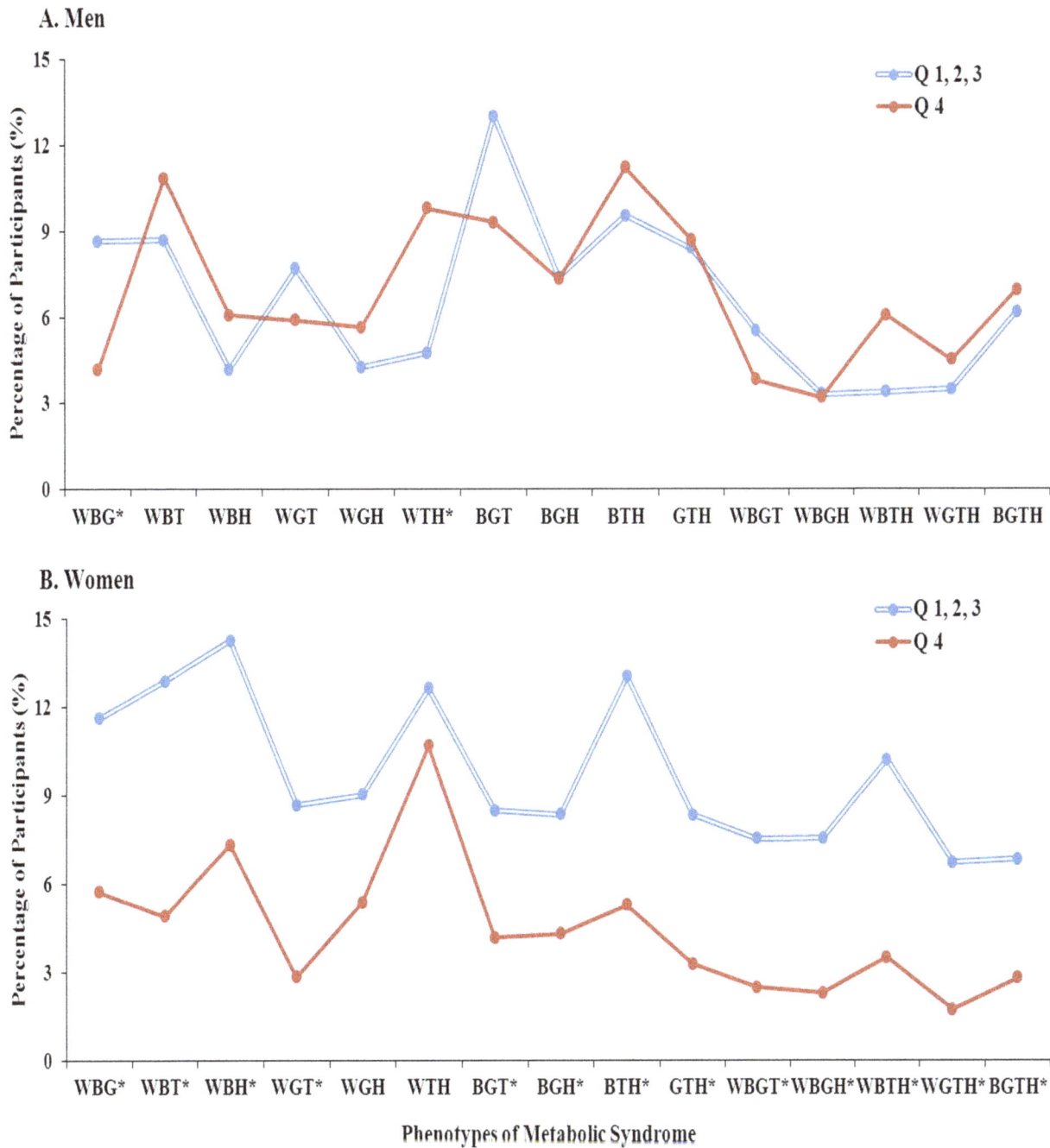

Figure 2. Participant distribution among metabolic syndrome phenotypes and serum zinc level quartiles. *p value<0.05, W: elevated waist circumference, B: elevated blood pressure, G: elevated fasting glucose, H: reduced HDL-cholesterol, T: elevated triglycerides.

In experimental study with mice, the expression of zinc transporter gene, which plays a critical role in the hypozincemia, was up-regulated by inflammation [46], and in an experiment with HL-60 cells, the oxidative stress released zinc from metallothionein, one of cellular zinc buffering systems, and increased the availability of cellular zinc, therefore, it resulted in a cellular zinc deficiency [47], suggesting that as part of MetS, chronic inflammation or oxidative stress negatively affect to body zinc status, and then, the decreased zinc status may play an important role in the development or aggravation of MetS. To date, studies on the effects of zinc intake in adults with MetS are scarce, and have reported inconsistent

results; therefore, further studies on the dietary intake or supplementation of zinc are warranted to associate with the status of chronic inflammation or oxidative stress, and to help reduce the prevalence or improve the manifestation of MetS.

The strengths of this study were that the data were collected through a representative nationwide survey of the South Korean population and that this is the first study in Korean adults to investigate the associations among serum zinc levels, MetS, and its metabolic risk factors. However, this study had certain limitations. First, it was conducted using a cross-sectional design. Second, dietary patterns and the kind of food as sources of zinc intake were not included as a covariate in this study, because dietary zinc intake was not estimated in the KNHANES. Zinc is highly concentrated in the organs and flesh of mammals, fowl, fish, and crustaceans. However, the bioavailability of zinc is determined mostly by the amount of zinc in the diet and phytate, which is a major inhibitor of zinc absorption, so not only total zinc intake but also the types of foods or dietary patterns should be considered when assessing dietary zinc intake [48]. Although zinc intake in the South Korean population was adequate in the data provided by 188 countries to the Food and Agriculture Organization of the United Nations [49], further studies are warranted to clarify the association between dietary zinc intake, serum zinc levels that represent body zinc status, and MetS. Third, we did not consider other trace elements, such as copper, that might affect serum zinc levels, since the trace elemental minerals were not measured in the KNHANES.

References

1. Tang X, Shay NF (2001) Zinc has an insulin-like effect on glucose transport mediated by phosphoinositol-3-kinase and Akt in 3T3-L1 fibroblasts and adipocytes. J Nutr 131: 1414–1420.
2. Haase H, Maret W (2005) Protein tyrosine phosphatases as targets of the combined insulinomimetic effects of zinc and oxidants. Biometals 18: 333–338.
3. Bryant NJ, Govers R, James DE (2002) Regulated transport of the glucose transporter GLUT4. Nat Rev Mol Cell Biol 3: 267–277.
4. Ilouz R, Kaidanovich O, Gurwitz D, Eldar-Finkelman H (2002) Inhibition of glycogen synthase kinase-3beta by bivalent zinc ions: insight into the insulin-mimetic action of zinc. Biochem Biophys Res Commun 295: 102–106.
5. McCall KA, Huang C, Fierke CA (2000) Function and mechanism of zinc metalloenzymes. J Nutr 130 5S Suppl: 1437s–1446s.
6. Prasad AS (2009) Zinc: role in immunity, oxidative stress and chronic inflammation. Curr Opin Clin Nutr Metab Care 12: 646–652.
7. Prasad AS (2008) Clinical, immunological, anti-inflammatory and antioxidant roles of zinc. Exp Gerontol 43: 370–377.
8. Grundy SM (2006) Metabolic syndrome: connecting and reconciling cardiovascular and diabetes worlds. J Am Coll Cardiol 47: 1093–1100.
9. Alberti KG, Eckel RH, Grundy SM, Zimmet PZ, Cleeman JI, et al. (2009) Harmonizing the metabolic syndrome: a joint interim statement of the International Diabetes Federation Task Force on Epidemiology and Prevention; National Heart, Lung, and Blood Institute; American Heart Association; World Heart Federation; International Atherosclerosis Society; and International Association for the Study of Obesity. Circulation 120: 1640–1645.
10. Alberti KG, Zimmet P, Shaw J (2005) The metabolic syndrome-a new worldwide definition. Lancet 366: 1059–1062.
11. Grundy SM (2008) Metabolic syndrome pandemic. Arterioscler Thromb Vasc Biol 28: 629–636.
12. Mozumdar A, Liguori G (2011) Persistent increase of prevalence of metabolic syndrome among U.S. adults: NHANES III to NHANES 1999–2006. Diabetes Care 34: 216–219.
13. Lim S, Shin H, Song JH, Kwak SH, Kang SM, et al. (2011) Increasing prevalence of metabolic syndrome in Korea: the Korean National Health and Nutrition Examination Survey for 1998–2007. Diabetes Care 34: 1323–1328.
14. Gill H, Mugo M, Whaley-Connell A, Stump C, Sowers JR (2005) The key role of insulin resistance in the cardiometabolic syndrome. Am J Med Sci 330: 290–294.
15. Roberts CK, Sindhu KK (2009) Oxidative stress and metabolic syndrome. Life Sci 84: 705–712.
16. Sutherland JP, McKinley B, Eckel RH (2004) The metabolic syndrome and inflammation. Metab Syndr Relat Disord 2: 82–104.
17. Bălăşoiu M, Bălăşoiu AT, Stepan AE, Dinescu SN, Avrămescu CS, et al. (2014) Proatherogenic adipocytokines levels in metabolic syndrome. Rom J Morphol Embryol 55: 29–33.
18. Ghasemi A, Zahediasl S, Hosseini-Esfahani F, Azizi F (2014) Gender differences in the relationship between serum zinc concentration and metabolic syndrome. Ann Hum Biol. doi:10.3109/03014460.2013.870228.
19. Yu Y, Cai Z, Zheng J, Chen J, Zhang X, et al. (2012) Serum levels of polyunsaturated fatty acids are low in Chinese men with metabolic syndrome, whereas serum levels of saturated fatty acids, zinc, and magnesium are high. Nutr Res 32: 71–77.
20. Arnaud J, de Lorgeril M, Akbaraly T, Salen P, Arnout J, et al. (2012) Gender differences in copper, zinc and selenium status in diabetic-free metabolic syndrome European population - the IMMIDIET study. Nutr Metab Cardiovasc Dis 22: 517–524.
21. Ghayour-Mobarhan M, Shapouri-Moghaddam A, Azimi-Nezhad M, Esmaeili H, Parizadeh SM, et al. (2009) The relationship between established coronary risk factors and serum copper and zinc concentrations in a large Persian cohort. J Trace Elem Med Biol 23: 167–175.

In conclusion, serum zinc levels were negatively associated with elevated fasting glucose levels and positively associated with elevated triglycerides in men. Serum zinc levels differed according to the number of MetS components in women, and serum zinc levels showed a decreasing trend as the number of MetS components increased in women with MetS. These findings suggest that serum zinc levels might be associated with MetS or metabolic risk factors. Further gender-specific studies are needed to evaluate the effects of dietary or supplemental zinc intake on the improvement of MetS.

Author Contributions

Conceived and designed the experiments: JAS SWS KH KJL HNK. Analyzed the data: JAS KH HNK. Contributed to the writing of the manuscript: JAS SWS KJL HNK.

22. Korean Centers for Disease Control and Prevention Korea National Health and Nutrition Examination Survey. Available: http://knhanes.cdc.go.kr.
23. Grundy SM, Cleeman JI, Daniels SR, Donato KA, Eckel RH, et al. (2005) Diagnosis and management of the metabolic syndrome: an American Heart Association/National Heart, Lung, and Blood Institute Scientific Statement. Circulation 112: 2735–2752.
24. Lee SY, Park HS, Kim DJ, Han JH, Kim SM, et al. (2007) Appropriate waist circumference cutoff points for central obesity in Korean adults. Diabetes Res Clin Pract 75: 72–80.
25. Matthews DR, Hosker JP, Rudenski AS, Naylor BA, Treacher DF, et al. (1985) Homeostasis model assessment: insulin resistance and beta-cell function from fasting plasma glucose and insulin concentrations in man. Diabetologia 28: 412–419.
26. Levey AS, Coresh J, Greene T, Marsh J, Stevens LA, et al. (2007) Expressing the Modification of Diet in Renal Disease Study equation for estimating glomerular filtration rate with standardized serum creatinine values. Clin Chem 53: 766–772.
27. World Health Organization (2010) Global recommendations on physical activity for health. Geneva, Switzerland: World Health Organization.
28. Gibson RS, Hess SY, Hotz C, Brown KH (2008) Indicators of zinc status at the population level: a review of the evidence. Br J Nutr 99 Suppl 3: S14–23.
29. Lowe NM, Fekete K, Decsi T (2009) Methods of assessment of zinc status in humans: a systematic review. Am J Clin Nutr 89: 2040s–2051s.
30. Hess SY, Peerson JM, King JC, Brown KH (2007) Use of serum zinc concentration as an indicator of population zinc status. Food Nutr Bull 28: S403–429.
31. Lowe NM, Woodhouse LR, Sutherland B, Shames DM, Burri BJ, et al. (2004) Kinetic parameters and plasma zinc concentration correlate well with net loss and gain of zinc from men. J Nutr 134: 2178–2181.
32. Kahn R, Buse J, Ferrannini E, Stern M (2005) The metabolic syndrome: time for a critical appraisal: joint statement from the American Diabetes Association and the European Association for the Study of Diabetes. Diabetes Care 28: 2289–2304.
33. Islam MR, Arslan I, Attia J, McEvoy M, McElduff P, et al. (2013) Is serum zinc level associated with prediabetes and diabetes?: a cross-sectional study from Bangladesh. PLoS One 8: e61776.
34. Vashum KP, McEvoy M, Milton AH, Islam MR, Hancock S, et al. (2014) Is serum zinc associated with pancreatic beta cell function and insulin sensitivity in pre-diabetic and normal individuals? Findings from the Hunter Community Study. PLoS One 9: e83944.
35. Eckel RH, Grundy SM, Zimmet PZ (2005) The metabolic syndrome. Lancet 365: 1415–1428.
36. Samuel VT, Liu ZX, Qu X, Elder BD, Bilz S, et al. (2004) Mechanism of hepatic insulin resistance in non-alcoholic fatty liver disease. J Biol Chem 279: 32345–32353.
37. Abiaka C, Olusi S, Al-Awadhi A (2003) Serum microminerals and the indices of lipid metabolism in an apparently healthy population. J Clin Lab Anal 17: 61–65.
38. Obeid O, Elfakhani M, Hlais S, Iskandar M, Batal M, et al. (2008) Plasma copper, zinc, and selenium levels and correlates with metabolic syndrome components of lebanese adults. Biol Trace Elem Res 123: 58–65.
39. Foster M, Petocz P, Samman S (2010) Effects of zinc on plasma lipoprotein cholesterol concentrations in humans: a meta analysis of randomised controlled trials. Atherosclerosis 210: 344–352.
40. de Oliveira Otto MC, Alonso A, Lee DH, Delclos GL, Bertoni AG, et al. (2012) Dietary intakes of zinc and heme iron from red meat, but not from other sources, are associated with greater risk of metabolic syndrome and cardiovascular disease. J Nutr 142: 526–533.

41. Roozbeh J, Hedayati P, Sagheb MM, Sharifian M, Hamidian Jahromi A, et al. (2009) Effect of zinc supplementation on triglyceride, cholesterol, LDL, and HDL levels in zinc-deficient hemodialysis patients. Ren Fail 31: 798–801.

42. Chevalier CA, Liepa G, Murphy MD, Suneson J, Vanbeber AD, et al. (2002) The effects of zinc supplementation on serum zinc and cholesterol concentrations in hemodialysis patients. J Ren Nutr 12: 183–189.

43. Farvid MS, Siassi F, Jalali M, Hosseini M, Saadat N (2004) The impact of vitamin and/or mineral supplementation on lipid profiles in type 2 diabetes. Diabetes Res Clin Pract 65: 21–28.

44. Partida-Hernandez G, Arreola F, Fenton B, Cabeza M, Roman-Ramos R, et al. (2006) Effect of zinc replacement on lipids and lipoproteins in type 2-diabetic patients. Biomed Pharmacother 60: 161–168.

45. Trayhurn P, Wood IS (2004) Adipokines: inflammation and the pleiotropic role of white adipose tissue. Br J Nutr 92: 347–355.

46. Liuzzi JP, Lichten LA, Rivera S, Blanchard RK, Aydemir TB, et al. (2005) Interleukin-6 regulates the zinc transporter Zip14 in liver and contributes to the hypozincemia of the acute-phase response. Proc Natl Acad Sci U S A 102: 6843–6848.

47. Zangger K, Oz G, Haslinger E, Kunert O, Armitage IM (2001) Nitric oxide selectively releases metals from the amino-terminal domain of metallothioneins: potential role at inflammatory sites. Faseb j 15: 1303–1305.

48. Hambidge KM, Miller LV, Westcott JE, Sheng X, Krebs NF (2010) Zinc bioavailability and homeostasis. Am J Clin Nutr 91: 1478s–1483s.

49. Wessells KR, Brown KH (2012) Estimating the global prevalence of zinc deficiency: results based on zinc availability in national food supplies and the prevalence of stunting. PLoS One 7: e50568.

Regulation of Insulin Degrading Enzyme Activity by Obesity-Associated Factors and Pioglitazone in Liver of Diet-Induced Obese Mice

Xiuqing Wei[1,2], Bilun Ke[1,2], Zhiyun Zhao[2], Xin Ye[2], Zhanguo Gao[2], Jianping Ye[2]*

1 Department of Digestive Disease, Third Affiliated Hospital, Sun Yet-Sen University, Guangzhou, China, 2 Antioxidant and Gene Regulation Laboratory, Pennington Biomedical Research Center, Louisiana State University System, Baton Rouge, Louisiana, United States of America

Abstract

Insulin degrading enzyme (IDE) is a potential drug target in the treatment of type 2 diabetes (T2D). IDE controls circulating insulin through a degradation-dependent clearance mechanism in multiple tissues. However, there is not sufficient information about IDE regulation in obesity. In this study, we test obesity-associated factors and pioglitazone in the regulation of IDE in diet-induced obese (DIO) C57BL/6 mice. The enzyme activity and protein level of IDE were increased in the liver of DIO mice. Pioglitazone (10 mg/kg/day) administration for 2 months significantly enhanced the enzyme activity (75%), protein (180%) and mRNA (100%) of IDE in DIO mice. The pioglitazone-induced changes were coupled with 50% reduction in fasting insulin and 20% reduction in fasting blood glucose. The mechanism of IDE regulation in liver was investigated in the mouse hepatoma cell line (Hepa 1c1c7 cells), in which pioglitazone (5 μM) increased IDE protein and mRNA in a time-dependent manner in an 8 h study. Free fatty acid (palmitate 300 μM) induced IDE protein, but reduced the mRNA. Glucagon induced, and TNF-α decreased IDE protein. Insulin did not exhibit any activity in the same condition. In summary, pioglitazone, FFA and glucagon directly increased, but TNF-α decreased the IDE activity in hepatocytes. The results suggest that IDE activity is regulated in liver by multiple factors in obesity and pioglitazone may induce IDE activity in the control of T2D.

Editor: Mengwei Zang, Boston University School of Medicine, United States of America

Funding: This work was supported by National Institutes of Health grant (DK068036 and DK085495) to JY, and National Opinion Research Center (NIH 2P30DK072476) center grants. The funders had no role in study design, data collection and analysis, decision to publish, or preparation of the manuscript.

* E-mail: yej@pbrc.edu

Introduction

Hyperinsulinemia is associated with obesity and is a risk factor for insulin resistance. Circulating insulin is determined by the balance of insulin clearance and secretion. A reduction in insulin clearance is a mechanism of hyperinsulinemia [1–3]. The role of insulin clearance is less investigated in the pathogenesis of hyperinsulinemia relative to insulin secretion in the obese models. There is controversy about the insulin clearance in obesity. In two recent studies, insulin clearance was enhanced in rodents by HFD in the first [4], but reduced in the second [5]. Insulin clearance was claimed as a target in the treatment of T2D given the role of hyperinsulinemia in the pathogenesis of insulin resistance [1–3]. Insulin resistance occurs after activation of the negative feedback loop of insulin receptor pathway in response to the high level insulin [1]. Serine kinases (Akt, PKC, mTOR, and S6K, etc) are involved in the feedback by inducing serine phosphorylation of insulin receptor substrates (IRSs) [1,6–8]. Induction of IDE activity is expected to prevent the negative feedback by lowering circulating insulin. However, there is not sufficient information about IDE regulation in obesity [9,10]. In this study, we investigated IDE activity in response to obesity-associated factors and pioglitazone.

IDE is a rate-limiting enzyme in the insulin degradation process [11]. It is an intracellular 110–kDa thiol zinc-metalloendopepti-

dase located in the cytosol, peroxisomes, endosomes, and cell surface. IDE catalyzes degradation of several small proteins including insulin, amylin, β-amyloid protein, etc. [12]. IDE enzyme activity is induced by zinc, inhibited by copper, aluminum [13], and nitric oxide [14]. Inactivation of IDE by gene knockout induces hyperinsulinemia and insulin resistance in mice [15]. Pioglitazone is an insulin sensitizing medicine that reduces blood insulin and improves systemic insulin sensitivity. It is generally believed that the control of hyperinsulinemia is a result of improved insulin sensitivity in the peripheral tissues [16,17]. Pioglitazone leads to insulin sensitization in liver and skeletal muscle by reducing circulating lipids through activation of PPARγ in the fat tissues [18], which stimulates adipocyte differentiation and small adipocyte generation in the subcutaneous fat pads. Although pioglitazone reduce circulating insulin, it is not clear if IDE is involved. To address this question, we investigated IDE (insulin) in the liver of DIO mice following pioglitazone treatment.

In this study, we observed that IDE enzyme activity and protein were induced in liver by HFD in DIO mice. In the obesity-associated factors, FFA and glucagon elevated, but TNF-α decreased IDE protein. The IDE activity was enhanced by pioglitazone in DIO mice, suggesting a new mechanism of thiazolidinedione action in the control of insulin resistance.

Methods

Reagents

Rabbit polyclonal antibody to insulin degrading enzyme (IDE, Cat. ab32216) and mouse monoclonal to β-Actin (Cat. ab6276) were from Abcam (1 Kendall Square, Suite B2304 Cambridge, MA 02139–1517, USA). Secondary antibodies include ECL Anti-rabbit IgG horseradish peroxidase linked whole antibody (from donkey, Cat. NA934V, and ECL Anti-mouse IgG horseradish peroxidase linked whole antibody (from sheep, Cat. NA931V, GE Healthcare UK limited, Little Chalfont Buckinghamshire, HP7 9NA UK). Immobilon-P^{SQ} PVDF Transfer Membranes (Cat. ISEQ 10100) and Chemiluminescence reagent Luminata Western HRP Substrate (Cat. WBLUF0100) were from Millipore (Billerica, MA 01821). The X-ray film was from Phenix Research (Cat. F-BX810, Candler, NC, USA).

Diet-induced Obese (DIO) Model

All animal experiments were approved by the Institutional Animal Care and Use Committee at the Pennington Biomedical Research Center. DIO model was generated as described elsewhere [19]. C57BL/6 mice of 6–8 weeks were purchased from Jax Lab and fed a high fat diet (HFD; 58% kcal in fat, D12331; Research Diets, New Brunswick, NJ) for six months to induce type 2 diabetes. Regular Chow diet was used in the control group. Pioglitazone (Actos, 10 mg/kg/day) was administrated through dietary supplement for 2 months after 4 month HFD-feeding. Mice were sacrificed after 4 hour fasting. The liver samples were collected and maintained at −80°C degrees. The serums were collected and maintained at −20°C degrees.

Cellular Model

The mouse hepatoma cell line (1c1c7) was obtained from American Type Cell Culture and maintained in our lab. Cells were cultured and maintained in Dulbecco's Modified Eagle's Medium (DMEM) with 10% fetal bovine serum (Cat. S11150, Atlanta Biologicals, Inc. Lawrenceville, GA, USA) and maintained at 37°C with 5% CO_2/air atmosphere. All the cells were passaged once per two days and routinely examined for mycoplasma contamination. When the cell reached a 90% confluence in the 10 cm plate, it was used in experiments.

5×10^5 cells were loaded to each well of the six-well plates 12 hours before experiments; then starved overnight in Dulbecco's Modified Eagle's Medium (DMEM) containing 0.25% BSA. The cells were treated with 300 μM BSA-conjugated palmitic acid (Cat. P9767, Sigma) for 1, 2, 4, and 8 hours. BSA was used in the control. The cells were treated with 200 nM insulin (Cat. I9278, Sigma) or 5 μM pioglitazone (Cat. E6910, Sigma). DMSO was used 1:1000 in the control for pioglitazone.

IDE Activity Assay

Liver tissue extracts were prepared by homogenizing tissue in Cytobuster Protein Extraction Reagent (Cat. 71009-3, EMD Millipore, Billerica, MA 01821) according to the manufacturer's recommended protocol. IDE activity was assessed with the InnoZyme Insulysin/IDE Immunocapture Activity Assay Kit (Cat. CBA079, Calbiochem/Millipore) and was normalized to the value of control group. Relative IDE activity was expressed in this study.

Western Blotting

The protein preparation and the immunoblotting were described elsewhere [19,20]. Briefly, the whole-cell lysate was made in a lysis buffer under sonication, which breaks both cytoplasmic and nuclear membranes. All of the immunoblotting experiments were conducted at least three times. To make a compare, the intensity of the protein signal was analyzed quantitatively using Image J software (National Institutes of Health, Bethesda, MD). The ratio of IDE signal over the β actin signal was used to express the quantification result.

Quantitative Real-time RT-PCR (qRT-PCR)

TaqMan RT-PCR reaction was used to quantify mRNA of IDE. The total RNA was prepared from cell lysates or tissues with Trizol reagent (Cat. T9424, Sigma, St. Louis, MO) as described elsewhere [19,20]. The assay was conducted using the 7900 HT Fast real-time PCR System (Applied Biosystems, Foster City, CA). The target mRNA signal was normalized with ribosome 18S RNA. IDE (Mm00473077) primer and probe were from the Applied Biosystems.

Plasma Glucose and Insulin

The mice were fasted over night with free access to water. Blood glucose was monitored in the tail vein blood using the FreeStyle blood glucose monitoring system (TheraSense, Phoenix, AZ). Insulin was determined using a Mouse Serum Adipokine multiplex Kit (Cat. MADPK-71K, Millipore) according to the manufacturer's instruction.

Statistical Analysis

Student-t test was performed in data analysis with significance at $P < 0.05$.

Results

Induction of Hepatic IDE by HFD

We investigated insulin clearance in DIO model by examining hepatic IDE activity. Liver is a primary organ in insulin clearance and it is responsible for removal of 70% secreted insulin from islet. A reduction in the insulin clearance function contributes to hyperinsulinemia. IDE is a major rate-limiting enzyme for insulin clearance. Inactivation of IDE activity leads to hyperinsulinemia in gene knockout mice [15]. Hyperinsulinemia is a character of DIO mice, and the role of IDE in the hyperinsulinemia remains largely unknown. To address this question, we examined IDE activity in enzyme function, protein and mRNA in the liver tissue of DIO mice. The enzyme activity was determined in the liver tissue using an enzyme assay kit. The activity was increased in the DIO mice by 186% (Fig. 1A). This change was associated with a 150% increase in IDE protein in a Western blot (Fig. 1B). However, mRNA of IDE was reduced by 65% in qRT-PCR test. The data suggest that IDE activity was enhanced by the high fat diet in the liver of DIO mice.

Induction of Hepatic IDE by Pioglitazone

Pioglitazone is a thiazolidinedione (TZD)-derived insulin-sensitizing medicine. It is generally believed that Pioglitazone reduces hyperinsulinemia through improvement of peripheral insulin sensitivity. However, one study suggests that rosiglitazone (a similar insulin-sensitizing medicine derived from TZD) may enhance insulin clearance in patients [21]. Unfortunately, IDE activity was not examined in the study. To address this issue, we examined IDE activity in the liver tissues of DIO mice after 2 month pioglitazone treatment at a dosage of 10 mg/kg/day. The enzyme activity of IDE was increased by 75% in the pioglitazone-treated mice (Fig. 2A). The IDE protein was enhanced by 190% (Fig. 2B) and mRNA was increased by 100% (Fig. 2C). Pioglitazone reduced fasting insulin, fasting glucose and HOMA-

A

B

C

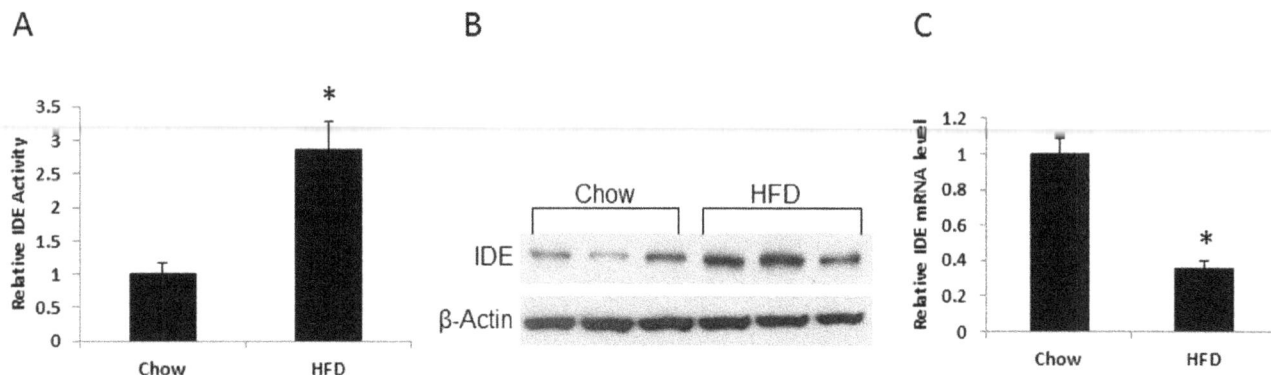

Figure 1. IED in liver tissue of DIO mice. The mice were on chow diet or high fat diet (HFD) for 6 months, and the samples were collected in 4 h fasting state. A. Enzyme activity of IDE. HFD increased enzyme activity of IDE that was determined via the InnoZymeTM Insulysin/IDE Immunocapture Activity Assay Kit (n = 10). B. IDE protein. HFD increased IDE protein level in Western blot. The experiment was performed three times with consistent results, and a representative blot is shown. C. IDE mRNA in liver (n = 4). *P<0.05 compared with the control.

IR index in DIO mice (Fig. 2, D–F), suggesting an improvement in insulin sensitivity. The data suggests that pioglitazone administration enhances IDE activity in the liver during improvement of insulin sensitivity.

Pioglitazone Induction of IDE Expression in Hepatic Cell Line

Cellular studies were conducted to understand the mechanism of IDE regulation in the liver. We examined IDE activity in the mouse hepatoma cell line 1c1c7 in cell culture after pioglitazone treatment. 1c1c7 is widely used as a model of hepatocytes. In this study, the cells were treated with 5 μM pioglitazone for 8 hours. IED protein and mRNA were determined at multiple time points in the time-course study. IDE protein was increased by

pioglitazone in a time-dependent manner in the first few hours with a peak at 4 hours (Fig. 3A). The increase disappeared thereafter at 8 hours. IDE mRNA exhibited an increase, but in a different time course. The mRNA was peaked at 1 hour and gradually reduced thereafter (Fig. 3B). This group of data suggests that pioglitazone directly induced IDE expression in hepatocytes in a time-dependent manner. The induction was observed in both IDE mRNA and protein.

Induction of IDE Protein by Free Fatty Acid (FFA)

IDE protein was enhanced in mouse liver by HFD in this study (Fig. 1). The mechanism was not known. We addressed this issue by testing IDE in 1c1c cells following the palmitic acid treatment as long chain fatty acids are the main component in HFD. IDE

A

B

C

D

E

F

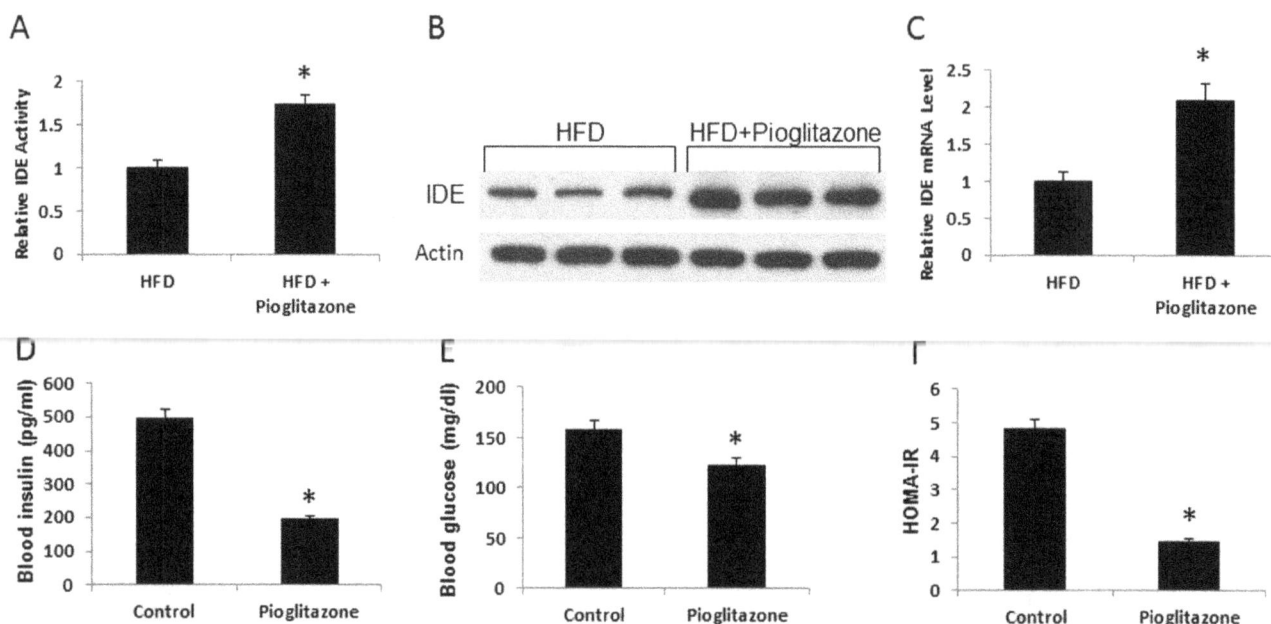

Figure 2. Regulation of liver IDE by pioglitazone. A. IDE enzyme activity. Liver tissue was collected from DIO C57BL/6J mice were treated with pioglitazone (10 mg/kg/d) for last 2 months in 6 month HFD feeding. The samples were collected in fasting state. The IDE enzyme activity was determined (n = 10). B. IDE protein. The protein level was determined in Western blot. The experiment was performed three times with consistent results, and a representative blot is shown. C. IDE mRNA. mRNA level was determined in qRT-PCR (n = 5). D. Fasting blood insulin. E. Fasting blood glucose. F. HOMA-IR index (n = 10). *P<0.05 compared with the control.

A

B

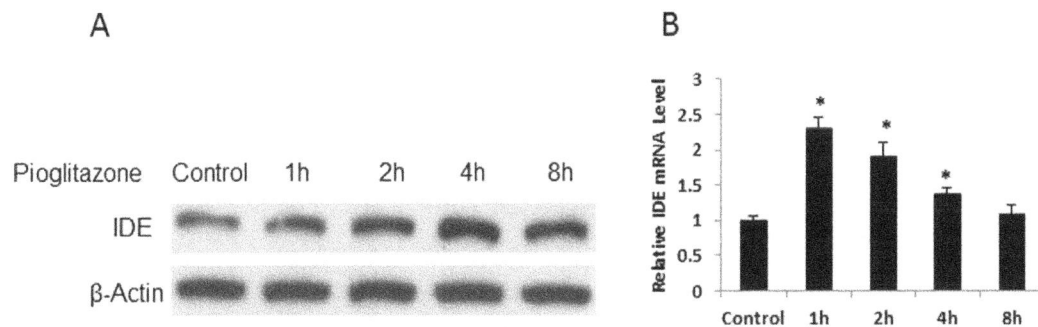

Figure 3. Regulation of IDE in hepatocytes by pioglitazone. A. IDE protein. Hepatocytes (1c1c7) were treated with pioglitazone (5 µM) for 8 hours. In the control, vehicle (DMSO) was added at 1:1000 into the culture medium for 8 hour treatment. The experiment was performed three times with consistent results, and a representative blot is shown. B. IDE mRNA. mRNA was determined by qRT-PCR (n = 3), *$P < 0.05$ compared with the control.

protein was increased in a time-dependent manner by the palmitate acid (300 µM) with the highest level at 8 hours (Fig. 4A). However, IDE mRNA was not increased in the same condition. Instead, mRNA was decreased at 4 and 8 hours in the presence of FFA (Fig. 4B). This pattern of changes resembles those observed in the liver of DIO mice. The data suggest that FFA may directly up-regulate IDE protein in hepatocytes.

Insulin did not Regulate IED in Hepatocytes

Regulation of IDE activity by insulin is of interesting as there is hyperinsulinemia in obesity. However, the relationship remains to be established. To address this question, we examined IDE activity in 1c1c7 cells after the insulin treatment. The cells were treated with 200 nM insulin for 8 hours. IDE activity was determined in protein and mRNA. No significant change was observed in IDE in the insulin-treated cells (Fig. 5, A and B), suggesting that insulin may not directly regulate IDE expression in hepatocytes.

Induction of IDE Protein by Glucagon and Forskolin

An increase in glucagon activity contributes to hyperglycemia in obesity [22]. There is no literature about IDE regulation by glucagon according to our knowledge. The glucagon activity was tested in 1c1c cells. IDE protein was induced by glucagon in a time-dependent manner in an 8 hour study. IDE protein was induced by 70% at 30 mins and a peak of increase at 100% was observed at 1 hour (Fig. 6A). The elevation was maintained for 4

hours and then decreased at 8 hours. A similar pattern of IDE protein increase was observed in the cells treated with forskolin, an activator of protein kinase A (PKA), suggesting that glucagon induced IDE protein through activation of the cAMP/PKA signaling pathway.

Inhibition of IDE Protein by TNF-α

Chronic inflammation is associated with obesity and liver is one of the inflammatory sites next to the white adipose tissue [23]. There is no study about regulation of IDE by inflammation in obesity models. We addressed this issue by testing IDE in hepatocytes following treatment with TNF-α, a representative pro-inflammatory cytokine. IDE protein was modestly increased by TNF-α at 1 hour and then decreased significantly thereafter in the 8 hour treatment (Fig. 7A). IDE mRNA was consistently reduced by TNF-α in hepatocytes. The data suggests that the major activity of TNF-α is to inhibit IDE expression in hepatocytes.

Discussion

Our study suggests that pioglitazone has a potential activity in the induction of IDE activity. IDE is a potential drug target in the treatment of type 2 diabetes. Up-regulation of IDE activity may help to control hyperinsulinemia in the disease. The liver removes 50% insulin peptide in the portal vein during the first passage [9]. Insulin removal is dependent on receptor-mediated uptake and

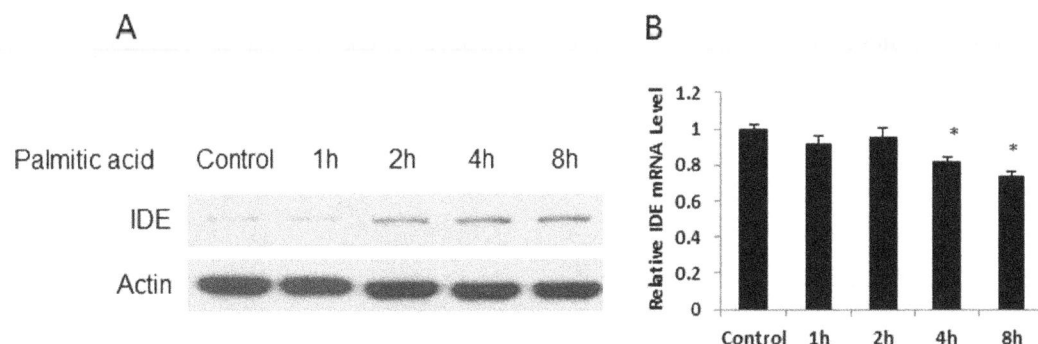

A

B

Figure 4. Regulation of IDE by free fatty acid. A. IDE protein. 1c1c7 cells were treated by palmitic acid (300 µM) for different times. In the control, cells were treated with BSA at the equal concentration for 8 hours. IDE protein was determined in whole cell lysate in Western blot. The experiment was performed three times with consistent results, and a representative blot is shown. B. IDE mRNA. IDE mRNA was in qRT-PCR (n = 3). *$P < 0.05$ compared with the control.

A

B

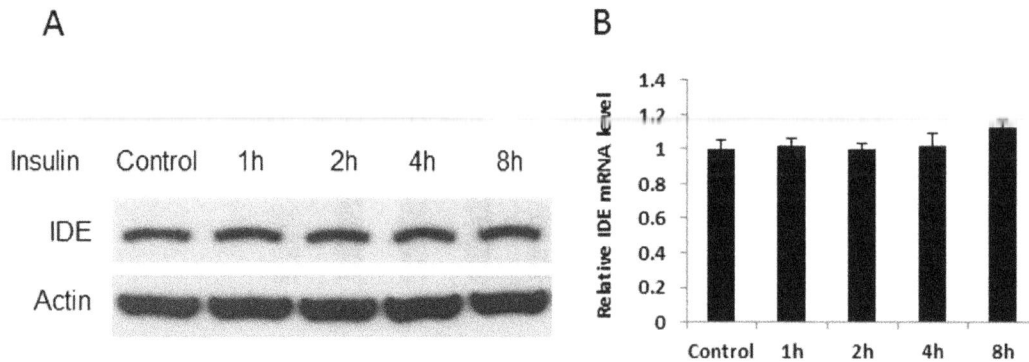

Figure 5. Regulation of IDE by insulin. A. IDE protein. 1c1c7 cells were treated by insulin (200 nM) for 8 hours. IDE protein was determined in the whole cell lysate in Western blot. In the control, PBS was added into the culture medium in the 8 hour treatment. The experiment was performed three times with consistent results, and a representative blot is shown. B. IDE mRNA. mRNA was determined by qRT-PCR (n = 3).

IDE-catalyzed degradation of insulin in several tissues, in which liver is a major one [9]. Insulin clearance is impaired in obesity [24] and a defect in IDE activity is proposed as a major factor [9]. Knockout of IDE gene leads to hyperinsulinemia in mice from impaired insulin clearance in multiple tissues [15,25]. IDE gene mutation is responsible for hyperinsulinemia and insulin resistance in the Goto–Kakizaki rats (a genetic model of non-insulin-dependent diabetes) [26]. Human studies suggest that polymorphisms of IDE gene is closely associated with a high risk for type 2 diabetes [27,28]. IDE malfunction contributes to insulin resistance and hyperglycemia in many cases although not all [9]. Up-regulation of IDE activity is an ideal approach in the treatment of insulin-mediated insulin resistance in T2D. Unfortunately, not much is known about IDE regulation in obesity [9].

We observed that pioglitazone induced IDE enzyme activity in the liver of DIO mice, which was associated with an increase in IDE protein and mRNA. Although IDE catalyzes degradation of insulin and β-amyloid peptide, current knowledge about IDE regulation is mostly derived from the study of β-amyloid peptide in the Alzheimer disease field. IDE takes care of β-amyloid clearance and IDE dysfunction is a critical factor in the pathogenesis of Alzheimer disease. In the current study, we observed that pioglitazone induced IDE protein and mRNA in vivo and in vitro. Consistently, the IDE gene promoter contains a PPARγ binding site, and PPARγ induces the gene transcription in neuronal cells [29]. Regulation of IDE expression represents a novel activity of pioglitazone in the pharmacological action. This activity suggests that pioglitazone may reduce hyperinsulinemia through accelerating clearance of insulin. Our study supports the role of PPARγ in the regulation of IDE expression. IDE gene transcription was reported to be induced by NRF1 [30] and reduced by Notch signaling proteins HES-1 or Hey-1 in neuronal cells [31]. In addition, pioglitazone may increase IDE through inhibition of TNF-α expression.

Our study suggests that FFA (palmitate) and glucagon induces IDE protein. We examined FFA, insulin and glucagon to understand IDE change in the liver of DIO model. Our data suggests that FFA and glucagon induce IDE protein. Early reports suggest that FFA reduces IDE activity and insulin clearance in cell cultures [32,33]. The FFA effect remains to be verified with well-designed experiments in vivo. Two human studies report opposite effects of high fat diet on insulin clearance. Cafeteria diet was reported to enhance the insulin clearance in the first study [4], but reduced in the second study [5], suggesting that the FFA activity remains unclear in vivo. In this study, we observed that IDE protein and enzyme activity were induced in the liver of DIO mice. However, IDE mRNA was reduced. FFA exhibited the same effect in cell culture, suggesting that FFA directly induces IDE protein in hepatocytes. The molecular mechanism of FFA activity remains to be identified. Gene expression may not involve as FFA did not induce IDE mRNA. Protein modification may play a role, and IDE protein is regulated by ubiquitin [34]. The FFA signaling pathway remains to be identified in the IDE regulation. FFA activates protein kinase C (PKC), JUN c-terminal kinase (JNK), and IkBα kinase (IKK) pathways [35]. The role of PKC, JNK and IKK pathways are not supported in IDE up-regulation due to the TNF-α inhibition of IDE protein and mRNA in this study. Glucagon induced IDE protein in this study. Activation of cAMP/

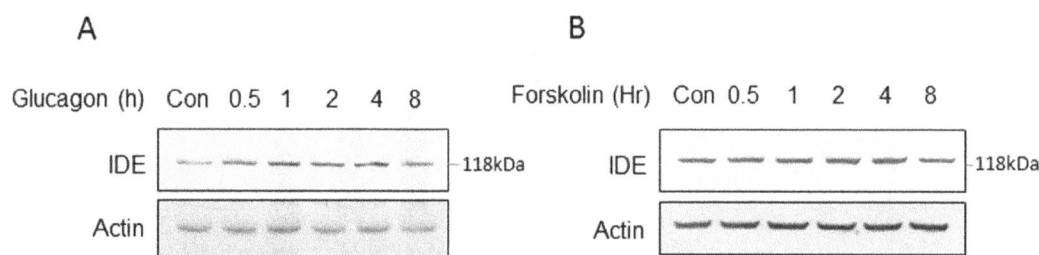

A

B

Figure 6. Regulation of IDE by glucagon. A. IDE protein induction by glucagon. 1c1c7 cells were treated with glucagon (100 ng/ml) for 8 hours. IDE protein was determined in the whole cell lysate at different times in Western blot. In the control, PBS was added into the culture medium in the 8 hour treatment. B. IDE protein induction by forskolin (10 μM). IED protein was determined in the whole cell lysate at different times in Western blot. The experiment was performed three times with consistent results, and a representative blot is shown.

A

B

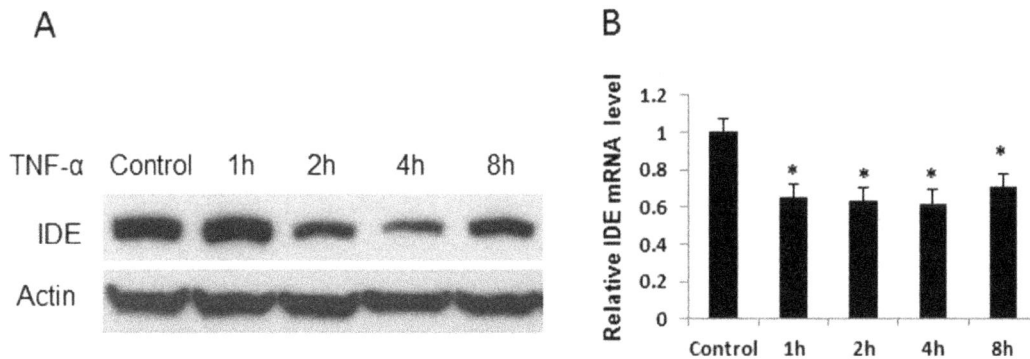

Figure 7. Regulation of IDE by TNF-α. A. IDE protein. 1c1c7 cells were treated with TNF-α (10 ng/ml) for 8 hours. Equal volume of PBS was added into the culture medium in the control for 8 hours. IDE protein was determined at different times as shown and the experiment was performed three times with consistent results. A representative blot is shown. B. IDE mRNA (n = 3). *$P<0.05$ compared with the control group.

PKA pathway by forskolin exhibited the same effect as glucagon. Therefore, the cAMP pathway is likely involved in IDE up-regulation by glucagon. The physiological significance is that IDE likely involve in a feedback regulation of glucagon. It was reported that IDE protein was induced by 25% by insulin in the primary hippocampal neurons [36]. However, such an effect was not observed in the liver cell line in the current study. Insulin was reported to inhibit IDE enzyme activity in an early study [37], but induce the activity in a later study [38]. We cannot exclude insulin activity in the regulation of IDE enzyme activity as it was not examined in this study.

Our data suggests that TNF-α inhibits IDE activity in 1c1c cells. The mechanism is not known. We propose that activation of NF-kB by TNF-α may play a role. NF-kB is known to suppress PPARγ function through multiple mechanisms [17,39]. Pioglitazone may antagonize the TNF-α activity by activation of PPARγ. In addition, inhibition of TNF-α expression by pioglitazone may be another mechanism of pioglitazone action. Thiazolidinediones including pioglitazone have anti-inflammatory effects in macrophages [40,41].

This is a preliminary study and the observations need to be confirmed with more sophisticated assays or model systems in the future. The assay used to measure IDE enzyme activity is a FRET-based assay using a 9 amino acid peptide. The activity remains to be tested using full length insulin as a substrate as IDE activity

toward insulin and small peptides is not the same [42]. We show that IDE levels and activity are altered by a number of stimuli. The results are based on mRNA and protein levels of IDE in cellular models, and the IDE enzyme activity remains to be tested in insulin degradation. In addition, different fatty acids such as mono-unsaturated fatty acid (oleic acid) and poly-unsaturated fatty acids (DHA and EPA) remain to be tested in the regulation of IDE.

In summary, we examined several factors in the regulation of IDE activity. In the multiple-step process of insulin clearance, IDE defect may impair insulin clearance and increase the risk for hyperinsulinemia. Fatty liver and chronic inflammation may contribute to the pathogenesis of T2D through impairing IDE activity. The IDE activity was induced by pioglitazone, suggesting a new action of the medicine in the treatment of T2D. Although the study was conducted in liver and hepatocytes, the observation may apply to IDE regulation in other tissues such as kidney, brain and fat tissues.

Author Contributions

Conceived and designed the experiments: JY. Performed the experiments: XW BK ZZ XY ZG. Analyzed the data: XW BK ZG. Contributed reagents/materials/analysis tools: JY. Wrote the paper: JY.

References

1. Ye J (2007) Role of insulin in the pathogenesis of free fatty acid-induced insulin resistance in skeletal muscle. Endocr Metab Immune Disord Drug Targets 7: 65–74.

2. Corkey BE (2012) Banting lecture 2011: hyperinsulinemia: cause or consequence? Diabetes 61: 4–13.

3. Ye J (2013) Mechanisms of insulin resistance in obesity. Front Med 7: 14–24.

4. Castell-Auvi A, Cedo L, Pallares V, Blay M, Ardevol A, et al. (2012) The effects of a cafeteria diet on insulin production and clearance in rats. Br J Nutr 108: 1155–1162.

5. Brandimarti P, Costa-Junior JM, Ferreira SM, Protzek AO, Santos GJ, et al. (2013) Cafeteria diet inhibits insulin clearance by reduced insulin-degrading enzyme expression and mRNA splicing. J Endocrinol 219: 173–182.

6. Lee YH, White MF (2004) Insulin receptor substrate proteins and diabetes. Arch Pharm Res 27: 361–370.

7. Gao Z, Zuberi A, Quon M, Dong Z, Ye J (2003) Aspirin Inhibits Serine Phosphorylation of Insulin Receptor Substrate 1 in Tumor Necrosis Factor-treated Cells through Targeting Multiple Serine Kinases. J Biol Chem 278: 24944–24950.

8. Zhang J, Gao Z, Yin J, Quon MJ, Ye J (2008) S6K Directly Phosphorylates IRS-1 on Ser-270 to Promote Insulin Resistance in Response to TNF-α Signaling Through IKK2. J Biol Chem 283: 35375–35382.

9. Duckworth WC, Bennett RG, Hamel FG (1998) Insulin degradation: progress and potential. Endocr Rev 19: 608–624.

10. Hulse RE, Ralat LA, Wei-Jen T (2009) Structure, function, and regulation of insulin-degrading enzyme. Vitam Horm 80: 635–648.

11. Valera Mora ME, Scarfone A, Calvani M, Greco AV, Mingrone G (2003) Insulin clearance in obesity. J Am Coll Nutr 22: 487–493.

12. Shen Y, Joachimiak A, Rosner MR, Tang WJ (2006) Structures of human insulin-degrading enzyme reveal a new substrate recognition mechanism. Nature 443: 870–874.

13. Grasso G, Pietropaolo A, Spoto G, Pappalardo G, Tundo GR, et al. (2011) Copper(I) and copper(II) inhibit Abeta peptides proteolysis by insulin-degrading enzyme differently: implications for metallostasis alteration in Alzheimer's disease. Chemistry 17: 2752–2762.

14. Cordes CM, Bennett RG, Siford GL, Hamel FG (2009) Nitric oxide inhibits insulin-degrading enzyme activity and function through S-nitrosylation. Biochem Pharmacol 77: 1064–1073.

15. Farris W, Mansourian S, Chang Y, Lindsley L, Eckman EA, et al. (2003) Insulin-degrading enzyme regulates the levels of insulin, amyloid beta-protein, and the beta-amyloid precursor protein intracellular domain in vivo. Proc Natl Acad Sci U S A 100: 4162–4167.

16. Berger J, Moller DE (2002) The mechanisms of action of PPARs. Annu Rev Med 53: 409–435.

17. Ye J (2008) Regulation of PPARg function by TNF-α. Biochem Biophys Res Commun 374 405–408.

18. Schoonjans K, Peinado-Onsurbe J, Lefebvre AM, Heyman RA, Briggs M, et al. (1996) PPARalpha and PPARgamma activators direct a distinct tissue-specific transcriptional response via a PPRE in the lipoprotein lipase gene. Embo J 15: 5336–5348.

19. Xu F, Gao Z, Zhang J, Rivera CA, Yin J, et al. (2010) Lack of SIRT1 (Mammalian Sirtuin 1) Activity Leads to Liver Steatosis in the SIRT1+/− Mice: A Role of Lipid Mobilization and Inflammation. Endocrinology 151 2504–2514.

20. Tang T, Zhang J, Yin J, Staszkiewicz J, Gawronska-Kozak B, et al. (2010) Uncoupling of Inflammation and Insulin Resistance by NF-kB in Transgenic Mice through Induction of Energy Expenditure. J Biol Chem 285: 4637–4644.

21. Osei K, Gaillard T, Schuster D (2007) Thiazolidinediones increase hepatic insulin extraction in African Americans with impaired glucose tolerance and type 2 diabetes mellitus. A pilot study of rosiglitazone. Metabolism 56: 24–29.

22. Sheng L, Zhou Y, Chen Z, Ren D, Cho KW, et al. (2012) NF-kappaB-inducing kinase (NIK) promotes hyperglycemia and glucose intolerance in obesity by augmenting glucagon action. Nat Med 18: 943–949.

23. Ye J, McGuinness OP (2013) Inflammation during obesity is not all bad: Evidence from animal and human studies. Am J Physiol Endocrinol Metab 304: E466–E477.

24. Erdmann J, Mayr M, Oppel U, Sypchenko O, Wagenpfeil S, et al. (2009) Weight-dependent differential contribution of insulin secretion and clearance to hyperinsulinemia of obesity. Regul Pept 152: 1–7.

25. Abdul-Hay SO, Kang D, McBride M, Li L, Zhao J, et al. (2011) Deletion of insulin-degrading enzyme elicits antipodal, age-dependent effects on glucose and insulin tolerance. PLoS One 6: e20818.

26. Fakhrai-Rad H, Nikoshkov A, Kamel A, Fernstrom M, Zierath JR, et al. (2000) Insulin-degrading enzyme identified as a candidate diabetes susceptibility gene in GK rats. Hum Mol Genet 9: 2149–2158.

27. Sladek R, Rocheleau G, Rung J, Dina C, Shen L, et al. (2007) A genome-wide association study identifies novel risk loci for type 2 diabetes. Nature 445: 881–885.

28. Marlowe L, Peila R, Benke KS, Hardy J, White LR, et al. (2006) Insulin-degrading enzyme haplotypes affect insulin levels but not dementia risk. Neurodegener Dis 3: 320–326.

29. Du J, Zhang L, Liu S, Zhang C, Huang X, et al. (2009) PPARgamma transcriptionally regulates the expression of insulin-degrading enzyme in primary neurons. Biochem Biophys Res Commun 383: 485–490.

30. Zhang L, Ding Q, Wang Z (2012) Nuclear respiratory factor 1 mediates the transcription initiation of insulin-degrading enzyme in a TATA box-binding protein-independent manner. PLoS One 7: e42035.

31. Leal MC, Surace EI, Holgado MP, Ferrari CC, Tarelli R, et al. (2012) Notch signaling proteins HES-1 and Hey-1 bind to insulin degrading enzyme (IDE) proximal promoter and repress its transcription and activity: implications for cellular Abeta metabolism. Biochim Biophys Acta 1823: 227–235.

32. Svedberg J, Bjorntorp P, Smith U, Lonnroth P (1990) Free-fatty acid inhibition of insulin binding, degradation, and action in isolated rat hepatocytes. Diabetes 39: 570–574.

33. Hamel FG, Upward JL, Bennett RG (2003) In vitro inhibition of insulin-degrading enzyme by long-chain fatty acids and their coenzyme A thioesters. Endocrinology 144: 2404–2408.

34. Grasso G, Rizzarelli E, Spoto G (2008) How the binding and degrading capabilities of insulin degrading enzyme are affected by ubiquitin. Biochim Biophys Acta 1784: 1122–1126.

35. Gao Z, Zhang X, Zuberi A, Hwang D, Quon MJ, et al. (2004) Inhibition of Insulin Sensitivity by Free Fatty Acids Requires Activation of Multiple Serine Kinases in 3T3-L1 Adipocytes. Mol Endocrinol 18: 2024–2034.

36. Zhao L, Teter B, Morihara T, Lim GP, Ambegaokar SS, et al. (2004) Insulin-degrading enzyme as a downstream target of insulin receptor signaling cascade: implications for Alzheimer's disease intervention. J Neurosci 24: 11120–11126.

37. Duckworth WC, Bennett RG, Hamel FG (1994) A direct inhibitory effect of insulin on a cytosolic proteolytic complex containing insulin-degrading enzyme and multicatalytic proteinase. J Biol Chem 269: 24575–24580.

38. Pivovarova O, Gogebakan O, Pfeiffer AF, Rudovich N (2009) Glucose inhibits the insulin-induced activation of the insulin-degrading enzyme in HepG2 cells. Diabetologia 52: 1656–1664.

39. Gao Z, He Q, Peng B, Chiao PJ, Ye J (2006) Regulation of Nuclear Translocation of HDAC3 by IkBa Is Required for Tumor Necrosis Factor Inhibition of Peroxisome Proliferator-activated Receptor {gamma} Function. J Biol Chem 281: 4540–4547.

40. Ogawa S, Lozach J, Benner C, Pascual G, Tangirala RK, et al. (2005) Molecular Determinants of Crosstalk between Nuclear Receptors and Toll-like Receptors. Cell 122: 707–721.

41. Pascual G, Fong AL, Ogawa S, Gamliel A, Li AC, et al. (2005) A SUMOylation-dependent pathway mediates transrepression of inflammatory response genes by PPAR-gamma. Nature 437: 759–763.

42. Song ES, Juliano MA, Juliano L, Hersh LB (2003) Substrate activation of insulin-degrading enzyme (insulysin). A potential target for drug development. J Biol Chem 278: 49789–49794.

Lower Fetuin-A, Retinol Binding Protein 4 and Several Metabolites after Gastric Bypass Compared to Sleeve Gastrectomy in Patients with Type 2 Diabetes

Mia Jüllig[1,2], Shelley Yip[3], Aimin Xu[4], Greg Smith[5], Martin Middleditch[1,2], Michael Booth[6], Richard Babor[7], Grant Beban[8], Rinki Murphy[3]*

1 Maurice Wilkins Centre for Molecular Biodiscovery, University of Auckland, Auckland, New Zealand, 2 School of Biological Sciences, University of Auckland, Auckland, New Zealand, 3 Department of Medicine, University of Auckland, Auckland, New Zealand, 4 Department of Medicine, Department of Pharmacology and Pharmacy, The University of Hong Kong, Hong Kong, Special Administrative Region, China, 5 Department of Pharmacology, University of New South Wales, Sydney, New South Wales, Australia, 6 Department of Surgery, North Shore Hospital, Auckland, New Zealand, 7 Department of Surgery, Middlemore Hospital, Auckland, New Zealand, 8 Department of Surgery, Auckland City Hospital, Auckland, New Zealand

Abstract

Background: Bypass of foregut secreted factors promoting insulin resistance is hypothesized to be one of the mechanisms by which resolution of type 2 diabetes (T2D) follows roux-en-y gastric bypass (GBP) surgery.

Aim: To identify insulin resistance-associated proteins and metabolites which decrease more after GBP than after sleeve gastrectomy (SG) prior to diabetes remission.

Methods: Fasting plasma from 15 subjects with T2D undergoing GBP or SG was analyzed by proteomic and metabolomic methods 3 days before and 3 days after surgery. Subjects were matched for age, BMI, metformin therapy and glycemic control. Insulin resistance was calculated using homeostasis model assessment (HOMA-IR). For proteomics, samples were depleted of abundant plasma proteins, digested with trypsin and labeled with iTRAQ isobaric tags prior to liquid chromatography-tandem mass spectrometry analysis. Metabolomic analysis was performed using gas chromatography-mass spectrometry. The effect of the respective bariatric surgery on identified proteins and metabolites was evaluated using two-way analysis of variance and appropriate post-hoc tests.

Results: HOMA-IR improved, albeit not significantly, in both groups after surgery. Proteomic analysis yielded seven proteins which decreased significantly after GBP only, including Fetuin-A and Retinol binding protein 4, both previously linked to insulin resistance. Significant decrease in Fetuin-A and Retinol binding protein 4 after GBP was confirmed using ELISA and immunoassay. Metabolomic analysis identified significant decrease of citrate, proline, histidine and decanoic acid specifically after GBP.

Conclusion: Greater early decrease was seen for Fetuin-A, Retinol binding protein 4, and several metabolites after GBP compared to SG, preceding significant weight loss. This may contribute to enhanced T2D remission observed following foregut bypass procedures.

Editor: Pankaj K. Singh, University of Nebraska Medical Center, United States of America

Funding: This work was supported by the Jens Henrick Jensen fund and the NovoNordisk Diabetes grant fund. The funders had no role in study design, data collection and analysis, decision to publish, or preparation of the manuscript.

* E-mail: R.Murphy@auckland.ac.nz

Introduction

The success of bariatric surgery in obtaining remission of type 2 diabetes (T2D) varies with the type of surgery performed, with generally higher rates observed after gastric bypass (GBP) or biliopancreatic diversion, than with purely restrictive operations such as gastric banding [1,2]. This is not explained by the difference in overall weight loss achieved by the different procedures, because weight loss achieved is not significantly associated with T2D outcome in individuals and there is no difference in weight loss between patients with remission of T2D and non-remission between or within bariatric procedures [3]. One of the mechanisms by which procedures involving intestinal rearrangement such as GBP and biliopancreatic diversion normalize glycaemia is through greater improvement in insulin resistance, seen to a lesser extent following non diversionary surgeries such as sleeve gastrectomy (SG) or gastric banding [4,5].

To explain the rapid and sustained impact of GBP on improving glycaemia in patients with type 2 diabetes, two hypotheses have been proposed: The hindgut hypothesis suggests that the rapid transit of nutrients to the distal bowel improves glucose metabolism by stimulating secretion of the incretin hormone GLP-1 from the ileum and colon L-cells [6]. Indeed, prandial GLP-1 secretion acts to increase glucose-stimulated insulin secretion and improves post-prandial glycaemia, however this does not explain the rapid normalization of fasting glycaemia seen following GBP [7]. The foregut hypothesis proposes that nutrient bypass of the upper gut leads to reduction in secretion of an unidentified gut peptide which promotes insulin resistance [8,9]. Identification of such a gut peptide could yield insights into the pathophysiology of obesity associated T2D and new thera-peutic targets.

Proteomics refers to the identification and/or quantification of the proteins expressed in a tissue, and is used for both inter- and intra-individual comparisons of samples [10]. Early proteomic studies often relied on two-dimensional polyacrylamide gel electrophoresis [11] while newer proteomic approaches e.g. isobaric tagging of peptides separated by liquid chromatography and analyzed using tandem mass spectrometry have been developed to overcome limitations associated with gel electropho-resis and allow more rapid and accurate proteomic analysis of complex proteinaceous samples. New opportunities for discovery in biofluids have also opened up with the development of selective depletion strategies for highly abundant proteins which otherwise tend to dominate the analysis, obstructing the analysis of biomarkers and other key proteins that are often in low abundance [11]. Complementing proteomic techniques, metabolomic analysis offers a highly sensitive means to profile a large number of metabolites in various metabolic pathways [12] and provides useful information on activity of metabolic pathways e.g. lipid and carbohydrate metabolism [13,14].

In this study we combined proteomic and metabolomic approaches to explore the foregut hypothesis. We aimed to identify proteins as well as metabolites which were decreased following GBP (foregut bypassed from nutrient flow), but not after SG (foregut intact with nutrient flow), with special focus on molecules already linked to insulin resistance. The post-operative time point (3 days post-operatively) was carefully chosen in order to place focus on cause rather than effect. Three days after surgery the greater expected T2D remission following GBP than SG was still negligible, hence any significant differences found in the plasma proteomic and metabolomic profiles were unlikely resulting from T2D remission. The effect of bypassing the foregut on secretion of molecules should however be evident shortly after GBP. By performing within-patient comparisons of fasting plasma protein and metabolite profiles before and soon after either GBP or SG when post–surgical caloric intake and physical activity was equivalent and very little weight loss had occurred, we also avoided confounding effects of weight loss and differences in caloric intake.

Materials and Methods

A non-randomised, matched, prospective controlled interven-tion trial that compared the acute effect of GBP to SG, compared with matched caloric intake, on glycemia among obese patients with type 2 diabetes has been previously described with its inclusion and exclusion criteria [15]. Briefly, from 1 August 2010 to 31 March 2012, 21 obese patients with type 2 diabetes treated with oral glucose lowering therapies (but not incretin hormone therapies) were recruited by contacting patients on the bariatric

surgery waiting lists, 10 who were scheduled for SG and 11 who were scheduled for GBP. A total of 7 patients who had SG and 8 who had GBP, all treated with metformin monotherapy at baseline, were eligible for inclusion in this pilot proteomic and metabolomic study. Baseline and follow up assessments were conducted in the patients' homes at 3 pre- and post-operative days. The protocol, allocation and supporting TREND checklist for this study are available as supporting information (Checklist S1 and Protocol S1), and Figureô 1 for the allocation flow chart. All patients were prescribed a hypocaloric diet with three servings of Optifast (152 Calories) per day during the three weeks prior to surgery and were instructed to fast from midnight the night before surgery. Patients received general anaesthesia with atracurium and propofol or equivalent agents for both laparoscopic surgeries. The GBP consisted of a 100 cm antecolic Roux-limb with hand-sewn pouch-jejunostomy, a 60 cm bilio-pancreatic limb and a hand sewn small bowel anastomosis. The SG was performed by a longitudinal resection of the stomach against a 32 French bougie from just lateral to the angle to His to 2 cm proximal to the pylorus.

Post-operative IV fluids with Plasmalyte were administered until oral fluid intake was 1 litre per day (approximately 48 hours). Routine medications given for the first 48 hours included analgesia as required (paracetamol, tramadol and fentanyl), anti-emetics (ondansetron, cyclizine and metoclopramide), and subcu-taneous heparin as prophylaxis for venous thrombo-embolism. Metformin therapy was stopped from the day of surgery until the end of the study period. Standard post-operative oral intake instructions were as follows: Day 1, sips of water; Day 2-4, free oral fluids with clear soups, low fat smoothies or Optifast.

Approximately 3 days before surgery, and again 3 days after surgery, in both cases following fasting for at least 10 hours, blood samples were collected into EDTA tubes and centrifuged following

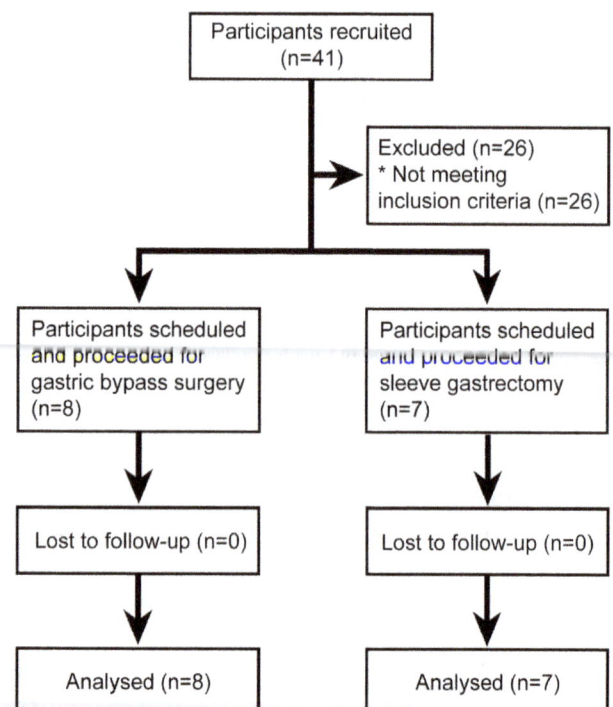

Figure 1. 2010 CONSORT flow diagram for the study.

routine procedures to yield plasma samples which were stored at −80°C until analysis.

Ethics statement

This prospective study was approved by the Northern X Regional Ethics Committee, New Zealand and was registered with the Australian New Zealand Clinical Trials Registry (ACTRN12609000679280). Informed, written consent was obtained from all patients.

Metabolic parameters

Serum insulin and glucose were quantified using the Human Metabolic Hormone Panel (Milliplex, Millipore) and Hitachi 902 auto-analyzer (Hitachi High Technologies Corporation), respectively. HOMA-IR was calculated as (fasting insulin in μU/ml x fasting glucose in mmol/L)/22.5.

Proteomic procedures

Plasma samples were subjected to immunodepletion of 20 highly abundant serum proteins (albumin, immunoglobulins (IgG, IgM, IgD), transferrin, fibrinogen, α-1-antitrypsin, α-2-antitrypsin, complements C3, C4, C1q, haptoglobin, apolipoproteins (A1, A2, B), acid-1-glycoprotein, ceruloplasmin, prealbumin, plasminogen) using a ProteoPrep 20 plasma immunodepletion centrifugal device (Sigma Aldrich, St Louis, MO, USA,) according to the manufacturer's instructions. Depleted samples were stored at −80°C until further processing. Sample volumes containing 40 μg total protein were reduced at 55°C for 15 minutes using 10 mM dithiothreitol, alkylated with 50 mM iodoacetamide (Sigma) at room temperature for 45 minutes in the dark and then digested at 40°C for 30 minutes with 2 μg of sequencing grade trypsin (Promega, Madison, WI, USA) in a chilled microwave (CEM Corporation, Matthews, NC, USA). Digests were cleaned up on 10 mg Oasis HLB SPE cartridges (Waters, Milford, MA, USA), eluted with 300 μl of 60% acetonitrile, dried in a vacuum centrifuge (Thermo Savant, Holbrook, NY, USA) and reconstituted with 20 μl of iTRAQ dissolution buffer (0.5 M triethylammonium bicarbonate at pH 8.5; Applied Biosystems, Foster City, CA, USA). Two samples from each subject (pre- and post- surgery) were derivatised with one of eight iTRAQ labels and combined in groups of eight. Pooled samples were separated by multidimensional liquid chromatography using a strong cation exchange column, followed by a reversed phase column (150 mm×300 um Zorbax SB 300A C-18 column, Agilent Technologies, Santa Clara, CA, USA). The column effluent was analyzed on a QSTAR-XL hybrid mass spectrometer (Applied Biosystems). A TOF-MS scan was made from m/z 300-1600 and the three most intense multiply-charged precursors isolated for fragmentation, with MS/MS spectra recorded from m/z 75-1600.

The patient samples were first analyzed in groups of eight as described above across four liquid chromatography-tandem mass spectrometry (LC-MS/MS) runs; an additional LC-MS/MS run containing selected samples from all four individual runs was then conducted to enable comparisons between runs.

The LC-MS/MS outputs were used to search the human IPI database (Version 3.87) using ProteinPilot software version 4.0 (Applied Biosystems) and protein matches with scores above the 1% false discovery rate threshold for each run were accepted for quantitative analysis. In cases where the software identified an unnamed or putative protein from the database, the amino acid sequence of the protein was used to conduct a BLAST search (available online at http://blast.ncbi.nlm.nih.gov/Blast.cgi) to gain a more meaningful identifier.

The ProteinPilot peptide summaries were used to manually calculate the abundance of each protein in each sample relative to a pre-GBP sample included in the same run as previously described [16]. By comparing in the additional run all pre-GBP samples that were used as reference samples within the previous runs, results obtained from separate LC-MS/MS runs could be scaled and effectively used to compare all samples across all runs. Finally, average ratios calculated in log space for each group were converted to linear space for presentation. Confidence intervals were calculated by converting to linear space the average ratios (ln) ± SEM (ln). Data files containing the complete proteomic output are available from the authors upon request.

Proteins of interest were validated using immunoassay or ELISA. Retinol Binding Protein 4 (RBP4) was measured as per manufacturer's protocol using the Human RBP4 Immunoassay Kit (AIS antibody and Immunoassay Services, Hong Kong). Fetuin-A were measured by a sandwich ELISA (BioVendor Laboratory Medicine, Brno, Czech Republic).

Metabolomics procedures

For each sample, a 300 μL aliquot of plasma was spiked with 20 μL of internal standard (10 mM d4-alanine; 2,3,3,3-d4-dl-alanine, 98 atom % D; Sigma-Aldrich), then lyophilised overnight before being extracted first with 500 μL of 50% methanol, then with 500 μL of 80% methanol. Extracted supernatants were pooled and freeze-dried. Dried samples were chemically derivatised by methyl chloroformate and analyzed by Gas Chromatography-Mass spectrometry (Agilent 7890A coupled with a 5975 inert Mass Spectrometry Detector). Chromatograms were processed using an in-house metabolite library and a custom-made R-software package, with manual checking and correction of information (GC-MS peak intensities). Metabolomic data for each sample were normalized using the internal standard prior to calculation of relative abundances of the separate metabolites in the four different groups.

Statistical analysis

All statistical calculations were performed using GraphPad Prism version 6.00 (GraphPad Software, La Jolla California USA).

Statistical significance of the effect of bariatric surgery on fasting glucose, fasting insulin and HOMA-IR was assessed using repeated measures, mixed model two-way ANOVA, pairing each post-operative sample with the pre-operative sample from the same patient.

Statistical analysis of the proteomic data was done after conversion of all ratios to their natural logs, as customary for iTRAQ data. The separate effect of surgery (post- versus pre-) as well as surgery group (GBP versus SG) were calculated for all identified proteins using repeated measures, mixed model two-way ANOVA paired as above. All proteins showing significant effect of bariatric surgery (p<0.05), were further evaluated using Sidak's multiple comparisons post-hoc test to test the specific effect of GBP and SG on protein levels.

The results of the immunoassay and ELISA validations were tested using two-tailed one sample t tests.

For metabolomic data, the separate effects of bariatric surgery as well as surgery type were calculated for all identified metabolites using repeated measures, mixed model two-way ANOVA. Metabolites showing significant effect of bariatric surgery (p<0.05) were further evaluated using Sidak's multiple comparisons post-hoc test to test the specific effect of GBP and SG on metabolite levels.

Correlation between selected proteins/metabolites and HOMA-IR was evaluated using Spearman correlations.

Results

Clinical characteristics

Fifteen obese subjects participating in a prospective bariatric surgery study [15] (8 scheduled for GBP, 7 for SG) were selected for this study based on similarity of baseline characteristics (Table 1). All patients were treated with metformin for T2D prior to surgery only. Despite cessation of metformin therapy post-operatively, mean fasting glucose and insulin levels, as well as insulin resistance (HOMA-IR) improved after both GBP and SG, although the differences did not reach statistical significance (Table 1).

Proteomic analysis

Of a total of 85 proteins identified with sufficient iTRAQ label and in three or more individuals per surgery group (Fig. 2), two-way ANOVA analysis showed significant effect of bariatric surgery for 32 proteins when time (before vs. after surgery) was plotted against surgery type (GBP vs SG). Of these, 23 proteins were significantly different also in post hoc tests, where the effects of the two surgery types were analyzed separately (Table 2). Summary statistics for all 85 identified proteins are available in Table S1. Specifically, six proteins were significantly lower and four significantly higher after both surgery types, four proteins increased and one decreased after SG only while only one protein increased after GBP. Seven proteins were significantly lower after GBP only and hence matched the main aim of the study. Of these, two (RBP4 and Fetuin-A) were previously reported in the context of insulin resistance. The significant decrease in RBP4 (decreased to 72% after GBP, p<0.01) and Fetuin-A (decreased to 75% after

GBP, p<0.05) as demonstrated by the iTRAQ proteomic study is detailed in Figure 3. Validation analysis by immunoassay and ELISA confirmed significant decrease of RBP4 ($-51.5\pm6.1\%$, p< 0.0001) and Fetuin-A ($-27.0\pm3.5\%$, p=0.0001) on day 3 after GBP (Fig. 4); consistent with the iTRAQ results. As shown in Table 3, the measured levels of both RBP4 and Fetuin-A showed significant correlation with HOMA-IR.

Metabolomic analysis

A total of 45 metabolites were detected, of which 19 were fatty acids and 20 were amino acids or amino acid derivatives. Eight metabolites showed significant (p<0.05) impact of bariatric surgery in the two-way ANOVA; post hoc analysis detected significant effect of one or both specific surgery types for seven of these (Table 4). Figure 5 shows significantly affected and other relevant metabolites in their implicated pathways. Summary statistics for all 45 detected metabolites are available in Table S2.

Discussion

We hypothesized that key species promoting insulin resistance (proteins or their downstream metabolic targets) would be decreased following GBP, where the foregut is bypassed from nutrient flow, but not after SG, where the foregut remains intact to nutrient flow. To identify such causal metabolic factors, we chose to study subjects shortly after both types of surgery, specifically before significant weight loss had occurred and before differences in remission of diabetes between the two types of surgery were evident.

Table 1. Subject characteristics and effect of surgeries on fasting glucose, fasting insulin and HOMA-IR.

	GBP (n = 8)		SG (n = 7)	
Sex	Females: 8		Females: 6	
	Males: 0		Males: 1	
Age (yrs)	41.0±3.1		46.8±2.9	
Ethnicity	5 NZE		6 NZE	
	2 PI		1 PI	
	1 Asian			
Duration diabetes (yrs)	3.7±0.7		3.1±0.6	
BMI (kg/m²)	42.1±4.0		42.3±5.9	
HbA1c (%)	7.2±0.2		7.8±0.7	
(mmol/mol)	54.8±2.5		61.9±7.8	
Duration of surgery (hours)	2.60±0.08		2.14±0.01	
	Baseline	Day 3 post surgery	Baseline	Day 3 post surgery
Fasting glucose (mmol/L)	6.9±0.7	5.9±0.5	7.0±0.7	6.1±0.6
p (pre Vs post bariatric surgery): 0.06				
p (SG Vs GBP): 0.82				
Fasting insulin (µIU/mL)	17.5±6.9	10.8±2.7	20.6±5.6	16.9±6.0
p (pre Vs post bariatric surgery): 0.15				
p (SG Vs GBP): 0.53				
Log HOMA-IR	1.07±0.45	0.75±0.32	1.64±0.25	1.26±0.31
p (pre Vs post bariatric surgery): 0.18				
p (SG Vs GBP): 0.23				

Data are shown as mean ± S.E.M.; p values are derived from Mixed Model Repeated Measures Two-Way ANOVA. Abbreviations: NZE, NZ European; PI, Pacific Islander; HOMA-IR, insulin resistance calculated by homeostatic model assessment.

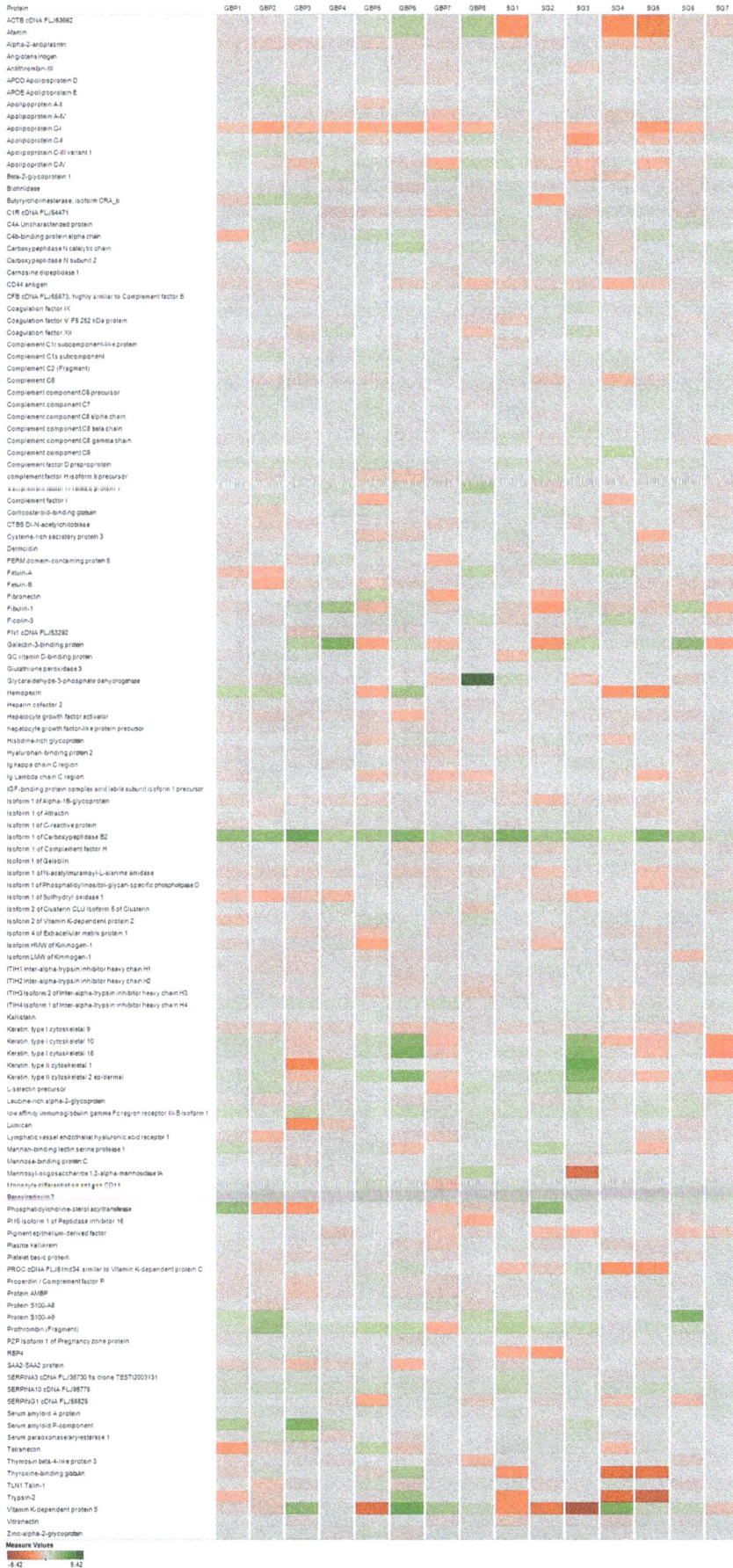

Protein	GBP1	GBP2	GBP3	GBP4	GBP5	GBP6	GBP7	GBP8	SG1	SG2	SG3	SG4	SG5	SG6	SG7
ACTB cDNA FLJ6366Z															
Afamin															
Alpha-2-antiplasmin															
Angiotensinogen															
Antithrombin-III															
APOD Apolipoprotein D															
APOE Apolipoprotein E															
Apolipoprotein A-II															
Apolipoprotein A-IV															
Apolipoprotein C-I															
Apolipoprotein C-II															
Apolipoprotein C-III variant 1															
Apolipoprotein C-IV															
Beta-2-glycoprotein 1															
Biotinidase															
Butyrylcholinesterase, isoform CRA_b															
C1R cDNA FLJ54471															
C4A Uncharacterized protein															
C4b-binding protein alpha chain															
Carboxypeptidase N catalytic chain															
Carboxypeptidase N subunit 2															
Carnosine dipeptidase 1															
CD44 antigen															
CFB cDNA FLJ56673, highly similar to Complement factor B															
Coagulation factor IX															
Coagulation factor V, FS 252 kDa protein															
Coagulation factor XII															
Complement C1r subcomponent-like protein															
Complement C1s subcomponent															
Complement C2 (Fragment)															
Complement C6															
Complement component C6 precursor															
Complement component C7															
Complement component C8 alpha chain															
Complement component C8 beta chain															
Complement component C8 gamma chain															
Complement component C9															
Complement factor D preproprotein															
complement factor H isoform a precursor															
complement factor I isoform a protein 1															
Complement factor I															
Corticosteroid-binding globulin															
CTBS Di-N-acetylchitobiase															
Cysteine-rich secretory protein 3															
Dermcidin															
FERM domain-containing protein 5															
Fetuin-A															
Fetuin-B															
Fibronectin															
Fibulin-1															
Ficolin-3															
FN1 cDNA FLJ53292															
Galectin-3-binding protein															
GC vitamin D-binding protein															
Glutathione peroxidase 3															
Glyceraldehyde-3-phosphate dehydrogenase															
Hemopexin															
Heparin cofactor 2															
Hepatocyte growth factor activator															
hepatocyte growth factor-like protein precursor															
Histidine-rich glycoprotein															
Hyaluronan-binding protein 2															
Ig kappa chain C region															
Ig Lambda chain C region															
IGF-binding protein complex acid labile subunit isoform 1 precursor															
Isoform 1 of Alpha-1B-glycoprotein															
Isoform 1 of Attractin															
Isoform 1 of C-reactive protein															
Isoform 1 of Carboxypeptidase B2															
Isoform 1 of Complement factor H															
Isoform 1 of Gelsolin															
Isoform 1 of N-acetylmuramoyl-L-alanine amidase															
Isoform 1 of Phosphatidylinositol-glycan-specific phospholipase D															
Isoform 1 of Sulfhydryl oxidase 1															
Isoform 2 of Clusterin CLU Isoform 5 of Clusterin															
Isoform 2 of Vitamin K-dependent protein Z															
Isoform 4 of Extracellular matrix protein 1															
Isoform HMW of Kininogen-1															
Isoform LMW of Kininogen-1															
ITIH1 Inter-alpha-trypsin inhibitor heavy chain H1															
ITIH2 Inter-alpha-trypsin inhibitor heavy chain H2															
ITIH3 Isoform 2 of Inter-alpha-trypsin inhibitor heavy chain H3															
ITIH4 Isoform 1 of Inter-alpha-trypsin inhibitor heavy chain H4															
Kallistatin															
Keratin, type I cytoskeletal 9															
Keratin, type I cytoskeletal 10															
Keratin, type I cytoskeletal 16															
Keratin, type II cytoskeletal 1															
Keratin, type II cytoskeletal 2 epidermal															
L-selectin precursor															
Leucine-rich alpha-2-glycoprotein															
low affinity immunoglobulin gamma Fc region receptor III-B isoform 1															
Lumican															
Lymphatic vessel endothelial hyaluronic acid receptor 1															
Mannan-binding lectin serine protease 1															
Mannose-binding protein C															
Mannosyl-oligosaccharide 1,2-alpha-mannosidase IA															
Monocyte differentiation antigen CD14															
Neprilysin-2															
Phosphatidylcholine-sterol acyltransferase															
PI16 Isoform 1 of Peptidase inhibitor 16															
Pigment epithelium-derived factor															
Plasma kallikrein															
Platelet basic protein															
PROC cDNA FLJ61nd34, similar to Vitamin K-dependent protein C															
Properdin / Complement factor P															
Protein AMBP															
Protein S100-A8															
Protein S100-A9															
Prothrombin (Fragment)															
PZP Isoform 1 of Pregnancy zone protein															
RBP4															
SAA2-SAA2 protein															
SERPINA3 cDNA FLJ36730 fis clone TESTI2003131															
SERPINA10 cDNA FLJ96778															
SERPING1 cDNA FLJ66826															
Serum amyloid A protein															
Serum amyloid P-component															
Serum paraoxonase/arylesterase 1															
Tetranectin															
Thymosin beta-4-like protein 3															
Thyroxine-binding globulin															
TLN1 Talin-1															
Trypsin-2															
Vitamin K-dependent protein S															
Vitronectin															
Zinc-alpha-2-glycoprotein															

Measure Values

-8.42   8.42

Figure 2. Heat map showing patient specific changes of all detected proteins. Each protein is represented on an individual row with data from each patient stacked in columns (GBP1 to GBP8 for GBP, SG1-SG7 for SG). Intensity of color corresponds to the degree of change from red (decrease) to green (increase) after surgery.

Amongst other findings, our proteomic analysis showed a significant decrease in two proteins involved in insulin resistance, RBP4 and Fetuin-A, [17,18], three days after GBP but not SG. Notably, although insulin resistance had not improved significantly three days after bariatric surgery, the statistically significant correlations between the levels of RBP4 and Fetuin-A with HOMA-IR support a direct relationship between lower levels of these proteins and improved insulin resistance in our dataset.

RBP4 is a vitamin A (retinol) transport protein secreted by hepatocytes and adipocytes into the bloodstream. This protein carries retinol to peripheral tissues where it is converted into ligands for nuclear hormone receptors and regulates gene transcription. In recent years, RBP4 has been proposed to be a cardiometabolic risk factor associated with T2D, obesity and hyperlipidaemia [19] and it appears to induce insulin resistance in skeletal muscle, liver and adipose tissue in vitro [20]. The regulation of RBP-4 is unclear, however RBPR2 was recently identified as a high affinity RBP4 receptor expressed primarily in liver and small intestine and induced in adipocytes of obese mice [21]. Studies show that RBP4 is decreased with hypocaloric diet

[22] as well as weight loss achieved by lifestyle [23] or weight loss achieved by SG bariatric surgery [12,24].

Fetuin-A is produced in the liver and has a role in the inhibition of insulin-receptor tyrosine kinase, which attenuates insulin signalling and triggers insulin resistance [25,26] and also down-regulates adiponectin, a known insulin sensitizer secreted by adipose tissue [27]. Fetuin-A has recently been shown to be an endogenous ligand for Toll-like receptor 4 (TLR4) through which it has a critical role in stimulating adipose tissue inflammation resulting in insulin resistance [28]. The regulation of Fetuin-A is thought to be through pro-inflammatory cytokines [29,30]. Studies suggest that those with high Fetuin-A levels have increased risk of myocardial infarction [31], stroke [32], and incident diabetes [17]. Fetuin-A levels have also been reported to decrease after weight

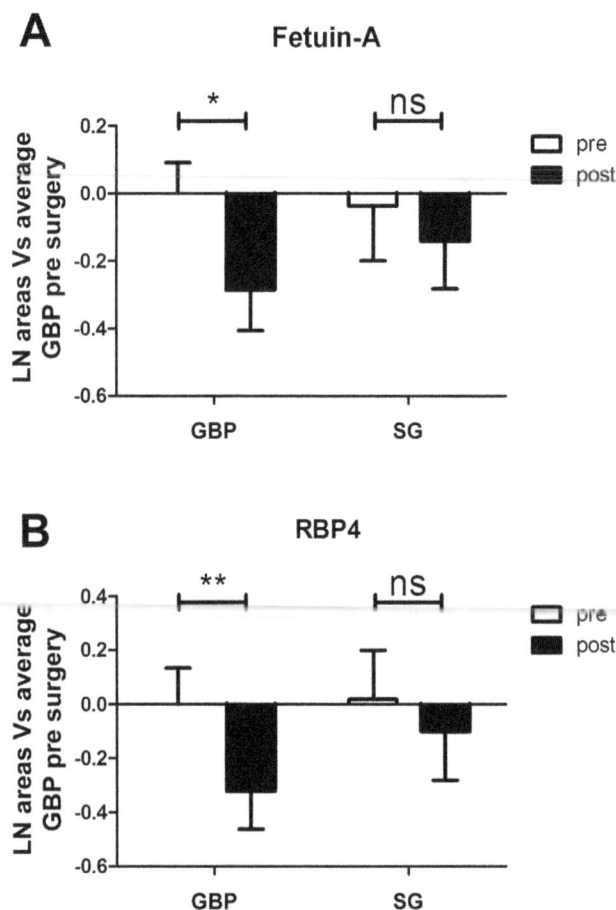

Figure 3. Proteomic results for Fetuin-A and RBP4. Relative abundance pre and post GBP and SG for Fetuin-A (A), and RBP4 (B) as per iTRAQ proteomic study, showing significant decrease after GBP but not after SG for both proteins. Abbreviations: *, p<0.05; **, p<0.01.

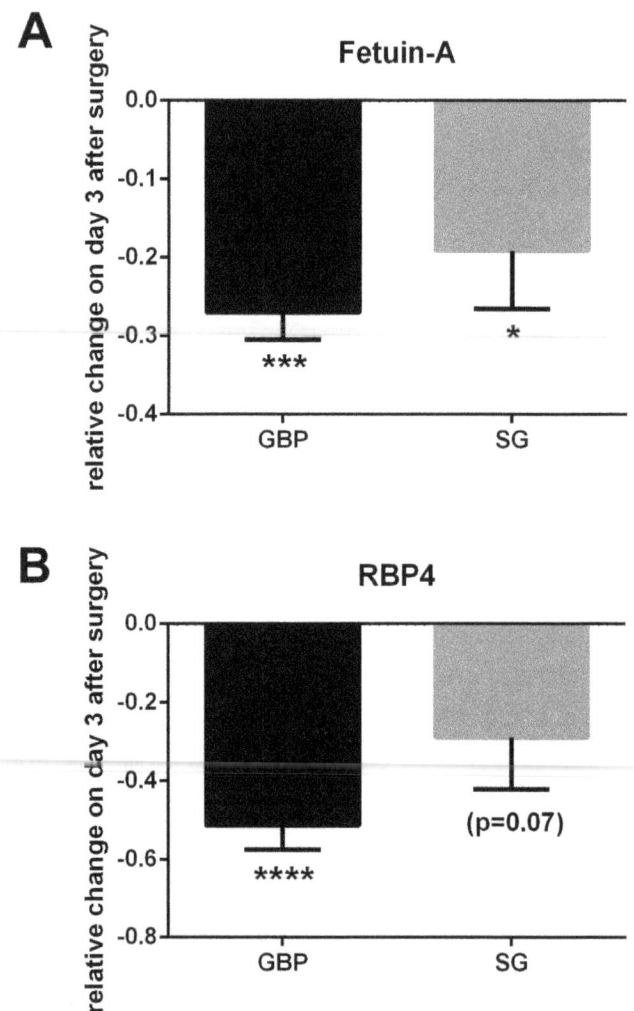

Figure 4. Validation of proteomic results for Fetuin-A and RBP4. Panel A: Fetuin-A levels were found by ELISA to decrease to some extent after both surgery types, however a more dramatic decrease was found after GBP. Panel B: significantly lower levels of RBP4 were detected by immunoassay after GBP only. Abbreviations: *, p< 0.05; ***, p<0.001; ****, p<0.0001.

Table 2. Proteins displaying post-operative changes in relative abundance (3 days after GBP and/or SG compared to 3 days prior to surgery) according to the proteomic study.

Protein name (Accession No)	pre GBP/pre GBP	post GBP/pre GBP	pre SG/pre GBP	post SG/pre GBP
Significant change after GBP only				
Isoform 2 of Inter-alpha-trypsin inhibitor heavy chain H3 (IPI00876950.1)	1.00	**1.33 **	1.15	**1.29** (n.s.)
	(0.88–1.14)	(1.16–1.54)	(1.00–1.32)	(1.09–1.53)
RBP4 (retinol-binding protein 4) (IPI00844536.2)	1.00	**0.72 **	1.02	**0.90** (n.s.)
	(0.87 –1.14)	(0.63–0.83)	(0.85–1.22)	(0.75–1.09)
Alpha-2-HS-glycoprotein (= Fetuin-A) (IPI00953689.1)	1.00	**0.75 ***	0.96	**0.87** (n.s.)
	(0.91–1.10)	(0.67–0.85)	(0.82–1.13)	(0.75–1.00)
Coagulation factor X (IPI00019576.1)	1.00	**0.83 ***	1.07	**0.98** (n.s.)
	(0.87–1.14)	(0.71–0.96)	(0.87–1.32)	(0.78–1.23)
Coagulation factor XII (IPI00019581.2)	1.00	**0.88 ***	0.96	**0.87** (n.s.)
	(0.87–1.15)	(0.75–1.03)	(0.84–1.10)	(0.76–1.00)
Heparin cofactor 2 (IPI00879573.1)	1.00	**0.74 ****	1.18	**1.03** (n.s.)
	(0.90–1.11)	(0.67–0.82)	(1.04–1.35)	(0.89–1.19)
Inter-alpha-trypsin inhibitor heavy chain 2 (IPI00645038.1)	1.00	**0.81 **	1.05	**0.97**(n.s.)
	(0.94–1.06)	(0.74–0.89)	(1.01–1.08)	(0.91–1.04)
Tetranectin (IPI00009028.2)	1.00	**0.80 ***	0.90	**0.82** (n.s.)
	(0.91–1.10)	(0.75–0.85)	(0.80–1.02)	(0.76–0.89)
Significant change after SG only				
Complement C5 (IPI00032291.2)	1.00	**1.07** (n.s.)	1.00	**1.21 ***
	(0.92–1.08)	(0.99–1.15)	(0.91–1.09)	(1.11–1.31)
Complement component C8 alpha chain (IPI00011252.1)	1.00	**1.06** (n.s.)	1.03	**1.24 ***
	(0.91–1.10)	(0.97–1.16)	(0.94–1.12)	(1.11–1.39)
CFB cDNA FLJ55673, (highly similar to Complement factor B) (IPI00019591.2)	1.00	**1.04** (n.s.)	0.98	**1.17 ***
	(0.93–1.08)	(0.97–1.12)	(0.91–1.07)	(1.07–1.29)
Isoform 1 of Inter-alpha-trypsin inhibitor heavy chain H4 (IPI00896419.3)	1.00	**1.04** (n.s.)	0.97	**1.14 **
	(0.93–1.07)	(0.98–1.10)	(0.90–1.04)	(1.08–1.20)
N-acetylmuramoyl-L-alanine amidase (IPI00163207.1)	1.00	**0.89** (n.s.)	1.09	**0.85 **
	(0.88–1.14)	(0.77–1.04)	(0.96–1.23)	(0.73–0.98)
Significant change after both surgery types				
Isoform 1 of C-reactive protein (IPI00022389.1)	1.00	**7.79 *****	0.78	**4.32 *****
	(0.82–1.22)	(6.07–9.99)	(0.61–1.01)	(3.47–5.37)
SERPINA3 (highly similar to alpha-1-antichymotrypsin) (IPI01025667.1)	1.00	**1.61 *****	0.92	**1.46 *****
	(0.76–1.31)	(1.24–2.10)	(0.68–1.24)	(1.04–2.06)
Complement component C9 (IPI00022395.1)	1.00	**1.43 ****	0.90	**1.42 ****
	(0.92–1.09)	(1.34–1.51)	(0.80–1.00)	(1.36–1.49)
Leucine-rich alpha-2-glycoprotein (IPI00224174)	1.00	**1.70 ****	0.80	**1.23 ****
	(0.91–1.10)	(1.51–1.91)	(0.70–0.91)	(1.12–1.34)
Apolipoprotein A-IV (IPI00304273.2)	1.00	**0.40 *****	0.85	**0.49 ****
	(0.86–1.16)	(0.34–0.46)	(0.78–0.93)	(0.42–0.55)
Insulin-like growth factor-binding protein complex acid labile subunit (IPI00925635.1)	1.00	**0.81***	0.81	**0.63 **
	(0.95–1.05)	(0.75–0.86)	(0.76–0.87)	(0.57–0.69)
Beta-Ala-His dipeptidase (Carnosine dipeptidase 1) (IPI00064667.5)	1.00	**0.75 **	1.11	**0.74 ****
	(0.91–1.10)	(0.67–0.84)	(0.98–1.25)	(0.65–0.84)
Kallistatin (IPI00328609.3)	1.00	**0.70 ****	1.11	**0.90 ***
	(0.95–1.05)	(0.66–0.75)	(1.01–1.22)	(0.85–0.95)
Gelsolin (IPI00026314.1)	1.00	**0.74 ****	0.89	**0.69 **
	(0.94–1.07)	(0.68–0.80)	(0.81–0.98)	(0.68–0.70)

Table 2. Cont.

Protein name (Accession No)	pre GBP/pre GBP	post GBP/pre GBP	pre SG/pre GBP	post SG/pre GBP
Afamin (IPI00019943.1)	1.00	0.76 ***	1.05	0.80 **
	(0.94–1.07)	(0.70–0.82)	(0.97–1.14)	(0.74–0.88)

All listed proteins displayed significant (p<0.05) effect of surgery (SG and GBP) as tested by two-way analysis of variance. IPI numbers in brackets refers to accession numbers in the human IPI database; asterisks following ratios denote significant effect of the indicated surgery type according to post-hoc test;
*, p<0.05;
**, p<0.01;
***, p<0.001;
****, p<0.0001; n.s., not significant. Values in brackets refer to confidence intervals.

loss achieved by lifestyle [33] and after GBP [34].

The greater decrease of both Fetuin-A and RBP4 seen after GBP than after SG is consistent with an impact of foregut exclusion on reducing these proteins. In the case of RBP4, this may be because diversion of nutrient absorption past the duodenum resulted in reduced foregut absorption of retinol and expression of RBRP2 [21]. Alternatively, altered gut microbiota, which has been reported to occur after both types of surgery [35,36,37], may influence the levels of these plasma proteins. For example, distinct gut microbiota functional changes after GBP may produce less circulating endotoxin levels and thereby incite lower levels of Fetuin-A [37]. Further studies are required to document the functional evolution of gut microbiota after foregut excluding GBP compared to restrictive types of bariatric surgery such as SG in order to test these hypotheses.

Our metabolomic analysis highlighted several metabolites which responded differently to the two types of bariatric surgery. Specifically after GBP, we detected significantly lower levels of the glucogenic amino acids histidine and proline, as well as of citrate and decanoic acid. This response is consistent with improved metabolic status based on several points. Enhanced post-prandial disposal of amino acids and more complete beta-oxidation of fatty acids has been reported following GBP compared with caloric restriction [38]. Elevated free fatty acids are well known to be associated with insulin resistance [39] and decreased decanoic acid after GBP may be a result of a greater uptake of long chain fatty acid into adipocytes [40]. Elevated histidine [41,42] and citrate [43,44,45,46] levels have been linked with insulin resistance and T2D. Although we did not find any correlation between these four metabolites and insulin sensitivity at this early stage, it is possible they may be predictive of future improvements.

Conversely, after SG we detected marked elevation of the branched-chain amino acid catabolite 3-methyl-2-oxo-pentanoic acid, accompanied by a non-significant tendency towards increased levels of all branched-chain amino acids. The latter is a well-known phenomenon in insulin resistance [47]. Also substantially elevated following SG was 2-hydroxybutyrate, which

has been proposed as a plasma biomarker for early stages of diabetes [48] and insulin resistance [49].

Together, the differential early changes in the above metabolites following GBP and SG suggest a more favourable metabolic profile associated with greater insulin sensitivity early after GBP compared with SG. Since both surgery groups were of similar obesity and diabetes status as well as similar in terms of reduced caloric intake at the post-operative time-point, these differences are likely directly linked to the types of bariatric surgery performed.

This study has two major limitations. Firstly, it is limited by small sample size. The subjects were however well matched for baseline clinical characteristics before two relatively similar laparoscopic bariatric surgical procedures with well-matched post-operative protocols for analgesia, fluid replacement and caloric intake. Secondly, the immunodepletion method used in the proteomic analysis improved detection of moderately abundant proteins but had limited ability to prime the samples for detection of proteins of very low abundance in plasma. Depletion techniques targeting a larger number of proteins [50] would allow a more comprehensive analysis in the search for additional novel biomarkers of insulin resistance. Nonetheless, our proteomic study identified significant decreases in RBP4 and Fetuin-A concentrations after GBP but not after SG, which was confirmed using other analytical methods. The metabolomic analysis was also limited to a relatively moderate number of metabolites and future investigations will benefit from the use of more powerful equipment.

Although we were unable to obtain a clear connection between our proteomic and metabolomics findings, by using these two complementary analytical approaches, we managed to identify a number of potentially important changes in key metabolic pathways as well as proteins with known or putative roles in the development of insulin resistance.

In summary, our findings suggest greater lowering of multiple proteins including RBP4, Fetuin-A as well as several metabolites associated with insulin resistance following GBP compared with SG prior to diabetes remission.

Table 3. Assessment of correlation between selected proteins and metabolites (showing greater decrease after GBP than SG) with insulin resistance (estimated by HOMA-IR).

	Fetuin-A	RBP4	Proline	Citrate	Histidine	Decanoic acid
HOMA-IR	0.36	0.48	0.10	0.06	−0.04	−0.07
p	(<0.05)*	(0.006)**	(0.61)	(0.74)	(0.85)	(0.72)

The values shown are Spearman rank correlation coefficients with two-tailed p values for significance of correlation in brackets. Asterisks highlights significant correlations (*, p<0.05; **, p<0.01).

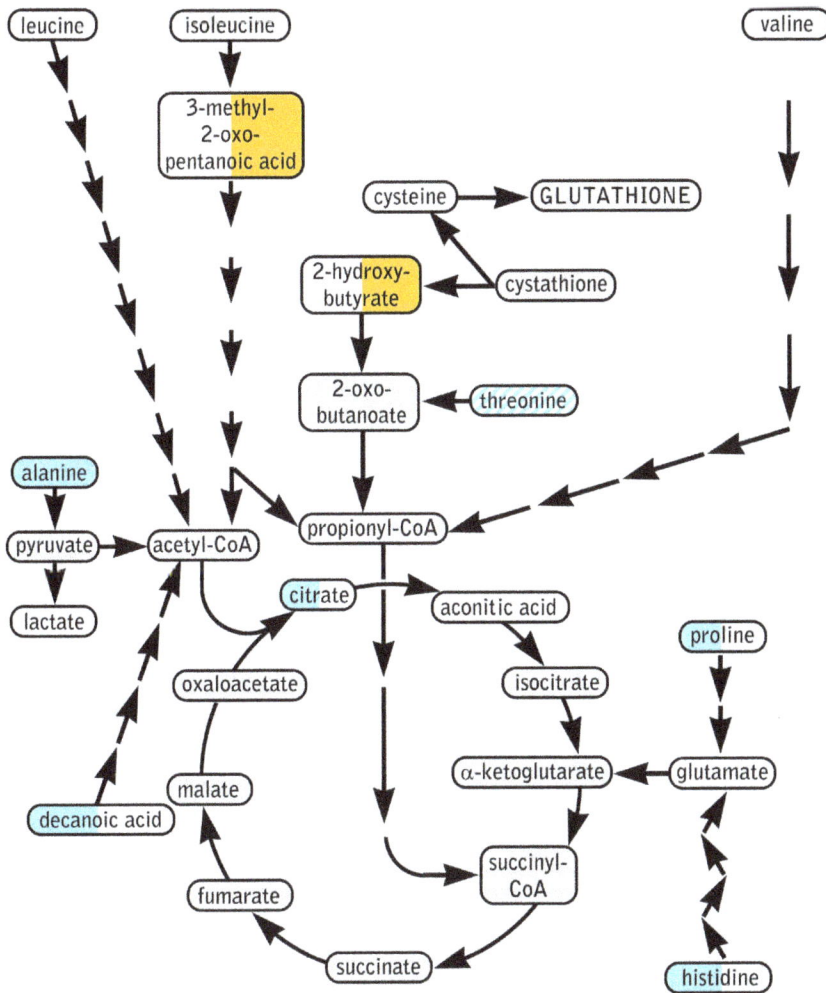

Figure 5. Schematic of implicated metabolic pathways based on metabolomics results (selected metabolites only). Metabolites are inscribed in color coded ellipses with the effect of GBP in left half and effect of SG in right half. Color code: blue, significantly lower; orange, significantly higher; white, no significant effect of bariatric surgery; diagonal stripes, significant effect of surgery but not significant in post-hoc test. Grey highlights an undetected metabolite.

Table 4. Metabolites showing significant effect (p<0.05) of bariatric surgery in a Repeated Measures Mixed Model Two-Way ANOVA.

Metabolite	Pre-GBP	Post-GBP	Pre-SG	Post-SG	Effect of surgery (p)
	Mean ± SEM	Mean ± SEM	Mean ± SEM	Mean ± SEM	
Alanine	1.00±0.09	0.52±0.04*	1.27±0.19	0.68±0.06**	0.0001
Proline	1.00±0.12	0.56±0.09*	1.00±0.18	0.71±0.11	0.0046
Histidine	1.00±0.12	0.72±0.07*	0.78±0.10	0.68±0.07	0.0073
Threonine	1.00±0.16	0.84±0.10	0.80±0.14	0.78±0.08	0.0452
Citric acid	1.00±0.10	0.76±0.07*	1.00±0.07	0.88±0.07	0.0095
Decanoic acid	1.00±0.12	0.67±0.08*	0.86±0.07	0.77±0.07	0.0232
2-Hydroxybutyric acid	1.00±0.14	1.16±0.17	0.97±0.12	2.01±0.39*	0.0359
3-Methyl-2-oxopentanoic acid	1.00±0.11	0.93±0.14	0.81±0.12	1.57±0.24**	0.0428

Values given are scaled to mean pre-GBP to enable comparison between all groups. Asterisks denote significant difference compared to baseline for the specific surgery type (Sidak's multiple comparisons test);
*, p<0.05;
**, p<0.01.

Supporting Information

Table S1   Summary statistics for all identified proteins.
Relative abundance, confidence intervals and outcome of statistical analysis are shown for the 85 proteins identified with sufficient confidence and iTRAQ label in at least 3 within patient comparisons as well as the final LC-MS/MS run combining samples from all previous runs. Entries in bold showed significant effect of surgery according to the Two-way ANOVA; *, $p<0.05$; **, $p<0.01$; ***, $p<0.001$, ****, $p<0.0001$; t, trending ($p<0.10$); n.s., $p>0.10$.

Table S2   Summary statistics for all identified metabolites.
Abundance (relative to averaged pre-operative GBP samples), S.E.M. and outcome of statistical analysis (Two-Way ANOVA followed by Sidak's post-test) are shown for all 45 metabolites identified. Abbreviations: *, $p<0.05$, **, $p<0.01$; ***, $p<0.001$, ****, $p<0.0001$; n.s., $p>0.05$.

Checklist S1   TREND Checklist used in this study.

Protocol S1   Proteomic sub-study protocol detailing patient recruitment, exclusion criteria and study protocol.

Acknowledgments

We would like to thank the participants.

Author Contributions

Conceived and designed the experiments: MJ SY AX MB RB GB RM. Performed the experiments: SY MJ GS RM. Analyzed the data: SY MJ GS RM. Contributed reagents/materials/analysis tools: RM. Wrote the paper: MJ SY RM. Criticial revision of the manuscript: AX GS MM MB RB GB.

References

1. Buchwald H, Estok R, Fahrbach K, Banel D, Jensen MD, et al. (2009) Weight and type 2 diabetes after bariatric surgery: systematic review and meta-analysis. Am J Med 122: 248256 e245256 e245.
2. Sjostrom L (2008) Bariatric surgery and reduction in morbidity and mortality: experiences from the SOS study. Int J Obes (Lond) 32 Suppl 7: S93–97.
3. Abbatini F, Rizzello M, Casella G, Alessandri G, Capoccia D, et al. (2010) Long-term effects of laparoscopic sleeve gastrectomy, gastric bypass, and adjustable gastric banding on type 2 diabetes. Surg Endosc 24: 1005–1010.
4. Rao RS, Yanagisawa R, Kini S (2012) Insulin resistance and bariatric surgery. Obes Rev 13: 316–328.
5. Wickremesekera K, Miller G, Naotunne TD, Knowles G, Stubbs RS (2005) Loss of insulin resistance after Roux-en-Y gastric bypass surgery: a time course study. Obes Surg 15: 474–481.
6. Cummings DE (2009) Endocrine mechanisms mediating remission of diabetes after gastric bypass surgery. Int J Obes (Lond) 33 Suppl 1: S33–40.
7. Peterli R, Wolnerhanssen B, Peters T, Devaux N, Kern B, et al. (2009) Improvement in glucose metabolism after bariatric surgery: comparison of laparoscopic Roux-en-Y gastric bypass and laparoscopic sleeve gastrectomy: a prospective randomized trial. Ann Surg 250: 234–241.
8. Rubino F, Gagner M, Gentileschi P, Kini S, Fukuyama S, et al. (2004) The early effect of the Roux-en-Y gastric bypass on hormones involved in body weight regulation and glucose metabolism. Ann Surg 240: 236–242.
9. Cummings DE, Overduin J, Foster-Schubert KE, Carlson MJ (2007) Role of the bypassed proximal intestine in the anti-diabetic effects of bariatric surgery. Surg Obes Relat Dis 3: 109–115.
10. Blonder J, Issaq HJ, Veenstra TD (2011) Proteomic biomarker discovery: it's more than just mass spectrometry. Electrophoresis 32: 1541–1548.
11. Millioni R, Tolin S, Puricelli L, Sbrignadello S, Fadini GP, et al. (2011) High abundance proteins depletion vs low abundance proteins enrichment: comparison of methods to reduce the plasma proteome complexity. PLoS One 6: e19603.
12. Oberbach A, von Bergen M, Bluher S, Lehmann S, Till H (2012) Combined serum proteomic and metabonomic profiling after laparoscopic sleeve gastrectomy in children and adolescents. J Laparoendosc Adv Surg Tech A 22: 184–188.
13. Friedrich N (2012) Metabolomics in diabetes research. J Endocrinol 215: 29–42.
14. Mutch DM, Fuhrmann JC, Rein D, Wiemer JC, Bouillot JL, et al. (2009) Metabolite profiling identifies candidate markers reflecting the clinical adaptations associated with Roux-en-Y gastric bypass surgery. PLoS One 4: e7905.
15. Yip S, Signal M, Smith G, Beban G, Booth M, et al. (2014) Lower glycemic fluctuations early after bariatric surgery partially explained by caloric restriction. Obes Surg 24: 62–70.
16. Jullig M, Chen X, Middleditch MJ, Vazhoor G, Hickey AJ, et al. (2010) Illuminating the molecular basis of diabetic arteriopathy: a proteomic comparison of aortic tissue from diabetic and healthy rats. Proteomics 10: 3367–3378.
17. Stefan N, Fritsche A, Weikert C, Boeing H, Joost HG, et al. (2008) Plasma fetuin-A levels and the risk of type 2 diabetes. Diabetes 57: 2762–2767.
18. Graham TE, Yang Q, Bluher M, Hammarstedt A, Ciaraldi TP, et al. (2006) Retinol-binding protein 4 and insulin resistance in lean, obese, and diabetic subjects. N Engl J Med 354: 2552–2563.
19. Christou GA, Tselepis AD, Kiortsis DN (2012) The metabolic role of retinol binding protein 4: an update. Horm Metab Res 44: 6 11.
20. Yang Q, Graham TE, Mody N, Preitner F, Peroni OD, et al. (2005) Serum retinol binding protein 4 contributes to insulin resistance in obesity and type 2 diabetes. Nature 436: 356–362.

21. Alapatt P, Guo F, Komanetsky SM, Wang S, Cai J, et al. (2013) Liver retinol transporter and receptor for serum retinol-binding protein (RBP4). J Biol Chem 288: 1250–1265.
22. Janke J, Engeli S, Boschmann M, Adams F, Bohnke J, et al. (2006) Retinol-binding protein 4 in human obesity. Diabetes 55: 2805–2810.
23. Gomez-Ambrosi J, Rodriguez A, Catalan V, Ramirez B, Silva C, et al. (2008) Serum retinol-binding protein 4 is not increased in obesity or obesity-associated type 2 diabetes mellitus, but is reduced after relevant reductions in body fat following gastric bypass. Clin Endocrinol (Oxf) 69: 208–215.
24. Oberbach A, Bluher M, Wirth H, Till H, Kovacs P, et al. (2011) Combined proteomic and metabolomic profiling of serum reveals association of the complement system with obesity and identifies novel markers of body fat mass changes. J Proteome Res 10: 4769–4788.
25. Ou HY, Yang YC, Wu HT, Wu JS, Lu FH, et al. (2011) Serum fetuin-A concentrations are elevated in subjects with impaired glucose tolerance and newly diagnosed type 2 diabetes. Clin Endocrinol (Oxf) 75: 450–455.
26. Gunduz FO, Yildirmak ST, Temizel M, Faki Y, Cakmak M, et al. (2011) Serum visfatin and fetuin-a levels and glycemic control in patients with obese type 2 diabetes mellitus. Diabetes Metab J 35: 523–528.
27. Mori K, Emoto M, Inaba M (2012) Fetuin-A and the cardiovascular system. Adv Clin Chem 56: 175–195.
28. Pal D, Dasgupta S, Kundu R, Maitra S, Das G, et al. (2012) Fetuin-A acts as an endogenous ligand of TLR4 to promote lipid-induced insulin resistance. Nat Med 18: 1279–1285.
29. Li W, Zhu S, Li J, Huang Y, Zhou R, et al. (2011) A hepatic protein, fetuin-A, occupies a protective role in lethal systemic inflammation. PLoS One 6: e16945.
30. Wang H, Zhu S, Zhou R, Li W, Sama AE (2008) Therapeutic potential of HMGB1-targeting agents in sepsis. Expert Rev Mol Med 10: e32.
31. Weikert C, Stefan N, Schulze MB, Pischon T, Berger K, et al. (2008) Plasma fetuin-a levels and the risk of myocardial infarction and ischemic stroke. Circulation 118: 2555–2562.
32. Tuttolomondo A, Di Raimondo D, Di Sciacca R, Casuccio A, Bivona G, et al. (2010) Fetuin-A and CD40 L plasma levels in acute ischemic stroke: differences in relation to TOAST subtype and correlation with clinical and laboratory variables. Atherosclerosis 208: 290–296.
33. Reinehr T, Roth CL (2008) Fetuin-A and its relation to metabolic syndrome and fatty liver disease in obese children before and after weight loss. J Clin Endocrinol Metab 93: 4479–4485.
34. Brix JM, Stingl H, Hollerl F, Schernthaner GH, Kopp HP, et al. (2010) Elevated Fetuin-A concentrations in morbid obesity decrease after dramatic weight loss. J Clin Endocrinol Metab 95: 4877–4881.
35. Kong LC, Tap J, Aron-Wisnewsky J, Pelloux V, Basdevant A, et al. (2013) Gut microbiota after gastric bypass in human obesity: increased richness and associations of bacterial genera with adipose tissue genes. Am J Clin Nutr 98: 16–24.
36. Patil DP, Dhotre DP, Chavan SG, Sultan A, Jain DS, et al. (2012) Molecular analysis of gut microbiota in obesity among Indian individuals. J Biosci 37: 647–657.
37. Aron-Wisnewsky J, Dore J, Clement K (2012) The importance of the gut microbiota after bariatric surgery. Nat Rev Gastroenterol Hepatol 9: 590–598.
38. Khoo CM, Muehlbauer MJ, Stevens RD, Pamuklar Z, Chen J, et al. (2013) Postprandial Metabolite Profiles Reveal Differential Nutrient Handling After Bariatric Surgery Compared With Matched Caloric Restriction. Ann Surg.
39. Groop LC, Saloranta C, Shank M, Bonadonna RC, Ferrannini E, et al. (1991) The role of free fatty acid metabolism in the pathogenesis of insulin resistance in obesity and noninsulin-dependent diabetes mellitus. J Clin Endocrinol Metab 72: 96–107.

40. Petrescu O, Fan X, Gentileschi P, Hossain S, Bradbury M, et al. (2005) Long-chain fatty acid uptake is upregulated in omental adipocytes from patients undergoing bariatric surgery for obesity. Int J Obes (Lond) 29: 196–203.

41. Huffman KM, Shah SH, Stevens RD, Bain JR, Muehlbauer M, et al. (2009) Relationships between circulating metabolic intermediates and insulin action in overweight to obese, inactive men and women. Diabetes Care 32: 1678–1683.

42. Fiehn O, Garvey WT, Newman JW, Lok KH, Hoppel CL, et al. (2010) Plasma metabolomic profiles reflective of glucose homeostasis in non-diabetic and type 2 diabetic obese African-American women. PLoS One 5: e15234.

43. Cupisti A, Meola M, D'Alessandro C, Bernabini G, Pasquali E, et al. (2007) Insulin resistance and low urinary citrate excretion in calcium stone formers. Biomed Pharmacother 61: 86–90.

44. Isken F, Schulz TJ, Mohlig M, Pfeiffer AF, Ristow M (2006) Chemical inhibition of citrate metabolism alters glucose metabolism in mice. Horm Metab Res 38: 543–545.

45. DeVilliers DC, Jr., Dixit PK, Lazarow A (1966) Citrate metabolism in diabetes. I. Plasma citrate in alloxan-diabetic rats and in clinical diabetes. Metabolism 15: 458–465.

46. Li H, Xie Z, Lin J, Song H, Wang Q, et al. (2008) Transcriptomic and metabonomic profiling of obesity-prone and obesity-resistant rats under high fat diet. J Proteome Res 7: 4775–4783.

47. Adeva MM, Calvino J, Souto G, Donapetry C (2012) Insulin resistance and the metabolism of branched-chain amino acids in humans. Amino Acids 43: 171–181.

48. Li X, Xu Z, Lu X, Yang X, Yin P, et al. (2009) Comprehensive two-dimensional gas chromatography/time-of-flight mass spectrometry for metabonomics: Biomarker discovery for diabetes mellitus. Anal Chim Acta 633: 257–262.

49. Gall WE, Beebe K, Lawton KA, Adam KP, Mitchell MW, et al. (2010) alpha-hydroxybutyrate is an early biomarker of insulin resistance and glucose intolerance in a nondiabetic population. PLoS One 5: e10883.

50. Merrell K, Southwick K, Graves SW, Esplin MS, Lewis NE, et al. (2004) Analysis of low-abundance, low-molecular-weight serum proteins using mass spectrometry. J Biomol Tech 15: 238–248.

21

Lactoferrin Dampens High-Fructose Corn Syrup-Induced Hepatic Manifestations of the Metabolic Syndrome in a Murine Model

Yi-Chieh Li, Chang-Chi Hsieh*

Department of Animal Science and Biotechnology, Tunghai University, Taichung, Taiwan

Abstract

Hepatic manifestations of the metabolic syndrome are related obesity, type 2 diabetes/insulin resistance and non-alcoholic fatty liver disease. Here we investigated how the anti-inflammatory properties of lactoferrin can protect against the onset of hepatic manifestations of the metabolic syndrome by using a murine model administered with high-fructose corn syrup. Our results show that a high-fructose diet stimulates intestinal bacterial overgrowth and increases intestinal permeability, leading to the introduction of endotoxin into blood circulation and liver. Immunohistochemical staining of Toll-like receptor-4 and thymic stromal lymphopoietin indicated that lactoferrin can modulate lipopolysaccharide-mediated inflammatory cascade. The important regulatory roles are played by adipokines including interleukin-1β, interleukin-6, tumor necrosis factor-α, monocyte chemotactic protein-1, and adiponectin, ultimately reducing hepatitis and decreasing serum alanine aminotransferase release. These beneficial effects of lactoferrin related to the downregulation of the lipopolysaccharide-induced inflammatory cascade in the liver. Furthermore, lactoferrin reduced serum and hepatic triglycerides to prevent lipid accumulation in the liver, and reduced lipid peroxidation, resulting in 4-hydroxynonenal accumulation. Lactoferrin reduced oral glucose tolerance test and homeostasis model assessment-insulin resistance. Lactoferrin administration thus significantly lowered liver weight, resulting from a decrease in the triglyceride and cholesterol synthesis that activates hepatic steatosis. Taken together, these results suggest that lactoferrin protected against high-fructose corn syrup induced hepatic manifestations of the metabolic syndrome.

Editor: Silvia C. Sookoian, Institute of Medical Research A Lanari-IDIM, University of Buenos Aires National Council of Scientific and Technological Research (CONICET), Argentina

Funding: This work was supported, in whole or in part, by grants from the Ministry of Science and Technology, Taiwan, R.O.C. (NSC 99-2622-E-029-002-CC3, NSC 100-2221-E-029-004). The funders had no role in study design, data collection and analysis, decision to publish, or preparation of the manuscript.

Competing Interests: The authors have declared that no competing interests exist.

* E-mail: cchsieh@thu.edu.tw

Introduction

Hepatic manifestations of the metabolic syndrome (HMMS) are associated with obesity, type 2 diabetes/insulin resistance, non-alcoholic fatty liver disease (NAFLD), and progression to non-alcoholic steatohepatitis (NASH) [1]. NAFLD is a common liver disease usually occurring in patients that do not habitually consume alcohol and manifesting as an excessive accumulation of triglycerides in the liver, leading to fat build-up and an increase in total liver weight of over 5%. The prevalence of fatty liver in obese and diabetic patients can reach 70–90% [2]. Fatty liver occurs either as simple steatosis (hepatic steatosis) or in combination with non-alcoholic liver inflammation. The resultant inflammation and liver cell damage may develop into liver fibrosis and progress to cirrhosis and even hepatocarcinoma. Histological changes in non-alcoholic and alcoholic fatty liver lesions mainly occur in the hepatic lobule, including fatty acid degeneration of liver cells, and fat accumulation of pathological features of the clinical symptom [3]. Sugar consumption has increased very rapidly in recent years in developed countries, and the prevalence of obesity and diabetes has parallely increased at an alarming rate. High-fructose corn syrup (HFCS) is used extensively in sugary drinks, especially in cola, soda, artificial juices, and other beverages. The hepatic metabolism of fructose begins with its phosphorylation by fructokinase. Fructose then directly enters the glycolytic pathway, bypassing the major control point by which glucose enters glycolysis. This unregulated carbon source provides glycerol-3-phosphate and acetyl-CoA for hepatic lipogenesis, increasing the hepatic pool of free fatty acids [4–6]. In addition, fructose neither suppresses ghrelin nor stimulates insulin or leptin to inhibit appetite [7]. According to a previous study, the prevalence of NAFLD in Taiwan ranges from 11–41%. Of the NAFLD patients, 6–13% were diagnosed with NASH. NAFLD has a severe impact on health that substantially increases when combined with obesity, diabetes, and the metabolic syndrome [8]. The presence of HFCS in beverages plays an important role in the progression of hepatic manifestations of the metabolic syndrome, including obesity, insulin resistance, NAFLD, and NASH.

In 1998, Day and James proposed the "double hit" hypothesis [9]. The first hit refers to the abnormal accumulation of lipids, especially triglycerides, in the liver. With the dysregulation of liver lipid homeostasis, free fatty acids (FFA) continue to be transported to the liver, resulting in a decreased capacity for β-oxidation of fats. In addition, most studies suggest that NASH is related to inflammation and insulin resistance. Further studies have shown that insulin resistance may lead to overexpression of the lipoprotein lipase (LPL) gene, thereby enabling continuous generation of free fatty acids in the liver [10]. Most patients may simply have a fatty liver with no associated inflammation. However, the "second hit" induces inflammatory responses, including abnormal inflammatory cytokine production and oxidative stress response [9]. Reactive oxygen species (ROS) activate redox-sensitive kinases, thereby activating IkappaB kinase beta (IKKβ), inducing nuclear factor-κB (NF-κB) activation, and further increasing the expression of TNF-α and production of cytokines by other inflammatory cells, leading to inflammation of the liver [11,12]. Therefore, improvement of hepatic lipid metabolism and accumulation in "first-hit" and alleviating inflammation, insulin resistance and oxidative stress in "second-hit" have been shown the therapeutic potential in preventing the progression of HMMS.

Lactoferrin (Lf) is a single-chain glycoprotein consisting of 700 amino acid residues, with a molecular weight of 76–80 kD. It plays a variety of physiological roles, and mediates antibacterial, antiviral, and anti-inflammatory effects [13]. Lactoferrin exerts an antibacterial effect by binding iron ions, which reduces the iron-dependent growth of bacteria such as E. coli [13]. However, lactoferrin also acts as an iron donor to promote the growth of beneficial bacteria, such as Lactobacillus and Bifidobacterium [14,15]. Inflammation or infection due to stimulation of phagocytes and release of cytokines further increases neutrophil infiltration. Lactoferrin is able to bind lipopolysaccharides (LPS), and is thereby able to reduce the LPS-driven inflammatory response [16]. It can also significantly reduce blood triglyceride and cholesterol levels and the peripheral fat mass in mice [17,18]. In this study, we attempted to use lactoferrin to improve HFCS-induced HMMS including hepatic steatosis, insulin resistance, inflammation and oxidative stress in a murine model.

Materials and Methods

Reagents, ELISA Kits

Lactoferrin (90.5% pure with 16% iron saturation) was obtained from Westland Milk Products (Hokitika, New Zealand). Double-antibody sandwich ELISA kits to identify TNF-α, IL-1β, IL-4, IL-6, IL-13, IL-33, MCP-1, and TSLP (ELISA Ready-SET-Go; eBioscience, San Diego, CA, USA) were purchased. In addition, adiponectin (Mouse Adiponectin/Acrp30 DuoSet; R&D Systems Inc., Minneapolis, MN, USA), insulin (Ultrasensitive Mouse Insulin ELISA; Mercodia Inc., Winston, Salem, NC, USA), endotoxin (lipopolysaccharide) (ToxinSensor Chromogenic LAL Endotoxin Assay Kit; GenScript USA Inc., Piscataway, NJ, USA), and bovine lactoferrin (Bethyl Laboratories Inc., Montgomery, TX, USA) ELISA kits were purchased and according to the instruction to detect serum or hepatic homogenate.

Animals and treatments

Fifty male C57BL/6JNarl mice (National Laboratory Animal Center, Taipei, Taiwan) were individually housed and maintained under environmentally controlled conditions (temperature 22–25°C, 12 h/12 h light/dark cycle, 45–60% humidity). The mice received a standard sterile rodent chow diet (Altromin Maintenance Irradiated Diet 1324 TFP, Altromin Spezialfutter GmbH & Co. KG, Lage, Germany) and distilled water ad libitum. The mice entered the experimental regimen at 6 weeks of age and were allowed 2 weeks to adapt. At 8 weeks of age, the mice were divided into 5 groups at the start of the experiments: naïve group: untreated; control group: HFCS-induced murine HMMS administered with distilled water; Lf treatment groups: HFCS-induced murine HMMS administered with lactoferrin at 50, 100, or

200 mg/kg/day. The body weight and food intake of each mouse was monitored on a weekly basis. After 8 weeks of treatment, all the mice were to fast for 8 h prior to measurement of blood glucose. Animals were anesthetized by isoflurane inhalation, and blood was collected via orbital sinus and centrifuged for 10 min at $3000 \times g$ at 4°C to obtain serum, which was stored at −80°C until analysis. After blood collection, the mice were sacrificed using cervical dislocation and the livers removed, weighed, snap frozen in liquid nitrogen, and stored at −80°C. The experiment was performed in accordance with the Taiwan Animal Protection Act (2011), and the experimental protocol was approved by the Animal Welfare Committee of Tunghai University, Taichung, Taiwan (permit number: 101-6). All the surgeries were performed under isoflurane anesthesia, and all efforts were made to minimize suffering.

Liver lipid extraction

Approximately 0.1 g of dissected liver was added to a 2-mL chloroform/methanol (2:1, v/v) mixture and ground at room temperature for 1 h. The upper lipid layer was removed by centrifugation at $5,000 \times g$ for 10 min. The lipid layer was further extracted by adding 0.2 volumes of 0.9% saline. After centrifugation at $5,000 \times g$ for 5 min, the extract was dried under nitrogen at 55°C. The dry pellet was resuspended in 1 mL tert-butyl alcohol/Triton X-100/methanol (2:1:1, v/v) solution, collected, and stored at −20°C for subsequent analysis.

Determination of alanine aminotransferase, cholesterol, and triglyceride levels

A 50-μL sample of serum was obtained from blood by centrifugation at $1700 \times g$ for 10 min at 4°C. Serum alanine aminotransferase (ALT), cholesterol, and triglyceride levels were measured using clinical kits (Roche Diagnostics, Mannheim, Germany) and a spectrophotometric system (Cobas Mira; Roche, Rotkreuz, Switzerland). Liver lipid extracts were measured using the same method.

Oral glucose tolerance test

At the end of dietary intervention, an oral glucose tolerance test (OGTT) was performed after an overnight fast. Each mouse was intragastrically administered with a dose of 2 g/kg body weight of D-glucose. Blood samples (5 μL) were obtained from the caudal vein to measure blood glucose levels at 0, 30, 60, 90, and 120 min using a CareSens II Blood Glucose Monitoring System and Test Strips (i-SENS Inc., Seoul, Korea).

Estimation of cytokines, insulin, endotoxin, and bovine lactoferrin in homogenized liver and serum

To study the effect of lactoferrin on liver and serum cytokines in HFCS-induced NASH mice, double-antibody sandwich ELISAs (for TNF-α, IL-1β, IL-4, IL-6, IL-13, IL-33, MCP-1, TSLP, adiponectin, insulin, endotoxin, or bovine lactoferrin) were performed according to the manufacturers' instructions. The frozen liver was thawed, and approximately 0.1 g of liver tissue removed and homogenized in 1 mL of buffer (1.15% KCl/Tris-EDTA pH 8.9 acetic acid 3:2:1.5 v/v), followed by centrifugation at $4500 \times g$ for 10 min at 4°C. The supernatant was collected and stored at −80°C for subsequent analysis. Capture antibodies were added to 96-well plates and incubated overnight at 4°C. Each sample well was washed three times, blocked for 60 min at room temperature, and washed three more times. Standards and samples at dilutions of 1:10–1:100 were then added to the wells. After a 2-h incubation at room temperature, the wells were washed five times. After applying the detection antibodies and incubating for 1–2 h, the wells were washed seven times to remove non-specific binding. Substrate solution (TMB) was added to each well, and following incubation in the dark at room temperature for 15 min, stop solution was added to terminate enzyme activity. Absorbance was measured at 450 nm, with 570 nm as the reference wavelength, using an ELISA reader (Multiskan Spectrum, Thermo Electron Corporation, San Jose, CA, USA).

Insulin Sensitivity Test

Homeostasis model assessment-insulin resistance (HOMA-IR) was determined using the steady-state blood glucose and insulin concentrations in a feedback interaction loop. HOMA-IR was calculated using the relationship between the blood glucose and insulin levels, according to the following formula:

HOMA-IR = Insulin (μU/L) × Blood glucose (mM)/22.5 [19]

Pathological examination

After formalin fixation, tissue samples were sliced (5-μm sections), embedded in the standard manner, and stained with hematoxylin & eosin (HE). Fatty liver was graded according to the method of Kleiner et al., 2005 [20], and using a low- to medium-power evaluation of standard HE-stained liver parenchyma to measure percentage parenchymal involvement by steatosis, graded as follows: grade 0, <5% steatosis; grade 1, 5–33% steatosis; grade 2, 33–66% steatosis; grade 3, >66% steatosis. To avoid sampling errors, all the biopsies were performed on the same lobe, and the semi-quantitative grades were assigned without knowledge of the sample treatment.

Frozen liver sections (10-μm) were embedded in FSC 22 Frozen Section Media (Surgipath, Leica Biosystems, Richmond Inc., IL, USA) and stained with Oil Red O to visualize hepatic lipids. Images of the red-stained lipid areas were enhanced with Adobe Photoshop CS6, and the size and number of lipid droplets were analyzed using ImagePro Plus 5.0, as previously described [21,22]. A minimum of 5 separate microscopic fields of view were used to measure the lipid droplet area of each section, at a magnification of 400×.

Immunohistochemical staining

The expression and localization of 4-hydroxynonenal (4-HNE), Toll-like receptor-4 (TLR-4), and thymic stromal lymphopoietin (TSLP) in the liver were determined by immunohistochemical staining, as described previously [23]. For primary staining of 4-HNE, TLR-4, and TSLP, deparaffinized tissue sections were incubated with polyclonal anti-4-HNE (MyBioSource, Inc., San Diego, CA, USA), anti-TLR-4, or anti-TSLP (Biosis, Inc., Woburn, MA, USA) antibodies. A secondary antibody (HRP conjugated mouse anti-goat immunoglobulin G fragment antibody) was added, and the specific staining was visualized using an immunodetection kit and a 3,3-diaminobenzidine chromogen (Novolink Max Polymer Detection System, Leica Biosystems Newcastle Ltd, Newcastle Upon Tyne, United Kingdom).

Statistical analysis

Results were expressed as mean ± SD. One-way ANOVA was used for multiple group comparisons, and Duncan's test was used for post hoc examination. Data for steatosis histopathological scores were presented as means and were analyzed using the non-parametric test, followed by a Mann–Whitney U-test to compare group differences. Differences with $P<0.05$ were considered significant.

Results

Body, liver, and spleen weight

The basic physiological data for 30% (v/v) HFCS-induced HMMS are shown in Table 1. After eight weeks, the control group (HFCS without lactoferrin) showed significant increases in body, liver, and spleen weight, as well as a body weight gain ($P<0.05$). The lactoferrin treatment groups (50, 100, and 200 mg/kg) showed significantly lower body, liver, and spleen weights, as well as body weight gain ($P<0.05$). The control group exhibited significant swelling, and further increase in portal hypertension induced spleen swelling.

Fatty liver and hepatic damage

After eight weeks of lactoferrin administration (50, 100, and 200 mg/kg) to mice with HFCS-induced HMMS, the mice were sacrificed, and their livers subjected to gross and microscopic examination. Mice from the control group (no lactoferrin) had fatty livers, while lipid accumulation was markedly reduced in the groups administered with lactoferrin (Figure 1). HE staining of paraffinized sections showed oil droplet vacuoles in the control group that were reduced in the lactoferrin treatment groups. A similar effect was shown in the frozen sections stained with Oil Red O (Figure 1). The control group's histopathological steatosis score was significantly higher than naïve group (Table 2; $P<0.001$). The lactoferrin treatment groups (50, 100, and 200 mg/kg) had significantly lower histopathological steatosis scores than the control group (Table 2; $P<0.01$). In the measurement of Oil Red O stain, lipid droplet area (%) and numbers were significantly lower in the lactoferrin-treated groups (Table 3; $P<0.05$). The hepatic homogenate was analyzed to measure fat accumulation. Hepatic triglyceride (hTG) and serum triglyceride (sTG) levels were significantly reduced in the lactoferrin treatment groups compared to the control group (Table 4, 5; $P<0.05$). In addition, serum concentrations of total cholesterol (sCHOL) were significantly increased in the HFCS-induced NASH control group (Table 4; $P<0.05$). Administration of lactoferrin (50, 100, and 200 mg/kg) significantly reduced sCHOL levels compared to the control group (Table 4; $P<0.05$). Severe lipid accumulation results in lipid peroxidation and inflammation. 4-HNE is an important indicator of lipid peroxidation, and immunohistochemical staining showed that 4-HNE staining in the liver tissue of the control group was significantly higher, but significantly reduced by lactoferrin treatment (Figure 2). In the control group, sALT increased significantly (Table 4; $P<0.05$), but reduced by lactoferrin administration (Table 4; $P<0.05$). These data indicate that lactoferrin was significantly reduced oil droplet accumulation and liver damage.

Inflammatory adipokines in liver damage

Inflammatory adipokines including cytokines, chemokines and acute phase proteins that are involved in adipocyte development. The liver contains a variety of cell types, which play roles in defense and detoxification, or which help form the structural matrix. Hepatic IL-1β (hIL-1β), hTNF-α, and hMCP-1 are primarily produced by Kupffer cells and neutrophils. In our present results, these inflammatory adipokines were significantly increased in the control group compared to the naïve group (Table 5; $P<0.05$), but not in the lactoferrin-treated groups (Table 5; $P<0.05$). Compared to the naïve group, levels of hIL-4 and hIL-13 were significantly increased in the control group (Table 5; $P<0.05$), but not in the lactoferrin-treated groups (Table 5; $P<0.05$). Epithelial cell-derived cytokines, including IL-33 and TSLP, modulate inflammation; hIL-33 and hTSLP levels

Table 1. Effects of lactoferrin on body, liver, and spleen weights, and weight gain in HFCS-induced murine HMMS.

	Naïve	HFCS-induced murine HMMS			
		Control, DW	Lf, 50 mg/kg	Lf, 100 mg/kg	Lf, 200 mg/kg
Pre-treatment body weight (Pre-BW), g	23.24±1.12	24.63±1.90	24.35±1.71	24.10±1.60	24.85±1.08
Post-treatment BW (Post-BW), g	24.90±1.14 [a]	33.23±2.44 [c]	27.71±2.29 [b]	28.14±2.00 [b]	27.63±1.96 [b]
Weight gain, g	1.66±0.35 [a]	8.60±1.75 [d]	3.36±0.84 [bc]	4.04±0.87 [c]	2.78±1.34 [b]
Liver weight (LW), g	0.94±0.08 [a]	1.37±0.12 [b]	1.08±0.06 [a]	0.96±0.31 [a]	1.00±0.16 [a]
Spleen weight (SW), mg	62.83±5.47 [a]	94.01±8.84 [d]	77.21±9.76 [bc]	80.34±11.64 [c]	70.75±10.42 [ab]
LW/Post-BW, %	3.80±0.30 [ab]	4.12±0.17 [b]	3.91±0.36 [ab]	3.39±1.10 [a]	3.62±0.41 [ab]

Following 8 weeks of lactoferrin administration (0, 50, 100, and 200 mg/kg), body, liver, and spleen weights, and weight gain were significantly higher in the control group than in the naïve group ($P<0.05$). Body, liver, and spleen weights, and weight gain were significantly lower in the lactoferrin-treated groups than in the control group ($P<0.05$). Data are presented as mean ± SD (n = 10), and were analyzed using one-way ANOVAs and Duncan's multiple range test. [a–d]: Different letters in the same row indicate a significant difference ($P<0.05$).

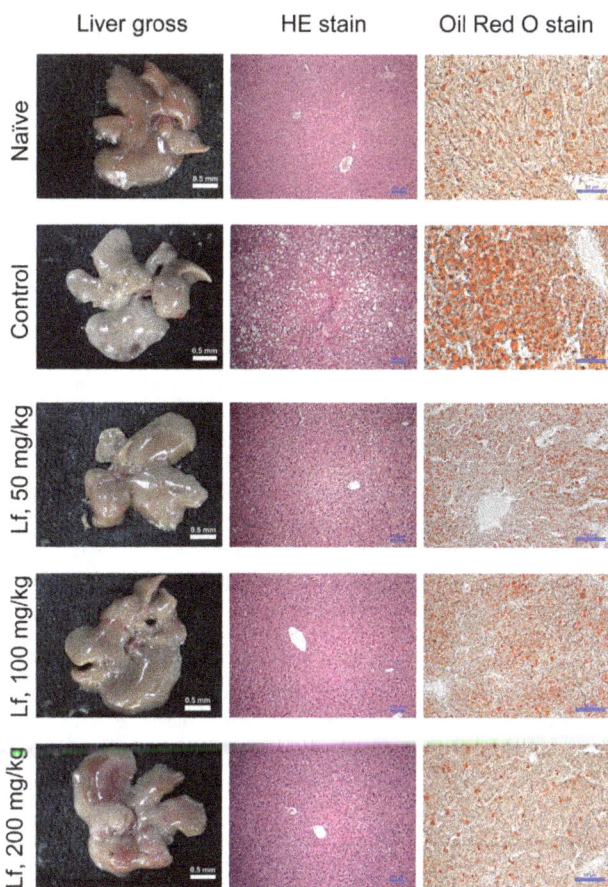

Figure 1. Gross and microscopic evaluation of the effect of lactoferrin on lipid accumulation by the mouse liver after HFCS challenge. Liver sections (5 µm) were prepared using HE and Oil Red O stains to determine lipid accumulation. Lipid accumulation around the vein was minimal in normal mice (naïve group). Lipid accumulation was marked in HMMS mice (control group). Treatment with lactoferrin at 50, 100, and 200 mg/kg markedly suppressed lipid accumulation. The scale bar represents 0.5 mm in liver gross, 100 µm in HE-stained sections, and 50 µm in Oil Red O stained sections.

were significantly increased in the control group compared to the naïve group (Table 5; $P<0.05$), but not in the lactoferrin-treated groups (Table 5; $P<0.05$). Finally, adiponectin (Adn) antagonizes adipocyte maturation, and the hAdn level was significantly reduced in the control group (Table 5; $P<0.05$) but not in the 100 and 200 mg/kg lactoferrin-treated groups (Table 5; $P<0.05$). TLR-4 and TSLP had been detected in inflammatory tissue by immunohistochemical staining and were significantly increased in the control group relative to the naïve group, but not in the lactoferrin-treated groups (Figure 2).

Endotoxin and bovine lactoferrin (bLf) levels in liver and blood

Endotoxin levels were significantly increased in the liver and blood of mice with HFCS-induced HMMS (Table 4, 5; $P<0.05$). After administration of various doses of bLf (50, 100, and 200 mg/kg), endotoxin levels in murine liver and blood significantly decreased ($P<0.05$). Lactoferrin therefore plays a role in scavenging endotoxins, such that the liver and blood levels in HFCS-induced NASH mice were not significantly different from that in naïve control mice. Oral administration of bLf (50, 100, and 200 mg/kg) resulted in significant increases in bLf levels in liver homogenates and serum (Table 4, 5; $P<0.05$).

HMMS-related insulin resistance

The hepatic manifestations of the metabolic syndrome are fatty liver and/or hepatic steatosis linked to insulin resistance. Type 2 diabetes is also a chronic inflammatory condition characterized by elevation of concentrations of ROS and endotoxins. As shown in Figure 3A, measurements of serum glucose by OGTT demonstrated that compared to the naïve group, the control group had higher blood glucose concentrations after fasting and 30, 60, 90, and 120 min after oral glucose administration (Figure 3A; $P<0.05$). The lactoferrin-treated groups showed significantly lower blood glucose levels at all times compared to the control group. Area under curve (AUC) measurements from the OGTT indicated that glucose levels were significantly higher in the control group than in the naïve group, and that glucose levels were significantly lower in the lactoferrin-treated groups than in the control group (Figure 3B; $P<0.05$). Fasting insulin levels were significantly reduced in the lactoferrin-treated groups, in a dose-dependent manner (Figure 3C; $P<0.05$). The homeostatic model

Table 2. Effect of lactoferrin on hepatic steatosis scores.

Group	Numbers of mice with different steatosis scores				Mean	P
		+	++	+++		
Naïve	10	0	0	0	0	
HFCS-induced HMMS						
Control	0	0	2	8	2.8###	0.000
Lf, 50 mg/kg	0	2	6	2	2.0**	0.007
Lf, 100 mg/kg	0	3	7	0	1.7***	0.000
Lf, 200 mg/kg	0	6	4	0	1.4***	0.000

Following eight weeks of lactoferrin administration (0, 50, 100, and 200 mg/kg), the control group had a significantly higher histopathological steatosis score than the naïve group (### $P < 0.001$). The lactoferrin-treated groups had significantly lower steatosis scores than the control group (**$P < 0.01$, ***$P < 0.001$). Data are presented as means and were analyzed with non-parametric statistics followed by the Mann–Whitney U-test to compare group differences. Grade designations of the histological findings are: (−, 0) normal, (+, 1) slight, (++, 2) moderate, and (+++, 3) severe steatosis. Each value represents the number of animals that showed a change in grade during the experimental period.

assessment (HOMA) is a method used to determine insulin resistance (HOMA-IR). Our data indicate that the lactoferrin-administered groups had significantly reduced HOMA-IR (Figure 3D; $P < 0.05$), suggesting that lactoferrin can lower insulin resistance.

Discussion

In the western diet, long-term consumption of beverages containing HFCS contributes to the development HMMS, including obesity, insulin resistance, hypertriglyceridemia, NAFLD, and NASH, all of which are associated with an inflammatory state. Previous studies have indicated that administration of 15–54% aqueous solutions of HFCS can elevate fasting blood glucose concentrations and increase insulin resistance in murine models [24,25]. Inflammatory status indicates the progression of obesity, insulin resistance, NAFLD, and NASH [26]. In this study, gross examination of the livers of HFCS-administered mice showed lipid accumulation and a 45% increase in liver weight (1.37 g vs. 0.94 g; Table 1). Microscopic examination of liver sections revealed steatosis after HFCS administration, which was significantly reduced in a dose-dependent manner by lactoferrin treatment (Figure 1). After 8 weeks of HFCS induction, severe steatosis (>80%) was observed. However, there were no severe steatosis could be detected in mice administered with the higher doses of lactoferrin (100 and 200 mg/kg; Table 2). Oil Red O staining also showed that lactoferrin administration could significantly reduce lipid droplet accumulation. Serum and hepatic triglyceride (sTG and hTG) levels significantly increased after HFCS induction; lacto-

ferrin treatment lowered sTG and hTG levels to the normal range (naïve group; Tables 4, 5). High serum cholesterol, another HFCS-induced HMMS, could also be reduced by lactoferrin administration (Table 5). Previous studies using the murine model have shown that lactoferrin can also significantly reduce triglycerides and cholesterol in the plasma and fat tissue mass [18,27]. As mentioned earlier, the first hit described by the "double hit" hypothesis is triglyceride accumulation in the liver [9]. Ishimoto et al. used fructokinase (Ketohexokinase-A and -C) knockout mice (KHK-A/C KO) to demonstrate that fructokinase plays a central role in the first hit, via the development of steatohepatitis resulting from a high-fat and high-sucrose (Western) diet [28]. In the present study, sTGs and hTGs were reduced to normal levels in the lactoferrin-treated groups (Table 4, 5). Histopathological analysis of Oil Red O staining also indicated that administration of lactoferrin significantly reduced the area and number of lipid droplets (Table 3, Figure 1). These results indicated that lactoferrin or lactoferrin hydrolysate could alter the transformation of fructose to fructose-1-phosphate via antagonism of fructokinase activity. Johnson et al. developed a method for fructokinase inhibition screening (U.S. Patent application: US20130195886A1) that involves the provision of fructokinase-C and -A inhibitors, including (z)-3-(methylthio)-1- phenyl-N'-(((4-trifluoromethoxy)-phenyl)carbamyoyl) oxy)-1H-pyrazole-4-carboximidamide, 5-amino-3-(methylthio)-1-phenyl-1H-pyrazole -4-carbonitrile, and 2-(3-(methylthio)-1-phenyl-1H-pyranol-4-yl)-4-phenylthiazole, which are phenyl-ring enriched. The sequence of lactoferrin is rich in aromatic-ring peptides (phenylalanine, tyrosine, and tryptophan), which might be the functional peptides in the digestive hydrolysate. Fernández-Musoles et al. predicted that the functional oligo peptides

Table 3. Effect of lactoferrin on liver lipid droplets in Oil Red O stain.

	Naïve	HFCS-induced murine HMMS			
		Control	Lf, 50 mg/kg	Lf, 100 mg/kg	Lf, 200 mg/kg
Area, %	3.0±0.4 [a]	18.8±5.3 [c]	6.1±2.6 [b]	4.7±1.9 [ab]	4.2±1.3 [ab]
Number	29.6±2.7 [a]	146.6±12.4 [b]	36.3±6.1 [a]	30.8±4.7 [a]	30.1±4.0 [a]

Following eight weeks of lactoferrin administration (0, 50, 100, and 200 mg/kg), the area (%) and number of lipid droplets were significantly higher in the control group than the naïve group ($P < 0.05$). The area (%) and number of lipid droplets were significantly lower in the lactoferrin-treated groups than in the control group ($P < 0.05$). Data are presented as the mean ± SD (n = 10), and were analyzed using one-way ANOVAs and Duncan's multiple range test. [a-c]. Different letters in the same row indicate a significant difference ($P < 0.05$).

Table 4. Effects of lactoferrin on serum mediators in HFCS-induced murine HMMS.

	Naïve	HFCS-induced murine HMMS			
		Control	Lf, 50 mg/kg	Lf, 100 mg/kg	Lf, 200 mg/kg
sALT, U/L	16.50±6.26 [a]	75.50±39.89 [c]	40.50±7.98 [b]	31.00±21.32 [ab]	24.00±10.49 [ab]
sTG, mg/dL	26.90±13.26 [a]	61.15±7.13 [b]	35.40±14.13 [a]	32.65±15.11 [a]	34.85±9.66 [a]
sCHOL, mg/dL	57.50±8.90 [a]	94.00±15.06 [c]	75.00±19.86 [b]	75.50±21.79 [b]	74.50±16.91 [b]
sLPS, EU/mL	0.16±0.03 [a]	0.62±0.01 [d]	0.46±0.02 [c]	0.42±0.02 [b]	0.40±0.01 [b]
sbLf, µg/mL	1.99±0.36 [a]	2.24±0.40 [a]	4.38±0.38 [b]	7.70±0.92 [c]	12.04±2.64 [d]

Following eight weeks of lactoferrin administration (0, 50, 100, and 200 mg/kg), levels of serum LPS (sLPS), serum ALT (sALT), serum triglyceride (sTG), serum cholesterol (sCHOL), and serum bovine lactoferrin (sbLf) were significantly higher in the control group than in the naïve group ($P<0.05$). sLPS, sALT, sTG, and sCHOL were significantly lower in the lactoferrin-treated groups than in the control group ($P<0.05$). sbLf was significantly higher in the lactoferrin-treated groups than in the control group, in a dose-dependent manner. Data are presented as the mean ± SD (n = 10), and were analyzed using one-way ANOVAs and Duncan's multiple range test. [a–d]: Different letters in the same row indicate a significant difference ($P<0.05$).

(LIWKL and RPYL) of lactoferrin have antihypertensive activity, and subsequently demonstrated that the antihypertensive activity of RPYL (200 µM) is equal to that of valsartan (0.1 µM) [29]. We predict that oligopeptides with aromatic rings, including PEWF, PYFGY, PYKLRP, PQTHYY, FQLFGSPP, and VVWCAVGP, would be showed fructokinase-antagonistic activity; we are going to investigate these oligopeptides in the further studies. Elevated lipid peroxidation can be detected by measuring 4-HNE, which along with malondialdehyde, arises from increases in the oxidative stress chain reaction. HCFS increased the 4-HNE accumulation observed in tissue sections, and its production was significantly reduced by lactoferrin treatment (Figure 2). There were no previous study indicate that lactoferrin reduces 4-HNE formation in tissues under hyperoxidative stress conditions. However, the role of lactoferrin play a part of defense mechanism against lipid peroxidation may explain why sputum lactoferrin levels are higher in smokers than in non-smokers [30]. Our study presents the novel observation that lactoferrin can reduce the 4-HNE protein adducts produced by the oxidative stress chain reaction.

Hepatic manifestations of the metabolic syndrome caused by HFCS administration also include insulin resistance. Fasting insulin, blood glucose, and HOMA-IR were significantly increased in serum after HFCS induction for 7 weeks (Figure 3A, 3C, 3D). Fasting insulin and blood glucose did not fall to the levels observed in the naïve group after treatment with lactoferrin (Figure 3A, 3C). But HOMA-IR of lactoferrin-treated groups were reduced to the level as in the naïve group ($P>0.05$, Figure 3D). Examination of the OGTT, an indicator of insulin insensitivity, showed the lactoferrin groups had significantly lower glucose levels than the control group at 30, 60, 90, and 120 min. At 120 min after oral administration of 2% glucose to fasting mice, the lactoferrin groups had cleared glucose as efficiently as the naïve group.

Table 5. Effects of lactoferrin on hepatic mediators in HFCS-induced murine HMMS.

	Naïve	HFCS-induced murine HMMS			
		Control	Lf, 50 mg/kg	Lf, 100 mg/kg	Lf, 200 mg/kg
hTG, mg/g	9.9±4.4 [a]	33.4±9.0 [b]	10.4±3.5 [a]	10.8±6.1 [a]	13.9±5.3 [a]
hIL-1β, ng/g	53.3±30.5 [a]	132.4±63.9 [b]	54.7±16.0 [a]	57.8±24.3 [a]	40.6±19.0 [a]
hIL-6, ng/g	16.8±4.6 [a]	23.8±6.2 [b]	20.5±8.6 [ab]	15.8±4.6 [a]	18.8±3.6 [ab]
hTNF-α, ng/g	97.9±66.4 [a]	175.2±63.9 [b]	109.8±41.7 [a]	93.9±42.9 [a]	121.4±52.7 [a]
hMCP-1, ng/g	115.0±64.8 [a]	223.7±55.2 [b]	133.9±26.5 [a]	128.0±65.8 [a]	142.3±44.3 [a]
hIL-4, ng/g	50.9±26.9 [a]	117.5±41.1 [b]	76.8±16.7 [a]	66.9±31.0 [a]	60.1±23.2 [a]
hIL-13, µg/g	14.6±6.1 [a]	24.5±7.9 [b]	16.5±2.7 [a]	15.7±5.7 [a]	15.3±5.3 [a]
hIL-33, ng/g	276.3±124.1 [a]	431.8±192.8 [b]	266.6±73.0 [a]	233.2±96.7 [a]	261.7±100.8 [a]
hTSLP, ng/g	81.6±17.3 [a]	133.7±36.6 [b]	100.8±40.6 [a]	83.5±22.3 [a]	93.0±39.9 [a]
hAdn, mg/g	5.8±1.1 [c]	3.7±1.3 [a]	4.3±1.2 [ab]	4.9±0.7 [bc]	5.7±0.9 [c]
hLPS, EU/g	2.8±0.4 [a]	4.3±0.8 [b]	3.1±0.5 [a]	3.0±0.5 [a]	2.7±0.2 [a]
hbLf, µg/g	7.3±1.4 [a]	8.9±1.3 [a]	14.2±1.7 [b]	17.2±9.2 [b]	22.8±5.1 [c]

Following eight weeks of lactoferrin administration (0, 50, 100, and 200 mg/kg), levels of hepatic LPS (hLPS), hTG, hIL-1β, hIL-6, hTNF-α, hMCP-1, hIL-4, hIL-13, hIL-33, and hTSLP were significantly higher in the control group than in the naïve group ($P<0.05$). Hepatic adiponectin (hAdn) was significantly lower in the control group than in the naïve group ($P<0.05$). There was no significant difference in hepatic bovine lactoferrin (hbLf) between the control and naïve groups. hLPS, hTG, hIL-1β, hTNF-α, hMCP-1, hIL-4, hIL-13, hIL-33, and hTSLP were significantly lower in the lactoferrin treatment groups (50, 100, and 200 mg/kg) than the control group ($P<0.05$). hIL-6 was significantly lower than the control only in the lactoferrin group receiving 100 mg/kg. hAdn was significantly higher than the control group in the 100 and 200 mg/kg lactoferrin groups ($P<0.05$). hbLf was significantly higher in the lactoferrin groups than the control group, in a dose-dependent manner. Data are presented as the mean ± SD (n = 10), and were analyzed with one-way ANOVAs and Duncan's multiple range test. [a–d]: Different letters in the same row indicate a significant difference ($P<0.05$).

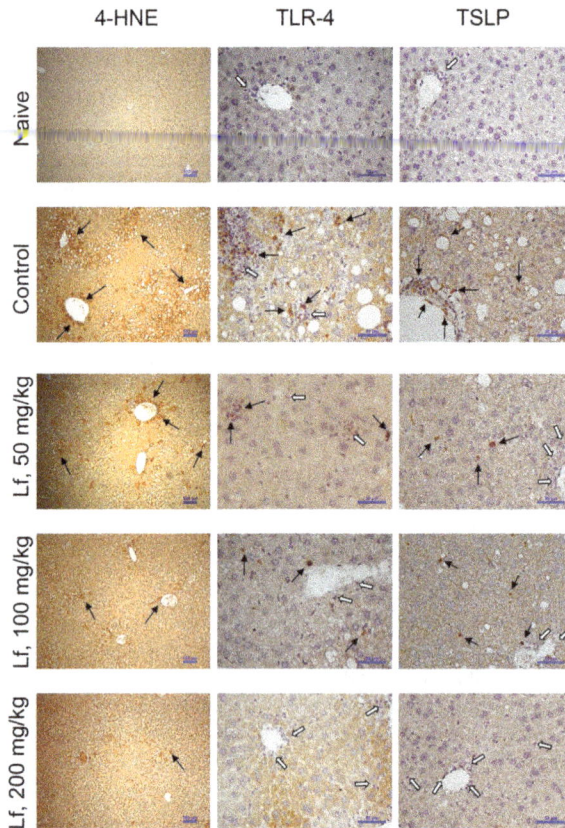

Figure 2. Treatment with lactoferrin improved the histology of livers of HFCS-induced HMMS mice. Immunohistochemical staining with 4-HNE, TLR-4, and TSLP show lipid peroxidation (4 HNE) and associated inflammatory markers (TLR-4 and TSLP). The control group showed lipid vascular accumulation and stained positive for 4-HNE, TLR-4, and TSLP, compared to the naïve group (indicated by arrows). Open arrows indicate negative staining for TLR-4 and TSLP, which indicate without infiltration of inflammatory cells. Treatment with lactoferrin at 50, 100, and 200 mg/kg markedly reduced 4-HNE, TLR-4, and TSLP expression. Scale bars represent 100 μm (4-HNE) and 50 μm (TLR-4 and TSLP).

Moreno-Navarrete *et al.* demonstrated that circulating lactoferrin was significantly decreased in patients with altered glucose tolerance and was negatively related to inflammatory markers [31]. In *ex vivo* experiments, a significant decrease in LPS-induced lactoferrin release from neutrophils was observed in subjects with type 2 diabetes [31]. Our study is the first observation in lactoferrin administration can improve insulin sensitivity as measured by OGTT and HOMA-IR.

HFSC stimulates overgrowth of intestinal microbiota, increasing intestinal permeability and leading to chronic inflammation [32]. In this study, HFCS (30%) induced overgrowth of fecal coliforms (data not shown) and higher serum LPS (Table 4). Our data indicate that lactoferrin altered the HFCS-induced imbalance in intestinal microbiota and reduced chronic inflammation. In previous studies, lactoferrin presents to exert anti-infectious and anti-inflammatory activities *in vivo*, and to inhibit LPS-induced IL-6 secretion in a human monocytic cell line [33]. This observation was extended with a demonstration that lactoferrin inhibits the expression of mRNA of proinflammatory cytokines, including TNF-α, IL-1, IL-6, and IL-8, and modulates the nuclear transcription factor kappa B (NF-κB) signaling cascade [34]. Lactoferrin has also been shown to downregulate IL-10 secretion

in LPS-stimulated macrophages [35]. In our study, serum and hepatic LPS levels significantly increased in HFCS-induced HMMS, and this increase was significantly reduced IL-10 by lactoferrin (Table 4, 5). Significantly, reduced expression of TLR-4 was also observed in lactoferrin-treated groups indicated the reducing inflammatory cascade signaling (Figure 2). Puddu *et al.* indicate bovine lactoferrin conteracts TLR mediated activation signals in monocyte-derived dendritic cells [36]. Serum ALT (sALT) is a direct indicator of hepatitis, and lactoferrin reduced sALT in a dose-dependent manner. Furthermore, cytokine measurements indicated that lactoferrin could significantly reduce hepatic IL-1β, TNF-α, and MCP-1 (Table 5). Previous studies have shown that lactoferrin can bind LPS from *E. coli* and *Salmonella typhimurium* and remove the glycolipid from the bacterial surface [37–39]. Lactoferricin, a peptide produced by hydrolysis of lactoferrin by a gastrointestinal digestive enzyme, plays a central role in scavenging LPS [40–42]. Analysis of the structural characteristics of lactoferricin identified a six-residue sequence responsible for binding LPS of *E. coli* or *Pseudomonas aeruginosa* [43–45]. Serum and hepatic lactoferrin were measured by ELISA, and no significant differences were observed between the naïve and control groups (Table 4, 5). Interestingly, lactoferrin can be detected in serum and liver homogenates in a dose-dependent manner. This indicates that orally administered bovine lactoferrin can be absorbed into the circulation. Fischer *et al.* showed that orally administered lactoferrin could be detected in the liver, kidneys, gall bladder, spleen, and brain of the mouse within 10–20 min [46].

When IL-33 and TSLP, which are both epithelial-related pro-inflammatory cytokines, are present in tissue matrix, polarization in a type 2-environment allows precursor substances (IL-4 and IL-13) to activate dendritic cells to stimulate Th2 cells differentiation [17]. Our data indicate that lactoferrin can significantly reduce levels of the epithelial cell-derived cytokines IL-33 and TSLP (Table 4). Examination of pathological tissue sections also indicated that TSLP was significantly reduced in the lactoferrin-treated groups (Figure 2). On the other way, the adipocyte-derived plasma protein adiponectin has been shown to be decreased by obesity and to inhibit TNF-α-induced expression of endothelial adhesion molecules [48]. Adiponectin acts as an anti-inflammatory and anti-atherogenic plasma protein. Adiponectin is a biologically relevant endogenous modulator of vascular remodeling, linking obesity and vascular disease [49]. Adiponectin may downregulate IL-6 and TNF-α expression from Kupffer cells, thereby inhibiting inflammatory progression in the liver [50,51]. Reducing visceral adipose tissue macrophages improves systemic glucose homeostasis, insulin sensitivity and increase adipnectin levels *via* CCR2/MCP-1 signaling in diet-induced obese mice [52,53]. Our data suggest that upregulation of adiponectin expression by lactoferrin is correlated with anti-inflammatory status (Table 5) in modulation of tissue specific macrophage.

Conclusions

In conclusion, treatment of mice with bovine lactoferrin had a twofold beneficial effect. Lactoferrin decreased the "first hit" by reducing serum triglyceride, cholesterol levels and retarding hepatic lipid accumulation. In addition, lactoferrin altered the "second hit" by and scavenging LPS in circulation to reduce the expression of hepatic inflammatory cytokines. As a natural substance, bovine lactoferrin contribute for the control of HFCS induced HMMS, including obesity, insulin resistance, hypertri glyceridemia, NAFLD and NASH.

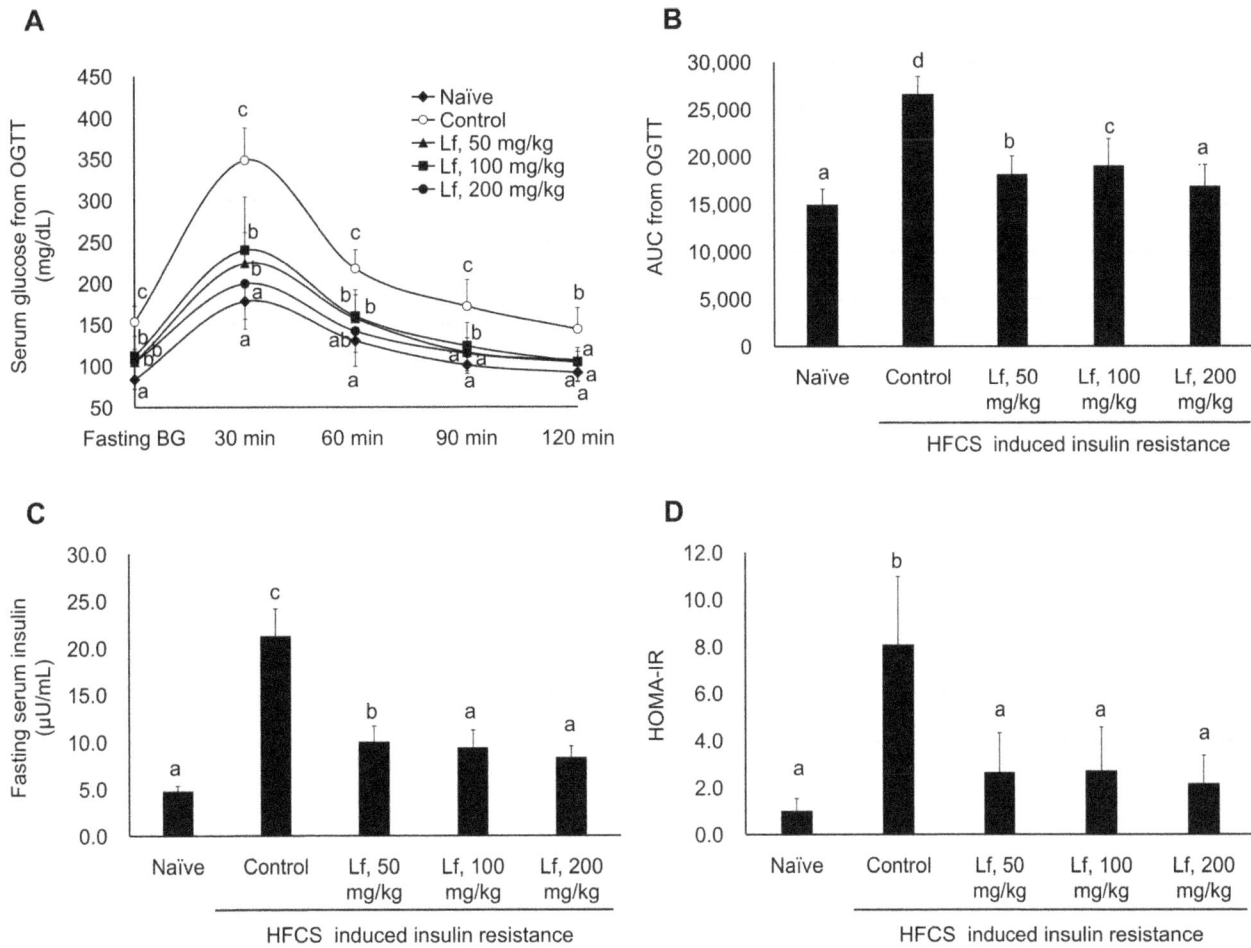

Figure 3. Insulin resistance and OGTT determination in HFCS-induced insulin resistance in the murine model. (A) Blood glucose determined by OGTT after oral administration of glucose (2%). (B) Area under curve (AUC) was calculated for the OGTT. The control group showed a significant increase compared to the naïve group, whereas lactoferrin at 50, 100, and 200 mg/kg markedly reduced the AUC. (C) Fasting serum insulin was determined by ELISA. Insulin levels were significantly increased in the control group compared to the naïve group, and lactoferrin at 50, 100, and 200 mg/kg markedly reduced blood insulin. (D) HOMA-IR insulin resistance calculated from fasting serum glucose and insulin levels. Lactoferrin at 50, 100, and 200 mg/kg markedly reduced blood insulin. Data are presented as mean $\pm$ SD (n = 10) and were analyzed using one-way ANOVAs and Duncan's multiple range test. [a–d]: Different letters indicate significant differences between groups (P<0.05).

Acknowledgments

We thank Professor Yun-Chu Wu for help with the statistical analysis. We further thank CCH Lab. team members, Hsin-Ya Chen and Jie-Yu Chen for their technical assistance.

Author Contributions

Conceived and designed the experiments: CCH. Performed the experiments: YCL CCH. Analyzed the data: YCL CCH. Contributed reagents/materials/analysis tools: CCH. Wrote the paper: CCH.

References

1. Baranova A, Randhawa M, Jarrar M, Younossi ZM (2007) Adipokines and melanocortins in the hepatic manifestation of the metabolic syndrome: nonalcoholic fatty liver disease. Expert Rev Mol Diagn 7: 195–205.
2. Castro GS, Cardoso JF, Vannucchi H, Zucoloto S, Jordão AA (2011) Fructose and NAFLD: metabolic implications and models of induction in rats. Acta Cir Bras 26 Suppl 2: 45–50.
3. Saito T, Misawa K, Kawata S (2007) 1. Fatty liver and non-alcoholic steatohepatitis. Intern Med 46: 101–103.
4. Basciano H, Federico L, Adeli K (2005) Fructose, insulin resistance, and metabolic dyslipidemia. Nutr Metab (Lond) 2: 1–14
5. Rutledge AC, Adeli K (2007) Fructose and the the metabolic syndrome: pathophysiology and molecular mechanisms. Nutr Rev 2007 65(6 Pt 2): S13–23.
6. Nseir W, Nassar F, Assy N (2010) Soft drinks consumption and nonalcoholic fatty liver disease. World J Gastroenterol 16: 2579–2588.
7. Cook GC (1969) Absorption products of D(-) fructose in man. Clin Sci 37: 675–687.
8. Hsu CS, Kao JH (2012) Non-alcoholic fatty liver disease: an emerging liver disease in Taiwan. J Formos Med Assoc 111: 527–535.
9. Day CP, James OF (1998) Steatohepatitis: a tale of two "hits"? Gastroenterology. 114: 842–845.
10. Keidar S, Kaplan M, Rosenblat M, Brook GJ, Aviram M (1992) Apolipoprotein E and lipoprotein lipase reduce macrophage degradation of oxidized very-low-density lipoprotein (VLDL), but increase cellular degradation of native VLDL. Metabolism 41: 1185–1192.
11. Petit JM, Bour JB, Galland-Jos C, Minello A, Verges B, et al. (2001) Risk factors for diabetes mellitus and early insulin resistance in chronic hepatitis C. J Hepatol 35: 279–283.
12. Rubbia-Brandt L, Giostra E, Mentha G, Quadri R, Negro F (2001) Expression of liver steatosis in hepatitis C virus infection and pattern of response to alpha-interferon. J Hepatol 35: 307–307.
13. Brock JH (2002) The physiology of lactoferrin. Biochem Cell Biol 80: 1–6.
14. Petschow BW, Talbott RD, Batema RP (1999) Ability of lactoferrin to promote the growth of Bifidobacterium spp. in vitro is independent of receptor binding capacity and iron saturation level. J Med Microbiol 48: 541–549.

15. Sherman MP, Bennett SH, Hwang FF, Yu C (2004) Neonatal small bowel epithelia: enhancing anti-bacterial defense with lactoferrin and Lactobacillus GG. Biometals 17: 285–289.
16. Valenti P, Antonini G (2005) Lactoferrin: an important host defence against microbial and viral attack. Cell Mol Life Sci 62: 2576–2587.
17. Takeuchi T, Shimizu H, Ando K, Harada E (2004) Bovine lactoferrin reduces plasma triacylglycerol and NEFA accompanied by decreased hepatic cholesterol and triacylglycerol contents in rodents. Br J Nutr 91: 533–538.
18. Morishita S, Ono T, Fujisaki C, Ishihara Y, Murakoshi M, et al. (2013) Bovine lactoferrin reduces visceral fat and liver triglycerides in ICR mice. J Oleo Sci 62: 97–103.
19. Matthews DR, Hosker JP, Rudenski AS, Naylor BA, Treacher DF, et al. (1985) Homeostasis model assessment: insulin resistance and beta-cell function from fasting plasma glucose and insulin concentrations in man. Diabetologia 28: 412–419.
20. Kleiner DE, Brunt EM, Van Natta M, Behling C, Contos MJ, et al. (2005) Nonalcoholic Steatohepatitis Clinical Research Network. Design and validation of a histological scoring system for nonalcoholic fatty liver disease. Hepatology 41: 1313–1321.
21. Fiorini RN, Kirtz J, Periyasamy B, Evans Z, Haines JK, et al. (2004) Development of an unbiased method for the estimation of liver steatosis. Clin Transplant 18: 700–706.
22. Yang J, Ren J, Song J, Liu F, Wu C, et al. (2013) Glucagon-like peptide 1 regulates adipogenesis in 3T3-L1 preadipocytes. Int J Mol Med. 31: 1429–1435.
23. Hsieh CC, Fang HL, Lin WC (2008) Inhibitory effect of Solanum nigrum on thioacetamide-induced liver fibrosis in mice. J Ethnopharmacol 119: 117–121.
24. Blakely SR, Hallfrisch J, Reiser S, Prather ES (1981) Long-term effects of moderate fructose feeding on glucose tolerance parameters in rats. J Nutr 111: 307–314.
25. Beck-Nielsen H, Pedersen O, Lindskov HO (1980) Impaired cellular insulin binding and insulin sensitivity induced by high-fructose feeding in normal subjects. Am J Clin Nutr 33: 273–278.
26. Schuppan D, Schattenberg JM (2013) Non-alcoholic steatohepatitis: pathogenesis and novel therapeutic approaches. J Gastroenterol Hepatol 28: 68–76.
27. Takeuchi T, Kitagawa H, Harada E (2004) Evidence of lactoferrin transportation into blood circulation from intestine via lymphatic pathway in adult rats. Exp Physiol 89: 263–270.
28. Ishimoto T, Lanaspa MA, Rivard CJ, Roncal-Jimenez CA, Orlicky DJ, et al. (2013) High-fat and high-sucrose (western) diet induces steatohepatitis that is dependent on fructokinase. Hepatology. 58: 1632–1643.
29. Fernández-Musoles R, Castelló-Ruiz M, Arce C, Manzanares P, Ivorra MD, et al. (2014) Antihypertensive Mechanism of Lactoferrin-Derived Peptides: Angiotensin Receptor Blocking Effect. J Agric Food Chem. 62: 173–181.
30. Rytilä P, Rehn T, Ilumets H, Rouhos A, Sovijärvi A, et al. (2006) Increased oxidative stress in asymptomatic current chronic smokers and GOLD stage 0 COPD. Respir Res 7: 1–10.
31. Moreno-Navarrete JM, Ortega FJ, Bassols J, Ricart W, Fernández-Real JM (2009) Decreased circulating lactoferrin in insulin resistance and altered glucose tolerance as a possible marker of neutrophil dysfunction in type 2 diabetes. J Clin Endocrinol Metab 94: 4036–4044.
32. Spruss A, Bergheim I (2009) Dietary fructose and intestinal barrier: potential risk factor in the pathogenesis of nonalcoholic fatty liver disease. J Nutr Biochem 20: 657–662.
33. Mattsby-Baltzer I, Roseanu A, Motas C, Elverfors J, Engberg I, et al. (1996) Lactoferrin or a fragment thereof inhibits the endotoxin-induced interleukin-6 response in human monocytic cells. Pediatr Res 40: 257–262.
34. Baeuerle PA (1998) Pro-inflammatory signaling: last pieces in the NF-kappaB puzzle? Curr Biol 8: R19–22.
35. Håversen L, Ohlsson BG, Hahn-Zoric M, Hanson LA, Mattsby-Baltzer I (2002) Lactoferrin down-regulates the LPS-induced cytokine production in monocytic cells via NF-kappa B. Cell Immunol 220: 83–95.
36. Puddu P, Latorre D, Carollo M, Catizone A, Ricci G, et al. (2011) Bovine lactoferrin counteracts Toll-like receptor mediated activation signals in antigen presenting cells. PLoS ONE 6: e22504.
37. Yamauchi K, Tomita M, Giehl TJ, Ellison RT III (1993) Antibacterial activity of lactoferrin and a pepsin-derived lactoferrin peptide fragment. Infect Immun 61: 719–728.
38. Ellison RT III, Giehl TJ, LaForce FM (1988) Damage of the outer membrane of enteric gram-negative bacteria by lactoferrin and transferrin. Infect Immun 56: 2774–2781.
39. Chapple DS, Hussain R, Joannou CL, Hancock RE, Odell E, et al. (2004) Structure and association of human lactoferrin peptides with Escherichia coli lipopolysaccharide. Antimicrob Agents Chemother 48: 2190–2198.
40. Bellamy W, Takase M, Wakabayashi H, Kawase K, Tomita M (1992) Antibacterial spectrum of lactoferricin B, a potent bactericidal peptide derived from the N-terminal region of bovine lactoferrin. J Appl Bacteriol 73: 472–479.
41. Chapple DS, Joannou CL, Mason DJ, Shergill JK, Odell EW, et al. (1998) A helical region on human lactoferrin. Its role in antibacterial pathogenesis. Adv Exp Med Biol 443: 215–220.
42. Farnaud S, Patel A, Odell EW, Evans RW (2004) Variation in antimicrobial activity of lactoferricin-derived peptides explained by structure modelling. FEMS Microbiol Lett 238: 221–226.
43. Chapple DS, Mason DJ, Joannou CL, Odell EW, Gant V, et al. (1998) Structure-function relationship of antibacterial synthetic peptides homologous to a helical surface region on human lactoferrin against Escherichia coli serotype O111. Infect Immun 66: 2434–2440.
44. Elass-Rochard E, Roseanu A, Legrand D, Trif M, Salmon V, et al. (1995) Lactoferrin-lipopolysaccharide interaction: involvement of the 28–34 loop region of human lactoferrin in the high-affinity binding to Escherichia coli 055B5 lipopolysaccharide. Biochem J 312: 839–845.
45. Xu G, Xiong W, Hu Q, Zuo P, Shao B, et al. (2010) Lactoferrin-derived peptides and Lactoferricin chimera inhibit virulence factor production and biofilm formation in Pseudomonas aeruginosa. J Appl Microbiol 109:1311–1318.
46. Fischer R, Debbabi H, Blais A, Dubarry M, Rautureau M, et al. (2007) Uptake of ingested bovine lactoferrin and its accumulation in adult mouse tissues. Int Immunopharmacol 7: 1387–1393.
47. Mjösberg J, Bernink J, Golebski K, Karrich JJ, Peters CP, et al. (2012) The transcription factor GATA3 is essential for the function of human type 2 innate lymphoid cells. Immunity 37: 649–659.
48. Ouchi N, Kihara S, Arita Y, Okamoto Y, Maeda K, et al. (2000) Adiponectin, an adipocyte-derived plasma protein, inhibits endothelial NF-kappaB signaling through a cAMP-dependent pathway. Circulation 102: 1296–1301.
49. Ouchi N, Kihara S, Funahashi T, Matsuzawa Y, Walsh K (2003) Obesity, adiponectin and vascular inflammatory disease. Curr Opin Lipidol 14: 561–566.
50. Wanninger J, Bauer S, Eisinger K, Weiss TS, Walter R, et al. (2012) Adiponectin upregulates hepatocyte CMKLR1 which is reduced in human fatty liver. Mol Cell Endocrinol 349: 248–254.
51. An L, Wang X, Cederbaum AI (2012) Cytokines in alcoholic liver disease. Arch Toxicol 86: 1337–1348.
52. Feng B, Jiao P, Nie Y, Kim T, Jun D, et al. (2011) Clodronate liposomes improve metabolic profile and reduce visceral adipose macrophage content in diet-induced obese mice. PLoS ONE 6: e24358.
53. Sullivan TJ, Miao Z, Zhao BN, Ertl LS, Wang Y, et al. (2013) Experimental evidence for the use of CCR2 antagonists in the treatment of type 2 diabetes. Metabolism 62: 1623–1632.

22

Role of Serum Vaspin in Progression of Type 2 Diabetes

Weixia Jian[1]◑, Wenhui Peng[2]◑, Sumei Xiao[3], Hailing Li[2], Jie Jin[1], Li Qin[1], Yan Dong[1], Qing Su[1]*

1 Department of Endocrinology, Xinhua Hospital, Shanghai Jiaotong University School of Medicine, Shanghai, China, 2 Department of Cardiology, Shanghai Tenth People's Hospital, Tongji University School of Medicine, Shanghai, China, 3 Department of Medicine, Faculty of Medicine, The University of Hong Kong, Pokfulam, Hong Kong

Abstract

Vaspin is a novel adipocytokine that has potential insulin-sensitizing effects. The aim of this study is to explore the role of vaspin in the progression of type 2 diabetes mellitus (T2DM) in humans through a longitudinal process. This was a 2-year follow-up study that included 132 patients with T2DM and 170 non-diabetic subjects. The serum vaspin and adiponectin levels were determined with ELISA. Anthropometric measurements, circulating glucose, hemoglobin A1c, insulin level, liver function, kidney function, and lipid profile were measured for each participant. The new onset of T2DM was counted in non-diabetic subjects and the glycemic control was analyzed in T2DM patients at follow-up. At enrollment, the serum vaspin and adiponectin levels were lower in T2DM patients compared with non-diabetic subjects. Significant positive correlation between serum vaspin and HDL-C levels (r = 0.23, $P = 0.006$) was observed in non-diabetic controls. The serum vaspin concentration was also significantly correlated with body mass index (BMI) (r = 0.19, $P = 0.028$), waist-hip ratio (WHR) (r = 0.17, $P = 0.035$) and homeostasis model assessment of insulin resistance (HOMA-IR) (r = 0.14, $P = 0.029$) in T2DM patients. In cohort analyses, it was found that lower serum vaspin [odds ratio (OR) = 0.52, 95% confidence interval (CI): 0.10–0.87, $P = 0.015$] and adiponectin (OR = 0.35, 95% CI: 0.20–0.72, $P = 0.015$) levels at baseline were risk factors for new onset of T2DM at follow-up. The percentage of insulin treatment in T2DM patients was higher in the sub-group with lower serum vaspin level than that in the sub-group with higher vaspin level at follow-up (55.3% vs. 44.7%, $P = 0.020$). Our study indicates that low serum concentration of vaspin is a risk factor for the progression of T2DM.

Editor: Amar Abderrahmani, University of Lille Nord de France, France

Funding: This study was supported by grant from National Natural Science Foundation of China (No. 30900699). The funder had no role in study design, data collection and analysis, decision to publish, or preparation of the manuscript.

Competing Interests: The authors have declared that no competing interests exist.

* E-mail: suqingxinhua@163.com

◑ These authors contributed equally to this work.

Introduction

Adipose tissue is not only an inert energy-storing tissue, but also an active endocrine organ [1], which secrets many kinds of adipocytokines, such as adiponectin, leptin, TNF-α and so on. Some adipocytokines are involved in the development of insulin resistance, which is an important pathological link among various metabolic dysfunctions, including obesity, diabetes and cardiovascular diseases [1]. Among the adipocytokines, adiponectin is one of the most-studied and proved to have beneficial effects on insulin resistance. Adiponectin ameliorates insulin sensitivity and stimulates fatty acid oxidation in skeletal muscle and also has anti-inflammatory effects in blood vessels [2–6]. Lower serum concentration of adiponectin also predicts higher risk of diabetes in human, suggesting an important role of adiponectin that links obesity, insulin resistance, and type 2 diabetes mellitus (T2DM) [7–9].

Vaspin (visceral adipose tissue-derived serine protease inhibitor), a novel adipocytokine, was firstly identified in obese OLETF rats. It has been suggested that vaspin has potential insulin-sensitizing effects [10]. Vaspin significantly improves glucose tolerance and insulin sensitivity in diet-induced obese mice. In db/db mice, vaspin treatment is associated with sustained glucose-lowering effects for at least 6 days after the injection [11]. In humans, vaspin expression in terms of mRNA was detected in human visceral and subcutaneous adipose tissue [12]. Recent studies also found that vaspin gene expression in human adipose tissue and circulating vaspin levels were positively associated with obesity-associated diseases and T2DM [13–16]. Furthermore, it is indicated that vaspin plays a role in adipoinsular axis, and may be associated with insulin resistance in obese subjects, including patients with T2DM and polycystic ovary syndrome [13]. Therefore, all these data suggest that vaspin may be involved in the glucose metabolism and the development of T2DM in human. Vaspin has been shown to significantly improve glucose tolerance and insulin sensitivity in murine and to be positively associated with obesity-related diseases in human [14], which seems to be conflicting with each other. Hida K's study demonstrated that vaspin was barely detectable in OLETF rat at 6 weeks and was highly expressed in adipocytes of visceral white adipose tissues at 30 weeks, the age when obesity, body weight, and insulin levels peak in OLETF rats. The tissue expression of vaspin and its serum levels decreased with worsening of diabetes and body weight loss at 50 wk [10]. These results indicate that the levels of serum vaspin may change with the progression of diabetes. Vaspin may increase at the beginning and decrease with worsening of diabetes in human. A significant correlation between serum vaspin and leptin concentrations supports previous human studies that serum vaspin concentration reflects body fat mass in human [17]. Vaspin may have a compensatory role in insulin resistance in human obesity-associated diseases. Up to date, all studies on roles of vaspin in human metabolic diseases were cross-sectional, but not cohort studies. Therefore, it is still unclear what the real role of vaspin is in the progression of diabetes in a longitudinal process.

Hypothetically, just like adiponectin, low vaspin level might be concomitant with poor glycemic control in diabetic patients because of its impact on insulin sensitivity and glucose metabolism. To our knowledge, the role of vaspin in glycemic control in diabetic patients has not been addressed in previous studies. In this 2.0-year follow-up study, our aims were to examine 1) whether serum vaspin levels are associated with adiposity and insulin-resistance; 2) whether non-diabetic subjects with lower serum vaspin levels are more susceptible to developing T2DM; 3) whether lower vaspin levels are concomitant with poorer glycemic control in T2DM.

Materials and Methods

Subjects

All subjects were local residents of Han ethnicity in Shanghai and consecutively recruited in Department of Endocrinology, Xinhua hospital, Shanghai Jiaotong University School of Medicine and Department of Cardiology, Shanghai Tenth People's Hospital, Tongji University School of Medicine from Oct 2009 to Mar 2010. T2DM was diagnosed according to 1999 WHO diagnostic criteria [18]. The non-diabetic subjects were recruited from those in-patients admitted to hospital due to hypertension or other mild cardiovascular symptoms. Subjects with mild cardiovascular symptoms were those with chief complaints including mild chest distress or chest pain, excluding acute coronary syndrome or acute myocardial infarction by simultaneous coronary angiography, electrocardiogram, and tests of myocardial enzymes. The diagnosis of type 1 diabetes (T1DM) was confirmed by c peptide level and presence of glutamic acid decarboxylase antibody. Patients with T1DM, severe kidney or liver diseases, severe cardiovascular diseases, chronic viral or bacterial infection, asthma, tumors, and connective tissue diseases were excluded. Non-diabetic subjects in our study were those simultaneously match the following three criteria: fasting plasma glucose (FPG) concentration less than 6.1 mmol/L; 2-hour postprandial plasma glucose (2h-PG) concentration less than 7.8 mmmol/L and glycosylated haemoglobin A1c (HbA1c) less than 6.0%. The clinical information and anthropometric indices for all subjects at baseline and follow up were obtained by standard methods.

The study was approved by the Human Ethical Review Committees, Xinhua Hospital and Shanghai Tenth People's Hospital, and performed in accordance with the Declaration of Helsinki. Written informed consent was obtained from all subjects.

Biochemical Assays

Blood samples for biochemical analysis were collected after overnight fasting for at least 10 hours, and immediately frozen in aliquots at −80°C until analysis. FPG, 2h-PG, serum liver and renal function and lipid profile were measured by using standard laboratory techniques on a Hitachi 7104 Analyzer (Hitachi, Tokyo, Japan). HbA1c was determined by using high-performance liquid chromatography (Hi-AUTO HA-8150, ARKRAY, Kyoto, Japan) method. Serum insulin concentrations were determined by commercially available radioimmunoassay in non-diabetic subjects

and insulin-naive T2DM patients (Linco Res., St. Charles, MO, USA). Insulin sensitivity index: homeostasis model assessment of insulin resistance (HOMA-IR) was calculated by the formula as reported before [19]. Serum vaspin and adiponectin levels were determined in all subjects at baseline. Serum vaspin (Adipogen, Seoul, South Korea) and total adiponectin (R&D Systems, Minneapolis, MN, USA) levels were analyzed by using commercially available ELISAs as indicated before [20]. The degree of precision of the ELISA system in terms of coefficient of variance (percent) of intra-assay was between 1.31% and 1.74%, and that of inter-assays was between 5.9% and 8.3%. Because Teshigawara S's study in Japanese population demonstrated that about 7% of higher vaspin levels more than 10 ng/ml was beyond the detection range of vaspin ELISA kit from Adipogen company [21], three subjects with vaspin levels more than 10 ng/ml in our sample were excluded.

Follow-up

At re-examination after two years, anthropometric indices, FPG, 2h-PG, HbA1c and lipid profile were measured in all subjects. Drug uses and concomitant diseases were also recorded at the same time. During the 2-year follow-up, FPG and HbA1c had been checked in diabetic patients every three months at clinic, and hypoglycemic agents were prescribed by experienced endocrinologists. For diabetic patients, during the stable therapeutical period of two years, insulin or oral antidiabetics (OAD) treatments were recorded. For non-diabetic controls, the incidence of T2DM was investigated, and the glucose levels and other metabolic indices were also analyzed at follow-up.

Statistical analysis

Statistical analysis was performed using the Statistical Package for the Social Sciences (SPSS v.11.0, SPSS Inc., Chicago, IL, USA). All datasets were examined for normal distribution using the Kolmogorov-Smirnov test. The traits that deviated significantly from normal distribution were approximately normalized by logarithmic transformation. Differences between groups were examined using an unpaired t test or covariance analysis for continuous variables and a χ^2 test for categorical variables. Pearson correlation coefficients were used to assess the associations of continuous variables with vaspin. Multiple stepwise logistic regression analysis was used to detect the risk factors for development of T2DM, with adjustment for potential confounding factors. Results are presented as mean (standard deviation) for continuous variables and as percentage for categorical variables. The serum vaspin and adiponectin concentrations were adjusted for sex in all analyses because of the higher levels of these hormones in women [22,23]. The baseline vaspin and adiponectin concentrations of the entire cohort were grouped into two subgroups in a sex-specific manner so that each subject was classified as being under or above the mean of vaspin and adiponectin level among individuals of the same sex. A 2-sided probability level of P≤0.05 was taken as significant.

Results

Clinical and biochemical characteristics of subjects at baseline

A total of 148 T2DM patients and 193 non-diabetic controls were included in the baseline analysis. Decreased vaspin levels were found in T2DM group compared with non-diabetic control group ($P=0.025$). The P value was 0.041 after adjusting for the confounding factors including gender, age and BMI. The median (interquartile range) level of vaspin was 0.425 ng/mL (0.160,

0.917 ng/mL) in non-diabetic group, and 0.353 ng/mL (0.191, 0.664 ng/mL) in T2DM group. Higher adiponectin [median (interquartile range): 10.525 μg/ml (5.977, 15.550) vs. 7.310 μg/ml (4.034, 13.113), $P = 0.05$] was found in non-diabetic controls when compared with T2DM group. The P value was not significant after adjusting for the confounding factors including gender, age and BMI. The serum fasting insulin level was significantly higher in T2DM group than that in control group ($P < 0.05$). In females with or without diabetes, both the serum vaspin and adiponectin levels were significantly higher than those in males (all $P < 0.05$). Detailed baseline clinical characteristics of all subjects were presented in Table S1. In control group, compared with subjects with lower vaspin levels, those with higher vaspin levels had significantly higher WHR (0.87 ± 0.05 vs. 0.80 ± 0.02, $P = 0.025$) and lower percentage of smokers (7.2% vs. 22.0% $P = 0.003$). In T2DM group, significantly higher HDL-C (1.2 ± 0.4 vs. 1.1 ± 0.3, $P = 0.043$) and HOMA-IR (2.49 ± 1.76 vs. 1.86 ± 0.90, $P = 0.004$) were found in sub-group with higher vaspin levels (Table 1).

Correlations between vaspin and anthropometric and biochemical indices

Significant positive correlation between vaspin and HDL-C ($r = 0.23$, $P = 0.006$) was found in controls. In T2DM group, vaspin was significantly positively correlated with BMI ($r = 0.19$, $P = 0.028$), WHR ($r = 0.17$, $P = 0.035$) and HOMA-IR ($r = 0.14$, $P = 0.029$). All results of Pearson correlation analysis were shown in Table 2. In either control or T2DM group, vaspin level did not correlate with glycemic measurements including FPG, 2h-PG and HbA1c. Vaspin level did not correlate with adiponectin level in either group.

Results of the follow-up study

In this study, 170 non-diabetic subjects and 132 T2DM patients were followed up for 2 years. Compared with baseline characteristics, T2DM patients had significantly lower HbA1c, higher HDL and higher percentage of insulin treatment at follow-up (data not shown).

1) Occurrence of T2DM in control group

Among 170 subjects without T2DM at baseline, 11 developed T2DM during follow-up. 3 and 6 subjects were diagnosed with impaired glucose tolerance (IGT) and impaired fasting glucose

Table 1. Basic clinical characteristics of all subjects at baseline.

	Control group (193)			T2DM group (148)		
	Low vaspin (82)	High vaspin (111)	P value	Low vaspin (66)	High vaspin (82)	P value
Age (years)	62±12	59±12	0.287	62±12	64±10	0.218
Male, n (%)	58 (70.7%)	50 (45.0%)	<0.001	41 (62.1%)	26 (39.4%)	0.009
Smoking, n (%)	18 (22.0%)	8 (7.2%)	0.003	23 (34.8%)	27 (24.2%)	0.182
Hypertension, n (%)	40 (48.8)	49 (44.1%)	0.523	28 (42.4%)	39 (47.6%)	0.533
Obesity, n (%)	13 (15.9%)	15 (13.5%)	0.648	11(16.7%)	19(23.2%)	0.328
Dislipidemia, n (%)	12 (14.6%)	13 (11.7%)	0.550	13 (19.7%)	18 (22.0%)	0.738
Duration of T2DM	-	-		9.2±7.4	8.8±7.4	0.654
BMI (kg/m^2)	24.6±3.4	23.7±3.5	0.320	25.0±4.1	27.0±5.2	0.054
WHR	0.80±0.02	0.87±0.05	0.025	0.92±0.07	0.93±0.08	0.593
SBP (mmHg)	143±25	138±20	0.056	135±18	141±22	0.059
DBP (mmHg)	82±13	81±13	0.333	79±11	81±11	0.281
BUN (mmol/L)	5.79±1.75	6.24±3.55	0.310	5.9±2.1	6.3±2.8	0.348
Creatinine (μmol/L)	68.3±22.0	70.9±44.7	0.508	68.4±23.6	66.4±26.4	0.640
TC (mmol/L)	4.5±1.1	4.8±0.9	0.090	4.6±1.0	4.8±1.1	0.375
TG (mmol/L)	1.6±1.5	1.5±0.6	0.189	1.9±1.6	2.5±4.0	0.269
HDL C (mmol/L)	1.1±0.3	1.2±0.3	0.580	1.1±0.3	1.2±0.4	0.043
LDL-C (mmol/L)	2.6±0.8	2.8±0.7	0.331	2.7±0.8	2.7±0.8	0.661
FPG (mmol/L)	5.2±0.9	5.1±0.6	0.660	8.1±3.1	7.9±2.6	0.580
2h-PG (mmol/L)	6.6±3.0	6.9±1.9	0.659	13.5±4.8	13.7±4.5	0.791
HbA1c (%)	5.4±1.2	5.5±1.1	0.872	8.7±2.1	8.7±2.0	0.953
Fasting insulin (mIU/L)	7.7±5.1	7.8±4.1	0.960	8.8±9.2	11.5±14.2	0.287
HOMA-IR*	1.90±1.30	1.81±0.95	0.812	1.86±0.90	2.49±1.76	0.004
Vaspin (ng/mL)*	0.15±0.09	2.35±3.30		0.19±0.09	0.81±0.54	
Adiponectin (μg/ml)*	12.57±10.25	12.25±10.31	0.819	10.10±6.71	7.68±4.59	0.187

BMI: body mass index; WHR: waist-hip ratio; SBP: systolic blood pressure; DBP: diastolic blood pressure; BUN: blood urea nitrogen; TC: total cholesterol; TG: triglycerides; HDL-C: high-density lipoprotein cholesterol; LDL-C: low density lipoprotein-cholesterol; FPG: fasting plasma glucose; 2h-PG: 2-h postprandial plasma glucose; HbA1c: glycosylated haemoglobin A1c; HOMA-IR: homeostasis model assessment of insulin resistance;
*logarithmically transformed before analysis.

Table 2. Results of Pearson correlations of vaspin with clinical and biomedical indices at baseline.

	Control group		T2DM group	
	r value	P value	r value	P value
Age	−0.01	0.876	0.10	0.263
Duration of T2DM	-	-	0.03	0.709
BMI	−0.10	0.298	0.19	0.028
WHR	0.21	0.682	0.17	0.035
TC	0.06	0.451	−0.01	0.924
TG	−0.03	0.711	0.10	0.242
LDL-C	−0.04	0.599	−0.13	0.126
HDL-C	0.23	0.006	0.15	0.090
FPG (mmol/L)	−0.04	0.589	0.03	0.688
2h-PG (mmol/L)	−0.03	0.857	0.07	0.431
HbA1c (%)	0.05	0.733	0.01	0.940
Fasting insulin	0.11	0.460	0.01	0.930
HOMA-IR*	0.03	0.843	0.14	0.029
adiponectin	0.13	0.101	−0.13	0.420

BMI: body mass index; WHR: waist-hip ratio; TC: total cholesterol; TG: triglycerides; HDL-C: high-density lipoprotein cholesterol; LDL-C: low density lipoprotein-cholesterol; FPG: fasting plasma glucose; 2h-PG: 2-h postprandial plasma glucose; HbA1c: glycosylated haemoglobin A1c; HOMA-IR: homeostasis model assessment of insulin resistance;
*logarithmically transformed before analysis.

(IFG) respectively. As were shown in Figure 1, higher percentage of new onset of T2DM was found in sub-group with low vaspin levels than in sub-group with high vaspin levels (11.0% vs. 2.3%, $P=0.021$). Similarly, higher percentage of new onset of T2DM was also found in sub-group with low adiponectin levels, compared with sub-group with high adiponectin levels. However, the statistical analysis was not significant (8.4% vs. 4.6%, $P=0.309$). It was found that higher FPG and BMI, lower serum vaspin and adiponectin levels at baseline were independent risk factors for the occurrence of T2DM during 2.0-year follow-up. Results of multiple stepwise logistic regression analysis were shown in Table 3, and the values of odds ratio of vaspin and adiponectin were 0.52 (95% CI: 0.10–0.87, $P=0.015$) and 0.35 (95% CI: 0.20–0.72, $P=0.015$), respectively.

2) Glucose levels in control and T2DM groups

For sub-group with low vaspin levels in control group, significantly increased FPG, 2h-PG and HbA1c at follow-up were found when compared with those at baseline ($P≤0.05$). At follow-up, FPG (5.1±0.8 vs. 6.4±1.4, $P=0.016$), 2h-PG (7.2±0.9 vs. 8.4±1.2, $P=0.025$) and HbA1c (5.6±0.8 vs. 6.3±1.2, $P=0.039$) were all significantly lower in sub-group with high vaspin levels than those in sub-group with low vaspin levels. In T2DM group, HbA1c was significantly lowered in sub-groups with either low or high vaspin levels at follow-up than baseline (both $P=0.008$). There was no significant difference of the glycemic control between sub-groups with low and high vaspin levels at follow-up. (Results were shown in Figure 2).

3) Insulin treatment in T2DM group

As were shown in Table 4, among 132 T2DM patients, 67 patients were administrated with insulin at baseline and 27

additional patients who were insulin-native at baseline had been administrated with insulin during follow-up. At baseline, there was no significant difference of percentages of insulin-treated patients between sub-groups with low and high vaspin levels. At follow-up, higher percentage of insulin treatment in T2DM patients was found in sub-group with low vaspin level than sub-group with high vaspin level (55.3% vs. 44.7%, $P=0.020$). Compared with sub-group with low adiponectin level, sub-group with high adiponectin level had less patients receiving insulin treatment both at baseline (37.3% vs. 62.7%, $P=0.009$) and follow-up (42.6% vs. 57.4%, $P=0.027$).

Discussion

Vaspin is a novel adipocytokine that is supposed to have insulin sensitizing effects [10]. However, the real role of vaspin on glucose dysregulation in humans is not well understood. Our longitudinal study analyzed the independent roles of vaspin and adiponectin in the incidence of T2DM in non-diabetic subjects and long-time glycemic control in patients with T2DM. We herein present novel evidence that decreased baseline serum vaspin is an independent risk factor for subsequent occurrence of diabetes in non-diabetic subjects and higher percentage of insulin treatment in diabetic patients.

Although results of animal studies indicate that vaspin is an insulin-sensitizing adipocytokine, the real role of vaspin in human insulin resistance is still unclear [23,24]. A study performed in adolescents found that the serum vaspin concentration increased with worsening insulin resistance and was acutely down-regulated following glucose provocation in insulin-resistant adolescents [25]. In overweight women with polycystic ovarian syndrome, vaspin was found to be positively associated with BMI and WHR. Furthermore, the expression of vaspin in omental adipose tissue was reduced by metformin treatment in accordance with the decrease in insulin resistance [13]. In another study performed in the morbidly obese women, the vaspin mRNA expression was significantly higher in both subcutaneous and visceral adipose tissue than lean controls [26]. However, inconsistent results were also found in other studies. In Youn's study, no difference was found in circulating vaspin levels between individuals with normal glucose tolerance and T2DM. T2DM seems to abrogate the correlation between circulating vaspin, BMI, and insulin sensitivity [24]. In another cross-sectional study performed in normal volunteers, glucose tolerance status and insulin sensitivity measured using euglycemic hyperinsulinemic clamp and HOMA-IR were not found to be associated with serum vaspin levels [27]. In our study, obese diabetic patients had a tendency of having increased serum vaspin, and increased HOMA-IR was found in diabetic patients with higher vaspin levels. In the correlation analysis, we have observed a significant positive association of vaspin with HOMA-IR in diabetic group and HDL-C in control group, which was consistent with the results from some other studies [23,28]. The latter studies found that circulating vaspin level was positively correlated with HDL-C in healthy subjects and negatively correlated with detrimental lipid parameters (TC, TG and LDL-C) in pregnant women. Results from the present and previous studies suggest that vaspin plays a role in human insulin resistance and lipid metabolism [29]. Vaspin may be a compensatory molecule in the pathogenesis of insulin resistance and obesity associated diseases [30]. It can be postulated that vaspin, as a serine protease inhibitor, inhibits a protease which plays a role in the degradation of a hormone or molecule with direct or indirect glucose and lipid lowering effects [11,31]. In our study, lower vaspin levels were found in T2DM patients than those in control

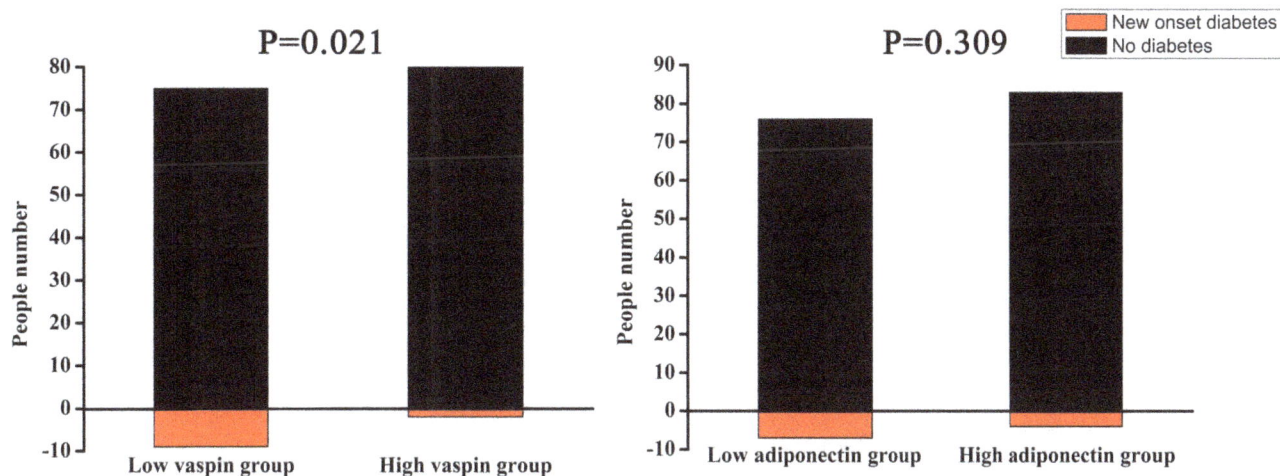

Figure 1. Percentages of new occurrences of T2DM in control subjects with low or high vaspin and adiponectin levels at follow-up. Red and black bars represent new onset diabetic patients and non-diabetic subjects in control group at follow-up, respectively χ² test was used to analyze the difference of percentage of new onset diabetic patients in sub-groups with low and high vaspin levels.

subjects. This result may be due to the long mean diabetes duration of our T2DM patients (10.5 years). The long diabetes duration and insulin treatment may affect the vaspin levels and thus induce the decrease of vaspin in our T2DM group than in non-diabetic group [10], [23].

Gulcelik's research found that serum vaspin levels in diabetic patients with chronic complications including neuropathy, retinopathy and nephropathy were lower than those without above complications [32]. Another study detected lower serum concentrations of vaspin in patients with carotid stenosis who experienced an ischemic event compared with asymptomatic patients [17]. The above results indicate that diabetic patients with lower vaspin levels may have poor outcomes and higher prevalence of micro- or macro-vascular complications during a long time. In our T2DM patients at follow-up, there were no significant associations between serum vaspin levels and glycemic controls. This result may be due to the confounding effects of drug administration during the follow-up. However, higher percentage of insulin administration at follow-up in diabetic patients was found in those with lower vaspin levels. In non-diabetic group, it was also found that lower vaspin level was associated with elevated glycemic levels and higher incidence of T2DM at follow-up. From above results, it could be speculated that low vaspin levels might be involved in poor glycemic control and other detrimental metabolic effects, and

thus play a role in development of chronic diabetic complications in T2DM patients.

In our study, it was found that adiponectin was an independent risk factor for new onset of T2DM in non-diabetic subjects at follow-up, which was accordant with some other studies [33,34]. Even though adiponectin and vaspin may both play beneficial roles in insulin resistance, the reported relationships between serum vaspin and adiponectin were controversial. In Giomisi's investigation, significant positive association between serum vaspin and adiponectin levels was detected in women of child-bearing age [28]. However, in a study performed in pubertal obese children and adolescents, vaspin levels were negatively correlated with adiponectin levels [35]. In another study performed in mice, it was found that increased expression of adiponectin was detected in high fat high sucrose chow ICR mice treated with vaspin [10]. In the correlation analysis of our study, the serum vaspin levels did not correlate with serum adiponectin levels. These results indicate that the relationship between serum adiponectin and vaspin levels can be affected by age, body weight and other metabolic status.

Several limitations should be considered before results interpretation. First, the control subjects were not normal people, but inpatients with hypertension or other mild cardiovascular diseases. This inclusion method can not exclude some confounding effects, including the effects of diseases itself and drugs treatment. However, people with high risk of T2DM constituted the control group, which might be partially responsible for the high occurrence of T2DM at follow-up and higher statistical power in small sample size. Second, the T2DM patients were not enrolled at the onset of the disease. The different duration of T2DM and different treatment in each patient may incorporate a possible source of selection bias. Third, the relatively small sample size in this study will decrease the statistical power, and further studies with larger sample size should be performed in the future to validate our results. Fourth, the relatively short follow-up period will weaken the effects of vaspin on glucose levels and chronic complications in T2DM group. Nevertheless, this cohort study provides support to the role of vaspin in glycemic control in non-diabetic people.

In conclusion, low circulating vaspin level, as well as adiponectin level can be used as risk factors for the progression

Table 3. Results of multiple stepwise logistic regression analysis for risk factors for new onset of T2DM in control group at follow-up.

	OR value	95% CI	P value
FPG	9.81	1.80–55.44	0.009
BMI	1.03	1.01–1.29	0.050
Adiponectin	0.35	0.20–0.72	0.015
Vaspin	0.52	0.10–0.87	0.015

FPG: fasting plasma glucose; BMI: body mass index.

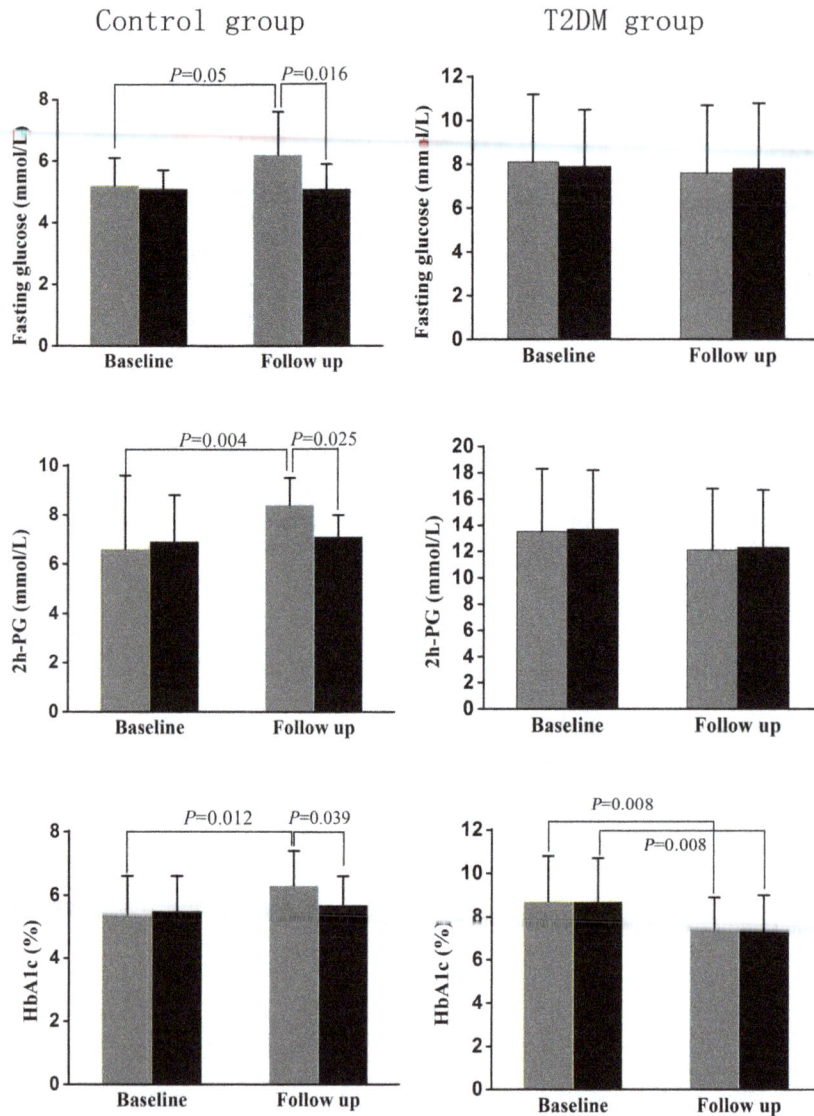

Figure 2. Glucose levels in groups with low and high serum vaspin concentrations. Gray and black bars represent diabetic patients with low and high vaspin levels, respectively. Fasting plasma glucose (FPG), 2-hour postprandial plasma glucose (2h-PG) and glycosylated haemoglobin A1c (HbA1c) were compared between those at baseline and follow-up in control and T2DM groups. Covariance analysis was used to analyze the differences between sub-groups.

Table 4. Medicine treatment in T2DM group with low or high vaspin and adiponectin levels at baseline and follow-up.

	Low vaspin	High vaspin	P value	Low adiponectin	High adiponectin	P value
Baseline hypoglycemic therapy						
One oral hypoglycemic agent	15 (41.7%)	21 (58.3%)		15 (40.5%)	21 (59.5%)	
Two or more oral hypoglycemic agents	16 (55.2%)	13 (44.8%)		9 (45.0%)	20 (55.0%)	
Insulin treatment	35 (52.2%)	32 (47.8%)	0.486	42 (62.7%)	25 (37.3%)	0.009
Follow-up						
One oral hypoglycemic agent	5 (22.7%)	17 (77.3%)		7 (31.8%)	15 (68.2%)	
Two or more oral hypoglycemic agents	9 (52.3%)	7 (47.7%)		5 (45.5%)	11 (54.5%)	0.027
Insulin treatment	52 (55.3%)	42 (44.7%)	0.020	54 (57.4%)	40 (42.6%)	

of T2DM. Further prospective observational studies are required to explain how a decrease in circulating vaspin level may be involved in the progression of T2DM.

Supporting Information

Table S1 Basic clinical characteristics of all subjects at baseline. Note: BMI: body mass index; WHR: waist-hip ratio; SBP: systolic blood pressure; DBP: diastolic blood pressure; BUN: blood urea nitrogen; TC: total cholesterol; TG: triglycerides; HDL-C: high-density lipoprotein cholesterol; LDL-C: low density lipoprotein-cholesterol; FPG: fasting plasma glucose; 2h-PG: 2-h postprandial plasma glucose; HbA1c: glycosylated haemoglobin A1c; HOMA-IR: homeostasis model assessment of insulin resistance;*logarithmically transformed before analysis. Adjusted

P values were from covariance analysis by adjusting for age, sex and BMI.

Acknowledgments

We are very grateful to all volunteers who participated in this study.

Author Contributions

Conceived and designed the experiments: QS WJ. Performed the experiments: WP WJ. Analyzed the data: SX YD LQ JJ. Contributed reagents/materials/analysis tools: HL SX YD LQ JJ. Wrote the paper: QS WJ.

References

1. Kershaw EE, Flier JS (2004) Adipose tissue as an endocrine organ. J Clin Endocrinol Metab 89: 2548–2556.
2. Cnop M, Havel PJ, Utzschneider KM, Carr DB, Sinha MK, et al. (2003) Relationship of adiponectin to body fat distribution, insulin sensitivity and plasma lipoproteins: evidence for independent roles of age and sex. Diabetologia 46: 459–469.
3. Kazumi T, Kawaguchi A, Sakai K, Hirano T, Yoshino G (2002) Young men with high-normal blood pressure have lower serum adiponectin, smaller LDL size, and higher elevated heart rate than those with optimal blood pressure. Diabetes Care 25: 971–976.
4. Matsubara M, Maruoka S, Katayose S (2002) Decreased plasma adiponectin concentrations in women with dyslipidemia. J Clin Endocrinol Metab 87: 2764–2769.
5. Spranger J, Kroke A, Mohlig M, Bergmann MM, Ristow M, et al. (2003) Adiponectin and protection against type 2 diabetes mellitus. Lancet 361: 226–228.
6. Lindsay RS, Funahashi T, Hanson RL, Matsuzawa Y, Tanaka S, et al. (2002) Adiponectin and development of type 2 diabetes in the Pima Indian population. Lancet 360: 57–58.
7. Berg AH, Combs TP, Du X, Brownlee M, Scherer PE (2001) The adipocyte-secreted protein Acrp30 enhances hepatic insulin action. Nat Med 7: 947–953.
8. Fruebis J, Tsao TS, Javorschi S, Ebbets-Reed D, Erickson MR, et al. (2001) Proteolytic cleavage product of 30-kDa adipocyte complement-related protein increases fatty acid oxidation in muscle and causes weight loss in mice. Proc Natl Acad Sci U S A 98: 2005–2010.
9. Yamauchi T, Kamon J, Waki H, Terauchi Y, Kubota N, et al. (2001) The fat-derived hormone adiponectin reverses insulin resistance associated with both lipoatrophy and obesity. Nat Med 7: 941–946.
10. Hida K, Wada J, Eguchi J, Zhang H, Baba M, et al. (2005) Visceral adipose tissue-derived serine protease inhibitor: a unique insulin-sensitizing adipocytokine in obesity. Proc Natl Acad Sci U S A 102: 10610–10615.
11. Kloting N, Kovacs P, Kern M, Heiker JT, Fasshauer M, et al. (2011) Central vaspin administration acutely reduces food intake and has sustained blood glucose-lowering effects. Diabetologia 54: 1819–1823.
12. Kloting N, Berndt J, Kralisch S, Kovacs P, Fasshauer M, et al. (2006) Vaspin gene expression in human adipose tissue: association with obesity and type 2 diabetes. Biochem Biophys Res Commun 339: 430–436.
13. Tan BK, Heutling D, Chen J, Farhatullah S, Adya R, et al. (2008) Metformin decreases the adipokine vaspin in overweight women with polycystic ovary syndrome concomitant with improvement in insulin sensitivity and a decrease in insulin resistance. Diabetes 57: 1501–1507.
14. Aktas B, Yilmaz Y, Eren F, Yonal O, Kurt R, et al. (2011) Serum levels of vaspin, obestatin, and apelin-36 in patients with nonalcoholic fatty liver disease. Metabolism 60: 544–549.
15. Cakal E, Ustun Y, Engin-Ustun Y, Ozkaya M, Kilinc M (2011) Serum vaspin and C-reactive protein levels in women with polycystic ovaries and polycystic ovary syndrome. Gynecol Endocrinol 27: 491–495.
16. Choi SH, Kwak SH, Lee Y, Moon MK, Lim S, et al. (2011) Plasma vaspin concentrations are elevated in metabolic syndrome in men and are correlated with coronary atherosclerosis in women. Clin Endocrinol (Oxf) 75: 628–635.
17. Aust G, Richter O, Rohm S, Kerner C, Hauss J, et al. (2009) Vaspin serum concentrations in patients with carotid stenosis. Atherosclerosis 204: 262–266.
18. Grimaldi A, Heurtier A (1999) Diagnostic criteria for type 2 diabetes. Rev Prat 49: 16–21.

19. Mills GW, Avery PJ, McCarthy MI, Hattersley AT, Levy JC, et al. (2004) Heritability estimates for beta cell function and features of the insulin resistance syndrome in UK families with an increased susceptibility to type 2 diabetes. Diabetologia 47: 732–738.
20. Ling Li H, Hui Peng W, Tao Cui S, Lei H, Dong Wei Y, et al. (2011) Vaspin plasma concentrations and mRNA expressions in patients with stable and unstable angina pectoris. Clin Chem Lab Med 49: 1547–1554.
21. Teshigawara S, Wada J, Hida K, Nakatsuka A, Eguchi J, et al. (2012) Serum vaspin concentrations are closely related to insulin resistance, and rs77060950 at SERPINA12 genetically defines distinct group with higher serum levels in Japanese population. J Clin Endocrinol Metab 97: E1202–1207.
22. Xu A, Chan KW, Hoo RL, Wang Y, Tan KC, et al. (2005) Testosterone selectively reduces the high molecular weight form of adiponectin by inhibiting its secretion from adipocytes. J Biol Chem 280: 18073–18080.
23. Seeger J, Ziegelmeier M, Bachmann A, Lossner U, Kratzsch J, et al. (2008) Serum levels of the adipokine vaspin in relation to metabolic and renal parameters. J Clin Endocrinol Metab 93: 247–251.
24. Youn BS, Kloting N, Kratzsch J, Lee N, Park JW, et al. (2008) Serum vaspin concentrations in human obesity and type 2 diabetes. Diabetes 57: 372–377.
25. Korner A, Neef M, Friebe D, Erbs S, Kratzsch J, et al. (2011) Vaspin is related to gender, puberty and deteriorating insulin sensitivity in children. Int J Obes (Lond) 35: 578–586.
26. Auguet T, Quintero Y, Riesco D, Morancho B, Terra X, et al. (2011) New adipokines vaspin and omentin. Circulating levels and gene expression in adipose tissue from morbidly obese women. BMC Med Genet 12: 60.
27. von Loeffelholz C, Mohlig M, Arafat AM, Isken F, Spranger J, et al. (2010) Circulating vaspin is unrelated to insulin sensitivity in a cohort of nondiabetic humans. Eur J Endocrinol 162: 507–513.
28. Giomisi A, Kourtis A, Toulis KA, Anastasilakis AD, Makedou KG, et al. (2011) Serum vaspin levels in normal pregnancy in comparison with non-pregnant women. Eur J Endocrinol 164: 579–583.
29. Genc H, Dogru T, Tapan S, Kara M, Ercin CN, et al. (2011) Circulating vaspin and its relationship with insulin sensitivity, adiponectin, and liver histology in subjects with non-alcoholic steatohepatitis. Scand J Gastroenterol 46: 1355–1361.
30. Wada J (2008) Vaspin: a novel serpin with insulin-sensitizing effects. Expert Opin Investig Drugs 17: 327–333.
31. Shaker OG, Sadik NA (2013) Vaspin gene in rat adipose tissue: relation to obesity-induced insulin resistance. Mol Cell Biochem 373: 229–239.
32. Gulcelik NE, Karakaya J, Gedik A, Usman A, Gurlek A (2009) Serum vaspin levels in type 2 diabetic women in relation to microvascular complications. Eur J Endocrinol 160: 65–70.
33. Fagerberg B, Kellis D, Bergstrom G, Behre CJ (2011) Adiponectin in relation to insulin sensitivity and insulin secretion in the development of type 2 diabetes: a prospective study in 64-year-old women. J Intern Med 269: 636–643.
34. Li Y, Yatsuya H, Iso H, Toyoshima H, Tamakoshi K (2012) Inverse relationship of serum adiponectin concentration with type 2 diabetes mellitus incidence in middle-aged Japanese workers: six-year follow-up. Diabetes Metab Res Rev 28: 349–356.
35. Suleymanoglu S, Tascilar E, Pirgon O, Tapan S, Meral C, et al. (2009) Vaspin and its correlation with insulin sensitivity indices in obese children. Diabetes Res Clin Pract 84: 325–328.

23

Whole-Body and Hepatic Insulin Resistance in Obese Children

Lorena del Rocío Ibarra-Reynoso, Liudmila Pisarchyk, Elva Leticia Pérez-Luque, Ma. Eugenia Garay-Sevilla*, Juan Manuel Malacara

Department of Medical Sciences, University of Guanajuato, Campus León, 20 de Enero 929, León Guanajuato, México

Abstract

Background: Insulin resistance may be assessed as whole body or hepatic.

Objective: To study factors associated with both types of insulin resistance.

Methods: Cross-sectional study of 182 obese children. Somatometric measurements were registered, and the following three adiposity indexes were compared: BMI, waist-to-height ratio and visceral adiposity. Whole-body insulin resistance was evaluated using HOMA-IR, with 2.5 as the cut-off point. Hepatic insulin resistance was considered for IGFBP-1 level quartiles 1 to 3 ($<$6.67 ng/ml). We determined metabolite and hormone levels and performed a liver ultrasound.

Results: The majority, 73.1%, of obese children had whole-body insulin resistance and hepatic insulin resistance, while 7% did not have either type. HOMA-IR was negatively associated with IGFBP-1 and positively associated with BMI, triglycerides, leptin and mother's BMI. Girls had increased HOMA-IR. IGFBP-1 was negatively associated with waist-to-height ratio, age, leptin, HOMA-IR and IGF-I. We did not find HOMA-IR or IGFBP-1 associated with fatty liver.

Conclusion: In school-aged children, BMI is the best metric to predict whole-body insulin resistance, and waist-to-height ratio is the best predictor of hepatic insulin resistance, indicating that central obesity is important for hepatic insulin resistance. The reciprocal negative association of IGFBP-1 and HOMA-IR may represent a strong interaction of the physiological processes of both whole-body and hepatic insulin resistance.

Editor: Rasheed Ahmad, Dasman Diabetes Institute, Kuwait

Funding: This work was supported by CONACYT GTO-2010-C02-145281 and in part by CONACYT grant CB 2007 – 84277. The funders had no role in study design, data collection and analysis, decision to publish, or preparation of the manuscript.

Competing Interests: The authors have declared that no competing interests exist.

* Email: marugaray_2000@yahoo.com

Introduction

Insulin resistance (IR) is an important metabolic alteration that is frequently associated with obesity and appears to be the primary mediator of metabolic syndrome [1]. IR and persistent hyperinsulinemia are found in a variety of other medical conditions, such as dyslipidemia and hypertension, mainly in obese children as early as 3 to 5 years of age [2].

IR is mediated by genetic and acquired pathophysiological factors. At early stages, IR appears to affect various molecular pathways, predominantly inflammation, at the cellular level in muscle, adipocytes, and endothelial cells [3]. Counter-regulatory hormone alteration is another factor involved in IR; in rodents, glucagon suppresses hepatic glucose production through activity regulated at the mediobasal hypothalamus through the vagus nerve [4].

IR has been considered to be either whole body or central (hepatic). The periphery IR consists of impaired glucose uptake and consumption mainly in muscle and fat and is measured by Homeostatic Model Assessment-IR (HOMA-IR) [5]. Hepatic IR

results in unrestrained liver glucose production [6]. The following heterogeneous signaling pathways participate in this process: liver cytohesin is required for insulin signaling and its inhibition by SecinH3 [7]; activation of NOTCH receptors results in lipolysis [8] and hepatic glucose production [9]; the target of rapamycin complex (TORC2) pathway also modulates glucose expenditure [10]; and sterol regulatory element-binding protein-1 (SREBP-1) mediates insulin's effect on fatty acid synthesis [11]. In a parallel process, saturated and unsaturated fats lead to hepatic accumulation of diacylglycerols, activation of protein kinase Cε (PKCε), and impairment of insulin-stimulated insulin receptor substrate 2 (IRS-2) signaling [12]. An important recently identified factor for hepatic IR is high glucose or fructose intake [13].

Insulin-like growth factor binding protein-1 (IGFBP-1) is secreted in the liver under insulin regulation and has been proposed as a specific marker of hepatic IR [14,15] and as a convenient and sensitive marker for hepatic IR in children [16].

Obesity is frequently associated with the development of non-alcoholic fatty liver disease (NAFLD) [17] and is a major factor in the pathogenesis of type 2 diabetes [18]. However, the association of NAFLD with hepatic or whole-body IR is not well defined.

In this work, we studied the factors associated with whole-body and hepatic IR as assessed by IGFBP-1 blood levels in obese children and the potential relationship with ultrasonographic assessment of NAFLD. For better estimation of the association between children's obesity and IR, we compared obesity metrics such as body mass index (BMI), visceral adiposity index (VAI), and waist-to-height ratio.

Materials and Methods

Between August 2011 and April 2012, we recruited 182 obese children, six to eleven years old, from grammar schools in the city of León in central Mexico, which is representative of the population of our region. The study group included children with BMI higher than the equivalent of 30 kg/m^2 for an adult after adjusting for gender and age according to the International Tables reported by Cole et al. [19]. The selected children did not have clinical evidence of hypothyroidism, chronic infections, or congenital or metabolic diseases.

Ethics Statement

The nature and purpose of the study was explained to the children and their parents. If both the children and parents or tutor accepted, the parents signed an informed consent form; confidentiality of individual results was guaranteed. The study was approved by the Ethics Committee of the Department of Medical Research. University of Guanajuato (CEDCM-2009-9).

Data collection

Data were collected by direct questioning of the children and at least one of their parents. We collected the family history of obesity and diabetes as well as the mother's BMI. Children's sleep duration and exercise levels were also recorded. Acanthosis nigricans was registered as a score from 0 to 4.

Weight and standing height were obtained with indoor clothing and without shoes using a roman-type scale and a Harpenden stadiometer in order to calculate the BMI. Waist girth was measured with indoor clothes using a non-extendible flexible tape at the midpoint of the last rib and the iliac crest. Waist-to-height ratio and VAI were calculated. The VAI formula was as follows: for boys = (waist girth/39.68+(1.88×BMI)) ×(triglycerides/1.03) × (1.31/HDL-cholesterol) and for girls = (waist girth/36.58+ (1.89×BMI)) ×(triglycerides/0.81) × (1.52/HDL-cholesterol) [20]. Skin fold thickness was obtained at bicipital, tricipital, suprailiac and subscapular sites to calculate body density as follows: for boys = 1.1533-(0.0643× log $\sum$ (4 measurements of skin fold thickness)) and for girls = 1.1369-(0.0598× log $\sum$ (4 measurements)) [21,22]. The percent body fat [23] was calculated as {4.95/body density - 4.5} ×100.

A venous blood sample was obtained after twelve hours of fasting to measure hormone and metabolite levels. Glucose, triglycerides, and cholesterol were measured by conventional methods. Insulin, leptin and adiponectin were measured by radioimmunoassay using a Millipore kit (St. Charles, Mo) with intra- and interassay variation coefficients of 4.4% and 6.0% for insulin, 3.4% and 3.6% for leptin, and 6.2% and 9.2% for adiponectin. Insulin-like growth factor I (IGF-I) and IGFBP-1 were measured by ELISA (Mediagnost, Reutlingen, Germany) with intra- and interassay variation coefficients of 5.1% and 6.8% for IGF-I and 6.2% and 7.4% for IGFBP-1.

Liver ultrasound

The presence of a fatty liver was assessed by ultrasound, which is considered an appropriate and practical method [24]. The procedure was carried out by an experienced physician radiologist using a General Electric Logic 400 MD Doppler Color with a convex transducer of 3.6 MHz. The results were assessed by two experienced radiologist and classified into the following four groups by the extent of liver steatosis: negative, slight, moderate and severe, according to Mittelstaedt [25].

Statistical Analysis

Data are shown as the means and standard deviations (SD). Whole-body IR was evaluated with HOMA-IR, taking 2.5 as the cut-off point as proposed for prepubertal children [26]. Considering that a low level of IGFBP-1 has been proposed to be a marker of hepatic IR [14], we took the 3rd quartile of IGFBP-1 as the cut-off point for hepatic IR. Groups with and without IR were compared by means of a two-tailed Student's t-test for independent samples or the Mann-Whitney U test when non-parametric data were obtained. The Chi-square test was used to analyze fatty liver and acanthosis nigricans scores.

We compared the groups of insulin resistance and **NAFLD groups** by ANOVA.

Factors associated with HOMA-IR and IGFBP-1 were analyzed by a generalized linear model with stepwise elimination of non-significant variables. Using the HOMA-IR results as the dependent variable, we tested the following candidate regressors: individual estimators of obesity (BMI, waist-to-height ratio, and VAI, successively), age, sex, fatty liver score, leptin, IGF-I, IGFBP-1, total cholesterol, triglycerides, adiponectin, sleep duration and mother's BMI. Using IGFBP-1 as the dependent variable, we tested the following candidate regressors: estimators of obesity, age, sex, leptin, adiponectin, HOMA, IGF-I, total cholesterol, triglycerides, mother's BMI, fatty liver score and hours of sleep. Statistica 7.0 for Windows (Statsoft, Tucson AZ) was used for the analyses. P<0.05 was considered significant.

Results

The 182 obese children had a mean age of 9.2±1.4 years, BMI 27.2±3.6, waist girth 89.0±11.5 cm, waist-to-height ratio 0.6±0.1, VAI 1.2±0.7, and percent body fat 38.3±2.8%. In regard to pubertal activation, only 7 girls from 10- to 11-year-old exhibited pubertal activation. HOMA-IR was 5.3±2.3, leptin 27.4±12.7 ng/ml, glucose 4.74±0.59 mmol/L, insulin 25.2±10.0 µIU/ml, IGF-I 26.9±14.2 nmol/L, and adiponectin 15.5±8.1 ng/ml. Overall, 18.4% of the children had at least one parent with a diagnosis of Type 2 Diabetes Mellitus (Type2 DM). A total of 167 (91.8%) obese children had HOMA-IR values higher than 2.5 and were therefore considered to have whole-body IR. IGFBP-1 was measured in 171 children with a mean value of 5.1±4.4 ng/ml. Among these children, 128 were considered to have hepatic IR (74.8%).

Comparison of groups with and without whole-body IR

As shown in table 1, subjects without whole-body IR (8.2%) were younger and had lower BMI, waist-to-height ratio, VAI, percent total body fat, triglycerides and leptin levels but increased IGFBP-1 levels. When comparing children with high HOMA-IR vs low HOMA-IR were found marginal differences for acanthosis nigricans, but unexpectedly there was no difference for fatty liver.

Table 1. Characteristics of the obese children with or without whole body IR (HOMA-IR cut off point 2.5).

	High HOMA-IR	Low HOMA-IR	t value	P value
	Mean±SD	Mean±SD		
	N = 167	N = 15		
Age, years	9.26±1.34	8.10±1.09	3.23	<0.002
BMI, kg/m²	27.44±3.58	24.28±2.62	3.33	<0.001
waist-to-height ratio	0.64±0.07	0.60±0.04	2.18	<0.03
VAI	1.30±0.75	0.69±0.31	3.16	<0.002
Percent body fat	38.61±2.70	35.17±2.20	4.80	<0.000003
Triglycerides, mmol/L	1.52±0.63	1.08±0.42	2.66	<0.009
Total cholesterol, mmol/L	3.95±0.74	3.96±0.77	−0.07	0.95
HDL cholesterol, mmol/L	1.06±0.24	1.15±0.22	−1.34	0.18
Leptin, ng/ml	28.19±12.80	18.00±6.04	3.05	<0.003
IGF-I, nmol/L	22.23±14.74	23.37±5.27	1.01	0.31
IGFBP-1, ng/ml	4.62±3.99	10.08±5.17	−4.93	<0.000002
Adiponectin, ng/ml	15.18±7.91	18.51±8.53	−1.50	0.13
Sleep, hours/day	9.16±1.01	9.47±1.14	−1.10	0.27
Exercise, min/week	222.88±225.53	263.33±217.18	−0.67	0.51
Mother's BMI	32.41±6.36	29.58±5.29	1.55	0.12
	N (%)	N (%)	Chi-square	p value
Without fatty liver	77 (57.46%)	8 (57.14%)	1.1	0.78
Slight	36 (26.87%)	5 (35.71%)		
Moderate	17 (12.69%)	1 (7.14%)		
Severe	4 (2.99%)	0 (0%)		
Without acantosis nigricans	45 (31.03%)	9 (75%)	9.74	<0.04
Grade 1	55 (37.93%)	2 (16.67%)		
Grade 2	28 (19.31%)	1 (8.33%)		
Grade 3	4(2.76%)	0 (0%)		
Grade 4	13(8.97)	0 (0%)		

Characteristics of obese children with or without whole-body IR (HOMA-IR cut off point 2.5). Body mass index (BMI), visceral adiposity index (VAI), insulin-like growth factor binding protein-1 (IGFBP-1), insulin-like growth factor I (IGF-I).

Comparison of groups with low and high IGFBP-1 values

The circulating levels of IGFBP-1 had a median of 4.33 ng/ml, lower quartile of 2.0 ng/ml and upper quartile of 6.67 ng/ml. We considered subjects with an IGFBP-1 value lower than 6.67 ng/ml as having hepatic IR. The comparison of children with low and high IGFBP-1 levels is shown in table 2. Similar to the group with high HOMA-IR, children with hepatic IR were older and had higher BMI, VAI, percent body fat and leptin. In contrast to the different triglyceride levels seen in the high vs low HOMA-IR groups, triglyceride levels were similar in children with and without hepatic IR. Children with hepatic IR had higher leptin, IGF-I and insulin levels and lower adiponectin and reduced sleep duration. Fatty liver and acanthosis nigricans were not associated with IGFBP-1 levels.

Factors associated with HOMA-IR

The generalized linear model tested three indices of adiposity and showed positive associations with mother's BMI, children's BMI, triglycerides and leptin levels and a negative association with IGFBP-1 levels. After testing for gender as a confounding variable, male gender was negatively associated with HOMA-IR levels in the total group (Table 3).

Factors associated with IGFBP-1 serum levels

The generalized linear model tested three indices of adiposity and showed negative associations with waist-to-height ratio, age, leptin, HOMA-IR and IGF-I levels (Table 4).

The triglyceride level was not independently associated with IGFBP-1; however, after repeating the analysis with HOMA-IR excluded, an association with triglycerides appeared (p<0.004).

Comparison of groups with high or low HOMA-IR and IGFBP-1

One hundred twenty-five children (73.1%) had high HOMA-IR and low IGFBP-1, interpreted as indicating whole-body insulin resistance and hepatic IR. Low HOMA-IR and high IGFBP-1 was found in 12 children (7.0%), consistent with the absence of both whole-body IR and hepatic IR. High HOMA-IR and high IGFBP-1, indicative of whole-body IR, was found in 31 children (18.1%). Three children (1.8%) had low HOMA-IR and low IGFBP-1, indicating only hepatic IR.

We compared these groups by ANOVA. The group without any form of IR were significantly younger (F = 7.11, p<0.0002) and had lower BMI (F = 5.74, p<0.0001), waist girth (F = 6.84, p<0.00002), VAI (F = 4.96, p<0.002), leptin (F = 5.82, p<0.003),

Table 2. Characteristics of the obese children with or without hepatic IR (IGFBP-1 cut off point 6.67 ng/ml).

	With Hepatic IR (three lowest quartiles) Mean±SD N = 128	Without Hepatic IR (highest quartile) Mean±SD N = 43	t value	P value
Age, years	9.34±1.26	8.37±1.35	4.24	<0.00004
BMI, kg/m²	27.51±3.41	25.48±3.15	3.40	<0.0008
Waist-to-height ratio	0.64±0.07	0.63±0.05	0.52	0.60
VAI	1.30±0.71	0.94±0.49	3.00	<0.003
Percent body fat	38.71±2.61	36.89±2.88	3.86	<0.0002
Glucose, mmol/L	4.75±0.60	4.65±0.53	0.95	0.34
Triglycerides, mmol/L	1.51±0.62	1.34±0.55	1.61	0.11
Total cholesterol, mmol/L	3.97±0.72	3.94±0.75	0.25	0.80
HDL cholesterol, mmol/L	1.07±0.24	1.08±0.25	−0.32	0.75
Leptin, ng/ml	29.24±13.22	21.28±8.63	3.69	<0.0003
Insulin, µIU/ml	27.27±9.21	17.74±8.09	6.05	<0.0000001
IGF-I, nmol/L	27.73±13.01	21.09±10.87	3.01	<0.003
Adiponectin, ng/ml	14.82±7.78	17.98±7.55	−2.31	<0.02
Sleep, hours/day	9.02±0.91	9.72±1.17	−4.06	<0.00007
Exercise, min/week	216.75±221.24	258.60±240.44	−1.05	0.3
Mother's BMI	32.39±6.63	31.29±5.65	0.83	0.41
	N (%)	N (%)	Chi-square	P value
Without fatty liver	57 (55.34%)	23 (62.16%)	1.11	0.77
Slight	28 (27.18%)	10 (27.03%)		
Moderate	15 (14.56%)	3 (8.11%)		
Severe	3 (2.91%)	1 (2.7%)		
Without acantosis nigricans	34 (30.36%)	19 (52.78%)	8.31	0.08
Grade 1	42 (37.50%)	8 (22.22%)		
Grade 2	24 (21.43%)	5 (13.89%)		
Grade 3	8 (7.14%)	4 (11.11%)		
Grade 4	4 (3.57%)	0 (0%)		

Characteristics of obese children with or without hepatic IR (IGFBP-1 cut off point 6.67 ng/ml). body mass index (BMI), visceral adiposity index (VAI), insulin-like growth factor binding protein-1 (IGFBP-1), insulin-like growth factor I (IGF-I).

compared with the group with both types of IR. The group without any type IR had lower waist girth (F = 6.84, p<0.04) than the group with only hepatic-IR. Additionally, the group without any type of IR had lower BMI (F = 5.74; p<0.02) and waist girth (F = 6.84, p<0.003), than the group with only whole-body IR. The group with only whole-body IR was younger (F = 7.11, p<0.002) and had lower VAI (F = 4.96, p<0.04), leptin (F = 5.82, p<0.005) and IGF-I levels (F = 3.42, p<0.002) than the group with both types of IR. (Table S1).

Comparison of NAFLD groups

We carried out a liver ultrasound in a total of 148 children and found that 85 did not have fatty liver, 41 had slight, 18 had moderate and four had severe fatty liver. Comparing the characteristics of these groups, we found that in children without fatty liver, had lower age (F = 3.49, p<0.02), BMI (F = 6.49, p< 0.0004), waist girth (F = 2.92, p<0.04) and leptin levels (F = 5.56, p<0.001). We did not find differences among the groups in terms of HOMA-IR, IGFBP-1, waist-to-height ratio, VAI, triglycerides, total cholesterol, HDL cholesterol and adiponectin. (Table S2).

Discussion

In this work, we compared whole-body and hepatic IR. The evaluation of hepatic IR was based on IGFBP-1 levels. There are currently no criteria for a cut-off point to discriminate between the different extents of low IGFBP-1 levels and diagnose hepatic IR. Intuitively, we proposed that at least three quarters of obese children have hepatic IR, so the upper quartile was considered not to have hepatic IR. These results should support further work to define a more appropriate cut-off point for hepatic IR diagnosis using IGFBP-1 levels.

IR is a metabolic disorder associated with metabolic syndrome [27]. The hormone and metabolic profile of our group of obese children is similar to those described in other reports [28]. Overall, 73.1% had whole-body and hepatic IR and only 7% had normal HOMA-IR and IGFBP-1 values, representing the expected profile for metabolically healthy subjects [29].

In univariate analysis, children without whole-body or hepatic IR were younger, as reported in a previous work [30]; this may indicate that the benign metabolic profile is transient and therefore

Table 3. Factors associated with HOMA-IR.

		Estimate±SD	Wald	P value
Testing the inclusion of waist-to-height ratio				
Triglycerides, mmol/L		0.002±0.0005	10.38	<0.001
Leptin, ng/ml		0.006±0.003	5.97	<0.01
IGFBP-1, ng/ml		−0.06±0.01	32.6	<0.0000001
Mother's BMI		0.01±0.004	12.08	<0.0005
Testing the inclusion of BMI				
BMI, kg/m²		0.02±0.008	7.96	<0.005
Triglycerides, mmol/L		0.001±0.0005	6.81	<0.009
IGFBP-1, ng/ml		−0.05±0.01	22.87	<0.000002
Mother's BMI		0.01±0.005	9.97	<0.002
Sex	boys	−0.07±0.03	4.59	<0.03
Testing the inclusion of VAI				
Triglycerides, mmol/L		0.002±0.0005	10.38	<0.001
Leptin, ng/ml		0.006±0.003	5.97	<0.01
IGFBP-1, ng/ml		−0.06±0.01	32.6	<0.0000001
Mother's BMI		0.01±0.004	12.08	<0.0005

Factors associated with HOMA-IR were analyzed by means of the generalized linear model, testing three different types of adiposity index. Body mass index (BMI), visceral adiposity index (VAI), insulin-like growth factor binding protein-1 (IGFBP-1).

more prevalent in younger children. Prospective studies are necessary to define the stability of insulin sensitivity.

In an attempt to understand the significance of hepatic IR, we compared factors associated with HOMA-IR and IGFBP-1. A reciprocal negative association of IGFBP 1 and HOMA-IR has also been reported in studies in children [31] and adults [32]. This represents the strong interaction between both physiopathological processes.

Other than the reciprocal association between both types of IR, leptin was the only factor associated with both whole-body IR and hepatic IR. The role of leptin in IR is a controversial subject. In our work, we found leptin was more strongly associated with hepatic IR. German et al. proposed that leptin improves hepatic sensitivity to insulin by means of hypothalamic signaling, an effect blocked by selective hepatic vagotomy [33]. Moreover, central leptin signaling stimulates fatty acid oxidation in white adipose

Table 4. Factors associated with IGFBP-1.

	Estimate±SD	Wald	p
Testing the inclusion of waist-to-height ratio			
Waist-to-height ratio	−2.15±0.88	5.92	<0.01
Age, years	−0.13±0.03	15.38	<0.00009
Leptin, ng/ml	−0.02±0.005	14.72	<0.0001
HOMA-IR	−0.15±0.025	34.82	<0.0000001
IGF-I, nmol/L	−0.004±0.0008	24.64	<0.000001
Testing the inclusion of BMI			
Age, years	−0.15±0.03	20.01	<0.0000001
Leptin, ng/ml	−0.02±0.005	17.26	<0.00003
HOMA-IR	−0.15±0.03	36.10	<0.0000001
IGF-I, nmol/L	−0.004±0.0008	20.59	<0.000006
Testing the inclusion of VAI			
Age, years	−0.15±0.03	20.01	<0.0000001
Leptin, ng/ml	−0.02±0.005	17.26	<0.00003
HOMA-IR	−0.15±0.03	36.10	<0.0000001
IGF-I, nmol/L	−0.004±0.0008	20.59	<0.000006

Factors associated with IGFBP-1 analyzed by means of the generalized linear model, testing three different types of adiposity index. Body mass index (BMI), visceral adiposity index (VAI), insulin-like growth factor binding protein-1 (IGFBP-1), insulin-like growth factor I (IGF-I).

tissue [34] thus controlling lipogenesis [35]. This effect has been implicated in the ability of leptin to improve peripheral insulin sensitivity by its actions in the hypothalamus. The association of leptin with HOMA-IR was marginal; some other studies also showed an association [36], but other reports in obese adults and adolescents did not find an association [37].

Another important factor related to IR is triglyceride levels, which were associated with HOMA-IR but not IGFBP-1. However, in the analysis of IGFBP-1, removal of HOMA-IR from the model permitted the association with triglycerides to emerge. This means that hypertriglyceridemia has a stronger association with whole-body IR than hepatic IR. One factor contributing to hypertriglyceridemia is the inability of insulin to inhibit the release of VLDL from the liver [38]. The contribution to hypertriglyceridemia by *de novo* fatty acid synthesis in other tissues such as fat, muscle and intestines requires peripheral IR [39]. Genetic factors also affect hypertriglyceridemia. The PNPLA3 I148M variant may determine triglyceride profiles independent of obesity, supporting the idea that the I148M variant hampers intrahepatocellular lipolysis rather than stimulates triglyceride synthesis [40].

Another explanation for the lack of association of serum triglyceride levels with hepatic IR is that Notch 1 activity increases the intracellular abundance of triglycerides without an effect on serum lipids or VLDL secretion [41].

We found a strong association of whole-body IR with the mother's BMI, as previously reported, and interpreted this association to mean that inheritance, as well as shared family environment and lifestyle, are important determinants of child adiposity [42].

In regard to gender, girls had higher HOMA-IR values, as reported in other studies [43]. The possible influence of pubertal activation could not be analyzed because only seven girls showed stage 2 thelarche.

We found a negative association of IGFBP-1 with IGF-I, probably as a result of the dynamics of hormone receptor interaction, but this process may also result from the proteolysis of IGFBP-1 [44].

In the univariate analysis, the group with hepatic IR reported fewer hours of sleep. A previous report showed an association between short sleep duration and increased BMI and adverse metabolic outcomes in school children [45] but not with actual obesity at adolescence [46]. Rehman et al. [47] found higher IGFBP-1 levels with increased sleep, irrespective of sleep timing, although sleeping during the day resulted in higher levels of IGFBP-1. Appropriate sleep preservation may be an important strategy to promote healthy metabolic conditions.

As expected, acanthosis nigricans was associated with HOMA-IR. This finding is in accordance with previous studies [48] This alteration may result from the interaction of increased insulin levels with IGF-1, triggering the proliferation of keratinocytes and fibroblasts [49].

NAFLD is associated with obesity. Overall, 42.6% of the children had ultrasonographic images showing a fatty liver. IR is considered an essential pathophysiological factor in the development of NAFLD [50]. Unexpectedly, in our study HOMA-IR was not associated with fatty liver. In agreement with this, a recent study reported that HOMA-IR was not independently associated with fatty liver in obese adolescents [51]. Furthermore, it has been suggested that steatosis is dissociated from insulin resistance in the I148M variant of PNPLA3 [52]. Therefore, we suggest that the direct association of fatty liver with HOMA-IR needs further investigation.

Previous studies showed that children with NAFLD have elevated leptin levels [53]. In our work, the analysis of variance showed higher leptin levels in children with fatty liver. We found that age associated with fatty liver. Kitajama et al. reported age associated with the severity of NAFLD in adults [54]. Waist girth was also associated with fatty liver as previously reported [55].

In this work, we also tested the interaction of three indices of adiposity with insulin resistance and associated factors. There is no agreement on the most appropriate estimator of obesity for metabolic evaluation in children. In adults, VAI is reported to be a good estimator of IR [56]. However, in children VAI seems to be inferior to BMI in terms of association with IR [57]. Some reports indicate that waist-to-height ratio is a sensitive marker of IR in children [58], but others indicate that this index is not superior to BMI in predicting metabolic or cardiovascular risk [59]. Our results are in agreement with the proposal that BMI is the best measure of adiposity associated with HOMA-IR in school children.

In the regression analysis, the waist-to-height ratio was the only index associated with IGFBP-1 levels. Previously, waist girdle was reported to be associated with low IGFBP-1 [60].

In summary, we found that 73.1% of obese children had whole-body and hepatic IR, indicating a strong interaction of these two physiopathological processes. These children were older than those without any type of IR. In regard to indices of adiposity, we found that BMI best predicts whole-body IR. In contrast, waist-to-height ratio seems to be the best index to predict hepatic IR, indicating that central obesity is critical for this condition. Leptin was the only factor associated with both whole-body and hepatic IR, but the significance of the association with hepatic IR was stronger. Triglyceride levels were related independently to whole-body IR. The mother's BMI was a predictor of children's HOMA-IR, showing the influence of genetic or early environment influences. IGF-I levels was another determinant of IGFBP-1. We did not find an independent association of fatty liver with IR in children.

Author Contributions

Conceived and designed the experiments: LRIR LP ELPL MEGS JMM. Performed the experiments: LRIR LP ELPL MEGS JMM. Analyzed the data: LRIR JMM. Contributed reagents/materials/analysis tools: LRIR LP ELPL MEGS JMM. Wrote the paper: LRIR LP ELPL MEGS JMM. Obtained grant for the study: MEGS JMM.

References

1. Yin J, Li M, Xu L, Wang Y, Cheng H, et al. (2013) Insulin resistance determined by Homeostasis Model Assessment (HOMA) and associations with metabolic syndrome among Chinese children and teenagers. Diabetol Metab Syndr 5: 71.

2. Bocca G, Ongering EC, Stolk RP, Sauer PJ (2013) Insulin resistance and cardiovascular risk factors in 3- to 5-year-old overweight or obese children. Horm Res Paediatr 80: 201–206.

3. Bornfeldt KE, Tabas I (2011) Insulin Resistance, Hyperglycemia, and Atherosclerosis. Cell Metab 14: 575–585.

4. Mighiu PI, Yue JT, Filippi BM, Abraham MA, Chari M, et al. (2013) Hypothalamic glucagon signaling inhibits hepatic glucose production. Nat Med 19: 766–772.

5. Pastucha D, Filipčíková R, Horáková D, Radová L, Marinov Z, et al. (2013) The incidence of metabolic syndrome in obese Czech children: the importance of early detection of insulin resistance using homeostatic indexes HOMA-IR and QUICKI. Physiol Res 62: 277–283.

6. Qureshi K, Clements RH, Saeed F, Abrams GA (2010) Comparative evaluation of whole body and hepatic insulin resistance using indices from oral glucose

tolerance test in morbidly obese subjects with nonalcoholic fatty liver disease. J Obes 2010: 1–7.

7. Hafner M, Schmitz A, Grüne I, Srivatsan SG, Paul B, et al. (2006) Inhibition of cytohesins by SecinH3 leads to hepatic insulin resistance. Nature 444: 941–944.

8. Pajvani UB, Qiang L, Kangsamaksin T, Kitajewski J, Ginsberg HN, et al. (2013) Inhibition of Notch uncouples Akt activation from hepatic lipid accumulation by decreasing mTorc1 stability. Nat Med 19: 1054–1060.

9. Pajvani UB, Shawber CJ, Samuel VT, Birkenfeld AL, Shulman GI, et al. (2011) Inhibition of Notch signaling ameliorates insulin resistance in a FoxO1-dependent manner. Nat Med 17: 961–967.

10. Koo SH, Flechner L, Qi L, Zhang X, Screaton RA, et al. (2005) The CREB coactivator TORC2 is a key regulator of fasting glucose metabolism. Nature 437: 1109–1111.

11. Fajas L, Schoonjans K, Gelman L, Kim JB, Najib J, et al. (1999) Regulation of peroxisome proliferator-activated receptor gamma expression by adipocyte differentiation and determination factor 1/sterol regulatory element binding protein 1: implications for adipocyte differentiation and metabolism. Mol Cell Biol 19: 5495–5503.

12. Galbo T, Perry RJ, Jurczak MJ, Camporez JP, Alves TC, et al. (2013) Saturated and unsaturated fat induce hepatic insulin resistance independently of TLR-4 signaling and ceramide synthesis in vivo. Proc Natl Acad Sci 110: 12780–12785.

13. Lecoultre V, Egli L, Carrel G, Theytaz F, Kreis R, et al. (2013) Effects of fructose and glucose overfeeding on hepatic insulin sensitivity and intrahepatic lipids in healthy humans. Obesity (Silver Spring) 21: 782–785.

14. Kotronen A, Lewitt M, Hall K, Brismar K, Yki-Järvinen H (2008) Insulin-like growth factor binding protein 1 as a novel specific marker of hepatic insulin sensitivity. J Clin Endocrinol Metab 93: 4867–4872.

15. Borai A, Livingstone C, Heald AH, Oyindamola Y, Ferns G (2013) Delta insulin-like growth factor binding protein-1 (ΔIGFBP-1): a marker of hepatic insulin resistance? Ann Clin Biochem 51: 269–276.

16. Motaghedi R, Gujral S, Sinha S, Sison C, Ten S, et al. (2007) Insulin-like growth factor binding protein-1 to screen for insulin resistance in children. Diabetes Technol Ther 9: 43–51.

17. Koo SH (2013) Nonalcoholic fatty liver disease: molecular mechanisms for the hepatic steatosis. Clin Mol Hepatol 19: 210–215.

18. Galbo T, Shulman GI (2013) Lipid-induced hepatic insulin resistance. Aging 5: 582, 583.

19. Cole TJ, Bellizzi MC, Flegal KM, Dietz WH (2000) Establishing a standard definition for child overweight and obesity worldwide: international survey. BMJ 320: 1240–1243.

20. Amato MC, Giordano C, Galia M, Criscimanna A, Vitabile S, et al. (2010) Visceral Adiposity Index: a reliable indicator of visceral fat function associated with cardiometabolic risk. Diabetes Care 33: 920–922.

21. Edwards DA, Hammond WH, Healy MJ, Tanner JM, Whitehouse RH (1955). Design and accuracy of calipers for measuring subcutaneous tissue thickness. Br J Nutr. 9: 133–43.

22. Durnin JV, Rahaman MM (1967) The assessment of the amount of fat in the human body from measurements of skinfold thickness. Br J Nutr 21(3): 681–9.

23. Brook CGD (1971) Determination of body composition of children from skinfold measurement. Archiv of Dis child 46: 182–184.

24. Saadeh S, Younossi ZM, Remer EM, Gramlich T, Ong JP, et al. (2002) Utility of radiological imaging in nonalcoholic fatty liver disease. Gastroenterology 123: 745–750.

25. Mittelstaedt CA (1992) General ultrasound, 1st edn. New York: Churchill Livingstone.

26. Madeira IR, Carvalho CN, Gazolla FM, de Matos HJ, Borges MA, et al. (2008) Cut-off point for Homeostatic Model Assessment for Insulin Resistance (HOMA-IR) index established from Receiver Operating Characteristic (ROC) curve in the detection of metabolic syndrome in overweight pre-pubertal children. Arq Bras Endocrinol Metabol 52: 1466–1473.

27. Turchiano M, Sweat V, Fierman A, Convit A (2012) Obesity, metabolic syndrome, and insulin resistance in urban high school students of minority race/ethnicity. Arch Pediatr Adolesc Med 166: 1030–1036.

28. Makkes S, Renders CM, Bosmans JE, van der Baan-Slootweg OH, Seidell JC (2013) Cardiometabolic risk factors and quality of life in severely obese children and adolescents in The Netherlands. BMC Pediatr 13: 62.

29. Vukovic R, Mitrovic K, Milenkovic T, Todorovic S, Soldatovic I, et al. (2013) Insulin-sensitive obese children display a favorable metabolic profile. Eur J Pediatr 172: 201–206.

30. Gayoso-Diz P, Otero-González A, Rodriguez-Alvarez MX, Gude F, García F, et al. (2013) Insulin resistance (HOMA-IR) cut-off values and the metabolic syndrome in a general adult population: effect of gender and age: EPIRCE cross-sectional study. BMC Endocr Disord 13: 47.

31. Street ME, Smerieri A, Montanini L, Predieri B, Iughetti L, et al. (2013) Interactions among pro-inflammatory cytokines, IGF system and thyroid function in pre-pubertal obese subjects. J Biol Regul Homeost Agents 27: 259–266.

32. Gokulakrishnan K, Velmurugan K, Ganesan S, Mohan V (2012) Circulating levels of insulin-like growth binding protein-1 in relation to insulin resistance, type 2 diabetes mellitus, and metabolic syndrome (Chennai Urban Rural Epidemiology Study 118). Metabolism 61: 43–46.

33. German J, Kim F, Schwartz GJ, Havel PJ, Rhodes CJ, et al. (2009) Hypothalamic leptin signaling regulates hepatic insulin sensitivity via a neurocircuit involving the vagus nerve. Endocrinology 150: 4502–4511.

34. Plum L, Rother E, Münzberg H, Wunderlich FT, Morgan DA, et al. (2007) Enhanced leptin-stimulated Pi3k activation in the CNS promotes white adipose tissue transdifferentiation. Cell Metab 6: 431–445.

35. Buettner C, Muse ED, Cheng A, Chen L, Scherer T, et al. (2008) Leptin controls adipose tissue lipogenesis via central, STAT3- independent mechanisms. Nat Med 14: 667–675.

36. Atwa M, Emara A, Balata M, Youssef N, Bayoumy N, et al. (2013) Serum leptin, adiponectin, and resistin among adult patients with acanthosis nigricans: correlations with insulin resistance and risk factors for cardiovascular disease. Int J Dermatol. doi: 10.1111/ijd.12340.

37. Aguilar MJ, González-Jiménez E, Antelo A, Perona JS (2013) Insulin resistance and inflammation markers: correlations in obese adolescents. J Clin Nurs 22: 2002–2010.

38. Malmström R, Packard CJ, Caslake M, Bedford D, Stewart P, et al. (1997) Defective regulation of triglyceride metabolism by insulin in the liver in NIDDM. Diabetologia 40: 454–462.

39. Zammit VA (2013) Hepatic triacylglycerol synthesis and secretion: DGAT2 as the link between glycaemia and triglyceridaemia. Biochem J 451: 1–12.

40. Hyysalo J, Gopalacharyulu P, Bian H, Hyötyläinen T, Leivonen M, et al. (2014) Circulating triacylglycerol signatures in nonalcoholic fatty liver disease associated with the I148M variant in PNPLA3 and with obesity. Diabetes 63: 312–322.

41. Czech MP (2013) Obesity Notches up fatty liver. Nat Med 19: 969–971.

42. Veena SR, Krishnaveni GV, Karat SC, Osmond C, Fall CH (2013) Testing the fetal overnutrition hypothesis; the relationship of maternal and paternal adiposity to adiposity, insulin resistance and cardiovascular risk factors in Indian children. Public Health Nutr 16: 1656–66.

43. Bugge A, El-Naaman B, McMurray RG, Froberg K, Nielsen CH, et al. (2012) Sex differences in the association between level of childhood interleukin-6 and insulin resistance in adolescence. Exp Diabetes Res 2012: 859186.

44. Kreitschmann-Andermahr I, Suarez P, Jennings R, Evers N, Brabant G (2010) GH/IGF-I Regulation in Obesity – Mechanisms and Practical Consequences in Children and Adults. Horm Res Paediatr 73: 153–160.

45. Seegers V, Petit D, Falissard B, Vitaro F, Tremblay RE, et al. (2011) Short sleep duration and body mass index: a prospective longitudinal study in preadolescence. Am J Epidemiol 173: 621–629.

46. Lytle LA, Pasch KE, Farbakhsh K (2011) The relationship between sleep and weight in a sample of adolescents. Obesity 19: 324–331.

47. Rehman JU, Brismar K, Holmbäck U, Akerstedt T, Axelsson J (2010) Sleeping during the day: effects on the 24-h patterns of IGF-binding protein 1, insulin, glucose, cortisol, and growth hormone. Eur J Endocrinol 163: 383–390.

48. Kluczynik CE, Mariz LS, Souza LC, Solano GB, Albuquerque FC, et al. (2012) Acanthosis nigricans and insulin resistance in overweight children and adolescents. An Bras Dermatol 87: 531–537.

49. Barbato MT, Criado PR, Silva AK, Averbeck E, Guerine MB, et al. (2012) Association of acanthosis nigricans and skin tags with insulin resistance. An Bras Dermatol 87: 97–104.

50. Pirgon Ö, Bilgin H, Çekmez F, Kurku H, Dündar BN (2013) Association between insulin resistance and oxidative stress parameters in obese adolescents with non-alcoholic fatty liver disease. J Clin Res Pediatr Endocrinol 5: 33–39.

51. Sayın O, Tokgöz Y, Arslan N (2014) Investigation of adropin and leptin levels in pediatric obesity-related nonalcoholic fatty liver disease. J Pediatr Endocrinol Metab 27: 1–6.

52. Amaro A, Fabbrini E, Kars M, Yue P, Schechtman K, et al. (2010) Dissociation between intrahepatic triglyceride content and insulin resistance in familial hypobetalipoproteinemia. Gastroenterology 139: 149–153.

53. Boyraz M, Çekmez F, Karaoglu A, Cinaz P, Durak M, et al. (2013) Serum adiponectin, leptin, resistin and RBP4 levels in obese and metabolic syndrome children with nonalcoholic fatty liver disease. Biomark Med 7: 737–745.

54. Kitajima Y, Hyogo H, Sumida Y, Eguchi Y, Ono N, et al. (2013) Severity of non-alcoholic steatohepatitis is associated with substitution of adipose tissue in skeletal muscle. J Gastroenterol Hepatol 28: 1507–1514.

55. Monteiro PA, de Moura Mello Antunes B, Silveira LS, Christofaro DG, Fernandes RA, et al. (2014) Body composition variables as predictors of NAFLD by ultrasound in obese children and adolescents. BMC Pediatr 14: 25.

56. Stepien M, Stepien A, Wlazel RN, Paradowski M, Rizzo M, et al. (2014) Predictors of insulin resistance in patients with obesity: a pilot study. Angiology 65: 22–30.

57. Al-Daghri NM, Al-Attas OS, Alokail M, Alkharfy K, Wani K, et al. (2014) Does Visceral Adiposity Index signify early metabolic risk in children and adolescents? Association with insulin resistance, adipokines and subclinical inflammation. Pediatr Res 75: 459–463.

Permissions

All chapters in this book were first published in PLOS ONE, by The Public Library of Science; hereby published with permission under the Creative Commons Attribution License or equivalent. Every chapter published in this book has been scrutinized by our experts. Their significance has been extensively debated. The topics covered herein carry significant findings which will fuel the growth of the discipline. They may even be implemented as practical applications or may be referred to as a beginning point for another development.

The contributors of this book come from diverse backgrounds, making this book a truly international effort. This book will bring forth new frontiers with its revolutionizing research information and detailed analysis of the nascent developments around the world.

We would like to thank all the contributing authors for lending their expertise to make the book truly unique. They have played a crucial role in the development of this book. Without their invaluable contributions this book wouldn't have been possible. They have made vital efforts to compile up to date information on the varied aspects of this subject to make this book a valuable addition to the collection of many professionals and students.

This book was conceptualized with the vision of imparting up-to-date information and advanced data in this field. To ensure the same, a matchless editorial board was set up. Every individual on the board went through rigorous rounds of assessment to prove their worth. After which they invested a large part of their time researching and compiling the most relevant data for our readers.

The editorial board has been involved in producing this book since its inception. They have spent rigorous hours researching and exploring the diverse topics which have resulted in the successful publishing of this book. They have passed on their knowledge of decades through this book. To expedite this challenging task, the publisher supported the team at every step. A small team of assistant editors was also appointed to further simplify the editing procedure and attain best results for the readers.

Apart from the editorial board, the designing team has also invested a significant amount of their time in understanding the subject and creating the most relevant covers. They scrutinized every image to scout for the most suitable representation of the subject and create an appropriate cover for the book.

The publishing team has been an ardent support to the editorial, designing and production team. Their endless efforts to recruit the best for this project, has resulted in the accomplishment of this book. They are a veteran in the field of academics and their pool of knowledge is as vast as their experience in printing. Their expertise and guidance has proved useful at every step. Their uncompromising quality standards have made this book an exceptional effort. Their encouragement from time to time has been an inspiration for everyone.

The publisher and the editorial board hope that this book will prove to be a valuable piece of knowledge for researchers, students, practitioners and scholars across the globe.

List of Contributors

Martin Pal, Claudia M. Wunderlich, Gabriele Spohn and F. Thomas Wunderlich
Max Planck Institute for Neurological Research, Institute for Genetics, University of Cologne and Cologne Excellence Cluster on Cellular Stress Responses in Aging-Associated Diseases (CECAD) and Center of Molecular Medicine Cologne (CMMC), Cologne, Germany

Hella S. Brönneke
Mouse Phenotyping Core Facility of Cologne Excellence Cluster on Cellular Stress Responses in Aging-Associated Diseases (CECAD), Cologne, Germany

Marc Schmidt-Supprian
Molecular Immunology and Signaltransduction, Max Planck Institute for Biochemistry, Munich, Germany

Xue-Qin Hao
Department of Pharmacy, College of Animal Science and Technology, Henan University of Science and Technology, Luoyang, PR China

Jing-Xia Du and Yan Li
Department of pharmacology, Medical College, Henan University of Science and Technology, Luoyang, PR China,

Meng Li
Luoyang Entry-Exit Inspection and Quarantine Bureau, Luoyang, PR China

Shou-Yan Zhang
Department of Cardiology, Luoyang Central Hospital Affiliated to Zhengzhou University, Luoyang, PR China

Eric Vounsia Balti
Diabetes Research Center, Faculty of Medicine and Pharmacy, Brussels Free University, Brussels, Belgium
National Obesity Center, Yaoundé Central Hospital and Faculty of Medicine and Biomedical Sciences, University of Yaoundé 1, Yaoundé, Cameroon

Jean Valentin Fogha Fokouo
National Obesity Center, Yaoundé Central Hospital and Faculty of Medicine and Biomedical Sciences, University of Yaoundé 1, Yaoundé, Cameroon

André Pascal Kengne
National Obesity Center, Yaoundé Central Hospital and Faculty of Medicine and Biomedical Sciences, University of Yaoundé 1, Yaoundé, Cameroon

NCRP for Cardiovascular and Metabolic Diseases, South African Medical Research Council and University of Cape Town, Cape Town, South Africa

Brice Enid Nouthé
National Obesity Center, Yaoundé Central Hospital and Faculty of Medicine and Biomedical Sciences, University of Yaoundé 1, Yaoundé, Cameroon
Department of Medicine, McGill University, Montreal, Quebec, Canada

Eugene Sobngwi
National Obesity Center, Yaoundé Central Hospital and Faculty of Medicine and Biomedical Sciences, University of Yaoundé 1, Yaoundé, Cameroon
Institute of Health and Society, Newcastle University, Newcastle, United Kingdom

Jung Eun Kim, Mi Hwa Lee, Deok Hwa Nam, Hye Kyoung Song, Young Sun Kang, Jin Joo Cha and Dae Ryong Cha
Department of Internal Medicine, Division of Nephrology, Korea University, Ansan City, Kyungki-Do, Korea

Ji Eun Lee and Hyun Wook Kim
Department of Internal Medicine, Division of Nephrology, Wonkwang University, Gunpo City, Kyungki-Do, Korea

Young Youl Hyun
Department of Internal Medicine, Division of Nephrology, Sungkyunkwan University, Seoul, Korea

Sang Youb Han and Kum Hyun Han
Department of Internal Medicine, Division of Nephrology, Inje University, Goyang City, Kyungki-Do, Korea

Jee Young Han
Department of Pathology, Inha University, Incheon City, Kyungki-Do, Korea

Sue Kim, Duk-Chul Lee and Ji-Won Lee
Department of Family Medicine, Severance Hospital, Yonsei University College of Medicine, Seoul, Korea

Ji-Young Kim and Justin Y. Jeon
Department of Sport and Leisure Studies, Yonsei University, Seoul, Korea

Hye-Sun Lee
Biostatistics Collaboration Units, Department of Research Affairs, Yonsei University College of Medicine, Seoul, Korea

Heather Kirk-Ballard, Gail Kilroy and Z. Elizabeth Floyd
Ubiquitin Biology Laboratory, Pennington Biomedical Research Center, Baton Rouge, Louisiana, United States of America

Priyanka Acharya
Ubiquitin Biology Laboratory, Pennington Biomedical Research Center, Baton Rouge, Louisiana, United States of America
Diabetes and Nutrition Laboratory, Pennington Biomedical Research Center, Baton Rouge, Louisiana, United States of America

Zhong Q. Wang, Xian H. Zhang, Yongmei Yu and William T. Cefalu
Diabetes and Nutrition Laboratory, Pennington Biomedical Research Center, Baton Rouge, Louisiana, United States of America

David Ribnicky
Department of Plant Biology and Pathology, Rutgers University, New Brunswick, New Jersey, United States of America

Haiyan Sun, Yifei Wang, Rui Liu and Yongde Peng
Department of Endocrinology, Shanghai First People's Hospital, Shanghai Jiao Tong University, Shanghai, China

Nengguang Fan
Department of Endocrinology, Shanghai First People's Hospital, Shanghai Jiao Tong University, Shanghai, China
Department of Endocrinology, Shanghai Songjiang Center Hospital, Shanghai, China

Lijuan Zhang and Zhenhua Xia
Department of Endocrinology, Shanghai Songjiang Center Hospital, Shanghai, China

Liang Peng, Yanqiang Hou and Weiqin Shen
Department of Laboratory Medicine, Shanghai Songjiang Center Hospital, Shanghai, China

Maarten Hulsmans, Benjamine Geeraert and Paul Holvoet
Atherosclerosis and Metabolism Unit, Department of Cardiovascular Sciences, KU Leuven, Leuven, Belgium

Thierry Arnould
Laboratory of Biochemistry and Cell Biology (URBC), NAmur Research Institute for LIfe Sciences (NARILIS), University of Namur (FUNDP), Namur, Belgium

Christos Tsatsanis
Department of Clinical Chemistry, School of Medicine, University of Crete, Heraklion, Greece

Lin-Huang Huang
Institute of Traditional Medicine, School of Medicine, National Yang-Ming University, Taipei, Taiwan,

Chia-Yu Liu, I-Ju Chen, Jung-Peng Chiu and Chung-Hua Hsu
Institute of Traditional Medicine, School of Medicine, National Yang-Ming University, Taipei, Taiwan
Department of Chinese Medicine, Branch of Linsen and Chinese Medicine, Taipei City Hospital, Taipei, Taiwan

Chien-Jung Huang
Department of Metabolism, Branch of Linsen and Chinese Medicine, Taipei City Hospital, Taipei, Taiwan

Neus Pueyo, Francisco J. Ortega, José M. Moreno-Navarrete, Monica Sabater, Wifredo Ricart and José M. Fernández-Real
Service of Diabetes, Endocrinology and Nutrition (UDEN), Institut d'Investigació Biomédica de Girona (IdIBGi), CIBER de la Fisiopatología de la Obesidad y la Nutrición (CIBERobn, CB06/03/0010) and Instituto de Salud Carlos III (ISCIII), Girona, Spain

Josep M. Mercader and Sílvia Bonàs
Joint IRB-BSC Program on Computational Biology, Barcelona Supercomputing Center, Barcelona, Spain

David Torrents
Joint IRB-BSC Program on Computational Biology, Barcelona Supercomputing Center, Barcelona, Spain
Institucio´ Catalana de Recerca i Estudis Avanc¸ats (ICREA), Barcelona, Spain

Patricia Botas and Elías Delgado
Hospital Central de Asturias, Oviedo, Spain

María T. Martinez-Larrad and Manuel Serrano-Ríos
Department of Internal Medicine II, Hospital Clínico San Carlos, CIBER de Diabetes y Enfermedades Metaboó licas Asociadas (CIBERDEM), Madrid, Spain

Yue Shen
Graduate School of Peking Union Medicine College, Beijing, People's Republic of China
Department of Epidemiology, Capital Institute of Pediatrics, Beijing, People's Republic of China

Lijun Wu, Xiaoyuan Zhao, Hong Cheng, Dongqing Hou and Jie Mi
Department of Epidemiology, Capital Institute of Pediatrics, Beijing, People's Republic of China

Bo Xi
Institute of Maternal and Child Health Care, School of Public Health, Shandong University, Shandong, People's Republic of China

Xin Liu and Xingyu Wang
Laboratory of Human Genetics, Beijing Hypertension League Institute, Beijing, People's Republic of China

Yun Gao, Attit Baskota, Tao Chen, Xingwu Ran and Haoming Tian
Department of Endocrinology and Metabolism, West China Hospital of Sichuan University, Sichuan, P. R. China

Fan Yang and Tianpeng Zheng
Department of Endocrinology and Metabolism, West China Hospital of Sichuan University, Sichuan, P. R. China
Department of Endocrinology and Metabolism, Affiliated Hospital of Guilin Medical University, Guangxi, P. R. China

Francilene B. Madeira
Physical Education Undergraduate Course, State University of Piauí, Teresina, Brazil

Antônio A. Silva and Helma F. Veloso
Department of Public Health, Federal University of Maranhão, São Luís, Brazil

Marcelo Z. Goldani
Department of Pediatrics and Puericulture, Faculty of Medicine, Federal University of Rio Grande do Sul, Porto Alegre, Brazil

Gilberto Kac
Department of Social and Applied Nutrition, Josué de Castro Nutrition Institute, Federal University of Rio de Janeiro, Rio de Janeiro, Brazil

Viviane C. Cardoso, Heloisa Bettiol and Marco A. Barbieri
Department of Puericulture and Pediatrics, Faculty of Medicine of Ribeirão Preto, University of São Paulo, Ribeirão Preto, Brazil

Linn Gillberg and Stine Jacobsen
Department of Endocrinology, Rigshospitalet, Copenhagen, Denmark
Steno Diabetes Center, Gentofte, Denmark

Allan Vaag
Department of Endocrinology, Rigshospitalet, Copenhagen, Denmark
Steno Diabetes Center, Gentofte, Denmark
Faculty of Health Sciences, University of Copenhagen, Copenhagen, Denmark

Trine W. Boesgaard
Steno Diabetes Center, Gentofte, Denmark
Hagedorn Research Institute, Gentofte, Denmark

Rasmus Ribel-Madsen and Anette Prior Gjesing
Section of Metabolic Genetics, The Novo Nordisk Foundation Center for Basic Metabolic Research, Faculty of Health Sciences, University of Copenhagen, Copenhagen, Denmark

Oluf Pedersen
Section of Metabolic Genetics, The Novo Nordisk Foundation Center for Basic Metabolic Research, Faculty of Health Sciences, University of Copenhagen, Copenhagen, Denmark
Hagedorn Research Institute, Gentofte, Denmark
Faculty of Health Sciences, University of Aarhus, Aarhus, Denmark

Torben Hansen
Section of Metabolic Genetics, The Novo Nordisk Foundation Center for Basic Metabolic Research, Faculty of Health Sciences, University of Copenhagen, Copenhagen, Denmark
Faculty of Health Sciences, University of Southern Denmark, Odense, Denmark

Charlotte Ling
Department of Clinical Sciences, Lund University, Malmoe, Sweden

Hong-Jun Ba, Hong-Shan Chen*, Zhe Su, Min-Lian Du, Qiu-Li Chen, Yan-Hong Li and Hua-Mei Ma
Pediatric Department, The First Affiliated Hospital, Sun Yat-sen University, Guangzhou, Guangdong Province, China

Manju Mamtani, Hemant Kulkarni, Thomas D. Dyer, Laura Almasy, Michael C. Mahaney, Ravindranath Duggirala, Anthony G. Comuzzie, John Blangero and Joanne E. Curran
Department of Genetics, Texas Biomedical Research Institute, San Antonio, Texas, United States of America

Christian H. C. A. Henning, Nana Zarnekow, Johannes Hedtrich and Sascha Stark
Institute of Agricultural Economics, University of Kiel, Kiel, Germany

Kathrin Türk and Matthias Laudes
Department of Internal Medicine 1, University of Kiel, Kiel, Germany

Jin-A Seo, Sang-Wook Song, Kyung-Jin Lee and Ha-Na Kim
Department of Family medicine, St. Vincent's Hospital, College of Medicine, The Catholic University of Korea, Seoul, Korea

Kyungdo Han
Department of Biostatistics, College of Medicine, The Catholic University of Korea, Seoul, Korea; Department of Preventive Medicine, College of Medicine, The Catholic University of Korea, Seoul, Korea

Xiuqing Wei and Bilun Ke
Department of Digestive Disease, Third Affiliated Hospital, Sun Yet-Sen University, Guangzhou, China Antioxidant and Gene Regulation Laboratory, Pennington Biomedical Research Center, Louisiana State University System, Baton Rouge, Louisiana, United States of America

Zhiyun Zhao, Xin Ye, Zhanguo Gao and Jianping Ye
Antioxidant and Gene Regulation Laboratory, Pennington Biomedical Research Center, Louisiana State University System, Baton Rouge, Louisiana, United States of America

Mia Jüllig and Martin Middleditch
Maurice Wilkins Centre for Molecular Biodiscovery, University of Auckland, Auckland, New Zealand School of Biological Sciences, University of Auckland, Auckland, New Zealand

Shelley Yip and Rinki Murphy
Department of Medicine, University of Auckland, Auckland, New Zealand

Aimin Xu
Department of Medicine, Department of Pharmacology and Pharmacy, The University of Hong Kong, Hong Kong, Special Administrative Region, China

Greg Smith
Department of Pharmacology, University of New South Wales, Sydney, New South Wales, Australia

Michael Booth
Department of Surgery, North Shore Hospital, Auckland, New Zealand

Richard Babor
Department of Surgery, Middlemore Hospital, Auckland, New Zealand

Grant Beban
Department of Surgery, Auckland City Hospital, Auckland, New Zealand

Yi-Chieh Li and Chang-Chi Hsieh
Department of Animal Science and Biotechnology, Tunghai University, Taichung, Taiwan

Weixia Jian, Jie Jin, Li Qin, Yan Dong and Qing Su
Department of Endocrinology, Xinhua Hospital, Shanghai Jiaotong University School of Medicine, Shanghai, China

Wenhui Peng and Hailing Li
Department of Cardiology, Shanghai Tenth People's Hospital, Tongji University School of Medicine, Shanghai, China

Sumei Xiao
Department of Medicine, Faculty of Medicine, The University of Hong Kong, Pokfulam, Hong Kong

Lorena del Rocío Ibarra-Reynoso, Liudmila Pisarchyk, Elva Leticia Pérez-Luque, Ma. Eugenia Garay-Sevilla and Juan Manuel Malacara
Department of Medical Sciences, University of Guanajuato, Campus León, 20 de Enero 929, León Guanajuato, México

Index

A

Adipokines, 42, 58, 65-67, 104, 128, 132, 135, 161, 180, 182, 187, 195, 202

Adiponectin, 29-32, 38-39, 42, 45, 58, 68-72, 74-81, 84-87, 110, 128, 132, 134, 141, 174, 180-181, 183, 185-186, 188-195, 197-199, 202

Adipose Tissue, 1, 11-12, 19, 29, 31, 34, 36-46, 50, 58-61, 63-73, 77-78, 96, 104, 108, 124-125, 127-128, 132, 135, 141, 161, 165, 174, 178, 186, 189, 192, 195, 202

Anthropometric Indexes, 136-139, 141

Apelin-12, 128-130, 132-134

Apolipoprotein A1, 80, 84-85

Aspartate Aminotransferase, 14-15, 17-19

Atherosclerosis, 27-29, 37, 68-70, 76-80, 87, 96, 112-113, 117-119, 142, 149, 160, 178, 195, 202

Atrogin-1, 46-57

B

Beta-cell, 19, 44, 57, 87, 109, 119, 127, 142, 160, 188

Bone Marrow-derived Macrophages, 68, 72, 75

C

Cardiorespiratory Fitness, 40-42, 44-45

Celastrol, 29-39

Chemokines, 29, 37, 39, 104, 182

Cjun N-terminal Kinase, 1

Creatinine, 16-18, 29-32, 38, 81, 84-85, 90, 106, 153, 160, 191

Cytokine Signaling 3, 58

D

Dexamethasone, 47, 49, 51, 59

Diastolic Blood Pressures, 24

Dyslipidemia, 14, 21, 29, 41-42, 68-69, 75, 80, 86-87, 96, 103, 105, 128, 134, 142, 152, 187, 195-196

E

Ectopic Fat, 42, 44

Epicatechin, 80, 82

Epididymal Fat, 5, 31, 36, 38

Epigallocatechin Gallate, 80, 82, 87

F

Fasting Plasma Glucose, 22, 29-32, 44-45, 57, 82, 87, 89, 103, 106, 115, 119, 123, 127-130, 132-133, 153, 160, 188, 190-195

Fenofibrate, 39, 68-79

Fetuin-a, 109, 171-172, 174-176, 178

G

Gastric Bypass, 169, 178

Glucagon-like Peptide 1, 80-81, 87, 188

Glucocorticoids, 129, 135

Glucokinase Regulator Protein, 98

Glucose Homeostasis, 1-2, 5-9, 14, 88, 96, 98, 179, 186

Glucose Phosphorylation, 100

H

Heparin-binding Growth Factor, 58, 67

Hepatoma Cell Line, 162-164

High-density Lipoproteins, 22

Hormone Peptides, 80-81, 84-85, 87

Hyperglycemia, 1, 53, 80, 86, 120, 128, 152, 165-166, 168, 202

Hyperinsulinemia, 9, 19, 29, 53, 111, 128-129, 134, 162-163, 165-168, 196

Hypertriglyceridemia, 53, 104, 111, 113, 117, 184, 186, 201

Hypothalamus, 11, 38, 128, 143, 150, 196, 201

I

Insulin Degrading Enzyme, 162-163, 168

Insulin Receptor Substrate, 1, 9, 12, 64, 67, 150, 167, 196

Insulin Resistance, 1-3, 5-7, 9-15, 17, 19-22, 24-26, 28-30, 32-33, 49, 55-58, 75, 77-78, 84, 95-100, 108-113, 126-130, 149-155, 160, 162, 172, 174, 176, 178-193, 201-202

Insulin Sensitivity, 2, 5-9, 11-12, 15, 19, 21-22, 24-26, 42, 44-45, 47, 51, 53, 56, 66-68, 72, 77-78, 96, 111, 113-114, 132, 134, 157, 160, 168, 176, 182, 186, 192, 195, 200-202

J

Joint Interim Statement, 21-22, 25, 27, 111-113, 117-119, 142, 160

K

Kb Kinase, 1

L

Lipopolysaccharide, 14, 16-20, 67, 88, 180-181, 188

Low-density Lipoprotein Cholesterol, 41, 59, 62, 128-129

M

Melanocortin-4-receptor, 143

Metabolic Syndrome, 1, 12-15, 19, 21-24, 26-29, 39-46, 56, 67-68, 78-79, 87-88, 102, 104-113, 117-119, 134-135, 137, 139, 152, 154-155, 178, 180, 183, 185, 187, 199, 201-202

Methylation, 120-127

Midkine, 58-59, 67

Monocyte Chemoattractant Protein-1, 39, 68

Muscle Ring Finger-1, 46

N

Neuropeptide Y, 38-39

Nonalcoholic Steatohepatitis, 180, 188

Normal Weight Obesity, 111, 114-119

O

Oleic Acid, 31, 36, 167

Oxidative Stress, 19, 29, 32, 36-39, 78, 119, 121, 152, 158-160, 181, 185, 188, 202

P

Pancreatic Islets, 120-121, 125

Peroxisome Proliferator-activated Receptor, 67-68, 78-79, 120, 168, 202

Pioglitazone, 162-167

Plasma Adiponectin Levels, 29-31

Plasma Dipeptidyl Peptidase 4, 104, 110

Plasma Glucose, 22, 29-32, 44-45, 57, 82, 86-87, 89, 103, 105-106, 113, 115, 119, 121-123, 127-130, 132-133, 137, 153, 160, 163, 188, 190-195

Plasma Lipids, 158

Proliferator-activated Receptor Gamma Coactivator 1 Alpha, 120

R

Resistin, 42, 45, 66-68, 128, 134-135, 202

Rosiglitazone, 39, 58-60, 62-63, 66, 68-79, 163, 168

S

Sarcopenic Muscle Loss, 46, 56

Serum Alanine, 14, 17, 20, 81, 180-181

Serum Zinc Levels, 152-155, 157-160

Single Nucleotide Polymorphism, 88, 90, 95

Sleeve Gastrectomy, 169, 178

Surfactant Protein-d, 88, 90, 93, 95-96

T

Thiazolidinedione, 39, 162-163

Triceps Skinfolds, 111, 114, 116-117

Triglycerides, 22-24, 41, 59, 62, 69-70, 72, 76-77, 86, 94, 98-100, 105, 108, 112-117, 122, 128-133, 135, 137-138, 142, 152-155, 157-160, 180, 184, 188, 191-192, 195-201

Tumor Necrosis Factor-alpha, 12, 67, 129

Type 2 Diabetes, 1, 12, 14, 19-20, 27-29, 38-39, 45-47, 53, 56, 58, 68-69, 78, 80-81, 86-93, 100, 111, 120, 123, 134-136, 145, 149, 158, 165-166, 178, 180, 183, 186, 195, 197, 202

U

Ubiquitin-proteasome System, 46-47, 53, 55-56

V

Vaspin, 128, 189-195

Vastus Lateralis, 120-121

Visceral Adiposity, 40-45, 196-200, 202

Visfatin, 68, 128, 135, 178

W

Waist Circumference, 22-24, 41-42, 44, 81, 83-86, 89, 108, 111-112, 116-117, 129, 135-136, 139, 141-142, 144, 153-155, 157, 159-160

www.ingramcontent.com/pod-product-compliance
Lightning Source LLC
Chambersburg PA
CBHW080648200326
41458CB00013B/4775